HEMATOLOGY/ ONCO SECRETS

HEMATOLOGY/ ONCOLOGY SECRETS

MARIE E. WOOD, M.D.

Assistant Professor of Medicine
University of Colorado School of Medicine
Staff, Denver General Hospital
Division of Hematology and Oncology
Denver, Colorado

PAUL A. BUNN, JR., M.D.

Professor of Medicine
University of Colorado School of Medicine
Director, University of Colorado Cancer Center
Denver, Colorado

JAYPEE BROTHERS
P.B. No. 7193, New Delhi, India

First Edition 1994

FIRST INDIAN EDITION 1994

© 1994 by Hanley and Belfus Inc.

ISBN   1-56053-072-3

Printed in India

Published by

Jitendar P. Vij
JAYPEE BROTHERS MEDICAL PUBLISHERS (P) LTD.
B-3, EMCA House, 23/23- B, Ansari Road, Daryaganj,
P.B. 7193, New Delhi-110 002, (India).

Branches :

- 1A, Indian Mirror Street, Wellington Square
  Calcutta 710 013, Ph: 2451926

- 202, Batavia Chambers, 8, Kumara Kruppa Road,
  Kumara Park East, **Bangalore** 560001, Ph: 2281761

Printed by
P.L. Printers, C-3/19, R.P. Bagh, Delhi-7.

CONTENTS

III. MALIGNANT HEMATOLOGY

IV. GENERAL CARE OF THE CANCER PATIENT

Contents

CONTRIBUTORS

Charles M. Abernathy, M.D.
Professor of Surgery, University of Colorado School of Medicine, Denver, Colorado

Dennis J. Ahnen, M.D.
Associate Professor of Medicine, University of Colorado School of Medicine; Associate Director, University of Colorado Cancer Center, Denver, Colorado

Edythe A. Albano, M.D.
Assistant Professor of Pediatrics, University of Colorado School of Medicine, Denver, Colorado

Steven B. Aragon, D.D.S., M.D.
Chief Resident, Otolaryngology-Head & Neck Surgery, University of Colorado School of Medicine, Denver, Colorado

Elizabeth L. Aronsen, M.D.
Instructor, Department of Medicine, University of Colorado School of Medicine, Denver, Colorado

Louis Bair, D.O.
Department of Family Practice, Presbyterian-St. Luke's Hospital, Denver, Colorado

Richard F. Bakemeier, M.D.
Professor of Medicine, University of Colorado School of Medicine; Associate Director, University of Colorado Cancer Center, Denver, Colorado

Scott I. Bearman, M.D.
Associate Professor of Medicine, and Clinical Director, Bone Marrow Transplant Program, University of Colorado School of Medicine, Denver, Colorado

Mona Bernaiche Bedell, R.N., B.S.N., O.C.N.
Oncology Clinical Nurse Specialist, Department of Medicine, Denver General Hospital, Denver, Colorado

Daniel H. Bessesen, M.D.
Assistant Professor of Medicine, University of Colorado School of Medicine, Denver, Colorado

S. Mark Bettag, M.D.
Fellow in Oncology, University of Colorado School of Medicine, Denver, Colorado

Mitchell A. Bitter, M.D.
Associate Professor of Pathology and Director of Hematopathology, University of Colorado School of Medicine, Denver, Colorado

Laura L. Boehnke, Pharm.D.
Clinical Pharmacy Specialist, Division of Pharmacy, The University of Texas MD Anderson Cancer Center, Houston, Texas

Elizabeth Brew, M.D.
Surgery Resident, University of Colorado School of Medicine, Denver, Colorado

Paul A. Bunn, Jr., M.D.
Professor of Medicine, University of Colorado School of Medicine; Director, University of Colorado Cancer Center, Denver, Colorado

Georgia Lee Caven, R.N., B.S., O.C.N.
HIV/Oncology Nurse Clinician, Denver General Hospital, Denver, Colorado

Justin D. Cohen, M.D.
Assistant Professor of Medicine, University of Colorado School of Medicine, Denver, Colorado

Allen L. Cohn, M.D.
Assistant Professor of Medicine, Division of Medical Oncology, University of Colorado School of Medicine, Denver, Colorado

Nicholas J. DiBella, M.D.
Associate Clinical Professor, Department of Medicine, Division of Oncology, University of Colorado School of Medicine, Denver, Colorado

Robert E. Donohue, M.D.
Professor of Surgery (Urology), University of Colorado School fo Medicine, Denver, Colorado

Kyle M. Fink, M.D.
Assistant Clinical Professor of Medicine, University of Colorado School of Medicine, Denver, Colorado

Kerry Scott Fisher, M.D.
Saint Joseph Hospital, Denver, Colorado

Helen L. Frederickson, M.D.
Director of Gynecologic Oncology, Saint Joseph Hospital, Denver, Colorado

Ann D. Futterman, Ph.D.
Assistant Professor of Psychiatry, University of Colorado School of Medicine, Denver, Colorado

David H. Garfield, M.D.
Associate Clinical Professor of Medicine, University of Colorado School of Medicine, Denver, Colorado

William J. Georgitis, M.D., COL, MC
Associate Clinical Professor of Medicine, University of Colorado School of Medicine, Denver; Assistant Chief, Endocrine Service, Fitzsimons Army Medical Center, Aurora, Colorado

L. Michael Glode, M.D.
Professor of Medicine, University of Colorado School of Medicine, Denver, Colorado

Brian S. Greffe, M.D.
Assistant Professor of Pediatrics, University of Colorado School of Medicine, Denver, Colorado

David S. Hanson, M.D.
Senior Associate Consultant in Medical Oncology, Mayo Clinic Jacksonville, Jacksonville, Florida

Kathryn L. Hassell, M.D.
Assistant Professor of Medicine, University of Colorado School of Medicine, Denver, Colorado

Fred D. Hofeldt, M.D.
Professor of Medicine, University of Colorado School of Medicine, Denver, Colorado

Stephen J. Hoffman, Ph.D., M.D.
Fellow, Department of Dermatology, University of Colorado School of Medicine, Denver, Colorado

Christine M. Holm, M.D.
Senior Fellow in Oncology, University of Colorado School of Medicine, Denver, Colorado

Lori Jensen, M.D.
Fellow in Hematology/Oncology, University of Colorado School of Medicine, Denver, Colorado

Madeleine Kane, M.D., Ph.D.
Associate Professor of Medicine, and Acting Head, Division of Medical Oncology, University of Colorado School of Medicine, Denver, Colorado

Robert S. Kantor, M.D.
Lutheran Medical Center, Lakewood, Colorado

James P. Kelly, M.D.
Assistant Professor of Rehabilitation Medicine and Neurology, Brain Injury Program, Rehabilitation Institute of Chicago and Northwestern University Medical School, Chicago, Illinois

Karen Kelly, M.D.
Assistant Professor of Medicine, Division of Medical Oncology, University of Colorado School of Medicine, Denver Colorado

Douglas Jerome Kemme, M.D.
North Colorado Medical Center, Greeley, Colorado

Catherine E. Klein, M.D.
Associate Professor of Medicine, University of Colorado School of Medicine, Denver, Colorado

Joyce S. Kobayashi, M.D.
Associate Professor of Psychiatry, University of Colorado School of Medicine; Director, Neuropsychiatric Consultation Services, Denver Health and Hospitals, Denver, Colorado

J. Fred Kolhouse, M.D.
Professor of Biochemistry and Medicine, University of Colorado School of Medicine, Denver, Colorado

Robin J. Kovachy, M.D.
Director of Medical Oncology Services, Swedish Hospital, Englewood, Colorado

Jill Lacy, M.D.
Associate Professor of Medicine, Yale University School of Medicine, New Haven, Connecticut

Peter A. Lane, M.D.
Director, Colorado Sickle Cell Treatment and Research Center, and Assistant Professor of Pediatrics, University of Colorado School of Medicine, Denver, Colorado

Jerry B. Lefkowitz, M.D.
Assistant Professor of Pathology, University of Colorado School of Medicine; Director, Coagulation laboratory, University Hospital, Denver, Colorado

James F. Lombardo, M.D.
Resident, Department of Pathology, University of Colorado School of Medicine, Denver, Colorado

Alice Luknic, M.D.
Instructor, Department of Medicine, Division of Medical Oncology, University of Colorado School of Medicine, Denver, Colorado

Henry T. Lynch, M.D.
Professor and Chairman, Department of Preventive Medicine, Creighton University School of Medicine, Omaha, Nebraska

Jane F. Lynch, B.S.N.
Instructor, Department of Preventive Medicine, Creighton University School of Medicine, Omaha, Nebraska

Richard A. Marlar, Ph.D.
Director, Special Coagulation Laboratory, Department of Pathology, Denver VA Medical Center/University of Colorado School of Medicine, Denver, Colorado

George Mathai, M.D.
Fellow in Oncology, University of Colorado School of Medicine, Denver, Colorado

Frank J. Mayer, M.D.
Fellow in Oncology/Urology, University of Colorado School of Medicine, Denver, Colorado

Michael T. McDermott, M.D.
Chief of Endocrinology, Fitzsimons Army Medical Center, Aurora, Colorado

Arlen D. Meyers, M.D., M.B.A.
Professor of Otolaryngology–Head & Neck Surgery, University of Colorado School of Medicine, Denver, Colorado

Jeanette Mladenovic, M.D.
Professor and Vice Chairman, Education, Department of Medicine, University of Colorado School of Medicine; Chief of Medicine, Denver General Hospital, Denver, Colorado

George E. Moore, M.D., Ph.D.
Professor of Surgery, University of Colorado School of Medicine, Denver, Colorado

Patrick L. Moran, M.D.
Assistant Clinical Professor of Medicine, University of Colorado School of Medicine, Denver, Colorado

Louis A. Morris, M.D.
Instructor of Medicine, University of Colorado School of Medicine, Denver, Colorado

Nathan A. Munn, M.D.
Chief Resident, Department of Psychiatry–Consultation Liaison, University of Colorado School of Medicine, Denver, Colorado

Adam M. Myers, M.D.
Associate Professor of Medicine (Oncology), University of Colorado School of Medicine; Chief, Hematology/Oncology, Denver General Hospital, Denver, Colorado

Lorrie F. Odom, M.D.
Director of Clinical Oncology, and Associate Professor of Pediatric Hematology/Oncology, The Children's Hospital and University of Colorado School of Medicine, Denver, Colorado

Michael T. Parra, M.D.
Clinical Instructor, University of Colorado School of Medicine, Denver, Colorado

Polly E. Parsons, M.D.
Associate Professor of Medicine, University of Colorado School of Medicine, Denver, Colorado

George K. Philips, M.D.
Clinical Fellow in Hematology/Oncology, University of Colorado School of Medicine, Denver, Colorado

Malcolm H. Purdy, M.D.
Instructor, Bone Marrow Transplant Program, Department of Medicine, University of Colorado School of Medicine, Denver, Colorado

George Rajan, M.D.
Fellow, Department of Medicine, Division of Hematology/Oncology, University of Colorado School of Medicine, Denver, Colorado

William A. Robinson, M.D., Ph.D.
Professor of Medicine, Division of Medical Oncology, University of Colorado School of Medicine, Denver, Colorado

Douglas K. Rovira, M.D.
Assistant Professor of Medicine, University of Colorado School of Medicine, Denver, Colorado

C. R. Santhosh-Kumar, M.D.
Instructor of Medicine, University of Colorado School of Medicine, Denver, Colorado

Scot M. Sedlacek, M.D.
Clinical Assistant Professor of Medicine, University of Colorado School of Medicine, Denver, Colorado

Paul A. Seligman, M.D.
Professor of Medicine, Division of Hematology/Oncology, University of Colorado School of Medicine, Denver, Colorado

Sally P. Stabler, M.D.
Associate Professor of Medicine, University of Colorado School of Medicine, Denver, Colorado

Stephen E. Steinberg, M.D.
Professor of Medicine and Surgery, University of Colorado School of Medicine, Denver, Colorado

Linda C. Stork, M.D.
Assistant Professor of Pediatrics, University of Colorado School of Medicine, Denver, Colorado

Lance S. Terada, M.D.
Assistant Professor of Medicine, Webb Waring Institute at the University of Colorado, Denver, Colorado

Miho Toi, M.D.
Fellow, Department of Medicine, Division of Medical Oncology, University of Colorado School of Medicine, Denver, Colorado

Russell C. Tolley, M.D.
Clinical Instructor, Department of Medicine, University of Colorado School of Medicine, Denver, Colorado

Amy W. Valley, Pharm.D., BCPS
Oncology Pharmacy Specialist, Department of Pharmacy, Audie L. Murphy Memorial Veterans Affairs Hospital, San Antonio; Clinical Assistant Professor, Clinical Pharmacy Programs, University of Texas Health Science Center at San Antonio, San Antonio, Texas

James Clifton Vestal, M.D.
Fellow, Department of Urology, University of Colorado School of Medicine, Denver, Colorado

Deborah A. Waitz, M.D.
Assistant Professor of Radiology, University of Colorado School of Medicine, Denver, Colorado

Patrick Walsh, M.D.
Instructor and Fellow in Mohs' Surgery, Department of Dermatology, University of Colorado School of Medicine, Denver, Colorado

Madeline J. White, M.D.
Clinical Associate Professor of Medicine, University of Colorado School of Medicine, Denver, Colorado

Ross Wilkins, M.D., M.S.
Medical Director, Institute for Limb Preservation, Presbyterian–St. Luke's Hospital, Denver, Colorado

Irene R. Willingham, M.D.
Clinical Instructor, Department of Neurosurgery, University of Colorado School of Medicine, Denver, Colorado

Vincent L. Wilson, Ph.D.
Associate Professor of Pathology, University of Colorado School of Medicine; Director, Molecular Genetics/Oncology, The Children's Hospital, Denver, Colorado

Marie E. Wood, M.D.
Assistant Professor of Medicine, University of Colorado School of Medicine; Staff, Denver General Hospital, Division of Hematology and Oncology, Denver, Colorado

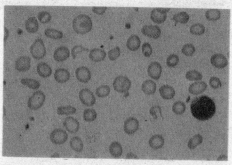

Figure 1. Peripheral blood film showing iron deficiency anemia. The red blood cells are small (compared to a lymphocyte nucleus) and hypochromatic. Notice the rare targets and absence of polychromatophilia. (See p. 19.)

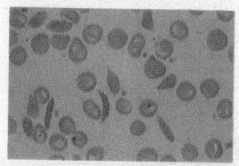

Figure 2. Bone marrow aspirate from a patient with megaloblastic anemia. Megaloblastic erythroid precursors may be mistaken for blasts by the inexperienced morphologist. (See p. 34.)

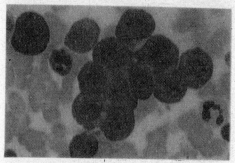

Figure 3. Peripheral blood film showing sickle cell anemia. Sickled erythrocytes are prominent. Polychromatophilia suggests a reticulocytosis and functional hyposplenia is indicated by the presence of a Howell-Jolly body (nuclear remnant in erythrocyte [center]). (See p. 46.)

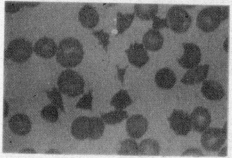

Figure 4. Peripheral blood film from a patient with thrombotic thrombocytopenic purpura. Fragmented cells are prominent. Platelets are decreased. This smear could also be seen in patients with disseminated intravascular coagulation, hemolytic uremic syndrome, malignant hypertension, prosthetic or pathologic heart valves, or large hemangiomas. (See pp. 18, 39, 61, 62.)

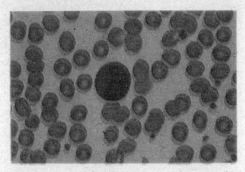

Figure 5. Peripheral blood film showing a reactive lymphocyte. Notice the large size, basophilic cytoplasm, and clumped chromatin. (See p. 110.)

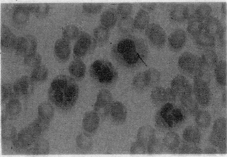

Figure 6. Peripheral blood film from a patient with a leukemoid reaction. Notice the toxic granulation (prominent cytoplasmic granules), and Döhle bodies (blue structures in cytoplasm) within neutrophils. The above findings, in addition to vacuolated polys (not seen in this field), are common in reactive neutrophilias. (See p. 28.)

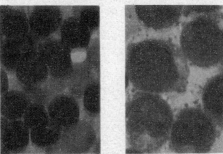

Figure 7. Bone marrow aspirate showing acute myelogenous leukemia (AML) *(left)* and acute lymphoblastic leukemia *(right)*. The myeloblasts are large with fine chromatin and moderate amounts of cytoplasm. An Auer rod *(bottom, center)* is virtually diagnostic of AML. Lymphoblasts are generally smaller with coarse chromatin and scant cytoplasm. (See p. 110.)

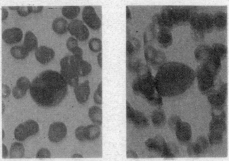

Figure 8. Peripheral blood film showing acute promyelocytic leukemia (APL) (FAB M3) usual form *(left)* and microgranular variant *(right)*. The typical APL cell on the left has a bilobed nucleus and prominent cytoplasmic granules. The microgranular variant (M3v) *(right)* shows cells with the same bilobed nucleus as is seen in the hypergranular form. However, the granules are below the resolution of the microscope and are therefore not visualized. (See p. 114.)

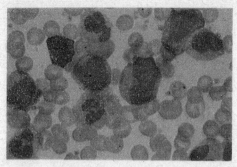

Figure 9. Peripheral blood film from a patient with chronic myelogenous leukemia. Neutrophils at various stages of maturation are seen. Thrombocytosis is common and basophilia is invariably seen. Basophilia can be very helpful in distinguishing this disorder from the leukemoid reaction. (See p. 123.)

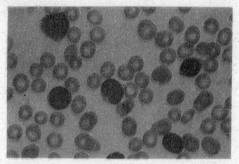

Figure 10. Peripheral blood film from a patient with chronic lymphocytic leukemia (CLL). A lymphocytosis is comprised of small, mature-appearing lymphocytes. Note the smudge cell (degenerated cell) in the lower right corner. Smudge cells are characteristic but not diagnostic of CLL. (See p. 119.)

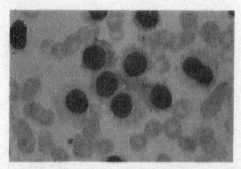

Figure 11. Peripheral blood film from a patient with hairy cell leukemia (HCL). The malignant cells show characteristic nuclear morphology and "hairy" cytoplasmic projections. This illustration is not typical of HCL because it is extremely unusual to find such large numbers of hairy cells circulating in the peripheral blood. (See p. 126.)

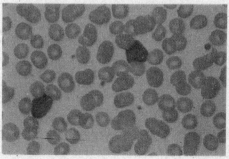

Figure 12. Peripheral blood film showing leukemic involvement by small-cleaved lymphoma. It is not uncommon to see small numbers of circulating lymphoma cells; however, overt leukemia is unusual. (See p. 135.)

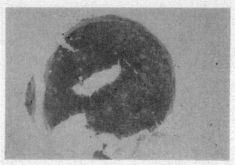

Figure 13. Lymph node showing follicular lymphoma. The neoplastic follicles are numerous and assume a back-to-back arrangement. (See p. 135.)

Figure 14. Lymph node from a patient with small, noncleaved (Burkitt's) lymphoma. Notice the prominent "starry sky" appearance. This finding is not limited to small noncleaved lymphoma, but is common in any high-grade lymphoma. (See p. 136.)

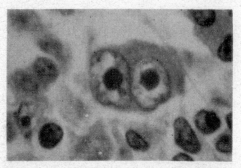

Figure 15. Lymph node from a patient with Hodgkin's disease. A Reed-Sternberg cell shows the typical "owl eye" nuclear appearance. (See p. 147.)

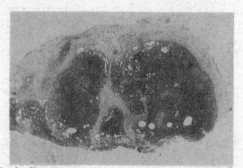

Figure 16. Lymph node showing Hodgkin's disease, nodular sclerosing type. Cellular areas are surrounded by dense fibrous bands. (See p. 148.)

I. General Concepts

1. EVALUATION OF A PALPABLE BREAST MASS

Charles M. Abernathy, M.D., and Elizabeth Brew, M.D.

1. What is one of the more difficult aspects of evaluating a woman with a palpable breast mass?

Determining whether an actual mass is present in the breast can be difficult. **Discrete** and **dominant** are two words that describe a mass that needs to be biopsied. Suspicious masses are three-dimensional, distinct from surrounding tissues, and generally asymmetrical in relation to the opposite breast. Only 10–20% of breast masses are initially discovered by the physician; therefore, an area that the patient feels is abnormal must be evaluated thoroughly. The examining physician must always err on the side of an actual mass being present.

2. Are there factors in the patient's history that are important in the evaluation of a breast mass?

The duration of the mass, related and referred pain, change in physical characteristics with variations in menstrual cycle, and preexisting risk factors for breast cancer (menstrual and family history, previous breast disease) are particularly important in the patient's history.

3. What characteristics of a breast mass are suggestive of cancer?

Masses that are firm, nontender, irregular with indistinct borders, immobile and fixed owing to skin or deep fascial attachments are suggestive of cancer. Skin dimpling and nipple retraction also are suspicious for carcinoma. Bloody nipple discharge and palpable enlarged lymph nodes also are worrisome findings.

4. What is the "gold standard" in the diagnosis of a palpable solid breast mass?

Excisional biopsy. "Perfection in diagnosis will require the removal of every solid mass. This can be expected to result in the biopsy of many benign lesions, but removal of many of them is desirable on other grounds. Although in some instances the probability of cancer may be exceedingly small, it is never zero. If biopsy is not recommended, the probability of cancer should be estimated so the patient can decide whether the level of risk is acceptable to her."[2]

Other biopsy techniques include **fine-needle aspiration** (see question 8), in which cells are aspirated and then smeared on a slide for cytologic analysis; **core-needle biopsy**, in which a core of tissue is withdrawn for pathologic evaluation; **incisional biopsy**, in which part of the mass is removed; and **excisional biopsy**, in which the entire mass is excised.

5. Does mammography play a role in the evaluation of a woman with a palpable breast mass?

It is absolutely critical to view mammography in proper perspective. The purpose of mammography is not primarily to characterize the mass but to evaluate the breasts for clinically occult lesions. A normal mammogram adds no information when evaluating a palpable breast mass. An abnormal mammogram may or may not be of any value, and even when a suspicious lesion is seen on a mammogram, it may not coincide with a palpable mass. Therapeutic decisions should *not* be based on a negative mammogram in a woman with a palpable breast mass.

6. Are mammograms necessary when evaluating a woman with a palpable breast mass?
Mammography is part of the examination of a woman with a breast mass, but it must be remembered that the function of mammography is primarily to evaluate other areas in the breast and contralateral breast for occult lesions and not to characterize the palpable mass. One study reported that when both palpation and mammography suggest that a mass is benign, the error rate is 3.7%—far too high to be acceptable to patients and their physicians.[3]

7. What are the sensitivity and specificity of mammography, physical examination, and combination of mammography and physical examination?

	SENSITIVITY (%)	SPECIFICITY (%)	OVERALL ACCURACY (%)
Combination mammography and physical exam	95	—	77
Mammography alone	94	55	73
Physical exam alone	88	71	81

From van Dam PA, et al: Palpable solid breast masses: Retrospective single and multimodality evaluation of 201 lesions. Radiology 166:435–439, 1988, with permission.

8. Discuss the role of fine-needle aspiration in the evaluation of a solid breast mass.
Fine-needle aspiration (FNA) of breast masses has become popular in recent years but is not always a substitute for open biopsy. However, the use of FNA has markedly diminished the need for open surgical biopsy of lesions that ultimately turn out to be benign. The false-negative rate (negative aspiration cytology in a patient with cancer) varies with the cytopathologist interpreting the results and ranges from 1–35%. This false-negative rate is the Achilles heel of FNA, which means that a negative FNA in the presence of a suspicious mass does *not* exclude cancer. The combination of physical examination, mammography, and FNA has a diagnostic accuracy of 95%.

The use of FNA in the diagnosis of cancer and subsequent determination of surgical therapy is controversial. However, an excisional biopsy can be done immediately prior to the operation to confirm a positive FNA.

9. Explain a "triple-negative diagnostic test."
The term triple negative refers to the combination of a "not suspicious" physical examination, a normal mammogram, and FNA cytology that is not suspicious for cancer. When all three of these tests are negative, the chance of the lesion being cancerous is reduced to <1%. This reduction from the higher false-negative rate of FNA alone is important to justify the use of aspiration cytology. Combined positive diagnostic test is a similar term used when physical examination, mammogram, and FNA all are suspicious for breast cancer.

10. How do you know if a palpable breast mass is a cyst?
Needle aspiration can be both diagnostic and therapeutic. Ultrasound may be necessary first if the patient will not permit aspiration or the mass is too small and deep for reliable aspiration. Even the most experienced examiner cannot distinguish a cystic from a solid lesion on physical examination.

11. What should be done with the fluid from a cyst aspiration?

The fluid may be discarded if it is not bloody, the mass disappears, and the mammogram is normal. Cytologic analysis of cyst fluid is recommended if the fluid is bloody or aspirated from a cyst in a postmenopausal woman. A follow-up mammogram is important to visualize tissue surrounding the collapsed cyst. If a residual mass remains, either FNA or biopsy is recommended.

12. If a cyst reappears after disappearing with the first aspiration, what should be done?

A cyst may be aspirated one or two times after the initial aspiration. With each repeat aspiration, the physician must review whether the mammogram is normal and the mass is completely disappearing. Statistically, less than 20% of cysts require repeat aspirations and less than 9% will reappear after two or three aspirations.

13. Discuss the role of stereotactic-guided core-needle biopsy in a woman with a palpable breast mass.

Once again, do not confuse the management of a palpable mass with the management of a mammographic lesion. A palpable mass can be evaluated without stereotactic or other radiologic guidance. If a mammographic lesion is present in the same breast, one must be certain that the mammographic lesion is coincident with the palpable mass.

14. Can a woman under the age of 30 have breast cancer?

Yes. A substantial number of women under the age of 30 have breast cancer; however, the chance of a breast mass being present in women under 25 years of age is essentially zero.

Pitfalls in the Management of Palpable Breast Masses

1. Assuming that mammography is "diagnostic."

Mammography seldom defines a mass well enough to avoid further diagnostic evaluation (FNA or excisional biopsy). Thus the value of mammography in managing a palpable breast mass is really quite minimal (detection of occult or multifocal disease). Remember that 10–15% of mammograms performed on women with known breast cancer will be negative.

2. Assuming that the radiographic lesion seen on mammography is the same as the palpable lesions.

If there is any question about this correlation, further evaluation is essential. A follow-up mammogram should be obtained 3 or 4 months after biopsy of all mammographically diagnosed lesions to determine that the suspicious mass was actually excised. This mammogram also serves as a new baseline mammogram, showing the changes after biopsy.

3. Letting a negative or nonsuspicious mammogram influence the judgment of whether a palpable mass needs to be biopsied.

Again, the decision to biopsy or aspirate should be made on physical examination criteria.

4. Assuming that a benign aspiration cytology is definitive.

BIBLIOGRAPHY

1. Bland KI, Copeland EM III (eds): The Breast: Comprehensive Management of Benign and Malignant Diseases. Philadelphia, W.B. Saunders, 1991.
2. Donegan WL: Evaluation of a palpable breast mass. N Engl J Med 327:937–942, 1992.
3. Layfield LF, Glasgow BJ, Cramer H: Fine-needle aspiration in the management of breast masses. Pathol Ann 24(part 2):23–62, 1989.
4. Van Dam PA, Van Goethem MLA, Kersschot E, et al: Palpable solid breast masses: Retrospective single and multimodality evaluation of 201 lesions. Radiology 166:435–439, 1988.
5. Zitarelli J, Burkhart LL, Weiss SM: False negative breast biopsy for palpable mass. Surg Oncol 52:61–63, 1993.

2. EVALUATION OF A LUNG MASS

Elizabeth L. Aronsen, M.D., and Polly E. Parsons, M.D.

1. What are the etiologies of a lung mass?
There are benign and malignant etiologies of lung masses. Although there are many other causes, benign masses are often granulomas or hamartomas. The frequency of benign disease depends on the patient population studied but may represent 75% of lung masses in some series of solitary pulmonary nodules. Young age, nonsmoking status, stable (small) size of the mass over 2 years, and calcification in the mass all favor a nonmalignant etiology. Metastases from a nonpulmonary site, especially breast, head and neck, or colon, constitute up to 30% of malignant lung masses. The remainder of the malignant lung masses are due to primary bronchogenic cancer or to malignant transformation of other tissues (such as thymus or lymph nodes) within the thorax.

2. How do patients with malignant lung masses present?
Patients with primary bronchogenic cancer generally present in one of four ways:
1. **Asymptomatic.** Fifteen percent of all patients with lung cancer are asymptomatic at the time of their diagnosis. Their disease is discovered by routine chest roentgenograph (CXR).
2. **Local disease.** These patients present with symptoms referable to the primary tumor itself or to local invasion of adjacent structures such as bronchi, vessels, or mediastinal structures. Symptoms include cough, dyspnea, chest pain, hemoptysis, wheezing, hoarseness, recurrent pneumonia, pleural effusion, dysrhythmias, dysphagia, Horner's syndrome, and superior vena cava (Hunter's) syndrome.
3. **Metastatic disease.** Some patients with metastatic lung cancer present with complaints dependent on the site of the extrapulmonary metastasis. Examples of this might be cerebrovascular accident, hepatomegaly, bone pain, and anemia. Fatigue, anorexia, and malaise, which occur in 20% of patients with lung cancer, are nonspecific systemic symptoms that are not necessarily associated with metastatic disease.
4. **Paraneoplastic syndromes.** A large number of paraneoplastic syndromes are associated with lung cancer, particularly squamous cell lung cancer (hypercalcemia) and small cell lung cancer (syndrome of inappropriate secretion of antidiuretic hormone and hypercortisolemia). The importance of correctly diagnosing a patient's symptoms as part of a paraneoplastic syndrome lies in the fact that the syndrome does not represent metastatic disease and, unlike metastatic disease, does not prevent the patient from pursuing a curative surgical therapy.

3. What other paraneoplastic syndromes are associated with lung cancer?
Endocrine and metabolic. Gene deregulation results in polypeptide release by the tumor and many endocrinologic and metabolic manifestations of paraneoplastic syndromes, including:

Hypercalcemia	Hypophosphatemia
Hyponatremia	Hyperthyroidism
Acromegaly	Hypercalcitonemia
Hypercortisolemia	

Neurologic. A number of neurologic paraneoplastic syndromes associated with small cell lung cancer have autoimmune mechanisms, including:

Eaton-Lambert myasthenia	Subacute peripheral sensory neuropathy
Limbic encephalitis	Chronic intestinal pseudo-obstruction
Necrotizing myelopathy	

Cutaneous
Clubbing
Hypertrophic pulmonary osteoarthropathy
Acanthosis nigricans
Tylosis

Hematologic
Anemia
Polycythemia
Coagulopathy

Renal
Membranous glomerulonephritis
Nephrotic syndrome

4. What are risk factors for lung cancer?

By far the biggest risk for lung cancer is tobacco abuse. Smoking causes approximately 85% of the 170,000 lung cancers diagnosed in Americans each year. According to the Surgeon General, 5000 of the 145,000 deaths due to lung cancer each year occur in patients exposed to passive smoke. Other risk factors that increase the incidence of lung cancer include occupational exposures to asbestos, arsenic, radon, ionizing radiation, chloromethyl methyl ether, and chromium. Tobacco abuse is synergistic to these other exposures. There may also be an increased incidence of lung cancer in males and in blacks independent of smoking history.

5. Discuss diagnostic procedures that can be used to determine the histology of a lung mass.

There are several ways to obtain tissue for diagnosis of a lung mass:

Sputum cytology. This is most helpful in central lesions, often due to squamous cell carcinoma. Sensitivity and specificity are affected by the method of obtaining the specimen (spontaneous vs. induced), the care taken in preserving the specimen, primary tumor size and location, and the skill of the pathologist in interpreting the results. Both false-negative and false-positive specimens are obtained. A negative sputum cytology from a patient with a lung mass on CXR does *not* rule out malignancy, and further workup must be done.

Transbronchial biopsy (TBBx). Many lung masses are central and large enough to be accessible through the fiberoptic bronchoscope. Diagnostic yield decreases considerably for small peripheral lesions. In addition, the operator must be able to see the peripheral lesion in two views by fluoroscopy, which limits the utility of this procedure for masses less than 1–2 cm. TBBx is augmented by bronchial brushing and bronchial washing during the procedure. This approach offers the additional advantage of visualization of the airways to look for endobronchial involvement and to determine proximity of the mass to the carina, which is important in staging the tumor. Central tumors often have squamous cell or small cell histologies.

Percutaneous transthoracic fine-needle aspiration (PTFNA). Peripheral lesions, especially those abutting the chest wall, are amenable to computed tomography (CT) or fluoroscopy-guided PTFNA. The histology of these tumors is most frequently adenocarcinoma or large cell carcinoma.

Open lung biopsy (OLBx). Small peripheral lung masses without evidence of nodal involvement or metastatic disease, termed solitary pulmonary nodules (SPN), are often removed entirely during OLBx through thoracotomy or thoracoscopy. The advantage of this approach is that the surgery is not only diagnostic but frequently curative.

Biopsy of a peripheral metastatic lesion. Lung cancer can metastasize to sites such as the supraclavicular lymph nodes or skin where the tissue becomes readily accessible to biopsy.

Thoracentesis. A pleural effusion can be associated with lung masses of multiple etiologies. Thoracentesis can be diagnostic and often therapeutic for those patients presenting with shortness of breath. Two-thirds of malignant pleural effusions result from lymphoma or lung or breast cancer.

6. Why is the histology of a lung cancer important?
The major histologic types of primary bronchogenic cancer are small cell lung cancer (SCLC), which accounts for 20% of all lung cancers, and non-small cell lung cancer (NSCLC). NSCLC can be further divided into squamous cell (30%), adenocarcinoma (30%), large cell undifferentiated (15%), and broncholoalveolar (<5%) carcinomas. There are several reasons why knowing the histology of a lung mass is important:
   1. **To direct further workup.** For example, adenocarcinoma and SCLC metastasize to the central nervous system more frequently than other cell types. Some physicians argue that all patients with lung cancer due to one of these two cell types should undergo head CT as part of their workup.
   2. **To direct therapy.** Chemotherapy is considered primary therapy for SCLC, whereas early stages of NSCLC require surgical resection for definitive cure.
   3. **Paraneoplastic syndromes.** Specific cell types are often associated with specific paraneoplastic syndromes. Therefore, knowing the histology of the lung mass will alert the physician to be especially vigilant for those symptoms.

7. What is the TNM classification of lung cancer?
The American Joint Committee on Cancer first developed the TNM classification of lung cancer in 1959. Since then there have been several updates; the most recent was published in 1986. This classification is used for NSCLC and refers to the size and location of the primary *T*umor, the presence and location of *N*odal involvement, and the presence or absence of distant *M*etastases. For example, most solitary pulmonary nodules are classified as T1N0M0. A lower case prefix designates whether the extent of disease was determined clinically (c), from pathologic specimens obtained at the time of surgery (p), prior to retreatment of recurrent disease (r), or at autopsy (a). Lung cancer is staged using the TNM subsets. For further staging information, see chapter 64, Lung Cancer.

8. How would you stage occult lung cancer or carcinoma in situ?
Occult carcinoma, defined as a sputum cytology positive for malignant cells but without evidence of disease on CXR or evidence of clinical disease, would be defined as Tx, N0, M0. Carcinoma in situ, which could be found on bronchoscopic biopsy but again not evident clinically or on chest radiography, would be a stage 0 cancer (T_{IS}). For further staging information see chapter 64, Lung Cancer.

9. Why is it important to stage lung cancer?
   1. The stage of NSCLC is directly related to prognosis. For example, stage I disease is associated with a 5-year survival of 60 to 80%, whereas stage IV disease has an extremely poor prognosis with less than 5% survival at 5 years.
   2. The stage of lung cancer often dictates the type of therapy that can reasonably be offered the patient. For example, most centers would consider surgical resection as part of the therapy for clinical stage IIIa disease but not for stage IIIb disease.
   3. Careful staging of lung cancer allows comparison of different therapeutic regimens between institutions, and leads to more effective therapy for this devastating disease.

10. Who is a candidate for surgical resection of a lung mass?
Simply put, a patient with NSCLC at clinical stage IIIa or less is a surgical candidate. However, further workup must be done prior to recommending surgery. This includes assessing the patient's general ability to undergo surgery, evaluating the patient for pulmonary reserve sufficient to withstand resection of lung parenchyma, and determining the resectability of the tumor. There is controversy whether a patient with SCLC is ever a surgical candidate (see below).

11. What general and pulmonary-specific preoperative assessments should be done for a patient prior to recommending thoracotomy for a lung mass?

Preoperative assessment of a patient about to undergo thoracotomy for resection of a malignancy includes determining the general risks of surgery as well as predicting the pulmonary-specific morbidity associated with the planned operation. Obviously someone who is not a surgical candidate for reasons of health or because of insufficient pulmonary reserve does not need extensive workup to assess the resectability of his or her disease.

General assessment. Any patient undergoing anesthesia for surgery requires a thorough history and physical as part of the preoperative assessment. The patient with lung cancer often has a history of tobacco abuse that is associated with a higher risk of other diseases such as hypertension and cardiovascular disease that may increase the risk of the operation. Comorbid diseases need to be assessed and optimal medical therapy instituted prior to operation. Routine laboratory analysis includes complete blood count, creatinine and electrolyte analyses, coagulation studies, and liver function tests. All patients with risk factors for cardiovascular disease require electrocardiograms. Nutritional assessment should be done and every effort made to optimize the patient's performance status.

Pulmonary-specific assessment. Patients who will have parenchymal resection for a lung mass also need specific assessment of their pulmonary reserve. Spirometry is often the first pulmonary function test ordered. In general, a reasonable *post*operative goal is a forced expiratory volume in 1 second (FEV_1) of 0.8 liters (L). Those patients with a preoperative FEV_1 of greater than 2 L can ordinarily undergo resection, including pneumonectomy, without further testing. An FEV_1 of 0.8 L or less excludes virtually all patients from consideration of surgical therapy. For the majority of patients, additional workup includes differential ventilation or perfusion lung scanning to determine the contribution of the parenchyma planned for resection to the overall FEV_1. For example, a patient in whom 60% of his lung function is contributed by the right lung would likely be able to undergo total *left* pneumonectomy with a preoperative FEV_1 of approximately 1.3 L. However, the same patient would need a preoperative FEV_1 of at least 2 L to undergo total *right* pneumonectomy. Similar calculations can be made for smaller resections such as lobectomies or wedge resections. For indeterminate cases, many physicians would recommend further testing, including maximal voluntary ventilation (MVV) or exercise testing. Finally, hypercarbia is associated with a higher surgical risk (although many of these patients will also be excluded for insufficient pulmonary reserve), and most patients will need a preoperative arterial blood gas analysis.

12. What workup is necessary to assess the resectability of a chest malignancy?

Once it has been established that surgery is not contraindicated in a patient, then the resectability of the lung mass must be established within the limits of a clinical assessment. This is done in several ways:

Chest computed tomography (CT). Virtually all patients will have a chest CT. This procedure establishes the boundaries of the primary tumor and suggests the minimal extent of parenchymal resection required. Multiple nodules not visible on plain film are sometimes found this way. It also can suggest invasion of adjacent structures, lymph node involvement, and liver or adrenal metastasis.

Bronchoscopy. Patients who have not undergone bronchoscopy as part of their initia¹ workup of a lung mass should probably have this done as part of the staging. This is necessary to evaluate the endobronchium for metastatic lesions and to assess the extent of proximal bronchial involvement that may exclude the patient from consideration of surgical therapy.

Mediastinoscopy. In patients with lymph nodes larger than 1 cm diameter by chest CT, mediastinoscopy with lymph node biopsy is often recommended to stage the disease. This is because enlarged lymph nodes are not specific for locally metastatic disease and do not necessarily exclude the patient from surgical resection. In contrast, for the patient with borderline function, mediastinoscopy as an intermediate step to surgery may prove nonresectable disease and avoid the larger, more morbid procedure.

Thoracentesis. All patients with pleural effusions and lung cancer should have thoracentesis to rule out metastatic disease. The characteristic effusion associated with lung cancer is often hemorrhagic and exudative.

Brain CT. This often is recommended for all patients with lung cancer, especially those with adenocarcinoma or SCLC, but probably should be reserved for those patients with neurologic signs or symptoms.

Bone marrow aspirate and biopsy. This is done in patients with SCLC as part of the routine staging procedure and should be mandatory in all patients with SCLC being considered for surgical resection (see also Controversies below) to rule out extensive disease.

13. Which modalities besides surgery are available for treating lung cancer?
No therapy of lung cancer should be considered exclusive of combination modalities.

Chemotherapy. This remains the primary therapy for most, if not all, SCLC. Most regimens include cyclophosphamide and/or platinum combination chemotherapy. Chemotherapy is less successful for the more resistant NSCLC.

External beam radiation therapy (XRT). XRT is often used as palliative treatment, but there have also been reports of long-term survival with this therapy for both NSCLC and SCLC.

Photodynamic therapy (PDT). PDT is used with success most often for carcinomas in situ. Photosensitizing agents given intravenously are concentrated in the cancer cells. The bronchoscope directs an argon laser light (wavelength 630 nm) to the lesion where toxic oxygen radicals are formed causing cell death.

Laser therapy. The neodymium–yttrium–aluminum–garnet (Nd-YAG) laser (wavelength 1064 nm) induces photocoagulation and thermal necrosis in endobronchial lesions. Its primary use has been in palliative therapy of metastatic disease.

Brachytherapy. Endobronchial radiation therapy used in cases of carcinoma in situ as well as for endobronchial metastatic lesions.

Immunotherapy. Immunotherapy is likely to be used in the future as tumor-specific cell surface markers are identified.

CONTROVERSIES

14. Why not screen all high-risk patients for lung cancer with routine CXR and/or sputum cytology?
For:
1. The most curable lung cancer, i.e., stage I disease, is that which usually presents asymptomatically. Therefore, screening is the only method available for detection.
2. CXR and sputum cytology represent complementary, noninvasive methods of screening for a disease with high morbidity and mortality.
3. Prolonging even one life through early detection of lung cancer is worth whatever the cost.
Against:
1. The prevalence of lung cancer was less than 0.7% for all ages in a large multicenter study of high-risk patients screened by these methods. Screening these patients alone would represent an enormous economic burden on the health care system.
2. The vast majority of resectable lung masses have a benign etiology. The finding of an incidental lung mass on screening CXR will impel these patients to undergo further unnecessary but expensive and potentially morbid diagnostic procedures in order to reassure both patient and physician that the mass is not malignant.
3. Most lung cancer is associated with tobacco abuse. The money would be better spent in education to prevent smoking.

15. Should patients with limited SCLC be offered surgical therapy?

For:

1. About 4% of SPN are SCLC histologically. In these patients, surgical resection is potentially curative.

2. There is a high incidence of local recurrence after chemotherapy and/or radiotherapy, suggesting a role for adjuvant surgical therapy.

3. The primary tumor may be a mixed NSCLC and SCLC cell type, suggesting a role for combining surgical therapy with standard SCLC chemotherapy and/or radiotherapy. Others have suggested that a carcinoid SCLC subtype may be more favorable for surgical resection.

Against:

1. There are no controlled studies that demonstrate that patients with SCLC treated surgically have any survival advantage over those treated with chemotherapy and/or radiotherapy alone.

2. Most patients with SCLC, including those with SPN, have micrometastases at the time of diagnosis, suggesting that these patients must also receive adjuvant chemotherapy.

3. There is no evidence that partial resection of a primary SCLC tumor has any advantage for subsequent conventional chemotherapy or radiotherapy.

BIBLIOGRAPHY

1. Beckett WS: Epidemiology and etiology of lung cancer. Clin Chest Med 14:1–15, 1993.
2. Berlin NI, Buncher R, Fontana RS, et al: The National Cancer Institute Cooperative Early Lung Cancer Detection Program. Early lung cancer detection: Summary and conclusions. Am Rev Respir Dis 130:565–570, 1984.
3. Cortese DA, Edell ES: Role of phototherapy, laser therapy, brachytherapy, and prosthetic stents in the management of lung cancer. Clin Chest Med 14:149–159, 1993.
4. Cottrell JJ: Preoperative assessment of the thoracic surgical patient. Clin Chest Med 13:47–53, 1992.
5. Dunn WF, Scanlon PD: Preoperative pulmonary function testing for patients with lung cancer. Mayo Clin Proc 68:371–377, 1993.
6. Faber LP: Issues in the management of chest malignancies. Clin Chest Med 13:113–135, 1992.
7. Graham DL Jr, Balducci L, Khansur T, et al: Surgery in small cell lung cancer. Ann Thorac Surg 45:687–692, 1988.
8. Ianuzzi MC, Scoggin CH: State of the art: Small cell lung cancer. Am Rev Respir Dis 134:593–608, 1986.
9. Libshitz HI: Computed tomography in bronchogenic carcinoma. Semin Roentgenol 25:64–72, 1990.
10. Mehta AC, Marty JJ, Lee FYW: Sputum cytology. Clin Chest Med 14:69–85, 1993.
11. Midthun DE, Swensen SJ, Jett JR: Clinical strategies for solitary pulmonary nodule. Annu Rev Med 43:195–208, 1992.
12. Mountain CF: A new international staging system for lung cancer. Chest 89:225S–233S, 1986.
13. Patel AM, Davila DG, Peters SG: Paraneoplastic syndromes associated with lung cancer. Mayo Clin Proc 68:278–287, 1993.
14. Strauss G, Gleason RE, Sugarbaker DJ: Screening for lung cancer re-examined: A reinterpretation of the Mayo Lung Project Randomized Trial on Lung Cancer Screening. Chest 103(Suppl 4):337S–341S, 1993.
15. Tape TG, Mushlin AI: The utility of routine chest radiographs. Ann Intern Med 104:663–670, 1986.

3. EVALUATION OF A TESTICULAR MASS

Robert E. Donohue, M.D.

1. Name the structures normally palpated during the routine scrotal examination and the most common abnormality involving each structure.

The structures to be palpated are the testis, epididymis, the space between the testis and epididymis to allow localization of a mass, the vas deferens, the veins of the pampiniform plexus, if present, and the contents of the tunica vaginalis. The most common abnormality of each structure is:

  Testis: germ cell tumor; 6,000 new cases per year (diagram 2 below)
  Epididymis: epididymitis, lower pole (diagram 3)
  Space between the testis and epididymis: to distinguish a testicular from an epididymal mass (diagrams 1, 2, and 3)
  Vas: sperm granuloma from previous vasectomy (diagram 3)
  Spermatic veins: varicocele
  Tunica vaginalis: hydrocele (diagram 4)

My preference is to examine the patient supine first and then upright. The normal scrotal side should be examined first. The examination should be completed without gloves and any abnormality diagrammed and labeled as to side. The diagram is completed as if the patient were standing and turned 90 degrees.

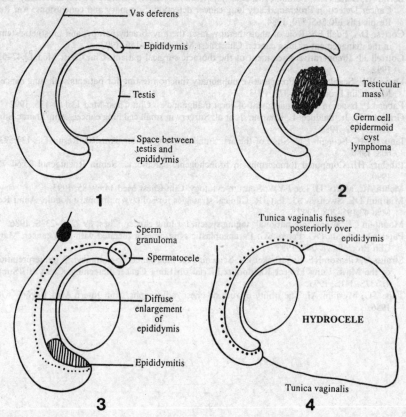

2. What are the significant events in the past history of a patient with a testicular mass thought to be a germ cell tumor?
The three significant events in the past history of a patient with a germ cell tumor are (1) cryptorchidism, either corrected or uncorrected, the age at correction being irrelevant, (2) testicular atrophy, most commonly from postpubertal mumps orchitis, and (3) recent trauma.

3. What percentage of intratesticular masses are germ cell tumors? Of these, what percentage are a single histologic type and what percentage are mixed tumors?
Ninety-seven percent of all intratesticular masses are germ cell tumors. Sixty percent of all germ cell tumors are a single histologic type, whereas 40% are mixed tumors.

4. Name the germ cell tumors and give their clinical incidence.
Seminoma: 40%   Teratocarcinoma: 25–30%
Embryonal cell carcinoma: 20–25%   Choriocarcinoma: 1%
Teratoma: 5–10%

5. What percentage of intratesticular masses are interstitial cell tumors and what are their names?
Two percent. Interstitial cell tumors are Leydig cell tumors and Sertoli cell tumors.

6. Which structures should be examined in a directed physical examination in a patient with a suspected testis tumor?
- The supraclavicular lymph nodes—metastatic spread of tumor filtered from the thoracic duct
- Breasts for gynecomastia—elevated human chorionic gonadotropin (hCG) from tumor leads to symmetric or asymmetric breast enlargement
- Upper abdomen, subxiphoid—first site of nodal metastases, the perirenal hilar area
- Lower abdomen for inguinal scars from previous surgery and masses—scars suggest a previous orchidopexy, hernia, or varicocele and possible altered lymphatic drainage to the inguinal nodes—a mass suggests inguinal adenopathy or tumor in an undescended testis
- Testis with the mass in it
- Opposite testis—the opposite testis may be the site of the tumor when the opposite testis was cryptorchid or the patient could have simultaneous bilateral tumors

7. If a testis tumor is suspected, what serum markers should be drawn preoperatively? What are the half-lives of these markers? Can their value after orchiectomy be of use?
The serum markers to be drawn are the alpha-fetoprotein (AFP), beta-chain human chorionic gonadotropin (β-hCG), and lactic dehydrogenase. The AFP half-life is 5–7 days; the β-hCG half-life is 24–36 hours. If the values of the markers decline with respect to their half-lives, it suggests that no other tumor is present in the patient.

8. Is age significant in the final histology of the patient with a testis tumor?
The three peak periods for testis tumors are the 20–40 age group, infancy, and late adulthood (>60 years). The testis tumor is the most common solid tumor in men between 20 and 35 years of age. Infants have benign teratomas, whereas preteens suffer from yolk sac tumors. Young adult males, aged 25 to 35, have embryonal cell carcinomas and teratocarcinomas (embryonal cell carcinomas with teratomas). Males aged 35 and older have a higher percentage of seminomas, whereas the most common testicular tumor in males over age 60 is lymphoma.

9. What is the initial treatment for a suspected testis tumor?
Radical inguinal orchiectomy is the treatment of choice. An inguinal incision is made with high ligation of the spermatic cord at the internal inguinal ring. If doubt exists as to the

diagnosis, the tunica vaginalis can be opened in the inguinal area and the testis examined directly.

10. How do you stage a testis tumor?
Staging of the diagnosed testis tumor consists of determining the extent of the tumor in the testis and surrounding structures, chest PA and lateral films, serum markers preoperatively and postoperatively, CT scan of the abdomen and possibly of the chest, and possibly a brain scan. Tumor stage is as follows:

Stage A: confined to scrotum
Stage B1:   <6 retroperitoneal lymph nodes: none larger than 2 cm
Stage B2:   >6 retroperitoneal lymph nodes: none larger than 5 cm
Stage B3:   palpable retroperitoneal nodes: nodes larger than 5 cm
Stage C: metastatic disease anywhere beyond the retroperitoneal lymph nodes—
            supraclavicular nodes, mediastinum, lung, liver, or brain metastases

11. If a testicular tumor is diagnosed and orchiectomy does not show the intratesticular mass to be a malignancy, what is the lesion, how common is it, and could it have been correctly diagnosed preoperatively?
The mass is an epidermoid cyst and its incidence is 1% of intratesticular masses. Fifty percent occur in the third decade of life. No diagnostic study at the present time short of orchiectomy allows the diagnosis to be made with certainty. The lesion may represent a monolayer teratoma and is benign.

12. Acute unilateral painful scrotal swellings associated with nausea and vomiting in a teenager or adult are most likely caused by what entity? What is the natural history of this entity?
The most likely entity is torsion of the spermatic cord. In any acute unilateral scrotal swelling, testicular torsion, testicular appendage torsion, epididymitis, epididymo-orchitis, and trauma must be considered.

The natural history of torsion of the spermatic cord is sudden onset of pain, often awakening the patient from sleep, with the pain peaking immediately, and associated with nausea and vomiting. Scrotal swelling occurs almost immediately. If asked, the patient often relates a history of multiple previous episodes. The spermatic cord torsion is produced by the heightened cremasteric reflex activity of puberty with a congenital abnormality of testicular fixation to the spermatic fascia of the scrotum.

Remember, the majority of patients with mumps orchitis have a preexisting parotid inflammation. Recall that mumps orchitis is a postpubertal infection of the testis.

13. What is the treatment of choice for acute spermatic cord torsion?
Immediate scrotal exploration and orchiectomy or orchidopexy (testicular fixation to the internal spermatic fascia) on the involved side and orchidopexy contralaterally must be accomplished.

14. How many hours of ischemia may elapse before the testis suffers irreversible ischemic damage and atrophies?
In our study, if the torsion of the spermatic cord was corrected by manual untwisting or surgical untwisting and fixation within 6 hours, none of our patients had any atrophy when examined from 6 months to 10 years after the acute episode. The opposite testis, also fixed at the original surgery, was used as the normal testis for each patient.

15. What time period must elapse after torsion of the spermatic cord and testicular fixation before the physician can state that the testis will undergo no atrophy or undergo no further atrophy?
Testis atrophy from the ischemic episode that results from torsion of the spermatic cord will usually occur within 6 months.

16. Name the three most common organisms that cause bacterial epididymitis.
Bacterial epididymitis is the most common type of epididymitis. The most common organisms causing this condition are *Chlamydia trachomatis* and *Neisseria gonorrhoeae* in males under 35 years of age and *Escherichia coli* in men over 35 years of age.

17. How does bacterial epididymitis present?
As a lower pole mass of the epididymis.

18. Name the most common lesion of the head of the epididymis.
A spermatocele.

19. Is unilateral absence of the vas a significant physical finding? What other scrotal abnormalities are associated with the absent vas?
Yes. Unilateral absence of the vas deferens is associated in 70% to 90% of cases with ipsilateral absence or agenesis of the kidney. The contralateral solitary kidney has a significant abnormality in 33% of patients. Associated scrotal and pelvic abnormalities include absence of the ipsilateral epididymis and seminal vesicle and an ipsilateral spermatocele.

20. What is a varicocele and how should it be examined?
The varicocele is caused by varicosities of the pampiniform plexus of the internal spermatic vein. It usually appears during puberty. Its incidence is about 15% on the left side and 1% on the right side. To examine the patient for a varicocele, stand the patient upright, examine the scrotum, and confirm the diagnosis. Have the patient perform a Valsalva maneuver if necessary. Place the patient supine and reexamine. The varicocele should collapse with elevation; the ipsilateral testis may be atrophied in up to 25% of adult males with a varicocele, the cause of which is unknown.

21. Is the sudden appearance of a varicocele in an adult a significant finding?
The sudden appearance of a varicocele suggests either intrinsic or extrinsic compression of the renal vein or inferior vena cava by a mass, which is most commonly malignant. The most common lesions are metastatic testicular carcinoma, lymphoma, renal cell carcinoma, and primary retroperitoneal malignancies. Abdominal ultrasonography should be performed to evaluate the patient initially. A CT scan of the abdomen may be required.

22. List the three most common entities that involve the tunica vaginalis.
1. Clear fluid within the tunica vaginalis from an inflammatory, ischemic, or traumatic testicular or epididymal event is a **hydrocele.**
2. Bloody fluid, usually after trauma, is a **hematocele.**
3. Small or large intestine or omentum entering into the scrotum via a patent processus vaginalis is an **incarcerated, indirect inguinal hernia.**

BIBLIOGRAPHY

1. Berger R, et al: Etiology, manifestations and therapy of acute epididymitis, a prospective study of 50 cases. J Urol 121:750–757, 1979.
2. Coolsaet B: The varicocele syndrome: Venography determining the optimum level for surgical management. J Urol 124:833–839, 1980.
3. Donohue R, et al: Torsion of the spermatic cord. Urology 11:33–37, 1978.
4. Donohue R, et al: Unilateral absence of the vas deferans—A useful clinical sign. JAMA 261:1180–1181, 1989.
5. Richie J: Neoplasms of the testis. In Walsh PC, et al (eds): Campbell's Urology, 6th ed. Philadelphia, W.B. Saunders, 1992, pp 1222–1266.
6. Vordermark J, et al: Epidermoid cysts of the testes and the role of sonography. Urology 41:75–78, 1993.
7. Whitmore WF: Testicular cancer in cryptorchids. Cancer 49:1023–1030, 1982.

4. INTRACRANIAL MASS LESIONS

Irene R. Willingham, M.D., and Lance S. Terada, M.D.

1. What are the signs and symptoms of an intracranial mass?
An intracranial mass can produce symptoms through mass effects, associated with increased intracranial pressure, and through local effects, associated with focal lateralizing neurologic deficits. Brain shifts may develop from the pressure of a mass; thus, lumbar puncture may pose a problem.

2. What imaging studies are best for demonstrating intracranial masses?
Computed tomography (CT) and magnetic resonance imaging (MRI) play important roles in the identification of intracranial masses. MRI appears to be slightly more sensitive than CT. Both studies require the administration of intravenous contrast material.

3. What can cause an intracranial mass?
Infection, tumors, and hemorrhage are common causes of central nervous system (CNS) masses.

4. How important is abscess as a cause of intracranial space-occupying lesions?
Of all intracranial masses, 1–2% are due to abscess. Microorganisms are introduced as a result of trauma, contiguous infection, or hematogenous spread. Hematogenous spread results in metastatic abscesses that often are multiple, whereas trauma and local infections tend to cause a single abscess collection.

5. Which microbiologic agents are most commonly responsible for brain abscesses?
Various parasites, fungi, and bacteria are capable of causing abscess. Aerobic or anaerobic streptcocci, pneumococci, *Staphylococcus aureus*, gram-negative bacteria, *Bacteroides* species, *Candida albicans*, and *Aspergillus* species are common causes of brain infection. *Toxoplasma gondii* is most often responsible for parasitic brain abscess.

6. Is metastatic cancer an important cause of intracranial mass?
Brain metastases develop in 15–20% of cancer patients.

7. Which primary tumors most commonly metastasize to the brain?
Tumors of the breast, lung, kidney, and colon, and melanoma.

8. What special diagnostic issues are present in patients who test positive for the human immunodeficiency virus (HIV)?
Neurologic disease is clinically evident in about 50% of HIV-positive patients. Progressive multifocal leukoencephalopathy, primary CNS lymphoma, and toxoplasmosis are the three most frequent causes of intracranial mass lesions.

9. Is biopsy of an intracranial mass in an HIV-positive patient always indicated?
Biopsy of tissue from the mass is the only definitive way to make the diagnosis. However, as more has been learned about intracranial mass lesions in the setting of HIV infection, certain diagnosis/treatment algorithms have been proposed. One approach is to treat with antibiotics for *T. gondii* if patients are seropositive for antibodies. Patients who are seronegative for *T. gondii* or who do not respond to antibiotic treatment are candidates for biopsy.

10. Can infarction behave as a mass lesion of the brain?
Brain infarction may behave as a mass lesion exerting local pressure or causing brain herniation. The signs and symptoms may be identical to those of brain neoplasms or

14

infection. The enhancement pattern and mass effect found on CT may mimic other types of mass lesions. MRI can add important information in the evaluation of ischemic brain disease. If the condition of the patient allows, serial imaging studies can be helpful in distinguishing between infarction and other mass lesions. It must be remembered that secondary hemorrhage may occur in infectious and neoplastic lesions.

11. How may cancer spread to the brain?
Cancer cells may gain direct access to the venous circulation or indirect access to the bloodstream through the lymphatic system. Cancers often metastasize to secondary sites, most commonly the lung and liver; from these sites tertiary metastasis may occur. An alternate means of metastases to the CNS may include venous channels that allow communication between the venous drainage of the thoracic and abdominal areas and the CNS. These venous channels are often called the venous plexus of Batson.

12. When is resection of an intracranial metastatic lesion considered?
The overall condition of the patient, including life expectancy and presence of other metastases, must be considered. Surgery is used most often in the treatment of metastases from radio-insensitive tumors such as those of the colon, thyroid, and kidney, and melanoma. The number of metastatic lesions and their location within the brain are also important factors in planning surgical excision.

13. Does age assist in forming the differential diagnosis of an intracranial mass?
Yes. The age of the patient may prove to be quite helpful, especially in the case of brain tumors. Certain brain tumors are more common in adults, including meningiomas, gliomas of the cerebral hemisphere, pituitary tumors, and metastatic tumors. Common tumors of childhood include pineal tumors, craniopharyngiomas, teratomas, granulomas, and primitive neuroectodermal tumors, as well as gliomas of the cerebellum, brainstem, and optic nerve.

14. What is a "drop met"? How does it occur?
Some primary CNS tumors, germinomas, and primitive neuroectodermal tumors develop secondary spread in the cerebrospinal fluid. This meningeal seeding may be referred to as a drop met, because the metastatic deposit seems to drop down the neural axis from the primary lesion.

15. Are cranial nerve palsies in a patient with leukemia an indication of intracranial mass?
Neurologic manifestations in the acute leukemias are common. Metastatic syndromes associated with leukemia include meningeal involvement resulting in cranial and spinal neuropathies, epidural compression, and hypothalamic invasion. Patients with high numbers of circulating blasts may develop hemorrhages within the brain.

16. How can the new technology of single-photon emission computed tomography (SPECT) help in the diagnosis of a CNS lesion?
SPECT is a technique of mapping the three-dimensional distribution of a radionuclide. SPECT scanning can be used to discriminate necrotic material from persistent or active tumor. It is most helpful in the setting of postradiation or postsurgical abnormalities found by CT or MRI. Patients who have relatively high thallium uptake on posttreatment SPECT images often have active tumor at the time of repeat biopsy, whereas low uptake is associated with non–tumor-related changes.

17. What percentage of brain tumors are primary CNS lymphomas?
Before the 1980s, primary CNS lymphoma was a rare disease, accounting for 1% of all primary brain tumors. With the advent of acquired immune deficiency syndrome (AIDS), the incidence of primary CNS lymphoma has increased significantly; 2% of patients with AIDS ultimately develop primary CNS lymphoma.

BIBLIOGRAPHY

1. Andrews B, Kenefick T: Neurosurgical management of acquired immune deficiency syndrome—An update. West J Med 158:249, 1993.
2. Baumgartner JA, Rachlin JR: Primary central nervous system lymphomas: Natural history and response to radiation therapy in 55 patients with acquired immuno-deficiency syndrome. J Neurosurg 73:206, 1990.
3. Haines SJ, Hall WA (eds): Infections in neurologic surgery. In Neurosurgery Clinics of North America, vol. 3. Philadelphia, W.B. Saunders, 1992.
4. Lunsford LD (ed): Stereotactic radiosurgery. In Neurosurgery Cinics of North America, vol. 3. Philadelphia, W.B. Saunders, 1992.
5. Rowland LP (ed): Merritt's Textbook of Neurology, 8th ed. Philadelphia, Lea & Febiger, 1989.
6. Wilkins RH, Rengachary SS (eds): Neurosurgery. New York, McGraw-Hill, 1985.

5. EVALUATION OF ANEMIA

Marie E. Wood, M.D.

1. Which laboratory tests are helpful in establishing the etiology of anemia?

The most important tools in the evaluation of anemia are the complete blood count (CBC), reticulocyte count, and microscopic examination of the peripheral smear. These three tests will help you to form a differential diagnosis; you can then decide on other confirmatory or diagnostic tests. Other tests should not be ordered before all three of the above are completed.

2. Define the red cell distribution width (RDW) and explain how it is used.

The RDW is a measure of the homogeneity of the red blood cell population. It is calculated by the Coulter counter as a percentage determined by dividing the standard deviation of the mean corpuscular volume (MCV) by the MCV and multiplying by 100. A normal RDW is $13.5\% \pm 1.5\%$. The RDW is elevated in deficiency states (iron, folate, and vitamin B12) and when there is a marked reticulocytosis. It can be very helpful in distinguishing anemia due to deficiency from thalassemia (see question 18).

3. Which tests should be ordered when the attending physician's instructions say to obtain "iron studies"?

Serum iron
Iron-binding capacity
Ferritin level

4. What do iron studies measure?

Ferritin is an iron storage protein. It exists mainly within cells; however, a small amount leaches into serum and it is this quantity that is measured. The serum ferritin level accurately reflects the total pool of storage ferritin. Ferritin also is an acute-phase reactant, and production will be stimulated by any inflammatory process; thus, it will appear as though the iron stores were elevated. However, the ferritin levels seen in iron overload states (>500 $\mu g/L$) are higher than commonly seen with any inflammatory state.

Total iron-binding capacity (TIBC) is a combined measurement of free iron in serum and iron bound to transferrin. When expressed as a percentage, it reflects the saturation of transferrin by iron. Normal transferrin saturation is 33%.

5. In which patients are iron studies falsely elevated or depressed?

Iron studies may be falsely elevated in individuals taking iron or in those who are vitamin B12 or folate deficient. This occurs because the bone marrow will decrease the utilization of iron for heme synthesis as heme synthesis is decreased in the deficient state.

Iron studies may be falsely low when there is a burst of eyrthropoiesis. This can happen when an individual previously deficient is placed on vitamin B12 or folate replacement, thereby restimulating erythropoiesis.

6. Is a bone marrow biopsy helpful in the evaluation of anemia?

Although it is true that a bone marrow biopsy is always helpful in the evaluation of anemia, it is important to remember that a bone marrow biopsy is a procedure associated with both risks and discomfort, and therefore consideration should be given to its usefulness in establishing the etiology of the anemia. In general, a bone marrow biopsy should be considered after the laboratory evaluation of anemia is completed.

7. When should a bone marrow biopsy be done early in the evaluation of anemia?

A bone marrow biopsy should be done early when a neoplastic process such as leukemia, lymphoma, carcinoma, myelodysplasia, or a myeloproliferative process is suspected, or if therapeutic intervention will alter the appearance or morphology of the bone marrow. This may happen in the treatment of nutritional deficiencies or hemolytic anemia.

The argument could be made that the bone marrow biopsy is not necessary and the patient could be treated empirically. However, if the empirical treatment is not successful, then the presumptive diagnosis may have been wrong and time will have been lost by not obtaining a bone marrow biopsy early.

8. What is the half-life of a red blood cell? When is it decreased?

The life span of a red blood cell is approximately 120 days in the systemic circulation. Therefore, the half-life is 60 days. Any process that causes hypersplenism causes shortened red blood cell survival owing to splenic sequestration. Probably the most important group of disorders that cause hypersplenism are the hemolytic anemias. In the past, red blood cell survival time was measured, but this is no longer considered useful.

9. Where is erythropoietin produced?

The majority of erythropoietin is produced in the kidney (approximately 90%), althoug the exact cell responsible for synthesis of erythropoietin remains unknown. The other 10% of erythropoietin is produced in the liver. Erythropoietin production by the liver is known to be much higher in the newborn as well as in the regenerating liver. Liver production of erythropoietin is not increased in response to renal disease or any other state causing inappropriately low erythropoietin levels.

10. In which disorders are erythropoietin levels increased or decreased?

High erythropoietin levels are seen in any disorder causing tissue hypoxia. This hypoxia can be due to decreased hemoglobin concentration from anemia or increased hemoglobin affinity for oxygen as seen with increased carbon monoxide levels or high-affinity hemoglobinopathies. Decreased oxygenation of hemoglobin also can cause an increased erythropoietin level, which can be due to lung disease, heart disease, or high altitude. Low erythropoietin levels are seen in renal disease and myeloproliferative states such as polycythemia vera. Therefore, the erythropoietin level can be used to distinguish primary from secondary erythrocytosis.

11. Explain how to evaluate a hemolytic anemia.

When evaluating a hemolytic anemia, it is important to determine whether it is a chronic or acute process. Individuals with acute hemolysis will be more symptomatic and show signs of cardiovascular stress such as tachycardia, tachypnea, dyspnea on exertion, and severe fatigue as well as dizziness and/or lightheadedness. These individuals require immediate treatment. Individuals with a chronic hemolytic process manifest relatively few symptoms often despite severe anemia.

The evaluation of a hemolytic anemia should begin with a CBC, reticulocyte count, and examination of the peripheral blood smear. Once the presence of a hemolytic process is established, evaluation of the etiology should proceed. This evaluation could include a disseminated intravascular coagulation (DIC) panel (thrombin time, fibrinogen level, and fibrin split products or the equivalent test), Coombs' testing (both direct and indirect), evaluation of red blood cell membrane stability (osmotic fragility and sucrose hemolysis), evaluation of hemoglobin stability (Heinz body prep, isopropanol or heat stability testing), and evaluation of the oxygen-hemoglobin dissociation curve.

12. Discuss how the reticulocyte count is "corrected" and tell why this is important.
The corrected reticulocyte count is obtained by multiplying the observed reticulocyte count by the quantity of the observed hematocrit divided by the normal hematocrit (45%). This becomes important when evaluating the appropriateness of the patient's bone marrow response to the level of anemia. For example, a reticulocyte count of 5.0% in an individual with a hematocrit of 20% should be corrected to 2.2% ([5 × (20/45)]). This suggests that the bone marrow is not responding as it should to the low level of hemoglobin. This occurrence should be further investigated.

13. Tell how to distinguish intravascular from extravascular hemolysis on the peripheral smear.
Intravascular hemolysis produces fragmented cells secondary to mechanical damage (as in DIC, thrombotic thrombocytopenic purpura, hemolytic-uremic syndrome, or shearing due to the presence of a prosthetic valve). (See Figure 4, Color Plates.) This damage is caused by red blood cells sticking to deposited fibrin and then breaking off. One can see helmet, triangular, and/or twisted cells. When the cells are broken and all hemoglobin is lost, the ghost cells will be seen on the peripheral smear.

Extravascular hemolysis occurs when cells or parts of cells are phagocytosed by the spleen. The result is the appearance of spherocytes, microspherocytes, or bite cells on the peripheral smear. Agglutinated red cells may also be seen if cold agglutination is occurring.

Whether intravascular or extravascular hemolysis occurs, there should be evidence of a bone marrow response on the peripheral smear. This will appear as polychromatophilic macrocytes, nucleated red blood cells, and a reticulocytosis.

14. How long does it take to become folate or vitamin B12 deficient?
Vitamin B12 deficiency takes years to develop (up to 12 years postgastrectomy). It is seen in individuals with impaired absorption (either gastric or intestinal) and may also occur in chronic abusers of nitrous oxide.

Folate deficiency, on the other hand, takes only weeks to develop, partly because of the small amount of folate stored in the body. These stores can easily be depleted, and folate deficiency is commonly seen when intake is decreased (as in alcoholism or tropical sprue) or demand for folate is high (as in pregnancy or chronic hemolytic anemia).

15. What can cause an "underproduction" anemia?
This type of anemia is seen when the bone marrow has been infiltrated with carcinoma, lymphoma, or leukemia. It can also be seen in anemia of chronic diseases or in nutritional deficiency states.

16. How can you distinguish anemia due to underproduction from anemia due to increased destruction?
Of course, a good history and physical examination are very important. Often the etiology or at least a good working differential diagnosis can be formed using the history and

physical examination alone. Probably the most important tools in distinguishing underproduction from increased destruction will be the reticulocyte count, bilirubin, and lactate dehydrogenase (LDH). Anemia due to increased destruction will generally be associated with an elevated reticulocyte count, whereas an underproduction anemia will have a normal or low reticulocyte count. The LDH and bilirubin in a hemolytic anemia should also be elevated. Caveats to this are:

1. The bilirubin and LDH can be elevated in vitamin B12 or folate deficiency.

2. If the reticulocytes are being destroyed by the hemolytic process, the reticulocyte count will be falsely low.

3. If the individual has become folate or iron deficient owing to a chronic hemolytic state, the reticulocyte count will again be falsely low.

17. Discuss the causes of anemia of chronic disease. How long does it take to develop?

Anemia of chronic disease is caused by an underlying medical disorder. Generally, this disorder must cause some sort of inflammatory reaction (i.e., infection or malignancy). If the inflammation is severe, as in an infectious process, the anemia can develop in as little as 2 weeks. Anemia of chronic disease is a normochromic/normocytic anemia characterized by a normal MCV, normal RDW, and normal but not elevated reticulocyte count. The ferritin is elevated, reflecting the increased bone marrow iron stores; however, the iron and TIBC are decreased. The bone marrow iron stores are not able to be properly mobilized in anemia of chronic disease; thus, the bone marrow does not respond to the decrease in hematocrit until the underlying problem is treated.

18. How can thalassemia be distinguished from nutritional deficiency anemia?

Thalassemia is a disorder of hemoglobin synthesis. The defect can be either with alpha- or beta-globin synthesis, resulting in a variety of clinical manifestations. All thalassemics will display impaired hemoglobin synthesis, resulting in defective erythropoiesis. This can be seen as a microcytic anemia (MCV 60 to 75 fl). Unlike iron deficiency, in microcytic anemia all cells will be of similar size, and therefore the RDW will be normal. (See Figure 1, Color Plates.) Other clues to a diagnosis of thalassemia include:

1. **Ethnic origin:** thalassemia is seen most commonly in individuals of Mediterranean or Southeast Asian background and less commonly in blacks.

2. **Hypersplenism:** the abnormal and excessive globin molecules will form tetramers that can precipitate intracellularly, resulting in inclusion bodies. In α-thalassemia, these inclusion bodies will form in the red blood cell precursors (erythroblasts) and be destroyed in the bone marrow, resulting in ineffective erythropoiesis. The erythroblasts may also be released prematurely into the circulation where they will be cleared by the spleen, resulting in hypersplenism. In β-thalassemia, the abnormal globin forms tetramers that precipitate only in the aged red blood cell. These aged red blood cells again will be cleared by the spleen, resulting in hypersplenism.

3. **Abnormal hemoglobin electrophoresis:** in β-thalassemia, there may be an increased amount of hemoglobin A2 (alpha$_2$, delta$_2$) or a persistence of fetal hemoglobin, resulting in increased hemoglobin F. In α-thalassemia, the hemoglobin electrophoresis can be normal.

19. Can hemoglobin affinity for oxygen cause anemia?

Yes. It can cause either an underproduction anemia when the abnormal hemoglobin has a low affinity for hemoglobin or a hemolytic anemia when there exists an unstable hemoglobin. These two causes of anemia are generally thought to be underrecognized and therefore underdiagnosed.

20. What causes abnormal hemoglobin affinity?

Disorders in hemoglobin affinity or stability collectively represent hemoglobinopathies. They arise from mutations in the hemoglobin molecule. These mutations cause an unstable hemoglobin or the formation of hemoglobin that has either a high or low affinity for oxygen and therefore a shifted oxygen dissociation curve. An unstable hemoglobin should be suspected when an individual is found to have a congenital hemolytic anemia. High-affinity hemoglobinopathies cause a polycythemic state, and, as mentioned, low-affinity hemoglobinopathies cause an underproduction anemia.

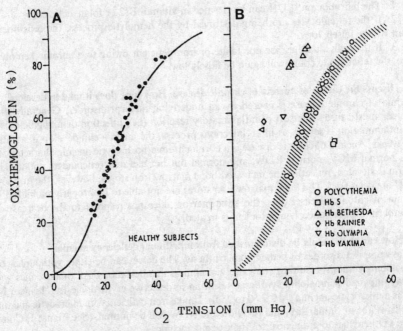

A, The percentage of hemoglobin as oxyhemoglobin at the antecubital venous P_{O_2}, corrected to pH 7.4, is shown for 38 healthy subjects. *B,* The shaded area depicts the normal range for healthy subjects. The circles represent observations in five subjects with hypoxic polycythemia and 10 with polycythemia vera. The triangles, squares, and diamonds represent observations in subjects with mutant hemoglobins with altered oxygen affinity. (From Lichtman MA, Murphy BS, Adamson JW: Detection of mutant hemoglobins with altered affinity for oxygen: A simplified technique. Ann Intern Med 84:517–520, 1976, with permission.)

21. How do you diagnose anemia due to abnormal hemoglobin affinity?

Diagnosing any one of these disorders can be difficult. They require sensitive assays of hemoglobin stability (either isopropanol or heat-stability tests) and a Heinz body preparation, looking for precipitated hemoglobin in the red blood cells. Hemoglobin electrophoresis can sometimes be helpful but may often be normal. Determination of the P_{50} may be the most practical test for this disorder. The P_{50} is the partial pressure of oxygen (mmHg) required to saturate 50% of the oxygen. It requires only a venous blood gas. The P_{50} is then calculated and compared with a normal control using the following equation:

$$P_{50} = \text{antilog}\left(\frac{\log 1/k}{n}\right)$$

where $1/k = \left[\text{antilog}\left(n \log P_{O_{2(7.4)}}\right)\right] \times \dfrac{100 - S_{O_2}}{S_{O_2}}$ and $n = 2.7$

This is a complicated formula. However, if it is used to assist in the evaluation of anemia or polycythemia, diagnoses will certainly be made that would not otherwise have been made.

22. In sickling diseases, how does the level of anemia assist in identifying the type of sickling disorder?

Sickling diseases represent a heterogeneous group of disorders with varying clinical pictures. The most severe disease is seen in patients who are homozygous for hemoglobin S (sickle cell disease). They tend to have the lowest hematocrit and the most severe clinical picture. Sickle cell trait, on the other hand, is associated with the mildest clinical picture and often a normal hemoglobin. Patients with either hemoglobin SC disease or sickle thalassemia have an intermediate clinical picture. Hemoglobin SC disease is associated with a fairly normal hematocrit. However, these individuals will be more symptomatic because of higher concentrations of hemoglobin (Hgb) S and higher intracellular Hgb concentration and thus an increased predisposition to sickling.

Individuals with thalassemia and Hgb S have various clinical pictures depending on the amount of globin chain synthesis present. Individuals with concurrent alpha-thalassemia will have a milder disease. The decreased production of alpha-globin chain ensures a higher concentration of Hgb A, as the alpha-globin chain has greater affinity for the normal beta-globin chain. Individuals who are double heterozygotes for sickle cell disease and β-thalassemia have a more severe clinical picture. The decreased production of the normal beta-chain leads to a higher percentage of Hgb S. It is important to remember that concurrent sickle cell disease and thalassemia should be suspected in patients with a positive sickle preparation and a low MCV (range 65–70).

The Principal Sickle Cell States

			MANIFESTATIONS	
DIAGNOSIS	β GENOTYPE	HEMOGLOBIN PATTERN	Hgb Level (g/dl)	Sickle Cell Crisis
Sickle cell trait	$\beta^A\beta^S$	Hgb A >Hgb S	>12	None
Sickle cell anemia	$\beta^S\beta^S$	Hgb S, no Hgb A	6–9	4+
SC disease	$\beta^S\beta^C$	Hgb S = Hgb C	10–12	2 to 4+
Sickle-thalassemia	$\beta^S\beta^O$	Hgb S, no Hgb A	7–10	4+
	$\beta^S\beta^+$	Hgb S >Hgb A	9–11	2 to 3+

The symbol β^O indicates a thalassemic gene that completely blocks beta-chain synthesis; the symbol β^+ indicates a thalassemic gene that limits but does not complete block beta-chain synthesis.
From Rapaport SI: Introduction to Hematology, 2nd ed. Philadelphia, J.B. Lippincott, 1987, with permission.

BIBLIOGRAPHY

1. Bessman JD, Gilmer PR, Gardner FH: Improved classification of anemias by MCV and RDW. Am J Clin Pathol 80:322–326, 1983.
2. Fairbanks VR: Laboratory testing for iron status. Hosp Pract 26:17–24, 1991.
3. Finch CA: Erythropoiesis, erythropoietin, and iron. Blood 60:1241–1246, 1982.
4. Hyun BH: Bone marrow examination. Hematol Oncol Clin North Am 2:(4), 1988.
5. Lichtman MA, Murphy MS, Adamson JW: Detection of mutant hemoglobins with altered affinity for oxygen, a simplified technique. Ann Intern Med 84:517–520, 1976.
6. Lindenbaum J: Aspects of vitamin B12 and folate metabolism in malabsorption syndromes. Am J Med 67:1037–1048, 1979.
7. Means RT, Krantz SB: Progress in understanding the pathogenesis of the anemia of chronic disease. Blood 80:1639–1647, 1992.
8. Rapaport S (ed): Introduction to Hematology, 2nd ed. Philadelphia, J.B. Lippincott, 1987.
9. Savage D, Lindenbaum J: Anemia in alcoholics. Medicine 65:322–338, 1986.
10. Strobach RS, Anderson SK, Doll DC, Ringenberg QS: The value of the physical examination in the diagnosis of anemia: Correlation of the physical findings and the hemoglobin concentration. Arch Intern Med 148:831–832, 1988.
11. Williams WJ, Beutler E, Ersley AJ, Lichtman MA (eds): Hematology, 4th ed. New York, McGraw-Hill, 1990.

6. EVALUATION OF THE PATIENT WITH A BLEEDING DIATHESIS

Kathryn Hassell, M.D.

1. What are the considerations in a patient who seems to bleed "too much"?
Excessive bleeding occurs when one or more components of the hemostatic mechanism are dysfunctional. The first step in the evaluation of a patient is to look carefully for areas of trauma or postoperative bleeding that may require mechanical repair. In the absence of obvious reasons for bleeding, function of the hemostatic system should be measured by assessing platelets, blood coagulation proteins, and breakdown products.

2. Are there any helpful questions to ask when taking a history to determine a bleeding risk?
The best predictors of bleeding risk can be found in taking a history. A patient should be asked about a personal history of bleeding. A lifelong history of easy bruising, nose bleeds, gum bleeding, or heavy menses may indicate a quantitative or qualitative platelet problem. Tonsillectomy and wisdom tooth extraction are two common surgeries that greatly stress the entire hemostatic system. If a patient has tolerated these procedures or other surgery/ trauma in the past, it is unlikely that he or she has a severe inherited bleeding disorder.

A careful family history should be taken for bleeding symptoms, because mild hemophilia and von Willebrand's disease are relatively common inherited mild bleeding disorders.

A careful medication history, including use of over-the-counter drugs, should be taken, because these can significantly alter hemostasis. Aspirin, nonsteroidal anti-inflammatory drugs, and some "cold" remedies (pseudoephedrine) can affect platelet function, as can many prescription medications. Heparin and coumadin (including prophylactic "low" doses) can also change test results and cause bleeding.

3. Are there any useful signs on physical examination to determine a bleeding disorder?
Petechiae (small purplish subcutaneous "spots" found especially on the dependent parts of the body) may indicate a quantitative or qualitative platelet disorder. Ecchymoses (bruises), especially in different stages of healing, can indicate either a platelet or blood coagulation protein disorder. Oozing or bleeding from old puncture sites or wounds may indicate inadequate platelets, inadequate blood coagulation factors, or an increase in fibrinolytic activity associated with disseminated intravascular coagulation (DIC).

4. What tests will assess platelets?
Both quantitative and qualitative abnormalities in platelets may cause excessive bleeding.

Quantitative testing is done using a platelet count. A normal platelet count is approximately 150,000–400,000/mm³; spontaneous bleeding in the absence of trauma is uncommon with a platelet count above 20,000/mm³, but a platelet count of 50,000–60,000/mm³ is necessary to maintain hemostasis postoperatively or with injury. Occasionally, patients with a very low platelet count (<20,000/mm³) may have immune-mediated thrombocytopenia (ITP). These patients produce young platelets with increased function, resulting in less bleeding than would be expected in a patient with a very low platelet count. In contrast, some patients with myeloproliferative disorders (where the bone marrow is producing excessive blood cells) may have platelet counts of up to 1,000,000/mm³, but the platelets function poorly, resulting in bleeding. When assessing the platelet count, a final consideration is pseudothrombocytopenia, which occurs because platelets from some patients will clump with EDTA (the anticoagulant used for the CBC "purple-top" tube); the peripheralblood smear will show this clumping and a repeat platelet count should be done using a heparinized ("green top" Vacutainer tube) blood sample.

Qualitative platelet function can be assessed by the bleeding time. In this test, a nick is made in the skin using a standardized template under standardized conditions, and the time to first formation of a blood clot is measured. The bleeding time can be prolonged by a number of factors other than qualitative platelet function, including platelet count, skin integrity, and blood vessel integrity, and needs to be interpreted with caution (see Controversies below). Platelet aggregation studies are done to assess responses to various agents that cause platelets to adhere and aggregate. These studies can be used to detect inherited or acquired platelet function disorders.

5. Which tests will assess the blood coagulation proteins?

Screening tests for abnormalities in the coagulation proteins include the prothrombin time (PT) and activated partial thromboplastin time (aPTT). Prolongation of these tests indicates either deficiencies of blood coagulation factors or interference with the function of these factors by an inhibitor. To determine whether an inhibitor or deficiency state exists, the prolonged test (PT or aPPT) is repeated by mixing the patient's plasma with normal plasma (1:1 mixing study). If the prolonged test corrects to normal, this indicates the patient is missing some factor that can be corrected by adding normal plasma. If it does not correct, the patient may have an inhibitor that blocks the function of factors when normal plasma is added. This mixing study is the first step to evaluate an abnormal PT or aPTT.

6. What does a prolonged PT mean?

The PT assesses the function of the extrinsic pathway (tissue factor, factor VII) and common pathway (factors X, V, II, fibrinogen) of coagulation. If any of these factors are low (<30–40% of normal), the PT will be prolonged. Although inherited deficiencies and inhibitors of these factors are rare, acquired deficiencies occur. Factors II, VII, and X require vitamin K and adequate liver function for production, so a patient with moderate to severe liver disease or poor vitamin K intake (from malabsorption, malnutrition, antibiotic therapy impairing gut production of vitamin K) will have a prolonged PT. Coumadin and rat poison, by inhibiting vitamin K metabolism, will also prolong the PT by inhibiting production of these factors. In very severe liver disease, all factors measured by the PT (including fibrinogen) will be decreased. Bleeding can occur in patients with only mild prolongation of the PT (1–2 seconds above the normal range) but is more common with more prolonged values (>3 seconds above normal).

7. What does a prolonged aPTT mean?

The aPTT assesses the function of the intrinsic pathway (factors XII, XI, IX, VIII) and common pathway (factors X, V, II, and fibrinogen) of coagulation. If any of these factors are low (<30–40% of normal), the aPTT will be prolonged. Inherited deficiencies of factor VIII (hemophilia A) and factor IX (hemophilia B) may be seen. In patients with mild hemophilia (factor levels of 10–30%), bleeding may occur only with trauma or surgery. Inherited deficiencies of other factors are rare.

Acquired deficiencies of these factors can be seen in severe liver disease (the site of production for the factors) and in long-term coumadin therapy (because factors II, IX, and X require vitamin K for production).

Von Willebrand's disease, an inherited disease that is characterized by low levels of factor VIII and von Willebrand's factor, with prolonged bleeding time due to platelet dysfunction, also can prolong the aPTT.

Specific inhibitors against factors VIII and IX are uncommon but result in severe bleeding disorders. *Nonspecific* inhibitors (e.g., lupus anticoagulant) can prolong the aPTT but are not associated with a bleeding diathesis. Bleeding can occur in patients with only mild prolongation of the aPTT (3–4 seconds above normal range) but is more common with more prolonged values (>5 seconds above normal).

8. Are there other tests that help evaluate the bleeding patient?
Measurement of the actual factor levels, including von Willebrand's factor, will confirm a deficiency or the activity of an inhibitor detected by the screening tests (PT, aPTT) or the 1:1 mixing study. Knowing that a specific factor is low may guide the choice of therapy; for example, the use of factor VIII concentrate in a hemophiliac, cryoprecipitate in a patient with a low fibrinogen or 1-deamino-8-D-arginine vasopressin (DDAVP) in a patient with von Willebrand's disease.

Measurement of fibrin split products (FSP), which accumulate when a large amount of clot has been formed and then broken down, can be useful. Increased FSP develop in disseminated intravascular coagulation (DIC), and in conjunction with an elevated PT or aPTT, low fibrinogen levels, and falling platelets help to make the diagnosis of DIC. In addition, elevated FSP can interfere with the measurement of the PT and aPTT, causing prolonged test results without necessarily increasing the risk of bleeding.

Assessment of hepatic and renal function is important. Because the liver makes all coagulation factors, liver enzymes (aspartate aminotransferase [AST], alanine aminotransferase [ALT], alkaline phosphatase) and liver function tests (total/direct bilirubin, albumin) should be measured. Blood urea nitrogen (BUN) and creatinine should be measured, because uremia affects platelet function.

9. In patients with a chronic bleeding problem, which diseases or conditions are likely?
A lifelong history of bleeding problems, especially if they began in childhood or at puberty, make an inherited condition more likely. Von Willebrand's disease, mild hemophilia, and qualitative platelet function disorders need to be considered, along with rare isolated factor deficiencies. If the problem is longstanding but has developed over time, an acquired disorder is more likely. Chronic liver disease, chronic renal disease, vasculitis with vascular damage, and chronic use of medications may affect hemostasis.

10. In patients with an acute bleeding problem, which diseases or conditions should be considered?
In the absence of a significant past history of bleeding, acquired disorders need to be considered. Consumption of platelets and coagulation factors can occur in instances of massive trauma, severe bleeding, overwhelming infection, severe liver disease, or because of DIC associated with any of these conditions. An isolated fall in platelets can be seen in ITP, thrombotic thrombocytopenia purpura/hemolytic uremic syndrome (TTP/HUS), or because of ingestion of a toxic drug. Finally, it is possible that a previously mild inherited disorder (e.g., von Willebrand's disease) has become apparent in the setting of a hemostatic stress (e.g., surgery, trauma).

CONTROVERSIES

11. Is the bleeding time of any value?
The bleeding time is affected by several hemostatic factors, including the qualitative function of platelets, the number of platelets, and the integrity of capillary vessels and of the skin itself. It is not specific to platelet function and may not correlate with the risk of bleeding from nonskin surfaces such as the mucosa, visceral organs, or other tissues that may sustain injury or surgical trauma. Several studies have shown it has no value in predicting the risk of bleeding in patients undergoing cardiac bypass surgery, gastrointestinal biopsy, percutaneous renal biopsy, or general surgery. Because it is nonspecific, it is unclear if an elevated bleeding time performed on a hospitalized patient who is acutely ill and on multiple medications indicates a bleeding diasthesis. The main use for a bleeding time

would be to screen for von Willebrand's disease or an inherited platelet defect; even in these diseases, the bleeding time is variable.

BIBLIOGRAPHY

1. Bennett JS, Kolodziej MA: Disorders of platelet function. Disease of the Month, 38:577, 1992.
2. Bick RL: Acquired platelet function defects. Hematol Oncol Clin North Am 6:1203, 1992.
3. Bloom AL: Von Willebrand factor: Clinical features of inherited and acquired disorders. Mayo Clin Proc 66:743, 1991.
4. Fareed J, et al: Drug-induced alterations of hemostasis and fibrinolysis. Hematol Oncol Clin. North Am 6:1229, 1992.
5. Galanakis DK: Fibrinogen anomalies and disease. A clinical update. Hematol Oncol Clin North Am 6:1171, 1992.
6. Kitchen CS: Approach to the bleeding patient. Hematol Oncol Clin North Am 6(5):983, 1992.
7. Mammen EF: Coagulation abnormalities in liver disease. Hematol Oncol Clin North Am 6:1247, 1992.
8. Rodgers RPC, et al: A critical reappraisal of the bleeding time. Semin Thromb Hemost 16:1, 1990.
9. Violi F, et al: Clotting abnormalities in chronic liver disease. Dig Dis 10(3):162, 1992.
10. Wu KK: Endothelial cells in hemostasis, thrombosis, and inflammation. Hosp Pract 27(4):145, 1992.

7. EVALUATION OF ADENOPATHY

George Philips, M.D., and Catherine E. Klein, M.D.

1. What is the differential diagnosis of a swelling in the neck?
Not all lumps in the neck are lymph nodes. Abscesses (particularly periodontal), infections in salivary glands, thyroid cysts, or thyroglossal duct cysts may present as masses in the neck. Many of these entities are midline, whereas nodes are usually lateral, or may move in conjunction with the thyroid during swallowing. These observations may help to differentiate the mass from true adenopathy.

2. What entities cause swelling in the groin?
Enlarged lymph nodes in the groin are common, often resulting from minor infections in the feet. Inguinal hernias and vascular aneurysms occasionally may be mistaken for adenopathy.

3. When should a posterior cervical lymph node raise concern?
Careful examination of the patient with isolated cervical adenopathy usually reveals an infection as the cause. The most common infections are viral or bacterial and involve the face or oropharynx. Infectious mononucleosis may present with posterior cervical adenopathy, but a careful search usually reveals mild splenomegaly and other swollen nodes as well as the typical pharyngitis. With the recent increase in mycobacterial disease, related in part to its associations with infection by the human immunodeficiency virus (HIV) and with the immigrant Asian population, more patients present with tuberculous cervical adenopathy. Other less common infections include cat-scratch fever, toxoplasmosis, histoplasmosis, and cytomegalovirus (CMV). Hodgkin's disease and other lymphomas present only rarely as isolated posterior cervical adenopathy.

4. Can drugs cause adenopathy?
Phenytoin is associated with a hypersensitivity reaction that gives the picture of pseudo-lymphoma. A small portion of these patients develop a true lymphoma. Antithyroid agents and isoniazid are also associated with occasional adenopathy.

5. What benign conditions cause generalized adenopathy?
Conditions associated with widespread adenopathy are systemic in nature. Many are infectious (Epstein-Barr virus [EBV], CMV, tuberculosis, histoplasmosis, syphilis, HIV infection, brucella, leptospirosis). Rheumatologic diseases, such as lupus, and widespread skin diseases, such as eczema, drug eruptions, and psoriasis, also may present with diffuse adenopathy. Occasionally patients with thyrotoxicosis, lipidoses, or sarcoidosis have generalized adenopathy.

6. What are the causes of adenopathy in the patient with accquired immunodeficiency syndrome (AIDS)?
Patients with AIDS frequently have generalized adenopathy of unclear etiology; for this condition, no therapy is needed. However, fungal and mycobacterial infections must be carefully excluded. The most common malignancies in patients with AIDS are Kaposi's sarcoma and lymphoma, both of which are associated with enlarged lymph nodes.

7. What are the common malignancies that cause adenopathy?
Cancerous lymph nodes may be either single or multiple, localized or widespread. The causes of widespread cancerous lymph ,,odes are usually systemic in nature—lymphoproliferative or, less commonly, myeloproliferative disorders. When the malignancy is solitary or localized to one or two lymph node groups, one should consider not only lymphomas and Hodgkin's disease but also metastatic carcinomas. Primary tumors of the head and neck often present with an abnormal node in the neck. Women with breast cancer may have detectable nodes in the axilla before the primary tumor has been diagnosed.

8. How does age affect the likelihood of finding tumor in an isolated enlarged node?
On average, 20% of patients under age 25 years who have a node biopsied are found to harbor a malignancy, whereas patients over age 50 years have an 80% probability of cancer at biopsy.

9. Are there characteristics of the node that should raise the suspicion of cancer?
Generally the larger the node, the greater the concern. Location is important: supraclavicular nodes are almost always malignant, whereas posterior cervical nodes are rarely malignant. Rock-hard nodes are highly worrisome for metastatic carcinoma. Painful nodes are less likley to be cancerous. Matted nodes, fixed to underlying structures and growing steadily over weeks to months, are suggestive of cancer. Of importance, none of these characteristics is diagnostic, and tissue for microscopic examination is required.

10. Which tests may be done to help to establish a diagnosis before the patient undergoes a lymph node biopsy?
Although not specific for any disease, the complete blood count (CBC) is frequently abnormal in patients with infections, malignancies, or rheumatologic disorders associated with adenopathy. A Venereal Disease Research Laboratory (VDRL) or rapid plasmin reagin (RPR) test may help to rule out syphilis and should be considered in any sexually active patient. HIV antibody testing in persons at risk is essential. In addition to liver function tests, serologic studies to detect the hepatitis virus (both B and C), EBV for infectious mononucleosis, antinuclear antibodies (ANA) for rheumatologic disease, and thyroid-stimulating hormone (TSH) for thyroid disease are probably warranted. A chest radiograph may be helpful in identifying mediastinal adenopathy in patients with sarcoidosis or lymphoma.

11. What is scrofula?
Scrofula is an old term referring to the presentation of mycobacterial disease as cervical adenopathy. Because of its worldwide prevalence, it is associated most commonly with *Mycobacterium tuberculosis*, even though *Mycobacterium scrofulaceum* is the organism most prone to present in this manner.

12. What is the best approach to making a diagnosis in a patient with adenopathy?
Not all patients with enlarged lymph nodes need histologic examination of tissue to establish a diagnosis. Many infectious diseases or rheumatologic disorders are better diagnosed from history, serologic examination, or cultures. In fact, the microscopic appearance of lymph nodes from these patients is often nonspecific. When suspicion of infection is high, a trial of antibiotics may be warranted, with reexamination in 2–3 weeks. For patients in whom the adenopathy does not regress as expected or in whom the likelihood of cancer is significant at presentation, tissue should be obtained for biopsy. The best specimen for histopathologic study is the excisional biopsy, in which the entire lymph node, fresh and in saline, is submitted to the pathologist for sectioning, staining, and culture. Sections are necessary to assess the architecture of the node, a fundamental part of the diagnosis of any lymphoma.

13. When should fine-needle aspiration be used?
Fine-needle aspiration of a node provides small samples for culture and cytologic examination. It can be useful when the patient is known to have cancer and is now suspected of having recurrent or metastatic disease. Fine-needle aspiration is also useful in the documentation of suspected new malignancy, although histologic specimens are generally preferred in this setting. When the aspiration is unrevealing, the next step is to biopsy the node.

14. What are the potential risks of fine-needle aspiration?
With proper sterile technique, the risk of infection is extremely low. Obviously there is a small risk of bleeding, particularly if a vascular structure is biopsied by mistake, but serious bleeding in patients with normal hemostatic function is rare. Of concern has been the possibility of seeding tumor cells along the tract of the needle, which may reduce the curability of some malignancies. This risk seems to be more theoretic than actual.

15. In the patient with multiple enlarged nodes, what should be biopsied?
In general, one diagnostic specimen is adequate, although more specimens may be required to document the exact stage of lymphoma. Biopsies of groin nodes are usually avoided because these nodes are commonly enlarged from other dermatopathic causes and are of low yield. Otherwise we look for large, readily accessible nodes. Nodes in the axilla, which often require more extensive dissection, are avoided if more superficial cervical nodes appear pathologically enlarged.

BIBLIOGRAPHY

1. Fijten GH, et al: Unexplained adenopathy in family practice: An evaluation of the probability of malignant causes and the effectiveness of the physicians' workup. J Fam Pract 27:373, 1988.
2. Friedberg J: Clinical diagnosis of neck lumps: A practical guide. Pediatr Ann 17:620, 1988.
3. Greenfield S, et al: The clinical investigation of lymphadenopathy in primary care practice. JAMA 240:1388, 1978.
4. Kline TS, et al: Lymphadenopathy and aspiration biopsy cytology: A review of 376 superficial nodes. Cancer 54:1076, 1984.
5. Kunitz A: An approach to peripheral lymphadenopathy in adult patients. West J Med 143:393, 1985.
6. Libman H: Generalized adenopathy: Clinical reviews. J Gen Intern Med 2:48, 1987.
7. Slap GB, et al: When to perform biopsies of enlarged peripheral lymph nodes in young patients. JAMA 252:1321, 1984.

8. EVALUATION OF LEUKOCYTOSIS

George Mathai, M.D., and William A. Robinson, M.D., Ph.D.

1. Define leukocytosis.
Leukocytosis is an elevation of the total white blood cell (WBC) count greater than two standard deviations above the mean, which in most laboratories is a total count >20,000 cells/mm³. This elevation may involve one or more subsets of the circulating white cells. Circulating leukocytes consist of neutrophils, monocytes, eosinophils, basophils, and lymphocytes. Each type of leukocyte is produced in response to specific growth factors. Neutrophilia is a specific elevation of the absolute neutrophil count and is the most common cause for leukocytosis.

2. What is a leukemoid reaction?
A leukemoid reaction is an elevation of the total WBC count >50,000 cells/mm³. This reaction is generally characterized by increased numbers of both mature neutrophils and band forms. (See Figure 6, Color Plates.) Immature cells and blast forms may be seen in a leukemoid reaction. A leukemoid reaction needs to be distinguished from chronic myelogenous leukemia (CML), acute leukemia, and a leukoerythroblastic reaction.

3. Are there different types of leukemoid reactions?
Yes. The most common is the myeloid leukemoid reaction, characterized by an elevation of mature neutrophils and band forms. One may also see a lymphoid leukemoid reaction, characterized by elevation predominantly of lymphocytes and caused most commonly by viral infections such as mononucleosis, hepatitis, or (in children) pertussis. Monocytic leukemoid reactions can also be identified, although they are less common than the other types. These reactions are generally caused by parasitic infections.

4. Discuss the steps in evaluating a patient with leukocytosis.
• Examine the peripheral blood smear and establish or confirm the diagnosis of leukocytosis.
• Determine the type and maturation of WBCs to aid in diagnosing the cause of leukocytosis.
• Evaluate the peripheral blood smear for concomitant abnormalities in red blood cells and platelets.
• Investigate symptoms suggestive of acute or chronic inflammatory disease. Relevant tests may include blood cultures (bacterial and fungal), viral cultures, smears, tissue biopsies, and radiologic tests.
• A leukocyte alkaline phosphatase score of neutrophils in peripheral blood will be high in a leukemoid reaction but low in CML.
• Parents' or siblings' blood counts may be examined to detect genetic or familial causes of leukocytosis.
• Bone marrow aspiration, core biopsy, and cytogenetics confirm the diagnosis of CML and other myeloproliferative disorders. A bone marrow biopsy also confirms leukoerythroblastosis and detects infiltrative marrow disease by cancer, inflammatory disorders, or fungal infections.

5. In which individuals should the bone marrow biopsy be performed early in the evaluation?
If the diagnosis of leukemia or myeloproliferative disorder is suspected on the basis of evaluation of the smear, prominent splenomegaly, or other findings, the bone marrow biopsy should be performed early. In an individual who tests positive for the human

immunodeficiency virus (HIV), the bone marrow may be done early to evaluate for lymphoma or to provide culture material.

6. What is a leukoerythroblastic reaction?
It is a reaction of the bone marrow to an infiltrating process, such as carcinoma (e.g., breast cancer, prostate cancer, lung cancer) or infection (e.g., tuberculosis, fungus). Leukoerythroblastic reaction can be identified on the peripheral smear by nucleated red blood cells, tear-drop shaped red cells, and early myeloid cells (i.e., promyelocytes and metamyelocytes).

7. How can a leukemoid reaction be distinguished from chronic or acute leukemia?
In **chronic myelogenous leukemia** (CML), the leukocyte alkaline phosphatase is low and generally the spleen is palpable. The blood smear often contains increased numbers of eosinophils and basophils. Most importantly, cytogenic evaluation of the bone marrow should reveal evidence of the Philadelphia chromosome in CML.

In **acute leukemia,** a higher percentage of blast forms may be seen on the peripheral blood smear. Again, a bone marrow examination should be performed to distinguish between acute leukemia and leukemoid reaction by identification of malignant clone cells in acute leukemia.

8. What causes the leukemoid reaction?
The exact cause is not clear. It may be due to elaboration of growth factors or tumor necrosis factor by certain malignancies or inflammatory processes. Release of endogenous epinephrine, cortisol, or histamine may also cause a leukemoid reaction.

9. Are there any drugs that cause an elevated white count?
Yes. Epinephrine and steroids are probably the most common causes. In patients treated with growth factors for neutropenia, the WBC count can become highly elevated if administration is not closely monitored. Psychiatric patients treated with lithium also demonstrate elevated WBC counts. Lithium appears to function as a growth factor on the bone marrow.

10. Can the white blood cell count be falsely elevated?
Yes. False elevation of the automated determination of the WBC count can be due to the presence of cryoglobulins, clotting, or platelet aggregation or to the presence of nucleated red cells or red cells that were not lysed, both of which are counted as WBCs.

11. What are the most common causes of a leukemoid reaction?
A leukemoid reaction is most commonly due to infection (bacterial or viral) or malignancy.

12. How should leukocytosis be treated? Should it be treated?
Treatment of leukocytosis depends on the underlying cause. In cases of congenital or idiopathic neutrophilia, treatment is not necessary because the elevated WBC count generally has no physiologic consequence.

13. How can congenital or idiopathic neutrophilia be identified?
Idiopathic neutrophilia, a cause of chronic neutrophilia, occurs in healthy individuals. Usually the WBC count is only moderately elevated (11,000–20,000 cells/mm^3). All other causes of leukocytosis must be excluded before this diagnosis can be made. Congenital neutrophilia is rare. It can be identified by examination of both the personal and family history. Leukemoid reactions (acute and chronic) can also be seen in Down's syndrome.

14. Does smoking cause leukocytosis?
Yes. It is known that nicotine can cause leukocytosis. One study identified the degree of leukocytosis among smokers as a risk factor for myocardial infarction.

15. Does leukocytosis predict the subsequent development of disease, such as CML?
No. Studies that followed patients with apparent idiopathic neutrophilia have shown that it does not predict the development of disease, specifically CML.

16. Is the level of leukocytosis helpful in distinguishing the diagnosis?
No studies correlate the level of leukocytosis with specific diagnoses. Even idiopathic neutrophilia, commonly associated with moderate elevation of the WBC count, can be associated with counts >40,000 cells/mm³.

BIBLIOGRAPHY

1. Brodeur GM, Dahl GV, Williams DL, et al: Transient leukemoid reaction and trisomy 21 mosaicism in a phenotypically normal newborn. Blood 55:691–693, 1980.
2. Dale DC, Fauci AS, Guerry D, Wolff SM: Comparison of agents producing a neutrophilic leukocytosis in man. J Clin Invest 56:808–813, 1975.
3. Herring WB, Smith LG, Walker RI, Herion JC: Hereditary neutrophilia. Am J Med 56:729–734, 1974.
4. McKee LC: Excess leukocytosis (leukemoid reactions) associated with malignant diseases. South Med J 78:1475–1482, 1985.
5. Walker RI, Willemze R: Neutrophil kinetics and the regulation of granulopoieses. Rev Infect Dis 2:282, 1980.
6. Ward HN, Reinhard EH: Chronic idiopathic leukocytosis. Ann Intern Med 75:193–198, 1971.
7. Zalokar JB, Richard JL, Claude JR: Leukocyte count, smoking, and myocardial infarction. N Engl J Med 304:465–468, 1981.

II. General Hematology

---

9. IRON DEFICIENCY ANEMIA

C.R. Santhosh-Kumar, M.D., and J. Fred Kolhouse, M.D.

---

1. What is the most common cause of iron deficiency anemia?
The most common causes are blood loss from the gastrointestinal (GI) tract in males and postmenopausal females and from the GI tract or owing to menstruation in premenopausal females. Iron deficiency in men always requires a search in the GI tract for a source of blood loss, whereas in women excessive menstrual blood loss as indicated by excessive use of menstrual pads or blood clots may be the explanation.

2. How sensitive is the stool Hemoccult test as an indication of excessive blood loss?
The stool Hemoccult test is useful only if it is positive. False-negative tests occur because of insensitivity of the test and because bleeding from the GI tract is frequently intermittent. False-positive tests may also occur with the ingestion of certain heme-containing foods.

3. Give the number of milligrams (mg) of reserve iron that humans have.
Men have from 500–2000 mg of reserve iron, whereas women have approximately 250 mg of reserve iron; 25% of premenopausal women in the United States have no reserve iron.

4. How many milligrams of iron are in a unit (500 ml) of blood?
Each milliliter of blood has 0.5 mg of iron in hemoglobin. Therefore, a 500-ml unit of blood has approximately 250 mg of iron. It is clear from this statement that the loss of an additional unit of blood can readily deplete normal iron stores in premenopausal females.

5. Loss of a unit of blood would be expected to produce what change in the hematocrit of a normal person?
The hematocrit decreases approximately 3 points and the hemoglobin decreases approximately 1 gm/dl for each unit of blood lost. Therefore, for each unit of blood loss and drop in the hematocrit of 3 points, approximately 250 mg of iron will be required to regenerate a normal hematocrit and hemoglobin in a normal person.

6. How often is the mean corpuscular volume (MCV) low in iron deficiency anemia?
Rarely is the MCV low in iron deficiency anemia. Approximately 10% of patients with severe iron deficiency (hematocrit <27%) will have a low MCV secondary to iron deficiency. Because iron deficiency is still the most common cause of anemia worldwide, the majority of individuals do not have a low MCV but will have anemia owing to iron deficiency.

7. Which disorders should you think of when the MCV is low and the hematocrit is >35%?
This situation can occur in several circumstances: (1) polycythemia treated with phlebotomies to induce an iron deficiency "anemia" that normalizes or lowers the hematocrit; (2) a patient with polycythemia vera, who has GI bleeding; and (3) a patient with beta-thalassemia. Interestingly, in beta-thalassemia, the free erythrocyte protoporphyrin (FEP) is normal.

8. Shortly after massive blood loss, what change in the hematocrit would you expect?
Minimal or no change in the hematocrit. This is because when blood loss occurs, equal volumes of plasma and red cells are lost simultaneously. Only after 48–72 hours will a nadir in the hematocrit occur as plasma volume is restored.

9. Is there a "gold standard" test for iron deficiency?
The bone marrow iron stores is an underutilized test for iron deficiency. No condition exists in which iron is present in the bone marrow and anemia is due to iron deficiency. It has been claimed that following treatment with iron-dextran, the bone marrow can still contain iron in macrophages as iron-dextran. The iron from iron-dextran is proposed to be nonutilizable by cells. With this exception, absent bone marrow iron is required for the diagnosis of iron deficiency anemia (i.e., the iron stain of the bone marrow aspirate will be negative). Bone marrow iron should always be determined before embarking upon an expensive diagnostic GI work-up for iron deficiency.

10. What pitfalls may be expected from a therapeutic trial of iron sulfate?
The hematocrit may fail to rise during a therapeutic trial of iron for presumed iron deficiency anemia because (1) the patient is noncompliant with the iron supplementation; (2) blood loss exceeds the ability to absorb increased iron from supplementation; and (3) the diagnosis of iron deficiency is in error. Regardless of whether a therapeutic trial of iron successfully increases the hematocrit, presumed iron deficiency requires further documentation and subsequent gastrointestinal tract evaluation for a source of blood loss.

11. Are there other tests that can be used to diagnose iron deficiency?
Numerous other tests are available for the evaluation of iron deficiency but none is without flaws. The FEP is normal in thalassemia but is elevated in both iron deficiency anemia and the anemia of chronic disorders. The serum ferritin is a very close indicator of total body iron stores, and when it is low, it is virtually diagnostic of iron deficiency. However, a normal or elevated ferritin does not in any way exclude iron deficiency. When the total iron binding capacity (TIBC) is high and the serum iron is low (creating a saturation of <10%), the patient very likely has iron deficiency. However, a very low serum iron may be associated with the anemia of chronic disorders, which also is usually acompanied by a low TIBC. In addition, the combination of the anemia of chronic disease and iron deficiency may be associated with a "normal" TIBC and low serum iron.

12. Describe the effect of iron deficiency on the level of A_2 hemoglobin.
Hemoglobin electrophoresis and quantitative hemoglobins (with an elevated A_2 hemoglobin) are frequently used to diagnose beta-thalassemia. Iron deficiency presents a picture that can complicate the diagnosis of beta-thalassemia. Iron deficiency *per se* can result in a low A_2 hemoglobin, and when present in conjunction with beta-thalassemia, A_2 hemoglobin may be normal or low (when an elevated A_2 hemoglobin is expected). Thus, a patient with beta-thalassemia who also has GI blood loss and iron deficiency will have at presentation a normal or low A_2 hemoglobin, but on replacement of iron, the hematocrit will increase *but not normalize* and the A_2 hemoglobin when repeated will be increased to above normal levels.

13. What consideration should be given when apparent iron deficiency anemia fails to respond to oral iron therapy?
As indicated in question 10, patients may fail to respond to a therapeutic trial of iron because of misdiagnosis or noncompliance. However, even in the compliant patient with the correct diagnosis, oral iron therapy may fail to correct the iron deficiency. In this setting, continued excessive blood loss and failure to absorb iron from ferrous sulfate (predominantly in the duodenum) may be the source of failure to respond to iron.

Failure to absorb oral iron can be tested by obtaining a fasting serum iron and a repeat serum iron 4 hours after a 320-mg tablet of ferrous sulfate. Normal absorption would be indicated by absorption of 6–7 mg of iron. The total iron absorbed is calculated by subtracting the fasting serum iron from the iron at 3 hours after ingestion of iron sulfate. This value is multiplied by 0.062, and 0.45 is added to the product. Because a 320-mg tablet of iron sulfate contains 60 mg of iron, a value of 6–7 mg (approximately 10%) is considered normal. If iron absorption is low, the physician should pursue the question of disease of the upper small intestine. Such a failure to absorb oral iron is an indication for parenteral (intravenous) iron-dextran therapy.

14. Describe the characteristic test abnormalities in the anemia of chronic disorders.
The diagnosis of anemia of chronic disorders is frequently considered a "wastebasket" diagnosis. However, the anemia of chronic disorders can be made as a positive diagnosis as well. In this disorder, certain conditions impair the utilization of iron by the body. Oral iron therapy in these individuals is of questionable or no benefit. This disorder is characterized by a reduced serum iron, a reduced TIBC, and frequently an elevated ferritin and sedimentation rate. Usually the etiology of these abnormalities is clear (active rheumatoid arthritis, osteomyelitis, pulmonary tuberculosis, neoplastic disease), but on occasion the patient may have to be followed and retested at intervals to establish the reason for having anemia of chronic disorders. Anemia of chronic disorders is a misnomer, because there are many anemias associated with chronic disorders that do not share this disorder's pathophysiology of failure to utilize iron stores (anemia of chronic renal failure, and so forth).

15. What is the major cause of anemia of chronic renal failure?
Although erythrocyte survival is slightly shortened, the major cause of the anemia of chronic renal failure is a lack of the hormone erythropoietin, which is produced by the kidneys. With everything else being normal, the anemia of chronic renal failure can be completely corrected by replacement therapy with erythropoietin. Because erythropoietin therapy is very expensive, a low serum erythropoietin level (<500) should always be ascertained prior to initiation of treatment.

16. Failure of the anemia of chronic renal failure to respond to erythropoietin is caused by what conditions?
Several possibilities should be considered. Nutritional deficiencies of either iron or folate may be found. Alternatively, aluminum toxicity (as in patients on long-term renal dialysis) may contribute to anemia. Recently, it has been suggested that the anemia of chronic renal failure may also fail to respond because secondary hyperparathyroidism in chronic renal failure induces a form of marrow fibrosis that impairs marrow response.

BIBLIOGRAPHY

1. Baer AN, Dessypris EN, Krants SB: The pathogenesis of anemia in rheumatoid arthritis: A clinical and laboratory analysis. Semin Arthritis Rheum 19:209–223, 1990.
2. Brown RG: Determining the cause of anemia. General approach, with emphasis on microcytic hypochromic anemias. Postgrad Med 89:161–164, 1991.
3. Cook JD: Clinical evaluation of iron deficiency. Semin Hematol 19:6–10, 1982.
4. Cook JD, Skikne BS: Iron deficiency: Definition and diagnosis. J Intern Med 226:349–355, 1989.
5. Farley PC, Foland J: Iron deficiency anemia. How to diagnose and correct. Postgrad Med 87:89–93, 96, 101, 1990.
6. Finch CA, Huebers H: Perspectives in iron metabolism. N Engl J Med 306:1520, 1982.
7. Green R: Disorders of inadequate iron. Hosp Pract 3:25–29, 1991.
8. Lipschitz DA: The anemia of chronic disease. J Am Geriatr Soc 38:1258–1264, 1990.
9. MacDougall IC, Hutton RD, Coles GA, Williams JD: The use of erythropoietin in renal failure. Postgrad Med 67:9–15, 1991.
10. Marsh WL, Nelson DP, Koening HM: Free erythrocyte protoporphyrin (FEP) II. The FEP test is clinically useful in classifying microcytic RBC disorders in adults. Am J Clin Pathol 79:661–666, 1983.

11. Massey AC: Mirocytic anemia: Differential diagnosis and management of iron deficiency anemia. Med Clin North Am 76:549–566, 1992.
12. Mohler ER Jr: Iron deficiency and anemia of chronic disease. Clues to differentiating these conditions. Postgrad Med 92:123–128, 1992.
13. Rao DS, Shih M, Mohini R: Effect of serum parathyroid hormone and bone fibrosis on the response to erythropoietin in uremia. N Engl J Med 328:171–175, 1993.
14. Van Wyck DB: Iron deficiency in patients with dialysis-associated anemia during eyrthropoietin replacement therapy: Strategies for assessment and management. Semin Nephrol 9:21–24, 1989.

10. MEGALOBLASTIC ANEMIA

C.R. *Santhosh-Kumar,* M.D., *and* J. *Fred Kolhouse,* M.D.

1. Are there features in the peripheral blood count that suggest megaloblastic anemia resulting from folate or cobalamin (vitamin B12) deficiency?

The peripheral blood counts in folate or cobalamin deficiency can range from normal (including a normal MCV) to anemia alone to pancytopenia. Classically, patients have mild pancytopenia with severe anemia and a very high mean corpuscular volume (MCV >120).

2. What changes in the elements of the blood smear suggest megaloblastic anemia?

There are numerous causes of an elevated MCV, including alcoholism, cigarette smoking, aplastic anemia, refractory anemia, and other causes related to intense erythropoietin stimulation. The macrocytosis in folate and cobalamin deficiency specifically reveals macro-ovalocytes (as opposed to macrocytes) and hypersegmented neutrophils. A predominance of five-lobed neutrophils and occasional six-lobed neutrophils is highly suggestive of cobalamin or folate deficiency. However, hypersegmentation may be seen in other conditions, including granulocyte leukemoid reactions.

3. Discuss the differential diagnosis of anemia with an elevated MCV.

Causes of a mild elevation of MCV (<110) include folate and cobalamin deficiency, but alcoholism with or without liver disease and smoking can cause a mild increase in MCV. The higher the MCV, the more likely the patient has folate or cobalamin deficiency or refractory anemia.

4. What is the characteristic bone marrow morphology of megaloblastic anemia?

The bone marrow is 95–100% cellular in megaloblastic anemias. Owing to the abnormal appearance of the cells in the marrow and because the marrow is packed, this diagnosis has been mislabeled as acute leukemia, particularly when only core biopsies are examined. (See Figure 2, Color Plates.) Thus, a bone marrow aspirate (which reveals marrow cytology) as well as a core biopsy (which reveals marrow cellularity) should always be obtained.

5. Define nuclear-cytoplasmic dissociation.

This form of myelodysplasia is the characteristic lesion of megaloblastic anemia. It refers to a dissociation between the maturation of the nucleus of cells (particularly erythroblasts) compared to the maturation of the cytoplasm. Normally, the nucleus of erythroid precursors in the bone marrow becomes more and more dense with maturation until it is a black dot, while the cytoplasm becomes more and more intensely pink as hemoglobin is synthesized. The presence of an immature nucleus which has open chromatin and is large with a mature cytoplasm is virtually diagnostic of the myelodysplasia that occurs with cobalamin or folate deficiency

6. What are the classic clinical findings of cobalamin deficiency?
Classically, patients with cobalamin deficiency have the signs and symptoms of a severe anemia and they also can have bleeding secondary to thrombocytopenia, although this is unusual. These patients have some of the lowest hemoglobins and hematocrits at presentation of any described with any disease. The hemoglobin and hematocrit become this low with relatively few symptoms probably because of the slow development of the anemia. Sometimes these patients have indications of icterus from indirect hyper-bilirubinemia.

Physical examination frequently reveals premature graying of the hair and a smooth tongue (glossitis). Neurologic findings range from psychosis with or without depression to classic subacute combined degeneration of the spinal cord. The latter finding is evidenced predominantly by a loss of position sense and vibratory sense, particularly in the lower extremities. It is due to posterior column degeneration. However, patients can also have paralysis from motor tract disease. Patients may have the neurologic syndrome of cobalamin deficiency, including all of the above, with no abnormalities in their blood. Thus, occult cobalamin deficiency is an unusual cause of organic brain syndrome.

7. How are the clinical findings of folate deficiency different from those of cobalamin deficiency?
The clinical findings of folate deficiency closely resemble those of cobalamin deficiency. The major difference is that patients with folate deficiency do not develop posterior column disease or paralysis, although they may have symptoms of depression and psychosis.

8. What gastric abnormalities are associated with cobalamin malabsorption?
Patients with classic cobalamin malabsorption may have gastric achlorhydria and atrophy of the mucosal cells of the stomach. This atrophy results in reduced intrinsic factor secretion and malabsorption of cobalamin.

9. Why does pancreatic insufficiency result in cobalamin malabsorption?
Pancreatic enzymes, particularly trypsin and chymotrypsin, are required for the degradation of the salivary-gastric R-type cobalamin-binding protein. This cobalamin-binding protein binds cobalamin very tightly but is not involved in (and in fact will inhibit) absorption. The reason for the existence of this protein is currently unknown. When cobalamin is ingested in the diet, it is immediately bound to the R-type cobalamin-binding protein in the stomach, whereas intrinsic factor has no or little cobalamin bound to it. As the two proteins enter the duodenum, the R-type protein is degraded by pancreatic enzymes while intrinsic factor is unaffected. The cobalamin binding to the R-type protein is then weakened and the cobalamin is transferred from the R-type protein to intrinsic factor that is required for its absorption. In pancreatic insufficiency, this transfer does not occur because the R-type protein degradation does not occur.

10. Cobalamin deficiency is most commonly caused by what disorder?
In the United States, the most common cause of cobalamin deficiency is an autoimmune disorder referred to as pernicious anemia. In pernicious anemia, autoantibodies are produced against gastric parietal cells as well as intrinsic factor. These antibodies are both precipitating antibodies and antibodies that block the binding of cobalamin to intrinsic factor. Although this autoimmune disorder is considered the most common cause of cobalamin deficiency in the United States, other causes also are a relatively frequent culprit. The second most common cause is failure to absorb food cobalamin in older patients because of gastric achlorhydria, even though intrinsic factor is still being secreted. In this syndrome, all other tests are normal except for tests related to cobalamin deficiency, and it appears that the patient is unable to release the cobalamin bound to proteins in the ingested food.

11. What other organ dysfunction may be present in cobalamin deficiency when the cause is pernicious anemia?
As stated earlier, pernicious anemia is, in effect, an autoimmune disorder, and other polyendocrine disorders from autoantibodies may be associated. These include hypothyroidism, diabetes mellitus, and adrenal insufficiency. The vitiligo observed in some patients with pernicious anemia also is thought to be related to autoimmunity.

12. How much time is required to develop cobalamin deficiency from absent cobalamin in the diet?
Even in strict vegetarians where cobalamin is excluded from the diet, deficiency is very difficult to produce. If all cobalamin is taken out of the diet, approximately 12 years are required for the individual to develop cobalamin deficiency, because cobalamin stores (predominantly in the liver) are high.

13. How much time is required to develop folate deficiency from low folate in the diet?
In contrast to cobalamin deficiency, folate deficiency develops very rapidly. In a classic study, folate deficiency developed over several weeks in an individual who restricted his folate intake to less than 5 μg/day. The serum folate fell within a week and other parameters of folate deficiency developed over the ensuing 4 months. By 4 months, the individual was extremely depressed and had flagrant megaloblastic anemia secondary to folate deficiency.

14. What is the Schilling test?
The Schilling test was devised to determine whether absorption of ingested crystalline cobalamin is normal. In its simplest form, this test studies the absorption of orally administered radioactive cobalamin by measuring subsequent excretion into the urine. Patients missing intrinsic factor do not absorb significant amounts of the radiolabeled cobalamin and therefore urinary excretion is markedly reduced. To ensure adequate urinary excretion and to inhibit binding of recently absorbed cobalamin to plasma cobalamin-binding proteins (which would decrease excretion even with normal absorption), a large dose of 1 mg of nonradioactive cobalamin is admininstered parenterally with the test. Various modifications of this test have been carried out over the past number of years, including a two-phase test where radioactive cobalamin also is given already bound to intrinsic factor to confirm that the low absorption in the first test is indeed due to absent or abnormal intrinsic factor.

15. What can cause acquired cobalamin deficiency with a normal Schilling test?
Because crystalline radioactive cobalamin is always used for the standard Schilling test, individuals who cannot release cobalamin from ingested food will have cobalamin malabsorption (see above) but will have a normal Schilling test.

16. Name the two mammalian enzymes that require cobalamin as a cofactor.
In contrast to bacteria and other species of organisms, humans and mammals require cobalamin (Cbl) as a cofactor for only two enzymes: methylmalonyl–coenzyme A (CoA) mutase, which converts L-methylmalonyl-CoA to succinyl-CoA, and methionine synthase, which transfers the methyl group from 5-methyltetrahydrofolate to homocysteine to form methionine. Reduced activity of these two enzymes leads to an increase in methylmalonic acid and homocysteine, respectively. In cobalamin deficiency, both metabolites are increased, whereas in folate deficiency only homocysteine is increased, as would be predicted. These pathways then explain the elevation of homocysteine and methylmalonic acid found in patients with cobalamin and folate deficiency, and this is now a commonly used test to measure cobalamin and folate sufficiency in tissues. This observation is also of major importance because homocysteine itself may be a toxic amino acid resulting in accelerated atherosclerosis.

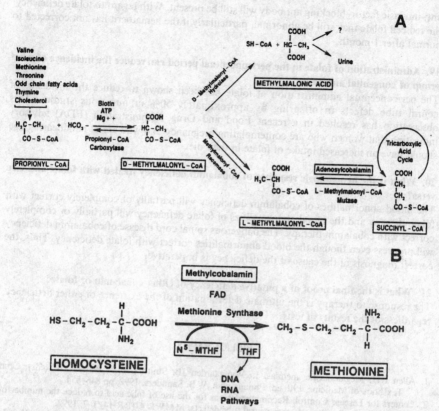

The metabolic pathways of mutase and methionine synthase. (A) The metabolic pathway leading from propionyl-CoA to succinyl-CoA. Note that mutase with its coenzyme, adenosylcobalamin, is the last step in this reaction and that D-methylmalonyl-CoA hydrolase results in the production of methylmalonic acid only from the D isomer. (B) The reaction leading from homocysteine to methionine that utilizes the enzyme methionine synthase. S-Adenosyl-methionine is thought to be required for the methylation of cobalamin during the first turnover, and subsequent methyl groups for transfer to homocysteine arise from 5-methyltetrahydrofolate (N⁵-MTHF) giving rise to tetrahydrofolate (THF). (From Kolhouse JF, Stabler SP, Allen RH: Identification and perturbation of mutant human fibroblasts based on measurements of methylmalonic acid and total homocysteine in the culture media. Arch Biochem Biophys 303:355–360, 1993, with permission.)

17. What tests will remain abnormal and diagnostic 24 hours after treatment of cobalamin or folate deficiency?

It depends to some extent on the parameters used to measure cobalamin and folate deficiency and their degree of abnormality. Although the abnormalities in the bone marrow begin to correct within hours after treatment with folate or cobalamin, they are rarely completely corrected by 24 hours. Depending on the initial elevation of the homocysteine and methylmalonic acid in serum, these two metabolites are rarely corrected after 24 hours.

18. Four weeks after treatment of cobalamin and folate deficiency, what tests will remain abnormal and diagnostic?

By 4 weeks, serum cobalamin, serum folate, and the homocysteine and methylmalonic metabolites will have corrected. However, in cobalamin deficiency due to abnormalities of intrinsic factor (as in pernicious anemia), the Schilling test will still be abnormal and the anti-intrinsic factor–blocking antibody will still be present. With regard to folate deficiency, the red cell folate may still be abnormal, particularly if the hematocrit has not corrected to normal after 1 month.

19. Administration of folate in the periconceptual period can reduce the incidence of what group of congenital anomalies?
The periconceptual administration of folate has been shown to reduce the incidence of neural tube defects in offspring by approximately 50% in numerous studies. This observation has resulted in a recent Food and Drug Administration (FDA) advisory indicating that women who are contemplating pregnancy and who are of childbearing age should have an increased intake of folate in their diet.

20. What is the hematologic response of cobalamin deficiency treated with folate and vice versa?
The blood abnormalities of cobalamin deficiency will partially or completely correct with folate therapy and the blood abnormalities of folate deficiency will partially or completely correct with cobalamin therapy. The dangerous spinal cord disease of cobalamin deficiency will progress even though the blood abnormalities correct with folate deficiency. Thus, the correct diagnosis of the cause of the deficiency is imperative.

21. What is the final proof of a putative deficiency of either cobalamin or folate?
The response to therapy is the ultimate determination of the existence of either deficiency, regardless of the results of tests.

BIBLIOGRAPHY

1. Allen RH: Megaloblastic anemias. In Wyngaarden JB, Smith LH Jr, Bennett JC (eds): Cecil Textbook of Medicine, 19th ed. Philadelphia, W.B. Saunders, 1992, pp 846–854.
2. Centers for Disease Control: Recommendations for the use of folic acid to reduce the number of cases of spina bifida and other neural tube defects. MMWR 41(RR-14):1–7, 1992.
3. Herbert V: Experimental nutritional folate deficiency in man. Trans Assoc Am Physicians 75:207–320, 1962.
4. Kolhouse JF, Stabler SP, Allen RH: Identification and perturbation of mutant human fibroblasts based on measurements of methylmalonic acid and total homocysteine in the culture media. Arch Biochem Biophys 303:355–360, 1993.
5. Morbidity and Mortality Weekly Report: Use of folic acid for prevention of spina bifida and other neural tube defects—1983-1991. JAMA 266:1190–1191, 1991.
6. Mulinare J, Cordero JF, Erickson JD, Berry RJ: Periconceptual use of multivitamins and the occurrence of neural tube defects. JAMA 260:3141–3145, 1988.
7. Stabler SP, Allen RH, Savage DG, Lindenbaum J: Clinical spectrum and diagnosis of cobalamin deficiency. Blood 76:871–881, 1990.

11. HEMOLYTIC ANEMIAS

C.R. Santhosh-Kumar, M.D., and J. Fred Kolhouse, M.D.

1. What two general causes of anemia result in a drop in the hemoglobin of more than 1 gm per week?
In the absence of hemolysis or excessive blood loss, the hemoglobin drops no more than 1 gm/week from failure of bone marrow erythropoiesis. Thus, a drop of >1 gm/week indicates excessive blood loss from bleeding or from hemolysis.

2. Name the test frequently used to measure the compensatory increase in erythrocyte production in anemia.

Reticulocyte count. This is a measure of new red blood cell production and is the most sensitive test to measure adequacy of bone marrow response to hemolysis or blood loss.

3. Discuss the chemistry laboratory tests that are useful in the diagnosis of hemolytic anemias.

Numerous tests are useful in the diagnosis of hemolytic anemia, but each has its own flaw. A common test used is the **serum haptoglobin**, which when saturated with hemoglobin from hemolysis will not bind radioactive hemoglobin and thus is reported as "absent." Approximately 2% of the population has congenitally absent haptoglobin. The **erythrocyte lactate dehydrogenase** (LDH) and **indirect reacting bilirubin tests** also are indicators of excess hemolysis. However, both of these tests may be elevated in megaloblastic anemias in which hemolysis is essentially occurring within the bone marrow. In addition, the LDH is elevated by numerous other factors in ill patients and the bilirubin elevation is somewhat dependent on liver function as well as red cell mass. It has been suggested by some that the total bilirubin (direct and indirect) be corrected for the reduced red cell mass that occurs in anemia (similar to correction of the reticulocyte count for the level of anemia), because the bilirubin predominantly evolves from the red cell mass. Applying such a correction in anemic patients frequently results in the indirect bilirubin being a more sensitive indicator of hemolysis. It should also be noted that the indirect bilirubin is frequently elevated in approximately 2% of the population who have Gilbert's disease.

4. Give the three general categories of abnormality of the erythrocyte that result in hemolytic anemia.

Three components that make up the erythrocyte that may be involved in hemolytic anemia are the erythrocyte membrane, the hemoglobin, and the intracellular erythrocyte enzymes that provide ATP energy and reducing equivalents for the hemoglobin of erythrocytes.

5. What are the two most important historical facts to obtain about a patient with a presumptive hemolytic anemia?

Patients who can be documented to have once had a normal hematocrit (particularly with a normal reticulocyte count) can be diagnosed as having an *acquired* hemolytic anemia as opposed to the numerous causes of *inherited* hemolytic anemia. The second question to ask is about a family history of anemia.

6. Discuss the two most common morphologic abnormalities of erythrocytes in patients with hemolytic anemia.

Patients with spherocytes or microspherocytes in the peripheral smear have hemolytic anemia. Numerous patients with hemolytic anemia do not have microspherocytes, but the presence of these cells indicates an underlying hemolytic process that can be from abnormalities of any of the above three components of the erythrocyte (see question 4). The other erythrocyte abnormality is microangiopathic erythrocytes (schistocytes or helmet cells). These cells occur in conjunction with intravascular hemolysis secondary to a vasculitis such as that which occurs with certain infections causing disseminated intravascular coagulation, thrombotic thrombocytopenic purpura, hemolytic-uremic syndrome, or vasculitis from malignant hypertension. (See Figure 4, Color Plates.)

7. Which test is used to determine the presence of an autoimmune hemolytic anemia?

The Coombs test is used to determine the presence of an autoimmune hemolytic anemia. Positivity of an indirect Coombs test with a negative-direct Coombs test is meaningless with regard to autoimmune hemolytic anemia. This situation frequently occurs in individuals who have been multiply transfused or in multiparous females. Indirect Coombs positivity causes difficulties with cross-match in the blood bank but has no other pathophysiologic significance. A positive direct Coombs test is very meaningful with regard to hemolytic anemia, although all patients with a positive direct Coombs test do not necessarily have an autoimmune hemolytic anemia. Approximately 90% of patients with an autoimmune hemolytic anemia have a positive direct Coombs test, whereas 10% of patients have undetectable antibody or complement on their red cell membrane but nevertheless have an autoimmune hemolytic anemia. Numerous methods have been used to diagnose this small proportion of patients, but no tests using elution of antibody have proved to be particularly beneficial.

8. What classes of antibodies are usually involved in autoimmune hemolytic anemias?
The two most common classes of antibodies involved in autoimmune hemolytic anemia are immunoglobulins (Igs) G and M. Certainly IgA has been associated with autoimmune hemolytic anemia, but this appears to be rare. As noted below (question 18), the pathophysiology and treatment of an autoimmune hemolytic anemia caused by IgG versus IgM are entirely different.

9. A Coombs test positive to "complement only" usually indicates which type of antibody in the pathophysiology of autoimmune hemolytic anemia?
Complement-only direct Coombs positivity is usually related to a cold-reacting IgM antibody. In this setting, the IgM is not present on the erythrocytes at the core body temperature. However, because IgM antibodies actively fix complement and the complement does stay on the erythrocytes, a complement-only positive Coombs test will be found in this disorder.

10. What is suggested when the direct Coombs test is positive for IgG and complement but no C'3d is present on the erythrocyte?
This usually means that the direct Coombs test is positive but the direct Coombs positivity and autoimmunity are not participating in the hemolysis. When complement is fixed on the erythrocyte membrane, C'3 is split into C'3a and C'3b, which is left on the erythrocyte surface. C'3b binds to specific receptors in the reticuloendothelial system, and an enzyme splits the C'3b into C'3d, which is left on the erythrocyte surface, and C'3c, which is left on the receptor surface. Thus, without cleavage of C'3b on the erythrocyte surface, hemolysis from this positive Coombs test is unlikely.

11. What is the most prominent inherited abnormality of the erythrocyte membrane that results in hemolysis?
Several proteins are involved in the submembrane surface of erythrocytes that help maintain a normal biconcave disk shape. These proteins are referred to as ankyrin, spectrin, and a protein named band 4.1. In hereditary spherocytosis, abnormalities exist in various families in spectrin, band 4.1, and ankyrin and in their interactions.

12. What possibilities are present when the mean corpuscular hemoglobin concentration (MCHC) is increased?
A true (nonartificial) elevation of the MCHC is seen in only one disorder in hematology—hereditary spherocytosis. Although the MCHC is increased in individual spherocytes in autoimmune hemolytic anemia, these rarely are a high enough percentage of the total erythrocytes to result in an overall increase in the MCHC. Only in hereditary spherocytosis, where approximately 40% of the erythrocytes are spherocytes, can the MCHC be increased enough to increase the overall blood MCHC. Cases of hereditary spherocytosis also occur with a normal MCHC. The MCHC is artificially increased in patients with cold agglutinin even when the concentration of the antibody is within normal limits. Thus, frequently the central hematology laboratory will note that the MCHC is vastly increased in a sample of blood. They will simply warm this blood to 37°C and rerun the sample on the automated counter to obtain a normal MCHC. Obviously, such a cold agglutinin can be of clinical importance if the titer is high enough.

13. Discuss the causes of a sudden drop in the hematocrit in hemolytic anemias.
When the hematocrit suddenly drops from increased hemolysis, the reticulocyte count should reveal whether the bone marrow is responding properly to a worsening hemolytic rate. If the hematocrit is dropping and the reticulocyte count is also decreasing, one must look immediately for causes of relative bone marrow failure resulting in the sudden drop of hematocrit. The drop in hematrocrit in each circumstance can be rather dramatic because the patients have an ongoing hemolytic anemia and are now not producing new erythrocytes. The cause of this may be (1) advancing chronic renal failure with a relative reduction in erythropoietin production (slower, gradual drop in hematocrit); (2) a reduction in micronutrients required for normal erythrocyte production (folate and iron); (3) an acute infection; (4) an infection of the bone marrow with parvovirus; or (5) drug suppression of the bone marrow. In this setting, the clinician usually orders a number of tests, including a bone marrow aspiration and biopsy, to determine a cause of the aplastic crisis.

14. Describe the characteristic features of the hemolytic anemia of paroxysmal nocturnal hemoglobinuria (PNH).
The reticulocyte count is usually elevated and the erythrocyte morphology on peripheral smear is normal; the direct Coombs test is negative and the patient will have characteristics of iron deficiency. The patient may be demonstrated to have excessive iron in the urine, absent haptoglobin, and absent bone marrow iron. In the setting of hemolytic anemia, with absent bone marrow iron, the diagnosis of PNH is presumed.

15. How is the diagnosis of PNH established?
The erythrocytes, leukocytes, and platelets of patients with PNH have an abnormally increased sensitivity to *normal* complement activation. The defect involves the cell membranes such that glycerophosphoinositol-anchored proteins that normally inactivate activated complement are missing on these cells. Thus, the PNH erythrocyte is far more sensitive to hemolysis after activation of normal complement in serum than are normal erythrocytes. The diagnosis of PNH may be established by artificially activating complement in the patient's serum compared with activation of complement in serum containing normal erythrocytes. Activation of serum complement may be produced by a mild acidification of the serum (the Ham acid hemolysis test) or reduction of the ionic strength of serum using sucrose to maintain tonicity (the sucrose hemolysis test).

16. What are the causes of death in patients with PNH?
Patients with PNH rarely have such severe hemolysis that they die from PNH alone. The vast majority of patients die from clotting abnormalities in unusual places such as the mesenteric veins, hepatic veins, and venous sinuses in the brain. Patients with PNH also can ultimately develop a myelodysplastic picture that can evolve into frank leukemia.

17. What are the causes of death in patients with autoimmune hemolytic anemias?
Approximately one-third of deaths are due to uncontrolled hemolysis, another one-third to the underlying secondary disorder (lymphomas and lymphocytic leukemias), and one-third to pulmonary embolus. As in PNH, thrombosis is very common in patients with auto-immune hemolytic anemias.

18. How is cold antibody hemolytic anemia treated differently compared with warm autoimmune hemolytic anemia?
Direct Coombs positivity to IgG alone or with complement in warm-mediated autoimmune hemolytic anemia results in removal of erythrocytes predominantly by the spleen. Thus, immunosuppression and splenectomy are very successful treatments for warm-mediated autoimmune hemolytic anemia, which can be severe and life-threatening. In contrast, cold antibody–mediated autoimmune hemolytic anemia is rarely as severe with regard to the anemia as warm-mediated autoimmune hemolytic anemia. Interestingly, splenectomy and

frequently immunosuppression are relatively ineffective because most of the erythrocytes are removed by the liver rather than the spleen. Immunosuppression may be of benefit if an underlying secondary malignancy, causing the cold-mediated autoimmune hemolytic anemia, is treated by this therapeutic maneuver or with chemotherapy.

19. What are the two most common causes of hemolytic anemia as a result of erythrocyte enzyme abnormalities?

The most common causes of hemolytic anemias of this component of erythrocytes are glucose-6-phosphate dehydrogenase deficiency and pyruvate kinase deficiency. Pyruvate kinase deficiency is observed almost entirely in the pediatric population, and severe hemolysis is present from birth on. In contrast, glucose-6-phosphate dehydrogenase (G-6-PD) deficiency is seen in approximately 10% of African-American men and is associated with an episodic hemolysis. G-6-PD deficiency follows a pattern of development in the malaria belt. It is a genetic polymorphism that protects individuals from death from malaria. In the rare Mediterranean form of G-6-PD deficiency, the hemolysis is persistent and chronic. In the United States, the episodic form of hemolysis is most common and is frequently induced by drugs that produce an excessive oxidant stress on erythrocytes. A classic example is the antimalarial primaquine, which produces an immediate drop in the hematocrit and a small rise in the reticulocyte count. Increasing the dose of primaquine results in a further drop in the hematocrit and a small further increase in the reticulocyte count. Thus, in the anemia induced by primaquine and other oxidant drugs in a patient with episodic hemolysis from G-6-PD deficiency, the hemolysis is dose related. This occurs because only the oldest erythrocytes are hemolyzed at a given dose. The older the erythrocyte, the less G-6-PD is available and thus the more sensitive are the cells. As the dose of the oxidant drug is increased, a greater and greater proportion of younger erythrocytes with greater amounts of G-6-PD are caused to hemolyze. This disorder is usually not associated with spherocytosis in the peripheral blood, but if the hemolysis is brisk enough, significant numbers of microspherocytes will be observed in the peripheral blood just as in the case of autoimmune hemolytic anemia.

20. By what mechanism can drugs result in anemia?

Drugs may produce immune-mediated hemolytic anemias or hemolytic anemia associated with G-6-PD deficiency, or they may suppress bone marrow production of reticulocytes—if the latter is severe enough, aplastic anemia will result.

BIBLIOGRAPHY

1. Beutler E: Glucose-6-phosphate dehydrogenase deficiency. In Stanbury JB, Wyngaarden JB, Fredrickson DS, et al (eds): Metabolic Basis of Inherited Disease, 5th ed. New York, McGraw-Hill, 1983, pp 1629–1653.
2. Curtis BR, Lamon J, Roelcke D, Chaplin H: Life-threatening, antiglobulin test-negative, acute autoimmune hemolytic anemia due to a non-complement-activating IgG1 kappa cold antibody with Pra specificity. Transfusion 30:838–843, 1990.
3. Davies KA, Lux SE: Hereditary disorders of the red cell membrane skeleton. Trends Genet 5:222–227, 1989.
4. Engelfriet CP, Overbeeke MA, von dem Borne AE: Autoimmune hemolytie anemia. Semin Hematol 29:3–12, 1992.
5. Frank MN, Schrieber AD, Atkinson JP, Jaffe CJ: NIH Conference: Pathophysiology of immune hemolytic anemia. Ann Intern Med 87:210–222, 1977.
6. Gibson J: Autoimmune hemolytic anemia: Current concepts. Aust NZ J Med 18:625–637, 1988.
7. Krantz SB: Diagnosis and treatment of pure red cell aplasia. Med Clin North Am 60:945–958, 1976.
8. Lubran MM: Hematologic side effects of drugs. Ann Clin Lab Sci 19:114–121, 1989.
9. Morse EE: Toxic effects of drugs on erythrocytes. Ann Clin Lab Sci 18:13–18, 1988.
10. Palek J, Lux SE: Red cell membranes skeletodefects in hereditary and acquired hemolytic anemias. Semin Hematol 20:189, 1983.

11. Pangburn MK, Schreiber RD, Muller-Eberhard HJ: Deficiency of an erythrocyte membrane protein with complement regulatory activity in a paroxysmal nocturnal hemoglobinuria. Proc Natl Acad Sci USA 80:5430, 1983.
12. Tabbara IA: Hemolytic anemias: Diagnosis and management. Med Clin North Am 76:649–668, 1992.
13. Valentine WN: The Stratton Lecture: Hemolytic anemia and inborn errors of metabolism. Blood 54:549–559, 1979.
14. Valentine WN, Paglia DE: Erythroenzymopathies and hemolytic anemia: The many faces of inherited variant enzymes. J Lab Clin Med 115:12–20, 1990.

12. APLASTIC ANEMIA

C.R. Santhosh-Kumar, M.D., and J. Fred Kolhouse, M.D.

1. Discuss the differential diagnosis of pancytopenia.
Pancytopenia may be caused by two basic mechanisms: (1) relative bone marrow failure and (2) excessive peripheral destruction of cells. Relative bone marrow failure may be caused by folate or vitamin B12 deficiency, which affects all three cell lines in the bone marrow but the marrow will always be vastly hypercellular. The marrow may also be very hypocellular, as in aplastic anemia, or may demonstrate myelofibrosis or severe myelodysplasia. An example of peripheral utilization is hypersplenism, which always requires a large (frequently massively enlarged) spleen.

2. Are splenomegaly and lymphadenopathy usually present in a patient with aplastic anemia at presentation?
No. Splenomegaly may develop after several blood transfusions, but in general the presence of splenomegaly and/or lymphadenopathy should raise a question as to the correct diagnosis.

3. Give the general categories of causes of aplastic anemia.
The causes of aplastic anemia may be divided into two categories that are of approximately equal incidence. In the first category, the aplastic anemia is caused by exposure to a toxin (benzene or other cleaning solvents), drugs (chloramphenicol, quinine derivatives), radiation, or infections. In the second category, patients have "autoimmune" aplastic anemia. In the first category, it has also been recognized that chemotherapy treatment results in short or prolonged pancytopenia and relative bone marrow aplasia, but this is usually reversible. The most common other drugs associated with aplastic anemia (in about 1:30,000 usages) are chloramphenicol and benzene derivatives. Chloramphenicol also has a reversible bone marrow suppression resulting in pancytopenia as its most common manifestation. The idiosyncratic aplastic anemia that is not dose related is much less frequent. Infections, particularly non-A, non-B hepatitis, are notoriously associated with severe aplastic anemia. In addition, other seemingly physiologic disorders such as pregnancy may be associated with aplastic anemia that appears at certain stages of pregnancy and each subsequent pregnancy in the individual. In the past few years, it has been increasingly recognized that a significant number of cases of aplastic anemia are due to aberration of the immune system (such as T-gamma lymphocytosis) resulting in agranulocytosis and pure red cell aplasia.

4. What is the appearance of the bone marrow in aplastic anemia?
The bone marrow is markedly hypocellular in aplastic anemia and the bone marrow space is occupied by fat. However, all degrees of aplastic anemia may be observed. In fact, a single

blood cell line may be reduced in the beginning of aplastic anemia, which if followed long enough will frequently develop full pancytopenia and the picture of aplastic anemia. Some physicians recommend bone marrow biopsy (the only way to accurately assess marrow cellularity) in at least two sites prior to establishing the diagnosis of aplastic anemia.

5. How is the severe form of aplastic anemia distinguised from the very severe form?
Although this may seem like a trivial question, it is an important one. Persons with early, very severe aplastic anemia that is not treated have a median survival of only a few months (3 to 6 months), whereas those with severe aplastic anemia may have a much more prolonged survival with some hope of spontaneous recovery or at least partial response to treatment. Very severe aplastic anemia is categorized as a granulocyte count of <500, a platelet count of $<20,000$, and a reticulocyte count of $<10,000/\mu l$ ($<0.1\%$). Patients with severe aplastic anemia who develop very severe aplastic anemia over the ensuing months have an equally grim prognosis. It is important to distinguish individuals with very severe aplastic anemia, because these patients should be treated as soon as possible with aggressive forms of therapy (see question 6).

6. Discuss the treatment of aplastic anemia.
All patients should be carefully questioned about exposure to drugs known to induce aplastic anemia (with the withdrawal of all drugs that are not absolutely necessary), and conditions in the workplace or home that could lead to aplastic anemia. Precautions with regard to gum damage with toothbrushing and stool softeners and anal care should be carefully monitored. Patients with moderate to severe aplastic anemia may be observed or placed on androgen therapy unless their blood counts begin to deteriorate. Patients with very severe aplastic anemia should be immediately considered for bone marrow transplantation if they are under the age of 40 years. In persons over the age of 40 years, difficulty with graft-versus-host reaction and other complications make bone marrow transplant an especially risky procedure. In older patients, therapy with antilymphocyte globulin should be initiated, which should be undertaken with particular caution because virtually every patient will develop serum sickness and a number of patients will develop anaphylactic reactions. Virtually all patients should receive this therapy while under observation in the hospital. Antilymphocyte globulin frequently produces a partial remission in aplastic anemia such that red cell transfusions are not required and the platelet count is adequate to prevent bleeding. The incidence of ultimate conversion of chronic moderate aplastic anemia to acute leukemia or a myelodysplastic syndrome may be very high. If a patient with aplastic anemia is a consideration for bone marrow transplantation, a major bone marrow transplant center should be contacted about the patient immediately so that the physician can receive instructions as to how to maximize the chances of a successful transplant with regard to transfusions and other management.

7. What blood abnormalities would suggest pure red cell aplasia?
As the name implies, pure red cell aplasia involves an aplastic anemia in the truest sense of the word *pure* because of the fact that leukocytes and platelets are normal. A patient with a very severe anemia with a normal leukocyte count and differential and platelet count and with a very low reticulocyte count is a candidate for the diagnosis of this unusual disorder. The diagnosis can be established by bone marrow biopsy where very few, if any, erythroid precursors would be observed in the marrow while the white cell precursors and megakaryocytes within the marrow are normal.

8. Explain the cause of idiopathic pure red cell aplasia.
Idiopathic pure red cell aplasia may represent an extreme example in the spectrum of the autoantibodies of autoimmune hemolytic anemia. In the case of pure red cell aplasia, the difficulty may be that the antibody is directed against an antigen on very early erythroid precursors. Clearly the disease is mediated by an antibody, based on elegant studies

performed by Sanford Krantz. The primary treatment of pure red cell aplasia involves immunosuppression with steroids and occasionally immunosuppressive agents. The majority of patients will respond rather dramatically to steroid therapy, but it is difficult to taper off steroids completely.

9. What is the typical mean corpuscular volume (MCV) in patients with aplastic anemia or pure red cell aplasia?
The MCV is typically elevated above 100 in patients with either aplastic anemia or pure red cell aplasia. This can sometimes cause some initial confusion and the suggestion that the patient may have a folate or B12 deficiency as a cause of their anemia. This question can be resolved by performing a bone marrow biopsy. The bone marrow of individuals with megaloblastic anemia secondary to folate or B12 deficiency is characteristically very cellular and sometimes confused with acute leukemia. Patients with severe anemia due to myelodysplasia will have myelodysplastic features in their bone marrow, whereas patients with aplastic anemia will have few or no bone marrow cells on bone marrow biopsy. The high MCV is presumably caused by early release of cells, because what few erythroid cells are produced are under intense stimulation by erythropoietin.

10. What is the cause of "secondary" pure red cell aplasia in patients with a chronic hemolytic anemia?
Patients with a chronic hemolytic anemia who develop aplastic crisis can have this crisis as a result of micronutrient deficiency, in which case significant numbers of erythroid precursors will be present, some of which may be megaloblastic. However, in secondary pure red cell aplasia and chronic hemolytic anemia, the culprit is frequently a parvovirus, which causes a severe depletion of erythroid precursors in the marrow with giant pronormoblasts. The diagnosis is established by the examination of the bone marrow morphology as well as serologies for B-19 antibody in serum.

BIBLIOGRAPHY

1. Camitta BM, Storb R, Thomas ED: Aplastic anemia: Pathogenesis, diagnosis, treatment and prognosis. N Engl J Med 306:645, 1982.
2. Camitta BM, Storb R, Thomas ED: Aplastic anemia: Pathogenesis, diagnosis, treatment and prognosis. N Engl J Med 306:712, 1982.
3. Camitta BM, O'Reilly RJ, Sensenbrenner L, et al: Antithoracic duct lymphocyte globulin therapy of severe aplastic anemia. Blood 62:883, 1983.
4. Clark CA, Dessypris EN, Krantz SB: Studies of pure red cell aplasia. IX: Results of immunosuppressive treatment of 37 patients. Blood 63:277, 1984.
5. Krantz SB, Kao V: Studies on red cell aplasia. I. Demonstration of a plasma inhibitor to heme synthesis and an antibody to erythroblastic nuclei. Proc Natl Acad Sci USA 58:493, 1967.
6. Najaen Y: For joint group for the study of aplastic and refractory anemia: Long-term follow-up in patients with aplastic anemia. A study of 137 androgen-treated patients surviving more than two years. Am J Med 71:543, 1981.
7. Smith MA, Ryan ME: Parvovirus infections: From benign to life-threatening. Postgrad Med 84:127-128, 131-134, 1988.

13. SICKLE CELL DISEASE AND THALASSEMIAS

Peter A. Lane, M.D.

SICKLE CELL DISEASE

1. What is the genetic basis of sickle cell disease?

Sickle cell disease is caused by an inherited mutation of adult hemoglobin in which glutamic acid is replaced by valine as the sixth amino acid of the beta-globin chain. Sickle disorders are inherited in an autosomal manner because the gene for beta-globin is located on chromosome 11. Persons heterozygous for sickle hemoglobin are asymptomatic carriers of sickle cell disease and are said to have sickle trait. Homozygosity for the sickle gene causes sickle cell anemia, which is the most common form of sickle cell disease. Other common forms of sickle cell disease occur in individuals who are compound heterozygotes for the sickle cell gene and a second beta-globin abnormality such as hemoglobin C or β-thalassemia.

2. Who is affected by sickle cell disease?

In the United States, sickle disorders are encountered most frequently in African-Americans. The sickle gene also occurs in high frequency in India, Saudi Arabia, Turkey, Greece, Southern Italy, and Sicily. Thus, sickle cell trait and sickle cell disease occur in both black and non-black Americans.

3. What two pathophysiologic processes are responsible for the clinical manifestations of sickle cell disease?

The signs and symptoms of sickle cell disease result from decreased red blood cell survival (hemolysis) and from the tendency of sickle cells to cause vaso-occlusion, especially in the microvasculature. Hemolysis causes varying degrees of anemia, jaundice, increased cardiac output (heart murmur and cardiomegaly), and delayed growth; it also predisposes patients to cholelithiasis and to anemic crises (aplastic and sequestration). (See Figure 3, Color Plates.) Vaso-occlusion causes tissue ischemia and organ dysfunction and frequently manifests as intermittent episodes of pain. Other important vaso-occlusive complications include pulmonary infarction, stroke, hepatic and renal dysfunction, aseptic necrosis of the femoral head, priapism, leg ulcers, and proliferative retinopathy.

4. Do all patients with sickle cell disease have anemia?

No. The severity of hemolysis varies among the different forms of sickle cell disease, and for each syndrome there is much individual heterogeneity. Some persons with sickle hemoglobin C disease and sickle β^+ thalassemia have mild hemolysis, and compensatory reticulocytosis prevents development of anemia (see table, following page). Thus, absence of anemia does not exclude sickle cell disease.

5. Describe the solubility test for sickle hemoglobin (Sickle Screen, Sickledex, or Sicklequik). What does a positive result indicate?

This test screens for the presence of sickle hemoglobin and is positive in persons with sickle cell trait as well as sickle cell diseases. Thus, a positive result does not differentiate persons with symptomatic disease from asymptomatic carriers. False negatives also occur, and the test does not identify carriers of β-thalassemia or hemoglobin C. Thus, hemoglobin electrophoresis is always necessary to evaluate the possibility of sickle cell disease or, in the context of genetic counseling, to identify persons at risk for having children with sickle cell disease.

6. How is sickle cell disease diagnosed?
The diagnosis of a sickle syndrome requires quantitative hemoglobin electrophoresis. Typical results for the common sickle cell diseases and for sickle cell trait are shown in the table below.

Common Sickle Syndromes: Estimates of Clinical Severity and Typical Hemoglobin Electrophoresis Results

SYNDROME	β-GLOBIN GENOTYPE	HEMOLYSIS	VASO-OCCLUSIVE COMPLICATIONS	HEMOGLOBINS (%)				
				A	A_2	F	S	C
Sickle cell diseases								
Sickle cell anemia	S-S	+ + + +	+ + + +	0	3	7	90	0
Sickle Hgb C disease	S-C	+	+ +	0	*	1	50	49
Sickle β^0-thalassemia	S-$\beta^{0\dagger}$	+ + +	+ + +	0	7	8	85	0
Sickle β^+-thalassemia	S-$\beta^{+\ddagger}$	+	+	20	6	7	67	0
Sickle trait	A-S	0	0	56	3	1	40	0

* Hgb A_2 cannot be quantitated in presence of Hgb C.
† β^0 denotes β-thalassemia mutation that causes absent production of beta-globin.
‡ β^+ denotes β-thalassemia mutation that causes decreased production of beta-globin.

7. Are persons with sickle cell disease at increased risk for bacterial infections?
Yes. Numerous immunologic defects have been described in patients with sickle cell disease. The most important of these is the development (often early in life) of functional asplenia. Fulminant sepsis with pneumococcal and other encapsulated bacteria is the leading cause of death in childhood and remains a significant risk in adults.

8. What is the rationale for neonatal screening for sickle cell disease?
Sickle cell anemia is frequently asymptomatic during the first 1 to 2 years of life. The first manifestation of the disease is often pneumococcal sepsis or splenic sequestration, which are both potentially fatal complications. Identification of sickle cell anemia at birth provides an opportunity to educate families and health care providers about the nature of sickle cell disease and to institute prophylactic penicillin and comprehensive care. These interventions have been shown definitively to reduce morbidity and mortality in early childhood.

9. How can pneumonia and pulmonary infarction be reliably differentiated in patients with acute respiratory symptoms?
They cannot be differentiated reliably. Patients with sickle cell disease are at increased risk for pneumonia as well as for pulmonary infarction. Both complications typically present with fever, cough, chest pain, tachypnea, hypoxemia, and the presence of a new infiltrate on the chest radiograph. The term "acute chest syndrome" is used to describe such illness. Medical treatment generally includes antibiotics for infection, as well as hydration, analgesia, oxygen, and sometimes exchange transfusion for vaso-occlusion.

10. What is the most commonly performed surgical procedure in persons with sickle cell disease?
Cholecystectomy. Most patients with sickle cell anemia develop cholelithiasis during childhood and adolescence. Many patients subsequently become symptomatic. Elective cholecystectomy for asymptomatic gallstones is often recommended.

11. Describe important therapeutic considerations in the management of patients with sickle cell disease who require general anesthesia.

General anesthesia for surgical procedures is associated with a significant risk of intraoperative and postoperative complications. These complications include acute chest syndrome, pain episodes, infection, stroke, renal failure, and death. Thus, the intraoperative and postoperative management of patients with sickle cell disease requires scrupulous efforts to prevent dehydration or overhydration, hypoxemia, acidosis, and pulmonary atelectasis. To prevent sickling complications, many institutions routinely perform exchange transfusion prior to surgery to obtain a hemoglobin level of ≥10 gm/dL and a percentage of sickle hemoglobin <30%. Other institutions recommend simple transfusion with packed red blood cells prior to general anesthesia. A multicenter study of preoperative transfusion therapy is currently being conducted.

12. What are the leading causes of death in adults with sickle cell disease?
- Cardiopulmonary disease (acute chest syndrome or chronic lung disease with cor pulmonale)
- Chronic renal failure
- Stroke
- Infection

13. Is sickle cell trait associated with any medical complications?

Persons with sickle cell trait are generally asymptomatic, and the diagnosis of sickle cell trait is important principally for genetic counseling implications. However, red blood cells in sickle trait may sickle under hypoxemic, acidotic, or hypertonic conditions. Persons with sickle cell trait often develop mild hyposthenuria, and some may have intermittent episodes of painless microscopic or macroscopic hematuria. Exposure to environmental hypoxia (unpressurized aircraft, high mountain altitudes) may occasionally precipitate splenic infarction, but an overwhelming majority of persons with sickle cell trait can participate in mountain recreation such as hiking and skiing without any adverse effects. Sickle cell trait is not a contraindication to participation in competitive athletics. Life expectancy is not altered by the presence of sickle cell trait.

THALASSEMIA

14. Define thalassemia.

Thalassemia syndromes constitute a heterogeneous group of genetic disorders whose clinical manifestations result from the decreased or absent production of normal globin chains of hemoglobin. These abnormalities result in hypochromic, microcytic anemias of varying severity. Alpha-thalassemia is caused by the decreased production of alpha-globin chains, and β-thalassemia by the decreased production of beta-globin chains.

15. Who is affected by thalassemia?

Thalassemia may be encountered in persons of all ethnic backgrounds. In the United States, the thalassemia syndromes occur with greatest frequency among persons whose ancestors originated from Africa, the Mediterranean Basin, the Middle East, southern and Southeast Asia, southern China, and the Pacific Islands.

16. With what disorder is thalassemia most often confused?

Iron deficiency. An almost universal manifestation of thalassemia is microcytosis (low mean corpuscular volume [MCV]). Thalassemia is the most common inherited cause of microcytosis, and iron deficiency is the most common acquired cause of microcytosis. Thus, thalassemia should always be suspected in a person with a low MCV, especially when iron deficiency has been excluded by laboratory tests or by failure to respond to therapeutic administration of iron.

17. Describe the genetic basis, clinical manifestations, and laboratory diagnosis of β-thalassemia minor.

Beta-thalassemia minor occurs in persons heterozygous for a β-thalassemia gene. Most are asymptomatic and many are not anemic, but their red blood cells are hypochromic and microcytic. The MCV is low unless the blood picture is clouded by coexistent folate or cobalamin deficiency. The diagnosis is confirmed by detecting elevated levels of hemoglobin A_2 and/or hemoglobin F by hemoglobin electrophoresis.

18. Since β-thalassemia minor is usually asymptomatic, why is it important to make this diagnosis?

Heterozygous β-thalassemia may have important genetic counseling implications. In addition, unnecessary administration of supplemental iron in a futile attempt to correct the microcytosis should be avoided. Women with β-thalassemia minor may also develop symptomatic anemia during pregnancy and rarely may require blood transfusion.

19. What is Cooley's anemia?

Cooley's anemia is homozygous β-thalassemia, or β-thalassemia major. Patients with Cooley's anemia develop a severe hypochromic microcytic anemia during the first year of life and require chronic blood transfusions with iron chelation or bone marrow transplantation for survival.

20. Describe the genetic basis of α-thalassemia.

Most α-thalassemia syndromes are due to deletions of the alpha-globin genes. Normal persons have four alpha-globin genes, two on each chromosome 16. Thus, the severity of α-thalassemia syndromes is related to the number of gene deletions present. The α-thalassemia syndromes have important genetic counseling implications because deletion of all four alpha-globin genes results in fetal hydrops, which is incompatible with life, and because such pregnancies are associated with significant maternal morbidity.

Alpha-Thalassemia Syndromes

USUAL GENOTYPES	α GENE NO.	CLINICAL FEATURES
αα/αα	4	Normal
α-/αα	3	Silent carrier
α-/α- or --/αα	2	α-Thalassemia trait
--/α-	1	Hemoglobin H disease
--/--	0	Fetal hydrops

α, presence of α gene; -, deletion of α gene.

21. What is α-thalassemia trait? How is it diagnosed?

Alpha-thalassemia trait is a mild, asymptomatic form of α-thalassemia caused by the deletion of two of four alpha-globin genes. The MCV is low but anemia may not be present. Hemoglobin electrophoresis results are normal, so the diagnosis is often a presumptive one based on the exclusion of iron deficiency and β-thalassemia trait. DNA studies are usually required for a definitive diagnosis and should be obtained in the context of genetic counseling or prenatal diagnosis.

22. What is hemoglobin H disease?

Hemoglobin H disease is a moderately severe form of α-thalassemia that is usually caused by deletion of three of four alpha-globin genes. Effected patients typically have a moderately severe hypochromic microcytic anemia (hemoglobin 7 to 9 g/dl) with an elevated reticulocyte count. Clinical manifestations may include jaundice, splenomegaly, and cholelithiasis. Hemoglobin electrophoresis of fresh blood shows hemoglobin H (a tetramer composed of four beta-globin chains), and incubation of blood with brilliant cresyl blue (hemoglobin H prep) shows red blood cell inclusions.

BIBLIOGRAPHY

1. Bunn HF, Forget BG: Hemoglobin: Molecular, Genetic and Clinical Aspects. Philadelphia, W.B. Saunders, 1986.
2. Charache S, Lubin B, Reid CD (eds): Management and Therapy of Sickle Cell Disease. U.S. Department of Health and Human Services, NIH Publication No. 89-2117, revised September 1989.
3. Consensus Development Panel: Newborn screening for sickle cell disease and other hemoglobinopathies. JAMA 258:1205, 1987.
4. Gaston NH, Verter JI, Woods G, et al: Prophylaxis with oral penicillin in children with sickle cell anemia: A randomized trial. N Engl J Med 314:1593, 1986.
5. Giardina PJ, Hilgartner MW: Update on thalassemia. Pediatr Rev 13:55, 1992.
6. Koshy M, Entsuah R, Koranda A, et al: Leg ulcers in patients with sickle cell disease. Blood 74:1403, 1989.
7. Mentzer WC, Wagner GM (eds): The Hereditary Hemolytic Anemias. New York, Churchill Livingstone, 1989.
8. Milner PF, Kraus AP, Sebes JI, et al: Sickle cell disease as a cause of osteonecrosis of the femoral head. N Engl J Med 325:1476, 1991.
9. Ohene-Frempong K: Stroke in sickle cell disease: Demographic, clinical, and therapeutic considerations. Semin Hematol 28:213, 1991.
10. Platt OS, Thorington BD, Brambilla DJ, et al: Pain in sickle cell disease: Rates and risk factors. N Engl J Med 325:11, 1991.
11. Powars DR, Elliott-Mills DD, Chan L, et al: Chronic renal failure in sickle cell disease: Risk factors, clinical course and mortality. Ann Intern Med 115:614, 1991.
12. Powars D, Weidman JA, Odom-Maryon T, et al: Sickle cell chronic lung disease: Prior morbidity and the risk of pulmonary failure. Medicine 67:66, 1988.
13. Rackoff WR, Kunkel N, Silber JH, et al: Pulse oximetry and factors associated with hemoglobin oxygen desaturation in children with sickle cell disease. Blood 81:3422, 1993.
14. Serjeant GR: Sickle Cell Disease, 2nd ed. Oxford, England, Oxford University Press, 1992.
15. Wayne AS, Kevy SW, Nathan DG: Transfusion management of sickle cell disease. Blood 81:1109, 1993.
16. West MS, Wethers D, Smith J, et al: Laboratory profile of sickle cell disease: A cross-section analysis. J Clin Epidemiol 45:893, 1992.
17. Zarkowsky HS, Gallagher D, Gill FM, et al: Bacteremia in sickle hemoglobinopathies. J Pediatr 109:579, 1986.

14. POLYCYTHEMIC STATES

Christine M. Holm, M.D., and Marie E. Wood, M.D.

1. What disease states should you think of when faced with a patient with polycythemia (elevated hemoglobin)?

Generally, it is useful to think of two diagnostic categories, relative (spurious) and real. The category of real polycythemia can be further divided into appropriate or inappropriate.

Individuals with **relative (or spurious) polycythemia** have normal red blood cell (RBC) mass and conditions that reduce the plasma volume, causing hemoconcentration. Examples include dehydration from high altitude, medications, decreased oral intake, burns, or stress (i.e., pheochromocytoma). A specific and common example of a relative polycythemia is Gaisbock's syndrome, which characteristically occurs in a hypertensive, obese male who smokes.

Individuals with **real polycythemia** have an elevated RBC mass (>36 ml/kg for males or >32 ml/kg for females). Generally, the hematocrit is >60% (without evidence of dehydration). Values less than this may need to be verified by red blood cell mass measurements.

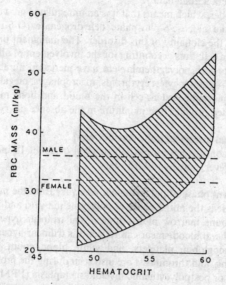

Range of red cell masses that may be seen in clinically stable patients with hematocrits in the range of 45–60 ml/dl. The interrupted, horizontal lines depict the upper limits of the normal range for men and women. Patients with hematocrits in the range of 48–58 may or may not have increased red cell mass. (From Murphy S: Polycythemia vera. Disease-a-Month 3:158–212, 1992, with permission.)

Erythropoietin levels in this group of disorders will generally be increased (except for polycythemia vera and high-affinity hemoglobinopathies). The erythropoietin level may be an appropriate response to tissue hypoxia, as is evident in individuals who have chronic obstructive pulmonary diseae (COPD), sleep apnea, cardiovascular shunts, elevated carboxyhemoglobin, or decreased 2,3-diphosphoglycerate (2,3-DPG) levels.

The erythropoietin level may be increased, causing a polycythemic state in individuals with erythropoietin-secreting tumors (i.e., renal or adrenal tumors, cerebellar hemangiomas, hepatomas, ovarian carcinoma). Erythropoietin levels may also be elevated owing to renal disease such as hydronephrosis, cysts and renal transplantation.

2. What clinical clues might help one to diagnose the cause of the polycythemic state?
The history and physical examination should focus on symptoms or signs of a secondary erythrocytosis such as mentioned above. A family history of polycythemic disorders (i.e., polycythemia vera, high-affinity hemoglobinopathies) is also important.

The patient with polycythemia vera often has symptoms of vascular congestion or occlusion, central nervous system (CNS) symptoms, headache, peripheral vascular disease (PVD), gout, and/or weight loss. Pruritus, especially after a hot shower, is often reported. The physical examination in patients with polycythemia vera may reveal ruddy cyanosis, hypertension, gout, a palpable spleen or liver, and findings of PVD. Signs or symptoms of infection should **not** be present.

3. How common is polycythemia vera?
It is quite common. The incidence is about 1:100,000, with men being affected slightly more often than women (1.2:1). The average age at diagnosis is 60 years. Less than 5% of

individuals with polycythemia vera are under 40 years old, and less than 0.1% are under 20. Few patients (0.4%) have a family history of polycythemia vera. Radiation exposure (i.e., atomic bomb fallout) may increase the risk for polycythemia vera.

4. Is polycythemia vera a malignancy?
Yes. It is a clonal disorder, which means that it is an unregulated growth of a malignant cell. Studies in heterozygote glucose-6-phosphate dehydrogenase (G-6-PD)-deficient women initially demonstrated the clonality of this disorder. The malignant precursor is thought to be the pluripotent stem cell, thus accounting for the involvement of all three cell lines in the bone marrow. Patients with polycythemia vera have increased numbers of CFU-GEMM (colony-forming units—granulocytes, erythroids, macrophages, megakaryocytes), a progenitor cell close to the pluripotent stem cell in the blood and bone marrow. CFU-GEMM demonstrate unregulated proliferation in culture in the absence of erythropoietin.

5. What is the natural history of polycythemia vera?
Historical untreated controls have a median survival of about 18 months from diagnosis. Treated patients, however, may live 10–15 years.

6. How does the spent phase of polycythemia vera vary from the proliferative phase?
The **proliferative phase** is the initial phase of polycythemia vera and is typified by effective hematopoiesis. The bone marrow biopsy may reveal trilinear hyperplasia and increased cellularity. The peripheral blood smear can reflect this trilinear hyperplasia, demonstrating elevation of the hemoglobin, platelets, and white blood count. Vascular congestion, splenomegaly, bleeding, and thrombosis are also seen during the proliferative phase.

The **spent phase** or postpolycythemic myeloid metaplasia (PPMM) is seen after about 10 years in only 5–15% of patients. It is characterized by a decreased need for cytoreductive treatment, a decreased red cell mass, and increasing splenomegaly. A leukoerythroblastic blood smear, pancytopenia, extensive bone marrow fibrosis, and ineffective hematopoiesis with extramedullary hematopoiesis are common features of PPMM. Anemia in these patients is due to increased splenic sequestration, iron deficiency, and bleeding secondary to platelet dysfunction. A decreased platelet count as well as platelet dysfunction may be observed. In PPMM, 20–50% of cases will transfrom to acute leukemia. The prognosis for this group of patients is poor, with only 30% alive at 3 years. Those who received ^{32}P or alkylating agents have the highest incidence of acute leukemia.

7. Is splenomegaly seen during the proliferative phase due to extramedullary hematopoiesis?
No. Hematopoiesis is effective at this stage. Splenomegaly results from increased platelet and red blood cell sequestration within the spleen. The spleen can contain two to three times the platelet count (as estimated by a CBC) and splenectomy may result in a dramatic and dangerous increase of the platelet count.

8. What are the complications of polycythemia vera?
The most common complications are hemorrhage, thrombosis, PPMM, and leukemic transformation. Thrombosis is the most frequent cause of mortality (30–40%). Unusual sites such as the splenic vein and hepatic artery and vein as well as portal vein thrombosis are common. About 10% of patients with the Budd-Chiari syndrome have underlying polycythemia vera. An elevated hematocrit with resultant viscous blood, an elevated platelet count, and abnormal platelet function all contribute to this thrombotic tendency. Surgery in polycythemia vera has an especially increased risk of thrombosis or hemorrhage. In untreated polycythemia vera, 79% of patients risk these complications, whereas in treated polycythemia, there is only a 28% risk of complications. Surgical complications consist of hemorrhage (52%), thrombosis (18%), or both (14%), as well as a postoperative mortality of 18%.[12]

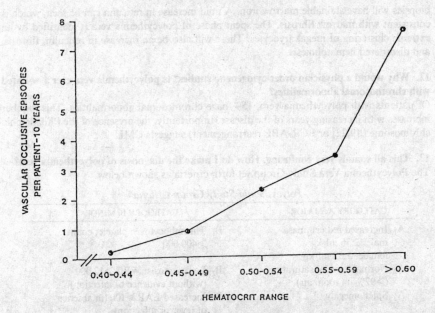

HEMATOCRIT RANGE

(From Pearson TC, Weatherley-Mein G: Vascular occlusive episodes and venous hematocrit in primary proliferative polycythemia. Lancet 2:1219–1222, 1978, with permission.)

9. Which laboratory tests would help isolate the cause of polycythemia?

1. **Secondary erythrocytosis:** Affected individuals will have evidence of tissue hypoxia (low Po_2 or local tissue hypoxia) or erythropoietin-secreting tumors. Both situations can be associated with elevated erythropoietin levels.

2. **High-affinity hemoglobinopathies:** Individuals with this diagnosis will have a decreased P_{50} on the oxygen dissociation curve (see question 14).

3. **Polycythemia vera:** Affected individuals will demonstrate an increased RBC mass (>36 ml/kg male; >32 ml/kg female) and may have evidence of the following:

   - Iron deficiency anemia
   - Leukocytosis (seen in 66% of patients). There should be no evidence of an infection.
   - Basophilia (one-third of patients)
   - Elevated leukocyte alkaline phosphatase (LAP) score. However, if the WBC is increased and the LAP <100, the diagnosis of chronic myelogenous leukemia (CML) should be considered.
   - Increased vitamin B12 (secondary to increased binding protein, transcobalamin I produced by white blood cells).
   - Increased uric acid and increased LDH (moderately increased in proliferative phase but may exceed 1000 mg/dl in postpolycythemic myeloid metaplasia).
   - Increased platelet count (50% of patients will have a platelet count >500,000; 10% will have a platelet count >1,000,000).

10. What does a "dry tap" refer to?

It is the inability to aspirate bone marrow in the patient when performing a bone marrow biopsy. This is commonly seen in polycythemia vera and may be due to hypercellularity or fibrosis of the bone marrow.

11. What are the bone marrow findings in the patient with polycythemia vera?

During the proliferative phase, the bone marrow is hypercellular, often demonstrating trilinear hyperplasia. One may see abnormal megakaryocytes, and <5% of bone marrow biopsies will have stainable marrow iron. A mild increase in reticulin can be seen, which is consistent with marrow fibrosis. The spent phase of polycythemia vera is identified by an extreme clustering of megakaryocytes. There will also be an increase in reticulin, fibrosis, and disordered hematopoiesis.

12. Why would a physician order cytogenetic studies? Is polycythemia vera ever associated with chromosomal abnormalities?
Of patients with polycythemia vera, 15% have chromosomal abnormalities. This number increases with increasing years of the disease. Importantly, the presence of the Philadelphia chromosome (t[9,22] or BCR-ABL rearrangement) suggests CML.

13. This all sounds very confusing. How do I make the diagnosis of polycythemia vera?
The Polycythemia Vera Study Group set forth criteria as shown below.

*Polycythemia Study Group Criteria**

CATEGORY A: MAJOR	CATEGORY B: MINOR
A₁ Increased red cell mass male: ≥36 ml/kg female: ≥32 ml/kg	B₁ Thrombocytosis: platelet count >400,000
A₂ Normal anterial saturation (>92% on room air)	B₂ Leukocytosis: WBC >12,000 (without evidence of infection)
A₃ Splenomegaly	B₃ Increased LAP >100 (in absence of fever or infection)
	B₄ Increased vitamin B12 (>900 pg/ml) or unbound vitamin B12 binding capacity >2200 pg/ml

*The diagnosis of polycythemia vera can be made if all three criteria from category A are present or with documentation of A₁ + A₂ + 2 criteria from category B.
From Berlin NJ: Diagnosis and classification of the polycythemias. Semin Hematol 12:339–351, 1975, with permission.

14. How should polycythemia vera be treated?
Control of the white blood cell count and hemoglobin and platelet counts will decrease the incidence of complications (hemorrhage and/or thrombosis). Treatment might include the following:
• Use of phlebotomy to maintain the hemoglobin <14 gm/dl in men and <12 gm/dl in women.
• If the platelet count is >500,000/μl and/or thrombosis is clinically evident, cyto-reductive drugs (i.e., hydroxyurea, interferon) should be used. This therapy can be used in addition to phlebotomy.

Therapy: Proliferative Phase

Phlebotomy → Hct ≤43
↓
Age ≥70 years or thrombotic manifestations
↓
Hydroxyurea or interferon

• ³²P and chlorambucil have been shown to be effective in the past, but the markedly increased incidence of leukemia associated with these drugs precludes their use except as a last resort.
• Pruritus may respond to myelosuppressive treatment.
• There is no effective treatment for PPMM and problem-oriented supportive care is generally offered.
• Secondary leukemic transformation responds poorly to standard regimens, and treatment decisions should be individualized for each patient.

15. In the following case history, what is the differential diagnosis and why?

A hematology consultation was requested for a patient with an elevated hemoglobin. The patient was a 19-year-old white man. He was admitted to the hospital with acute psychotic symptoms and a history of drug abuse. The patient denied any history of medical problems but stated he had a family history of polycythemia vera. His paternal aunt, paternal uncle, and father all had been told they had polycythemia vera.

On physical examination, the patient had mild rubor, no ecchymosis or petechiae, no cyanosis, no clubbing, and no adenopathy. His liver span was 14 cm, and he had a palpable spleen tip.

The laboratory evaluation revealed a white blood count of $5000/\mu l$, hemoglobin of 17 gm/dl with a normal mean corpuscular volume (MCV) and mean corpuscular hemoglobin concentration (MCHC). The platelet count was normal at $184,000/\mu l$. Electrolytes were normal and the erythropoietin level was 6 μ/ml (normal 0–50 μ/ml). A head CT scan was normal and an abdominal ultrasound revealed only splenomegaly.

One would suspect polycythemia vera or a high-affinity hemoglobinopathy. Consistent with the diagnosis of polycythemia vera, the patient had an elevated hematocrit, splenomegaly, and a positive family history for polycythemia vera. The erythropoietin level was normal, as is seen in polycythemia vera, and most secondary causes of polycythemia had been ruled out. Against the diagnosis of polycythemia vera was that no other blood cell lines were elevated (WBC or platelets). There was no personal or family history of bleeding or thrombosis, and the age of diagnosis would be young for polycythemia vera.

Thus, the support for the diagnosis of polycythemia vera was weak and another diagnosis was suspected, such as the presence of a high-affinity hemoglobin. High-affinity hemoglobinopathies are often a familial, autosomal dominant disorder. A strong family history is even more common, as heterozygotes also have clinical manifestations. The high-affinity hemoglobin releases a smaller percent of oxygen to the tissues than normal hemoglobin; thus, a higher volume of RBC is needed to stoichiometrically achieve the same oxygen delivery. At equilibrium erythropoietin is usually normal. The diagnosis is made by constructing an oxygen hemoglobin dissociation curve. Hemoglobin electrophoresis may identify some but not all increased-affinity hemoglobins. If the abnormal-affinity hemoglobin is unstable, signs and/or symptoms of chronic hemolysis are seen.

It is important to distinguish a high-affinity hemoglobin state from polycythemia vera, thus saving the patient and relatives from misdiagnosis and possibly inappropriate treatment.

CONTROVERSIES

16. Should iron-deficient patients with polycythemia vera be given exogenous iron?

For:

Iron deficiency has been implicated in pruritus and may contribute to fatigue.

Iron deficiency can make the red blood cell less deformable. Some would argue that this contributes to thrombosis.

Against:

The resulting erythrocytosis is often uncontrollable without excessive phlebotomy or addition of myelosuppressive drugs.

The increased hemoglobin is a definite predisposition to thrombosis.

Finally, according to Rector et al.,[9] the nonhematologic sequelae of iron deficiency in patients with polycythemia vera were relatively insignificant. Iron-deficient patients with polycythemia vera studied over 25 years were shown to have (1) treadmill performances similar to normal controls, (2) no dysphagia or esophageal changes, and (3) physical examinations that did *not* reveal the skin and nail changes described in other iron-deficient patients.

17. Should all patients with an elevated hemoglobin be phlebotomized regardless of the etiology?

Generally not. The hemoglobin is often increased in an attempt to compensate for the common denominator of tissue hypoxia. However, a hematocrit over 60% may cause such sludging that O_2 delivery is impaired despite the hemoglobin increase. Acutely, phlebotomy may be indicated for a patient with hematocrit >60–65% with signs of sludging and/or tissue hypoxia. Hydration should precede and follow careful phlebotomy, and O_2 should be given. In special patients with a high-affinity hemoglobin, acute difficulty from sludging, and impaired tissue oxygenation, one should consider phlebotomy and replacement with normal blood (exchange transfusion). Anticoagulation with coumadin may help avoid sludging in the patient with a high-affinity hemoglobin and mild sludging symptoms. However, most patients with high-affinity hemoglobin do not require treatment.

On a more chronic basis, oxygen should be administered to the patient with secondary polycythemia and hypoxia. Erythropoietin-secreting tumors should be resected.

Pitfalls

- Iron deficiency may mask an increased RBC volume.
- Folate or B12 deficiency may mask polycythemia.
- RBC volume determinations in the obese are somewhat imprecise.
- A patient with evidence of a secondary polycythemia (e.g., the hypoxic smoker) may also have polycythemia vera—both diseases are common. A clue would be an elevated WBC or an elevated platelet count in addition to the elevated hemoglobin.
- Splenectomy in an individual during the proliferative phase of polycythemia vera can cause dangerously high thrombocytosis from release of the large volume of pooled platelets.

BIBLIOGRAPHY

1. Adamson JW, Fialkow PJ, Murphy S, et al: Polycythemia vera stem-cell and probable clonal origin of the disease. N Engl J Med 295:913–916, 1976.
2. Berlin NJ: Diagnosis and classification of the polycythemias. Semin Hematol 12:339–351, 1975.
3. Hoffman R, Boswell S: Polycythemia vera. In Hoffman R, Beny E, Shaff S, et al (eds): Hematology Basic Principles and Practice. New York, Churchill Livingstone, 1991, pp 834–854.
4. Meytes D, Katz D, Ramot B: Prognostic parameters in myeloid metaplasia: Agnogenic vs. post polycythemic myelofibrosis. Isr Med J 12:534–542, 1976.
5. Modan B: An epidemiological study of polycythemia vera. Blood 26:657–667, 1965.
6. Murphy S: Polycythemia vera. Disease-a-Month 3:158–212, 1992.
7. Murphy S: Polycythemia vera. In Williams WJ, Beutler E, Egslev AJ, Lichtman (eds): Hematology, 4th ed. New York, McGraw-Hill, 1990, pp 193–202.
8. Pearson TC, Weatherley-Mein G: Vascular occlusive episodes and venous hematocrit in primary proliferative polycythemia. Lancet 2:1219–1222, 1978.
9. Rector WG, Fortuin NJ, Conley CL: Non-hematologic effects of chronic iron deficiency: A study of patients with polycythemia vera treated solely with venasections. Medicine (Baltimore) 61:382–398, 1982.
10. Silverstein MN, Lanier AP: Polycythemia vera 1935–1969. An epidemiologic survey in Rochester, Minnesota. Mayo Clin Proc 46:751–753, 1971.
11. Swolin B, Weinfeld A, Wostin J: A prospective long-term cytogenic study in polycythemia vera in relation to treatment and clinical course. Blood 72:386–395, 1988.
12. Wasserman LP, Gilbert HS: Surgery in polycythemia vera. N Engl J Med 269:1226–1230, 1963.
13. Weatherall DJ: Polycythemia resulting from abnormal hemoglobins. N Engl J Med 280:604–606, 1969.
14. Weinreb NJ, Shin CF: Spurious polycythemia. Semin Hematol 12:397–406, 1975.

15. IRON OVERLOAD

S. Mark Bettag, M.D., and Paul A. Seligman, M.D.

1. Define iron overload.

Iron overload is an excess amount of total body iron. In the normal individual, two thirds of the total body iron is found in red blood cells, making up about 2 grams (gm) of iron. The remaining one third is almost exclusively found in storage iron that is sequestered in the iron storage protein called ferritin. Conditions that result in excess storage iron (i.e., more than 1 gm of iron sequestered in ferritin) cause iron overload.

2. Name the pathologic entities responsible for iron overload.

Hemochromatosis and hemosiderosis. Hemochromatosis is defined as iron overload with resultant tissue damage, whereas hemosiderosis is iron overload that is not associated with tissue damage. Pathologically, hemochromatosis implies excessive iron deposition in various parenchymal cells of the body, besides deposition in cells associated with iron storage (i.e., macrophages). In hemosiderosis, the vast majority of excess iron is found in the macrophages.

3. Discuss the causes of iron overload.

Causes of iron overload are generally divided into genetic and acquired. The main genetic cause is hereditary hemochromatosis (see question 4). Other genetic causes include refractory anemias such as thalassemia major, hereditary sideroblastic anemia, and congenital hemolytic anemias. In most cases, the genetic causes of iron overload are associated with obvious hemochromatosis (deposition of excess iron in parenchymal cells).

Acquired causes include refractory anemias such as aplastic anemia necessitating transfusion, chronic ingestion of medicinal iron, or excessive red cell transfusion. The acquired causes of iron overload are at first associated with hemosiderosis. However, with increased ingestion of iron or increased transfusions, iron excess associated with hemosiderosis eventually results in "spillover" of iron so that hemochromatosis associated with tissue damage becomes evident.

4. What is the mode of inheritance of hereditary hemochromatosis?

Primary hereditary hemochromatosis is of autosomal recessive inheritance. Heterozygotes have no clinical expression associated with iron overload, but if affected with another condition such as hemolytic anemia, this mixed heterozygous state may show evidence of clinical disease. Hereditary hemochromatosis is one of the most common hereditary diseases in North America. The gene incidence is about 10%, 1 in 400 individuals are homozygotes, and most of these individuals will have subclinical disease. A form of hemochromatosis seen in blacks originally called African nutritional hemochromatosis may have a genetic basis not related to the gene defect seen in hereditary hemochromatosis.

5. If hereditary hemochromatosis is so common, why do the clinical manifestations have such a low incidence?

People with homozygous hemochromatosis have a defect in iron absorption that results in an accumulation of excess iron over decades. Because women generally have a negative iron balance during childbearing years, on average they accumulate much less excess iron than men. It has been estimated that about 20 gm of excess iron is necessary to cause clinically significant disease; therefore, individuals with homozygous hemochromatosis, particularly women, may never accumulate this much excess iron in the period of the average life span (i.e., 75 years).

Homozygous hemochromatosis is probably underappreciated in the clinical population, because diseases such as diabetes, arthritis, impotence, and congestive heart failure (which are manifestations of hemochromatosis) are so common. Individuals with homozygous hemochromatosis who have other reasons for organ system involvement may have exacerbation of their disease process owing to damage caused by iron. Based on these considerations, it is important to make a diagnosis of homozygous hemochromatosis.

6. Is there a best screening test for homozygous hemochromatosis?
Screening tests used for the detection of homozygous hereditary hemochromatosis are the serum ferritin and the transferrin saturation. The transferrin saturation is the best screening test, because a saturation value >62% predicts the homozygous state in 92% of cases. The serum ferritin value is generally increased only with iron overload. The transferrin saturation is increased even in individuals with homozygous hemochromatosis screened during childhood or early adulthood. Once homozygous hemochromatosis is suspected, it is important to make the pathologic diagnosis by obtaining a liver biopsy, staining specifically for iron and identifying excess iron deposition in hepatocytes. A separate piece of liver tissue should be sent to the laboratory for a quantitative iron in order to quantify the amount of excess iron.

7. When an individual is diagnosed as having hemochromatosis, should the rest of the family be evaluated?
Once an index case of homozygous hemochromatosis is found in a family, the presence of each hemochromatosis allele can be followed by performing HLA typing. A family member who has an identical HLA type as the index case is presumed to have both hemochromatosis alleles and therefore, by definition, homozygous hemochromatosis. If a family member has only one of the HLA haplotypes of the index case, it is presumed that this person is a heterozygote. Thus, family members can be screened by HLA typing and the diagnosis confirmed by transferrin saturation. All homozygotes with high serum ferritin values or evidence of liver disease should have a liver biopsy.

8. How does iron overload cause tissue damage?
It is thought that excess iron accumulation in parenchymal cells causes enhanced lysosomal fragility associated with increased iron-laden ferritin that is denatured to hemosiderin. Peroxidation of membrane lipids mediated by free radical formation, a reaction catalyzed by iron, may also occur. The parenchymal cells most damaged by excess iron correlate with the clinical signs of disease discussed below.

9. Discuss the early and late clinical features of iron overload.
The diagnosis of early hemochromatosis may be associated with only subtle findings. In many instances, the presenting finding may be hepatomegaly, mild diabetes mellitus, or mild arthritis, particularly of the large joints or the metacarpophalangeal (MCP) joints. The arthritis associated with hemochromatosis may be similar to that seen with osteoarthritis, or, in rarer instances, the classic findings of chondrocalcinosis are evident. In some cases, other endocrinologic findings may be evident, including impotence or hypothyroidism. Cardiomyopathy is usually not the presenting finding of hemochromatosis in older individuals. A rare young individual (20 to 30 years old) with markedly excessive iron accumulation may present with congestive heart failure as an early manifestation.

The clinical manifestations of the disease are due to parenchymal cell damage caused by iron overload in hepatocytes, pancreatic islet cells, or the pituitary gland. The late clinical manifestations of hemochromatosis such as the classic triad of cirrhosis, diabetes mellitus, and bronze skin (due to excessive melanin production) are rarely seen in patients who present with the disease in modern times.

10. How is hemochromatosis treated?
The best therapy for homozygous hemochromatosis is phlebotomy. Because these patients have marked iron overload, the removal of 1 or even 2 units of blood per week is generally

well tolerated unless the patient is severely ill. At least 20 gm of iron is associated with clinical manifestations of the disease. One unit of blood contains about 250 mg of iron. It should be anticipated, therefore, that at least 80 phlebotomies will be necessary to normalize the total body iron. During phlebotomy therapy, patients are monitored with blood counts to ensure that they have maintained an adequate hemoglobin level. Serial ferritin values follow the decrease in total body iron stores for individual patients receiving phlebotomy therapy. Once symptomatic patients have a normalized total body iron, a maintenance phlebotomy regimen of two to four phlebotomies per year may be adequate to maintain body iron stores at normal levels.

Patients who have hereditary or acquired anemia and hemochromatosis associated with transfusion therapy should receive treatment with an iron chelator such as deferoxamine (to remove excess iron). These individuals must receive adequate iron chelation therapy, particularly if transfusions are necessary to maintain their hemoglobin at an acceptable range.

11. What is the overall prognosis for patients with hemochromatosis?
Treated patients with hemochromatosis who present with mild clinical disease or subclinical disease generally have a normal life span if iron stores are maintained at optimal levels. Patients who already have cardiac damage or severe diabetes generally will have only partial reversal of their disease state with phlebotomy therapy and will have decreased survival based on these complications. Patients with hepatic cirrhosis also have decreased survival. Although it has been suggested that in some instances phlebotomy therapy may reverse this process, patients with cirrhosis even if treated with phlebotomy therapy are at risk for the development of hepatoma.

12. Is there a best treatment for patients with hemochromatosis acquired from transfusions?
Yes. Chelation therapy, usually with deferoxamine. In this instance, phlebotomy is not the best therapy because the patient is dependent on transfusions to keep the hemoglobin at an acceptable range.

13. Can hemochromatosis be cured?
At present, no. Hemochromatosis is similar to diabetes mellitus, a condition in which insulin is needed to keep the glucose in check. In hemochromatosis, maintenance therapy with phlebotomy and/or chelation is required to keep the iron from accumulating. In the future, gene therapy may be available to cure patients.

14. Where is the gene for hemochromatosis located?
The gene for hemochromatosis is located on the short arm of chromosome 6. It is closely linked to the HLA locus. In fact, approximately 70% of patients with hemochromatosis carry the HLA-A3 allele compared with only about one quarter of the general population. Although the HLA gene and the hemochromatosis gene are in close proximity, they are separate and distinct genes and one's expression does not affect the other.

BIBLIOGRAPHY

1. Adams P, et al: Long-term survival analysis in hereditary hemochromatosis. Gastroenterology 101:368–372, 1991.
2. Edwards C, et al: Prevalence of hemochromatosis among 11,065 presumably healthy blood donors. N Engl J Med 318:355–362, 1988.
3. Edwards C, Kushner J: Screening for hemochromatosis. N Engl J Med 328:1616–1620, 1993.
4. Fairbanks V, Baldus W: Iron overload. In Hoffman R, et al (eds): Hematology: Basic Principles and Practice. New York, Churchill Livingstone, 1991, pp 340–349.
5. Gordeck V, et al: Iron overload in Africa. N Engl J Med 326:95–100, 1992.
6. Nichols C, et al: Hereditary hemochromatosis: Pathogenesis and clinical features of a common disease. Am J Gastroenterol 84:851, 1989.
7. Powell L, et al: Expression of hemochromatosis in homozygous subjects. Gastroenterology 98:1625–1632, 1990.

8. Skinke B, Cook J: Screening test for iron overload. Am J Clin Nutr 46:840–843, 1987.
9. Weintraub L: The many faces of hemochromatosis. Hosp Pract 26(4):49–59, 1991.
10. Weintraub L, et al: Treatment of hemochromatosis by phlebotomy. Med Clin North Am 50:1579, 1966.

16. DISSEMINATED INTRAVASCULAR COAGULATION

Robin J. Kovachy, M.D.

1. What is disseminated intravascular coagulation (DIC)?

It is the widespread deposition of fibrin in small blood vessels that may cause tissue or organ damage from ischemia. Depletion of clotting factors and platelets result in a bleeding diathesis. Simultaneous activation of plasmin and resulting fibrinolysis also occurs. This has been reported in association with any severe illness or may be more insidious in certain chronic diseases.

2. How common is DIC?

DIC is second only to liver disease as a cause of *acquired* coagulopathy. In the hospitalized population, DIC may be as common as 1 per 1000 admissions.

3. What illnesses are associated with DIC?

Common illnesses associated with DIC include:

Obstetric complications: abruptio placentae, septic abortion, chorioamnionitis, amniotic fluid embolism, intrauterine fetal death, postpartum hemolytic-uremic syndrome, and severe eclampsia

Infections: viral; bacterial, especially meningiococcemia; gram-negative sepsis; rickettsial; mycotic; protozoal

Neoplasms: carcinoma of the prostate, pancreas, breast, lung, ovary, gastric, and others

Intravascular hemolysis (e.g., transfusion reaction)

Vascular disorders: aneurysms, giant hemangiomas, or vasculitis

Massive tissue injury and trauma

Miscellaneous: snake bite, anaphylaxis, drug reactions, hypothermia, transplant rejection, adult respiratory distress syndrome (ARDS), acidosis, acute pancreatitis

4. Describe the clinical picture of acute DIC.

The major clinical finding is generalized bleeding. Patients may ooze from venipuncture sites and have widespread ecchymoses and petechiae. Bleeding into the kidneys, lungs, gastrointestinal tract, or central nervous system (CNS) may occur as well. Evidence of thromboembolic phenomena may also be present. Acral cyanosis (gray to purple discoloration of the tips of the fingers and toes) is occasionally seen, especially in patients with shock.

5. Describe the clinical picture of chronic DIC.

Chronic DIC is usually manifested by bruising and mucosal bleeding. Thrombophlebitis is common and often occurs in unusual sites. Evidence of renal dysfunction or transient neurologic syndromes are common.

6. What laboratory tests are needed to make the diagnosis of DIC?

In acute DIC, usually the prothrombin time (PT), partial thromboplastin time (PTT), and thrombin time are prolonged. The platelet count is decreased. Fibrin degradation products are elevated. Multiple clotting factors, especially fibrinogen and factors V, VIII, and XIII, are usually depressed. In chronic DIC, the platelet count and clotting factor levels may be normal. However, fibrin degradation products will be evaluated. Review of the peripheral blood smear will show schistocytes (fragmented RBCs) in 50% of cases. (See Figure 4, Color Plates.)

7. Name two conditions that may be confused clinically with DIC and describe how they can be distinguished.

1. Severe liver disease can look the same with thrombocytopenia, prolonged PT and PTT, and elevated fibrin degradation products (FDPs). Usually factor VIII is normal or increased in liver disease, whereas it is more likely to be depressed in DIC.

2. Primary fibrinogenolysis is a *rare* disorder with hemorrhagic tendencies from increased breakdown of fibrinogen. The PT and PTT will be prolonged. Usually the platelet count is normal. Schistocytes are not seen on the peripheral blood smear.

8. What is the most important treatment of DIC?

Treatment of the underlying illness is the cornerstone of treatment. Spontaneous reversal of DIC often occurs if the underlying illness is successfully treated. Frequently patients require transfusions of red blood cells and aggressive management of shock. Platelets should be transfused if there is severe hemorrhage and the platelet count is <50,000.

CONTROVERSIES

9. Should clotting factor replacement be given?
For:
Cryoprecipitate, rich in fibrinogen, should be given when the fibrinogen level is <100 mg/dl, especially if there is hemorrhage. In most series, infusion of fresh frozen plasma or cryoprecipitate has not been associated with adverse effects.
Against:
Infusion of fibrinogen might add "fuel to the fire" and aggravate the deposition of fibrin in small blood vessels. Thromboembolic complications have been reported with replacement of clotting factors. With large volumes of blood products, the risk of hepatitis or acquired immunodeficiency syndrome (AIDS) increases.

10. Should heparin be used to treat DIC?
For:
Heparin activates antithrombin III, which neutralizes free thrombin and inhibits its further formation. Because DIC is the abnormal activation of the clotting pathway, heparin should improve the coagulation abnormalities. Heparin is considered useful when there are clinical signs of major thrombotic events, such as acral ischemia, or in chronic DIC such as seen with malignancies.
Against:
No randomized trials have shown improved outcome in acute DIC with the use of heparin. Beneficial effects of heparin have been reported mostly in situations in which DIC is self-limited and would be expected to resolve spontaneously anyway. Heparin might increase the bleeding tendency.

BIBLIOGRAPHY

1. Bick RL: Disseminated intravascular coagulation and related syndromes: A clinical review. Semin Thromb Hemost 14:299, 1988.
2. Djulbegovic B: Reasoning and Decision Making in Hematology. New York, Churchill Livingstone, 1992, pp 215–219.
3. Feinstein DI: Disseminated intravascular coagulation. J Crit Illness 4:21, 1989.
4. Lee GR, et al: Wintrobe's Clinical Hematology. Philadelphia, Lea & Febiger, 1993, pp 1480–1493.
5. Ratnoff OD: Disorders of Hemostasis, 2nd ed. Philadelphia, W.B. Saunders, 1991, pp 292–326.

17. THROMBOTIC THROMBOCYTOPENIC PURPURA AND HEMOLYTIC UREMIC SYNDROME

Kathryn Hassell, M.D.

1. What is thrombotic thrombocytopenia purpura (TTP)?
TTP is a clinical syndrome classically characterized by a pentad of signs and symptoms:
1. Low platelet count
2. Microangiopathic hemolytic anemia
3. Neurologic changes
4. Impaired renal function
5. Fever

In many cases, not all five of these characteristics are present, but this diagnosis should be considered in a patient with hemolytic anemia with schistocytes (broken RBCs) on the peripheral smear (see Figure 4, Color Plates), low platelet count, and a rising creatinine.

2. Are there other syndromes related to TTP?
Yes. Hemolytic uremic syndrome (HUS) is a disease characterized by renal failure, microangiopathic hemolytic anemia, and a low platelet count. It is considered to be part of a clinical spectrum of diseases which include TTP, and has major features similar to TTP.

Hemolytic anemia with Elevated Liver enzymes and Low Platelets (HELLP syndrome) is seen in pregnant women usually in the late second or third trimester. It can occur in conjunction with signs of preeclampsia (hypertension, proteinuria, edema) and is characterized by microangiopathic hemolytic anemia, low platelet count, and marked elevation in liver enzymes. HELLP is thought to represent another disease in the spectrum of TTP.

3. What mechanisms are at work in TTP and HUS?
The precise pathophysiologic changes that occur in TTP are not clear. Based on biopsy and autopsy material, the primary pathologic change appears to be platelet microthrombi in the small arterioles and capillaries of all organs (including kidneys, liver, brain). These microthrombi consume platelets and impede blood flow, resulting in tissue damage and organ dysfunction. In addition, these microthrombi impede passage of the red blood cells, resulting in fragmentation and hemolysis (microangiopathic hemolytic anemia).

The events that promote the initial platelet aggregation and microthrombi are not known. A great deal of work has centered on the observation that patients with relapsing TTP have an increased amount of high molecular weight von Willebrand's factor in the circulation that may promote platelet aggregation. Because TTP has occurred after viral illness, in human immunodeficiency virus (HIV)–infected patients, after use of certain medications, during pregnancy, and in conjunction with autoimmune diseases, the role of endothelial cell inflammation and/or an autoimmune "trigger" to this disease has been considered. It is not known why some organs (brain, kidney, liver) are affected more than others in these syndromes. Some childhood cases of HUS have been associated with toxins produced by infections with *Shigella* species and *Escherichia coli*.

4. Are there other diseases that are often confused with TTP/HUS?
TTP and its related diseases are diagnosed clinically, so other possible diagnoses need to be eliminated. Disseminated intravascular coagulation (DIC) has many features similar to TTP, especially in a patient who is septic. Patients with DIC have a microangiopathic

hemolytic anemia and a low platelet count due to the intravascular coagulation and may develop fever, mental status changes, and renal failure due to overwhelming infection. In DIC, however, the prothrombin time (PT) and activated partial thromboplastin time (aPTT) are elevated due to the consumption of coagulation factors; this does **not** occur in TTP.

Malignant hypertension may be associated with acute renal failure, mental status changes, and, when severe, with microangiopathic hemolytic anemia and thrombocytopenia, as is seen in HUS. Very high blood pressure (as seen in malignant hypertension) is not common in HUS, however, and the lowering of blood pressure should result in resolution of these changes if they are due to malignant hypertension.

Acute liver failure can complicate pregnancy characterized by marked elevations in liver enzymes and (in some cases) a fall in platelet count resembling HELLP. However, microangiopathic hemolytic anemia is not seen and must be present to consider the diagnosis of HELLP.

5. How is the diagnosis of TTP/HUS made?

Because it is a clinical diagnosis, TTP and related disorders may be diagnosed only by identifying typical features and ruling out other possible disorders. Thrombocytopenia, sometimes mild but often severe ($<30,000$ to $40,000/mm^3$), must be present. Microangiopathic hemolytic anemia is diagnosed by the presence of anemia, elevated reticulocyte count, schistocytes on the peripheral smear, elevated indirect bilirubin, lactate dehydrogenase (LDH), and aspartate aminotransferase (AST; SGOT), indicating red blood cell destruction. Elevations in creatinine may be mild in TTP but are characteristically higher in HUS. Neurologic changes range from minor mental status changes and headaches to seizures, stroke, and coma. Fever is not always present. Coagulation tests (PT, aPTT) should be checked and should be normal to exclude the diagnosis of DIC. Gingival biopsy looking for arteriolar microthrombi can be helpful, but when it is negative, it does not exclude the diagnosis of TTP. The same is true for the value of renal biopsy in HUS.

6. What is the treatment of TTP/HUS?

Two main approaches to treatment involve (1) an attempt to decrease the formation of microthrombi and (2) the use of plasma and plasmapheresis.

Because the primary pathophysiology appears to center on the development of platelet microthrombi, antiplatelet agents, including aspirin and dipyridamole, have been used during acute episodes of TTP. Steroids, usually prednisone (1–2 mg/kg), are given to reduce any possible role of autoimmunity or other inflammatory stimuli in the development of vasculopathy. Heparin and other anticoagulants have not shown any benefit.

Fresh frozen plasma (FFP) has been used both by simple transfusion and via plasmapheresis with plasma exchange. Initially, plasmapheresis with total plasma exchange was thought to be necessary to remove unknown factors in the patient's circulation that were promoting platelet aggregation, but some patients seemed to improve with simple transfusion of FFP. It is now thought that some regulatory product, present in donor FFP but missing in the patient, can be replaced with FFP transfusion. Currently, plasmapheresis using donor FFP for replacement is used to treat acute episodes of TTP and HUS in conjunction with prednisone with or without aspirin.

In refractory cases, vincristine (a chemotherapeutic agent that alters microtubular function and may impair platelet function) has been used. Intravenous gamma globulin and splenectomy have also been tried with mixed success.

HELLP syndrome, in contrast to TTP/HUS, is treated with steroids and termination of the pregnancy. Most cases of HELLP reverse spontaneously once the baby has been delivered; in cases in which the symptoms persist, a more typical TTP-like syndrome is suspected and the patient is treated as though she has TTP. Because TTP does not require termination of pregnancy, distinguishing it from HELLP is important but not easy. In TTP, severe liver disease is unusual and suggests the diagnosis of HELLP.

7. Is there any harm in transfusing platelets for a low platelet count?
Platelet transfusions should be avoided in TTP/HUS. Because the basic pathophysiology seems to be related to platelet aggregation, it is theoretically possible to worsen the course of TTP/HUS markedly by platelet transfusion. Anecdotal data suggest that increased microthrombi deposition with development of stroke, worsening hemolytic anemia, and renal dysfunction has occurred with platelet transfusions.

8. How are patients monitored to determine if treatment is working?
Successful therapy of TTP/HUS will be reflected in improvement in neurologic and renal function. Daily determination of hemoglobin/hematocrit, platelet count, reticulocyte count, LDH, and creatinine should be done. Over the course of several days, a fall in reticulocyte count with a rise in hemoglobin and a reduction in LDH and schistocytes herald improvement in the microangiopathic process. Daily plasmapheresis should not be discontinued until there are signs of improvement, and some series suggest that "tapering" plasmapheresis over several days to weeks may reduce the acute relapse rate. Prednisone should be continued until the episode is clearly remitted and then tapered slowly.

9. How successful is treatment?
Acute, severe episodes of TTP can be difficult to treat, with a mortality rate of up to 30–40% despite therapy. Early recognition and appropriate treatment may reduce this mortality. Response rates of up to 90% have been reported in episodes where fresh frozen plasma is used.

10. Is there a high relapse rate if a patient is successfully treated?
There is a subgroup of patients who appear to have a chronic, relapsing form of TTP, where episodes can be triggered by recognized stimuli (e.g., certain medications, viral illnesses) or occur without apparent cause. Some of these patients have a large amount of high molecular weight von Willebrand's factor in their circulation chronically. Patients who have had TTP or HELLP in association with pregnancy may be at risk for recurrence with another pregnancy.

CONTROVERSIES

11. Should aspirin be used in the treatment of TTP?
Because patients with TTP have low platelet counts and often have associated bleeding, there is hesitation to add aspirin, which will compromise the function of the few remaining platelets and increase the risk of bleeding. Nonetheless, because functional platelets are thought to contribute significantly to the underlying pathophysiology of the disease, aspirin should theoretically be used. More recent studies have suggested that aspirin does not alter the overall course of TTP and therefore should not be used. Some continue to advocate its use, however, especially if thrombocytopenia is mild, there is little clinical bleeding, and plasmapheresis is not immediately available.

12. Is simple transfusion with FFP enough or is plasmapheresis always necessary?
Plasma exchange has been done, in part, because the concept involved removing "negative factors" in the patient's blood that could be promoting platelet aggregation. Evidence now suggests that some regulatory factor may be missing from the patient's blood that is given back by transfusing FFP, and that this represents the main benefit of exchange. Some series do show an improvement in an episode of TTP with simple transfusion of FFP. Nonetheless, current practice still includes plasmapheresis with plasma exchange, although the patient is often treated initially with simple transfusion of FFP until plasmapheresis can be initiated.

13. Is there a relationship between TTP and human immunodeficiency virus (HIV) infection?

An unexpected number of cases of TTP have been reported in patients infected with HIV. Given the alterations in the immune system associated with HIV infection (e.g., autoimmune diseases such as idiopathic thrombocytopenic purpura, polyclonal gammopathy), some investigators have postulated a theoretical link between this abnormal immune response and TTP/HUS. Proof of this relationship, however, has not yet been found.

BIBLIOGRAPHY

1. Barton JR, Sibai BM: Care of the pregnancy complicated by HELLP syndrome. Obstet Gynecol Clin North Am 18:165, 1991.
2. Fitzpatrick MM, Dillon MJ: Current views on aetiology and management of haemolytic uraemic syndrome. Postgrad Med J 67:707, 1991.
3. Kelton JG, et al: The platelet aggregating factor(s) of thrombotic thrombocytopenic purpura. Prog Clin Biol Res 337:141, 1990.
4. Martin JN Jr, Stedman CM: Imitators of preeclampsia and HELLP syndrome. Obstet Gynecol Clin North Am 18:181, 1991.
5. Miller JM Jr, Pastorek JG II: Thrombotic thrombocytopenic purpura and hemolytic uremic syndrome in pregnancy. Clin Obstet Gynecol 34:64, 1991.
6. Moake JL: The role of von Willebrand factor (vWF) in thrombotic thrombocytopenic purpura (TTP) and the hemolytic-uremic syndrome (HUS). Prog Clin Biol Res 337:135, 1990.
7. Raniele DP, et al: Should intravenous immunoglobulin G be first-line treatment for acute thrombotic thrombocytopenic purpura? Case report and review of the literature. Am J Kidney Dis 18:264, 1991.
8. Rarick MU, et al: Thrombotic thrombocytopenic purpura in patients with human immunodeficiency virus infection: A report of three cases and review of the literature. Am J Hematol 40:103, 1992.
9. Rock G, et al: Comparison of plasma exchange with plasma infusion in the treatment of thrombotic thrombocytopenic purpura. Canadian Apheresis Study Group. N Engl J Med 325:7, 1991.
10. Ruggenenti P, Remuzzi G: Thrombotic thrombocytopenic purpura and related disorders. Hematol Oncol Clin North Am 4:219, 1990.
11. Stricker RB, et al: Thrombotic thrombocytopenic purpura complicating systemic lupus erythematosus. Case report and literature review from the plasmapheresis era. J Rheumatol 19:1469, 1992.
12. Thompson CE, et al: Thrombotic microangiopathies in the 1980s: Clinical features, response to treatment, and the impact of the human immunodeficiency virus epidemic. Blood 80:1890, 1992.

18. IDIOPATHIC THROMBOCYTOPENIC PURPURA

Robin J. Kovachy, M.D.

1. Define idiopathic thrombocytopenic purpura (ITP).

ITP is a condition in which patients have low platelets owing to immunoglobulin G (IgG) platelet antibodies, resulting in increased destruction of platelets. Platelet production in the bone marrow is increased. It is a relatively common cause of thrombocytopenia and the most common immunologic disorder in women of childbearing age.

2. What laboratory abnormalities other than a low platelet count might be noted on the complete blood count (CBC)?

Unless the patient has had severe enough bleeding to cause iron deficiency anemia, the CBC will be relatively normal. Occasionally, the mean platelet volume (MPV) will be increased. IgG platelet antibodies are positive in approximately 90% of patients.

3. What can cause a falsely low or elevated platelet count on an automated CBC machine?
Ethylenediamine tetraacetic acid (EDTA)-induced platelet clumping, paraproteinemias, hyperlipidemia, giant platelets counted as white blood cells, or fragmented red blood cells counted as platelets. All patients with decreased platelet counts should have a peripheral blood smear reviewed to confirm the automated count.

4. Name the single test that establishes the definitive diagnosis of ITP.
There is no such test. ITP is a diagnosis of exclusion. Platelet-associated antibodies are not sensitive or specific enough. There are many false positives and false negatives. Other causes of thrombocytopenia must be ruled out, particularly thrombocytopenia related to drugs, which may be indistinguishable from ITP.

5. How can ITP be distinguished from thrombotic thrombocytopenia purpura (TTP), hemolytic uremic syndrome (HUS), and disseminated intravascular coagulation (DIC)?
Review of the peripheral smear reveals normal red blood cells and white blood cells in ITP. HUS and TTP always have fragmented red blood cells on the peripheral blood smear. With DIC, usually the protime and partial thromboplastin time (PTT) will be prolonged, fibrinogen will be low, and fibrin split products will be elevated.

6. How can ITP be distinguished from disorders of the hematopoietic system such as aplastic anemia, acute leukemia, myelodysplastic syndromes, and myeloma?
Review the peripheral blood smear. In ITP, red blood cell morphology is usually normal. Bone marrow biopsy and aspiration will show increased megakaryocytes as the only abnormality. Other primary hematologic disorders will be obvious on the bone marrow biopsy.

7. Which infectious diseases may be associated with thrombocytopenia in which an immune mechanism is not thought to be implicated?
Viral infections, including herpes, pertussis, rubella, infectious mononucleosis, chickenpox, hepatitis, Colorado tick fever, and acquired immunodeficiency syndrome (AIDS); rickettsial infections such as Rocky Mountain spotted fever and typhus; bacterial infections, especially subacute bacterial endocarditis, meningococcemia, and gram-negative sepsis.

8. Name commonly used drugs that have been found to be associated with thrombocytopenia by presumed immune mechanism.

Acetaminophen	Gold salts	Quinidine
Cephalothin	Heparin	Quinine
Diazepam	Penicillin	Sulfisoxazole

9. How do patients with ITP usually present?
They usually feel reasonably well and have no systemic symptoms such as fatigue, weight loss, or fever. They often have minor bleeding such as epistaxis, menorrhagia, easy bruising, and petechiae. Hematuria, melena, and hematemesis are not common but can be presenting symptoms.

10. What are some of the clinical characteristics of acute ITP?
Acute ITP occurs most often in children, with the peak incidence being from 2–6 years of age. Usually the disorder starts abruptly with hemorrhagic complications and follows a history of a viral illness 1–3 weeks before the diagnosis. Spontaneous remission is common. There is no sex predilection.

11. What are some of the characteristics of chronic ITP?
This is the form that occurs primarily in adults, with the peak incidence being between the ages of 20 and 40. Women are three times more likely to be affected than men. A prior history of infection is unusual. Spontaneous remission is rare. The onset is somewhat more insidious than in acute ITP.

12. How often is ITP associated with splenomegaly?

In 10–20% of the patients, mild splenomegaly may be noted. More significant spleno-megaly (i.e., more than 2–3 cm below the left costal margin) should lead to consideration of other diseases of the spleen such as neoplastic infiltration and congestive or infectious splenomegaly.

13. Discuss the most serious complication of ITP and how it should be treated.

Spontaneous intracranial hemorrhage can be life threatening, but fortunately occurs in less than 1% of the patients afflicted with this disorder. This is unlikely to occur unless platelets are <10,000. Once intracranial bleeding is diagnosed, the patient should be given a large dose of gamma globulin, intravenous steroids and platelet transfusion. Neurosurgical consultation should be obtained and splenectomy should be considered.

14. Give the three main therapies for treatment of ITP.

Corticosteroids (usually at an initial dose of 60 mg/day), splenectomy, and high-dose gamma globulin. Most patients respond to steroids, although sometimes steroids need to be continued for 2 weeks before response is seen. Only 10–30% of patients maintain a long remission with steroid therapy only.

15. What are the indications for splenectomy in ITP?

Splenectomy should be considered when patients are unable to be tapered off of prednisone within a 3- to 6-month period of time. Complications from long-term steroids are more severe than from splenectomy. Patients who fail to respond to steroid therapy and patients with severe contraindications to steroid usage (i.e., steroid psychosis, brittle diabetes) should be offered splenectomy.

16. When is splenectomy contraindicated in ITP?

Splenectomy is contraindicated early in the first episode of ITP, as most patients will respond to steroids. It is especially contraindicated in children because of the frequent spontaneous remission. Children under 2 years of age have a much higher risk of overwhelming sepsis if the spleen has been removed. Splenectomy should be avoided in pregnant women and in patients with severe cardiac and pulmonary diseases who are at risk from any major surgery.

17. How effective is splenectomy? What is the mortality? How can response to splenectomy be predicted?

Approximately 80% of patients will respond initially to splenectomy and 60% will have a sustained remission. There is no way to predict who will respond to splenectomy. Mortality from splenectomy is <1%. All patients should be treated with pneumococcal vaccine several weeks prior to splenectomy to minimize complications from sepsis.

18. List other treatments that are used in refractory ITP.

Cyclophosphamide	Danazol	Colchicine
Vincristine	Azathioprine	Plasmapheresis

19. List other conditions associated with ITP.

Sarcoidosis	Chronic lymphocytic leukemia
Non-Hodgkin's lymphoma	Systemic lupus erythematosus
Hodgkin's lymphoma	Thyrotoxicosis

20. What are additional concerns in patients with ITP who are pregnant?

Usually these patients can be managed with prednisone and/or high-dose gamma globulin. Splenectomy is to be avoided if at all possible. In mothers with a prior history of ITP and increased levels of platelet IgG antibodies, severe thrombocytopenia may occur in the fetus, resulting in spontaneous bleeding.

BIBLIOGRAPHY

1. Abrams RA, et al: Intravenous gammaglobulin in refractory immune thrombocytopenia purpura: Efficiency with or without concomitant steroid therapy. Am J Hematol 18:85, 1985.
2. Berchtold P, et al: Therapy of chronic thrombocytopenia purpura in adults. Blood 74:2309, 1989.
3. Cortelazza S, et al: High risk of severe bleeding in aged patients with chronic idiopathic thrombocytopenic purpura. Blood 77:31, 1991.
4. Djulbegovic B: Reasoning and Decision Making in Hematology. New York, Churchill Livingstone, 1992, pp 195–200.
5. Lee GR, et al: Wintrobe's Clinical Hematology. Philadelphia, Lea & Febiger, 1993, pp 1329–1347.
6. Ratnoff OD: Disorders of Hemostasis, 2nd ed. Philadelphia, W.B. Saunders, 1991, pp 108–130.
7. Steinberg MH, et al: An aid in the classification of thrombocytopenic disorders. N Engl J Med 317:1037, 1987.

19. THROMBOCYTOSIS

Douglas Jerome Kemme, M.D.

1. What is a normal platelet count?
It ranges from 150 to 400 thousand platelets per microliter (K/μl).

2. What is thrombocytosis?
A platelet count >400 K/μl.

3. What are the two broad categories of thrombocytosis?
Reactive thrombocytosis is due to an increased production of platelets or decreased destruction of platelets from another process. **Primary thrombocytosis** is due to a primary bone marrow disease that causes increased production of platelets.

4. Name eight conditions that can cause reactive thrombocytosis.

1. Chronic inflammation
2. Acute or chronic infection
3. Recovery from alcohol or malnutrition
4. Acute stress
5. The postoperative state
6. Malignancy
7. Splenectomy
8. Iron deficiency

5. How do inflammatory and infectious diseases cause reactive thrombocytosis?
Both chronic inflammation and infections increase the production of white blood cells required for the inflammatory response. Megakaryocytic production of platelets also is increased, which causes thrombocytosis.

6. Can alcohol cause an increase as well as a decrease in the platelet count?
Yes. Alcohol may decrease the platelet count by a direct toxic effect on the megakaryocytes. Thrombocytosis is commonly observed as the patient recovers from this effect.

7. Can iron deficiency cause an increase as well as a decrease in the platelet count?
Yes. Children and elderly patients may develop thrombocytopenia with iron deficiency. Severe iron deficiency in adults may cause thrombocytopenia, although the majority of adults will develop thrombocytosis.

8. When are patients with reactive thrombocytosis at risk for thrombosis?
Very few patients with reactive thrombocytosis will develop thrombosis when the platelet count is <1,000 K/μl. Above that, the risk is proportional to the platelet count, with patients

with platelet counts >2,000 K/μl at highest risk. Management of these patients is difficult. After excluding primary thrombocytosis (see below), aspirin is usually sufficient prophylaxis until the platelet count returns to normal with correction of the underlying problem. Standard anticoagulation should be given to patients with proven thromboembolism.

9. When are patients with reactive thrombocytosis at risk for bleeding complications?
Bleeding is very rare in patients with reactive thrombocytosis and is usually related to the underlying disorder or its treatment.

10. What disorders are associated with primary thrombocytosis?
Patients with myeloproliferative disorders often have thrombocytosis. These myeloproliferative disorders are polycythemia vera, chronic myelogenous leukemia, and myelofibrosis with myeloid metaplasia, which are described elsewhere, and essential thrombocytosis, which is the topic of the remainder of this chapter.

11. What is essential thrombocytosis?
Essential thrombocytosis is a myeloproliferative disorder that causes primarily an increase in the number of abnormally functioning platelets.

12. What causes this increase in the platelet count?
The megakaryocyte precursors, known as megakaryocyte colony-forming units (CFU-MK), have been shown to be abnormal in this disorder. These cells appear to replicate in the absence of the normal growth factors, demonstrating the loss of a normal feedback system. The abnormal CFU-MK cells have been demonstrated to be clonally derived.

13. Why do other myeloproliferative disorders demonstrate increased platelet counts?
The abnormal clone causing increased growth of white blood cells in chronic myelogenous leukemia or red blood cells in polycythemia vera appears to be an early progenitor cell capable of differentiation to the CFU-MK as well.

14. In individuals with primary thrombocytosis, do the platelets function normally?
No. In addition to an increase in number of platelets, these platelets have multiple functional abnormalities. Thus, one individual may have both bleeding and clotting problems.

15. How do you make the diagnosis of essential thrombocytosis?
Individuals will have platelet counts in excess of 600 K/μl with no known disorder causing reactive thrombocytosis, a normal hematocrit, and a bone marrow biopsy demonstrating normal to increased numbers of megakaryocytes without evidence of the Philadelphia chromosome.

16. How can reactive thrombocytosis be excluded in these individuals?
This may be difficult in some patients, particularly those who may have two disorders occurring simultaneously. Abnormal platelet aggregation studies may suggest a myeloproliferative disorder. A few centers have demonstrated abnormal CFU-MK growth on bone marrow aspirate samples, but this is not a widely available test.

17. How can you eliminate the possibility of chronic myelogenous leukemia in these individuals?
This is an important distinction, as the treatment is radically different for chronic myelogenous leukemia. Careful examination of the bone marrow by a hematopathologist and chromosome analysis for the Philadelphia chromosome is mandatory. Some centers use polymerase chain reaction (PCR) amplification of DNA from bone marrow samples, looking for the gene rearrangement characterized by the Philadelphia chromosome. Although PCR is not universally available, it should be performed in any younger patient in whom the correct diagnosis of chronic myelogenous leukemia is critical.

18. Who may develop essential thrombocytosis?
This is a rare disorder affecting women and men equally around the age of 50–60 years.

19. What are common presenting symptoms of essential thrombocytosis?
Patients with essential thrombocytosis may develop both bleeding and clotting problems. Many patients are diagnosed prior to any complications of the increased platelet count. Commonly, the disorder is found incidentally during laboratory analysis for an unrelated reason.

20. What type of thromboembolic events may a patient experience?
Clotting problems may range from arterial clots such as cerebral or myocardial ischemia and/or infarction. Venous clots may occur in unusual locations such as hepatic veins (Budd-Chiari syndrome). Individuals commonly do not have risk factors for venous thromboembolism.

21. Define erythromyalgia.
Erythromyalgia is a painful red rash occurring in patients with primary thrombocytosis due to clotting within the skin. Response of this disorder to aspirin is diagnostic of primary thrombocytosis.

22. Discuss the type of bleeding problems that develop in patients with essential thrombocytosis.
These patients may develop gastrointestinal or skin bleeding but they are rarely life threatening.

23. Can patients have both clotting and bleeding problems?
Yes. It is important to realize that a patient with clotting problems may develop bleeding problems at any platelet level. This makes it very risky to treat a patient with essential thrombocytosis with aspirin.

24. How do you manage a patient with life-threatening thromboembolic situations due to essential thrombocytosis?
Platelet pheresis and/or hydroxyurea are commonly used to decrease the platelet count dramatically.

25. What is the goal in the treatment of essential thrombocytosis?
The goal is to decrease the bleeding or thromboembolic complications of the disease. The platelet count should be decreased, which is commonly done with the use of hydroxyurea. The optimal number of platelets is unknown, although most hematologists aim for the upper limit of normal ($400 \, K/\mu l$). Transient ischemic attacks and erythromyalgia respond well to aspirin; however, caution should be used, as this medication also increases the risk of bleeding complications, even in patients with no known history of bleeding.

26. Does anegralide have a role in the treatment of essential thrombocytosis?
Anegralide is a new drug that produces thrombocytopenia by an unknown mechanism. It has been used in patients who have become refractory to standard therapy with good results. As anegralide is not leukemogenic, whereas hydroxyurea may be, this medication has advantages that await further study.

27. Is there a role for interferon in the treatment of essential thrombocytosis?
Interferon has been shown to decrease the platelet count in patients with myeloproliferative diseases, but has more side effects than hydroxyurea. It may be useful in patients refractory to hydroxyurea.

28. What is the prognosis for patients with essential thrombocytosis?
Patients with well-controlled platelet counts may expect many quality years with this disease, with median survival generally exceeding 10 years. However, affected individuals remain at risk for developing other myeloproliferative disorders or acute leukemia.

BIBLIOGRAPHY

1. Buss DH, O'Connor ML, Woodruff RF, et al: Bone marrow and peripheral blood findings in patients with extreme thrombocytosis. Arch Pathol Lab Med 115:475–480, 1991.
2. Buss DH, Stuart JJ, Lipscomb GE: The incidence of thrombotic and hemorrhagic disorders in association with extreme thrombocytosis: An analysis of 129 cases. Am J Hematol 20:365–372, 1985.
3. Cololbi M, Radaelli F, Zocchi L, Maiolo AT: Thrombotic and hemorrhagic complications in essential thrombocythemia: A retrospective study of 103 patients. Cancer 67:2926–2930, 1991.
4. Gerwirtz AM, Hoffman R: Primary platelet production disorder. In Hoffman R, Benz EJ, Shattil SJ, et al (eds): Hematology: Basic Principles and Practice. New York, Churchill Livingstone, 1991, pp 881–889.
5. Hoffman R, Silverstom MN: Primary thrombocythemia. In Hoffman R, Benz EJ, Shattil SJ, et al (eds): Hematology: Basic Principles and Practice. New York, Churchill Livingstone, 1991, ppp 881–889.
6. Kurzrock R, Cohen PR: Erythromyalgia: Review of clinical characteristics and pathophysiology. Am J Med 91:416–422, 1991.
7. McIntyre KJ, Hoagland HC, Silverstein MN, Pettitt RM: Essential thrombocythemia in young adults. Mayo Clin Proc 66:149–154, 1991.
8. Scheffer MG, Michiels JJ, Simoons ML, Roelandt JRTC: Thrombocythemia and coronary artery disease. Am Heart J 122:573, 1991.
9. Silverstein MN, et al: Anagrelide, a therapy for thrombocythemic states: Experience in 577 patients. Am J Med 92:69–76, 1992.
10. Wadenvik H, Kutti J, Ridell B, et al: The effect of α-interferon on bone marrow megakaryocytes and platelet production rate in essential thrombocythemia. Blood 77:2103–2108, 1991.

20. HEMOPHILIA
Sally P. Stabler, M.D.

1. Define hemophilia.
The term "hemophilia" can be used in a general sense to refer to any of a number of congenital factor deficiencies that result in a bleeding diathesis or more specifically to refer to the two most common deficiencies: hemophilia A (factor VIII deficiency) and hemophilia B (factor IX deficiency). It is preferable to discuss these disorders by referring to the specific factor that is deficient.

Factor VIII deficiency, or classic hemophilia, is the most common severe congenital clotting deficiency. It cannot be distinguished from the second most common disorder, factor IX deficiency, without specific assays. Von Willebrand's disease is the most common mild disorder. In some populations (such as Ashkenazi Jews), factor XI deficiency is actually more common than either factor VIII or factor IX deficiency. Factor XI deficiency causes a much less serious bleeding diathesis than the other two. Seen much less frequently than the above-mentioned disorders but of clinical significance is factor VII deficiency. This is most commonly present in the milder probably heterozygous forms but occasionally presents as postoperative hemorrhage without a previously known coagulopathy. It is beyond the scope of this chapter to discuss these less common congenital bleeding diatheses, and attention is focused on hemophilias A and B instead.

2. What is the best screening test for hemophilia?

In evaluating a patient with a suspected factor deficiency, the first screening tests should be the prothrombin time (PT), activated partial thromboplastin time (aPTT), thrombin time (TT), fibrinogen, and bleeding time. In factor VIII and factor IX deficiencies, the aPTT is prolonged. In cases of mild deficiency, the aPTT may be prolonged only 1 to 4 seconds over the normal control. In general, the more prolonged the aPTT, the more severe the hemophilia. The rest of the above-mentioned screening tests are usually normal in hemophilia. An isolated elevated PT will be found in congenital factor VII deficiency. Factors XI and XII deficiencies will cause a prolonged aPTT similar to that found in patients with factor VIII and IX deficiencies.

The next step is to perform a mix of normal plasma with the patient's plasma. If the aPTT corrects in the mix, this suggests a factor deficiency. Specific factor assays would then be performed for factors VIII, IX, XI, and XII. If the factor VIII or IX level is 1% of normal or less, the patient has severe hemophilia. If the level is between 1% and 3%, it is considered moderate hemophilia. If it is above 5%, it is considered mild hemophilia. Normal levels are usually 60–120%.

3. List the clinical situations in which factor VIII levels are decreased.

1. Hemophilia A and the carrier state
2. Acquired factor VIII inhibitor (acquired hemophilia, which is an autoimmune disorder infrequently seen but devastating when it occurs)
3. Disseminated intravascular coagulation
4. von Willebrand's disease (all patients with a low factor VIII should also have von Willebrand's factor antigen and von Willebrand's ristocetin cofactor assayed)

4. Why don't women get hemophilia?

Hemophilia A and B are X-linked disorders. This means that the gene is on the X chromosome and females are carriers. Although previously the carriers were thought not to manifest bleeding tendencies, this has been shown not to be true. Because of lyonization of the X chromosome, some carrier females have low levels of either factor VIII or IX, which are often in the 30–50% range. These individuals can have major postoperative hemorrhage, although they do not bleed spontaneously. Each son of a carrier female has a 50:50 chance of having hemophilia. All of the daughters of a hemophilic male are obligatory carriers of hemophilia. All sons of a hemophilic male are normal. The sisters of a hemophiliac or of a hemophilic carrier each have a 50:50 chance of being carriers.

5. Does a negative family history preclude the diagnosis of hemophilia?

No. With new molecular biology techniques, it has been discovered that approximately one-third of all patients with hemophilia are either a new mutation themselves or the son of a female with a new mutation. This means that the population of hemophiliacs is constantly renewed and that the family history may be unreliable. In mild hemophilia, patients are often not diagnosed until after they experience postsurgical bleeding. In this case, all potential family members should be screened because it is very possible that there will be affected individuals (even elderly males) who have not had a hemostatic challenge that previously led to diagnosis.

6. What are the most common manifestations of hemophiliac bleeding?

Severe and moderately severe hemophiliacs (factor levels <3%) have frequent spontaneous hemorrhages into the joints and soft tissues. Untreated, these hemarthroses result in an arthropathy, leading to total destruction of the knees, elbows, ankles, and hips. In addition, hemophiliacs have frequent spontaneous intracerebral hemorrhages, renal bleeding, and retroperitoneal hemorrhages. Gastrointestinal hemorrhaging also is frequent and usually due to underlying peptic ulcer disease, Mallory-Weiss tears, or other pathology.

7. Should transfusion of clotting factors be avoided because of the risk of transmission of viral diseases?

No. At present, the factor VIII and factor IX products available have all been treated so that they are not contaminated with human immunodeficiency virus (HIV), hepatitis B, or hepatitis C. They are safer than fresh frozen plasma or cryoprecipitate from the blood bank that has not been virally inactivated. The choices of factor VIII products include recombinant factor VIII, monoclonally purified factor VIII from human plasma, or a less pure preparation of factor VIII. They are all virally safe, but the cost differs markedly between the different preparations. There is no recombinant factor IX product available, but monoclonally purified factor IX is available as well as prothrombin complex, which includes other vitamin K–dependent factors. Factor treatment should **never** be withheld because of a fear of infectious complications.

8. How and when does one decide on the amount of factor to give for a specific episode?

Always remember to transfuse immediately. There is no point in measuring a PTT prior to transfusion because hemophiliacs always have an elevated PTT. Appropriate doses for different clinical situations are given below. In general, patients are transfused to approximately 40% of normal levels for soft tissue hemorrhages and mild to moderate joint bleeding. In life-threatening situations and after surgery, we transfuse more aggressively to maintain normal levels of factor VIII and never let the trough level fall below 40–50% (lowest level). The half-life of factor VIII is about 12 hours. This means that patients are dosed every 12 hours in order to maintain adequate trough levels. The half-life of factor IX is longer (about 24 hours); thus a once-daily transfusion usually maintains adequate levels. However, twice as much factor IX is required to obtain the same levels as factor VIII.

*Required Doses of Factor in Bleeding Hemophiliacs**

EPISODE	FACTOR VIII DEFICIENCY	FACTOR IX DEFICIENCY
Soft tissue bleed or mild joint bleed	20 μ/kg × 1	40 μ/kg × 1
Severe joint or soft tissue bleed	40 μ/kg × 1, then 20 μ/kg q12h × 2	80 μ/kg × 1, then 40 μ/kg q24h × 1
Compartment syndrome	40 μ/kg × 1, then 20 μ/kg q12h until resolved	80 μ/kg × 1, then 40 μ/kg q24h until resolved
Laceration with sutures	20 μ/kg during suturing, then qod until sutures removed	40 μ/kg during suturing, then qod until sutures removed
Dental cleaning and restoration	20 μ/kg × 1	40 μ/kg × 1
Oral surgery	40 μ/kg × 1, then 20 μ/kg q24h × 2 amino-caproic acid (Amicar) 6 g q6h × 4–6 d	80 μ/kg × 1, then 40 μ/kg q24h × 1 amino-caproic acid (Amicar) 6 g q6h × 4–6 d
Central nervous bleeding	40 μ/kg prior to CT scan, then 20 μ/kg q12h until resolved, then q24h to finish 10–14 d	80 μ/kg prior to CT scan, then 40 μ/kg q24h until resolved, then qod to finish 10–14 d
Major surgery and joint synovectomy*	50 μ/kg on induction of anesthesia, then 20 μ/kg q12h for 14 d	80 μ/kg on induction of anesthesia, then 40 μ/kg q24h for 14 d

Table continued on following page.

Required Doses of Factor in Bleeding Hemophiliacs (Continued)*

EPISODE	FACTOR VIII DEFICIENCY	FACTOR IX DEFICIENCY
Major orthopedic surgery, especially joint replacement*	60 μ/kg on induction 20 μ/kg after 4 h in surgery, then 2 μ/kg/h IV drip × 72 h, then 20 μ/kg q12 h × 11 d, 20 μ/kg 24h × 7 d, then qod × 2 wk	100 μ/kg on induction 50 μ/kg q24h × 3 days, then 40 μ/kg × 11 d, then 40 μ/kg qod × 3 wk
Bronchoscopy, lumbar puncture, bone marrow biopsy, for example	40 μ/kg × 1, treat any hematoma again	80 μ/kg × 1, treat any hematoma again

*Postoperative factor levels are mandatory. Trough factor levels should be >60% in the first 48 hours postoperatively and thereafter >40%.

9. How long do I need to treat a patient with factor?
The length of time of treatment depends on the lesion being treated. One or two doses usually stops the bleeding for a mild joint bleed or soft tissue hemorrhage. In compartment syndromes and very severe soft tissue hemorrhage, treatment should continue until the entire area has softened and all hematomas have resolved. After surgery, treatment should continue until the wound has completely healed, which will be between 10 and 14 days for abdominal and chest surgery. In orthopedic surgery, adequate levels of factors frequently must be maintained for 3–6 weeks. Inexperienced physicians often discontinue factor replacement after surgery on the third or fourth postoperative day, resulting in hematoma formation at the edges of the wound and dehiscence. The wound then becomes infected because of the large amount of blood present and requires a prolonged period of factor coverage while healing by secondary intention.

10. What is the best treatment for mild factor VIII deficiency?
For female carriers of hemophilia A with factor VIII levels <50% and mild hemophiliacs with levels of >10%, 1-deamino-8-D-arginine vasopressin (DDAVP) is often the treatment of choice. DDAVP 0.3 μg/kg given intravenously over 15 minutes will usually raise factor VIII levels three to four times the baseline level. This is adequate for many minor procedures and in female carriers is usually adequate for major surgery. In life-threatening hemorrhage or surgery on mucosal surfaces, such as the nose or sinuses, tonsillectomy, transurethral resection of the prostate, or cone biopsy of the cervix, the levels obtained with DDAVP usually are not sufficient and recombinant or monoclonally purified factor VIII would be a better choice of treatment. DDAVP does not increase factor IX levels. .

11. What is an inhibitor to factor VIII?
Yes. The worst complication of hemophilia is the development of neutralizing IgG antibodies to factor VIII. This occurs after treatment in about 15% of patients with severe hemophilia A and rarely in those with hemophilia B. These inhibitors are measured in an assay in which the amount of residual factor VIII is determined in normal plasma after 2 hours of incubation with the patient's plasma. The amount of inhibition is assigned a titer known as the Bethesda unit (BU). Low-titer inhibitors, <5 BU, can usually be overwhelmed using either large amounts of human factor VIII or factor VIII purified from pig plasma known as porcine factor VIII. In the majority of patients, however, the Bethesda titers are high, >20 BU, and it is very difficult to overwhelm them with factor VIII. In this case, factor IX concentrate or an activated factor IX complex is employed. These products have some bypassing activity and may promote hemostasis of a bleeding lesion. The activated material is cleared quickly by the patient's liver; thus, the infusion has no lasting benefit

and rebleeding is common. Once patients have developed an inhibitor, they are in danger of sustaining a fatal central nervous system hemorrhage and should not undergo elective surgery. Minor surgical procedures or intramuscular injections in these patients can result in life- and limb-threatening hemorrhage and are contraindicated. New methods of suppression of the inhibitors are being developed but are quite expensive and still experimental.

12. How do you choose a factor IX product?
Because multiple doses of the standard factor IX containing concentrates can cause thrombotic complications, purified coagulation factor IX has been developed. For one-dose use, patients should receive standard factor IX concentrate, which also contains other vitamin K–dependent factors. For surgery, massive trauma, or in patients with severe liver disease, purified factor IX (coagulation factor IX) should be used instead.

13. Is hemophilia always hereditary or can it be acquired?
Acquired hemophilia is the development of an antibody to factor VIII in a person who does not have a history of hemophilia. This arises in patients with autoimmune diseases or lymphoproliferative illness, postpartum patients, the very elderly population, and patients who have had antibiotics or blood transfusions and often a complicated ICU course for an unrelated illness. The patient will have a prolonged PTT and evidence of hematomas at sites of mild trauma. The 1:1 mix with normal plasma may correct immediately, but the PTT will prolong after a 2-hour incubation. The factor VIII level will be low, usually <20%, and the Bethesda titer may range from 5–30 BU. These inhibitors respond well to prednisone, high-dose intravenous gamma globulin, and other forms of immunosuppression. Unfortunately, there is a 25% mortality from bleeding before the patient responds. The treatment of choice for hemorrhage is porcine factor VIII in high enough doses to overwhelm the inhibitor. These patients should never undergo surgical procedures until hemostasis can be guaranteed. The response to immunosuppression may be as prompt as 2 weeks. Even if there is no response to immunosuppression, these inhibitors usually remit spontaneously within several years. The care of these patients should be done by a hemophilia center or hematologist experienced in coagulation.

14. Even though the factor products are virally safe now, isn't it true that most hemophiliacs were infected with transfusion-related viruses?
Approximately 80–90% of adults with severe hemophilia were infected with HIV during the years 1979 to 1984. In addition to HIV, most hemophiliacs have evidence of past infection with hepatitis B and hepatitis C. Since this cohort of hemophiliacs became HIV positive at approximately the same time, 20–30% have died of HIV disease already and another 30–40% have AIDS. With the exception of Kaposi's sarcoma, hemophiliacs with HIV disease have manifestations of disease similar to those of other populations with HIV. Chronic liver disease due to hepatitis C and occasionally hepatitis B is another problem, with approximately 10–20% of patients dying of cirrhosis. Hepatic transplantation is an option for the HIV-negative patients, as it cures both the liver disease and the hemophilia.

15. What is a hemophilia center?
The United States is divided into 10 regions that each have a federally and state funded hemophilia center. All hemophiliacs are invited to have their care overseen by the center. All hemophiliacs are encouraged to learn home factor transfusion in order to expedite prompt care of bleeding. New patients with hemophilia should be referred to one of these centers.

BIBLIOGRAPHY

1. Blanchette VS, Vorstman E, Shore A, et al: Hepatitis C infection in children with hemophilia A and B. Blood 79:285, 1991.

2. Brettler DB, Forsberg AD, Levine PH, et al: The use of porcine factor VIII concentrate (Hyate:C) in the treatment of patients with inhibitor antibodies to factor VIII. Arch Intern Med 149:1381, 1989.
3. Colman RW, Hirsh J, Marder VJ (eds): Hemostasis and Thrombosis. Philadelphia, J.B. Lippincott, 1987.
4. Eyster ME, Gill FM, Blatt PM, et al: Central nervous system bleeding in hemophiliacs. Blood 51:1179, 1978.
5. Hilgartner MW: Hemophilic arthropathy. Adv Pediatr 21:139, 1975.
6. Hoffman R, Benz EJ, Shattil SJ (eds): Hematology: Basic Principles and Practice. New York, Churchill Livingstone, 1991.
7. Kasper CK: Incidence and course of inhibitors among patients with classic hemophilia. Thromb Diath Haemorrh 30:264, 1973.
8. Kasper CK: Postoperative thromboses in hemophilia B. N Engl J Med 289:160, 1973.
9. Kasper CK: The therapy of factor VIII inhibitors. Prog Hemost Thromb 9:57, 1989.
10. Kim HC, McMillan CW, White GC, et al: Purified factor IX using monoclonal immunoaffinity technique: Clinical trials in hemophilia B and comparison to prothrombin complex concentrates. Blood 79:568, 1992.
11. Mannucci PM: Desmopressin: A nontransfusional form of treatment for congenital and acquired bleeding disorders. Blood 72:1449, 1988.
12. White G, MacMillan C, Kingdon H, et al: Recombinant factor VIII. N Engl J Med 320:166, 1989.

21. ACQUIRED FACTOR DEFICIENCIES

Jerry B. Lefkowitz, M.D., and James F. Lombardo, M.D.

LIVER DISEASE

1. Which procoagulant (clot-forming) factors are produced in the liver?

The liver synthesizes all procoagulant proteins except von Willebrand factor (VWF), which is synthesized in megakaryocytes and endothelial cells.

2. How does liver disease affect the synthesis, circulating levels, clearance, and use of procoagulant factors?

In liver disease, the following may occur:

1. Decreased synthesis of procoagulant factors
2. Increased synthesis of acute phase reactants, i.e., factor VIII and fibinogen
3. Synthesis of qualitatively abnormal clotting factors
4. Decreased clearance of fibrin split products (FSP)
5. Decreased clearance of active or inactive products of coagulation reactions
6. Increased utilization of procoagulant factors

3. Discuss the effect of liver disease on the vitamin K-dependent coagulation proteins.

The vitamin K-dependent gamma-carboxylation step, which converts the precursor coagulation proteins (factors II, VII, IX, and X) to their functional forms, occurs in hepatocyte microsomes. With liver disease, improper use of vitamin K or premature release of proteins by diseased parenchymal cells may result in hypocarboxylated or uncarboxylated (des-gla) vitamin K-dependent coagulation factors. These improperly carboxylated forms are not functional. In addition, the overall synthetic capacity of the diseased liver is compromised, and the absolute amount of normal coagulant proteins is decreased. (See also the section on vitamin K.) (See figure, next page.)

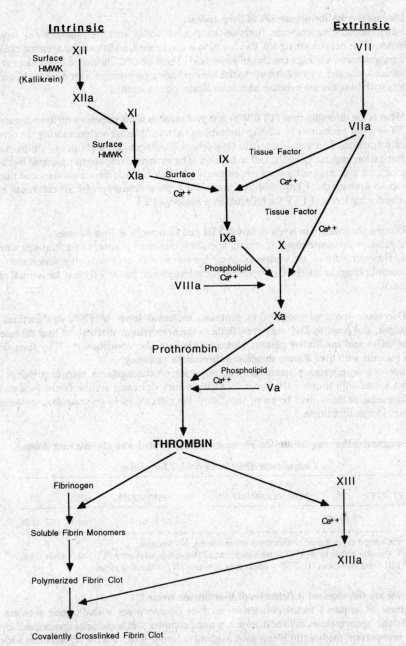

Intrinsic

XII

Surface
HMWK
(Kallikrein)

XIIa

XI

Surface
HMWK

XIa — Surface
Ca+

IX — Tissue Factor

IXa

Extrinsic

VII

VIIa

Tissue Factor
Ca++

Phospholipid
Ca++

VIIIa

X
Ca++

Xa

Prothrombin

Phospholipid
Ca++

Va

THROMBIN

Fibrinogen

Soluble Fibrin Monomers

Polymerized Fibrin Clot

Covalently Crosslinked Fibrin Clot

XIII

Ca++

XIIIa

Intrinsic and extrinsic pathways of coagulation.

4. Why may patients with early liver disease present with an isolated prolonged prothrombin time (PT)?

As depicted in the figure above, factor VIIa is a key enzyme in the extrinsic pathway of coagulation. This pathway is evaluated in vitro by the PT. Because factor VII has the shortest half-life of the procoagulant proteins, patients with early liver disease may present with an isolated prolonged PT.

5. Discuss the dysfibrinogenemia of liver disease.
Normally, hepatocyte enzymes function to remove sialic acid sidechains from large molecules. With hepatocyte injury, this function is diminished, and the fibrinogen molecule develops an excessively high content of sialic acid. These altered fibrinogen molecules may be dysfunctional and may contribute to the hemorrhagic symptoms of liver disease. Not all patients with liver disease produce abnormal fibrinogen molecules.

6. What is the thrombin time (TT)? Why is it prolonged in some patients with liver disease?
The TT is a test performed by adding thrombin to citrated plasma and measuring the time to clot formation. This test is sensitive to levels of fibrinogen, to inhibitors of fibrin clot polymerization (especially FSP), and to heparin. The abnormal fibrinogen produced by the compromised liver may not polymerize properly when cleaved to fibrin monomer and thus may act to prolong the TT. In addition, impaired hepatic clearance of FSP can result in high circulating levels of FSP, as reflected in a prolonged TT.

7. Discuss the changes in levels of factor VIII and fibrinogen in liver disease.
These proteins are acute phase reactants and show increased plasma concentrations with stress. However, late in the course of liver disease or with accompanying disseminated intravascular coagulation (DIC), the levels of fibrinogen and factor VIII may be normal or decreased.

8. Decreased levels of coagulation proteins, increased levels of FSP, dysfunctional fibrinogen, and possibly DIC may contribute to the hemorrhagic diathesis of liver disease. Quantitative and qualitative platelet abnormalities are also contributory. Why then do some patients with liver disease manifest a thrombotic tendency?
The liver also synthesizes plasminogen and physiologic anticoagulants, such as protein C, protein S, and antithrombin III. For individual patients, decreases in these fibrinolytic and anticoagulant proteins may be more significant than decreases in procoagulant proteins involved in clot formation.

9. Summarize the coagulation test abnormalities associated with chronic liver disease.

Coagulation Tests in Chronic Liver Disease

PT, PTT	TT	V, VII, II, IX, X ATIII, PLASMINOGEN	VIII, FIBRINOGEN	FSP	BT
↑	↑ or N	↓	↑ or N or ↓	↑ or N	↑ or N

↑ Prolonged or increased, ↓ shortened or decreased, N = normal.
PT = prothrombin time, PTT = activated partial thromboplastin time, TT = thrombin time, ATIII = antithrombin III, FSP = fibrin split products, BT = bleeding time.

10. How are the acquired deficiencies of liver disease treated?
Treatment of acquired factor deficiencies in liver disease poses a challenging problem. Hemostatic abnormalities in liver disease are quite complex and sometimes confounded by other intercurrent medical problems such as renal failure or DIC. Factor replacement with fresh frozen plasma (FFP) is the treatment of choice in the actively bleeding patient. If fibrinogen levels fall below 75–100 mg/dl, then cryoprecipitate also should be used. Vitamin K supplementation may be beneficial, but its effectiveness depends on residual hepatic synthetic capacity. The use of vitamin K–dependent factor concentrates (factor IX concentrates or prothrombin complex concentrates [PCC]) is **contraindicated** in liver disease because of reported thromboembolic phenomena in patients with liver disease after PCC infusions. The multifactorial nature of the coagulopathy of liver disease may make impossible the complete normalization of all coagulation parameters.

VITAMIN K: DEFICIENCY STATES AND ANTAGONISTS

11. List the forms and sources of vitamin K.
Vitamin K is a fat-soluble naphthoquinone. Vitamin K1 (phytonadione) occurs naturally in fruits and vegetables, and vitamin K2 (menaquinone) is synthesized by bacteria in the human digestive tract. Vitamin K3 (menadione) is available as a synthetic, water-soluble preparation.

12. What is the function of vitamin K?
Vitamin K is a necessary cofactor for the gamma-carboxylation of glutamic acid residues in the amino terminal region of the following coagulation proteins: factors II, VII, IX, and X, protein C, and protein S. The carboxylation enzyme system is localized to the hepatocyte microsomes. The uncarboxylated (des-carboxy or des-gla) forms of these coagulation proteins are not functional.

13. List several causes of vitamin K deficiency that result in decreases in the functional levels of the vitamin K–dependent coagulation proteins.
As a fat-soluble compound, vitamin K requires bile salts for absorption from the gastrointestinal tract. Obstruction of the biliary system or other causes of malabsorption (e.g., pancreatic insufficiency, dysentery, celiac disease, Crohn's disease, blind loop syndrome, short-bowel syndrome, and cystic fibrosis) may lead to deficiency. Malnutrition or unsupplemented intravenous hyperalimentation also can result in deficiency. Because the vitamin is produced in part by the gut bacterial flora. prolonged antibiotic therapy has been implicated as a cause of deficiency. Infants at birth often have low levels of vitamin K–dependent coagulation factors because of either (1) immaturity of the synthetic capacity of the neonatal liver or (2) a true state of vitamin K deficiency. It is common practice in the United States to administer vitamin K at birth.

14. What are the clinical and laboratory findings in vitamin K–deficient patients?
Patients with vitamin K deficiency can present with an unexplained bleeding diathesis. Laboratory findings include a prolonged PT and activated partial thromboplastin time (aPTT). Assays for factors II, VII, IX, and X show decreased functional levels. Vitamin K deficiency must be differentiated from other causes that decrease the levels of vitamin K–dependent coagulation factors (e.g., liver disease, ingestion of warfarin compounds [see below]).

15. How is vitamin K deficiency treated?
In the actively bleeding patient, transfusion with FFP is the initial treatment of choice. Administration of vitamin K compounds usually takes between 4 and 24 hours to have an effect on levels of the vitamin K–dependent proteins. In neonates and pregnant women, the preferred form of vitamin K replacement is phytonadione. In malabsorption syndromes, some physicians prefer the water-soluble form of menadione. However, high doses of menadione have been associated with hepatic injury and hemolytic anemia.

16. Which compounds act as antagonists to vitamin K and cause decreases in the functional levels of vitamin K–dependent proteins? Discuss the uses of these compounds.
Warfarin sodium and its derivatives are antagonists of vitamin K. Therapeutic oral anticoagulation with warfarin is a common cause of decreases in both the antigenic and functional forms of vitamin K–dependent proteins. Drug interactions and intentional or accidental overdose are causes of warfarin toxicity. Less commonly, intentional or accidental poisoning with so-called superwarfarin preparations results in severe and potentially life-threatening decreases in vitamin K–dependent factors. Superwarfarins such as brodifacoum or difenacoum are the active ingredients of commercially available rodenticides.

17. What are the clinical and laboratory findings in warfarin toxicity or rodenticide poisoning?

The patient presents with a bleeding diathesis (e.g., hematuria, gingival bleeding, soft-tissue hematomas, gastrointestinal hemorrhage and/or intracranial bleeding). Most patients do not have a prior bleeding history. Laboratory testing reveals a prolonged PT and a prolonged aPTT. Specific factor assays factors show depressed levels of factors II, VII, IX, and X. Serum assays for warfarin are negative in cases of superwarfarin poisoning. To confirm superwarfarin poisoning, specific tests for brodifacoum, difenacoum, or their congeners should be performed.

18. Why is it important to distinguish poisoning with a rodenticide from toxicity with therapeutic warfarins?

The half-life of warfarin is approximately 36–42 hours, whereas the half-life of rodenticides is measured in weeks. Unlike acute warfarin toxicity, appropriate therapy in cases of rodenticide poisoning may require months of vitamin K replacement.

19. What is the therapy for warfarin toxicity or rodenticide poisoning?

In the actively hemorrhaging patient, factor replacement in the form of FFP is the treatment of choice. In patients not actively bleeding, administration of vitamin K1 usually shows an effect on levels of functional coagulant proteins within 4–24 hours. Many physicians prefer to treat patients receiving warfarin for therapeutic anticoagulation with FFP, especially if warfarin therapy is to be reinstituted after the toxic episode. Vitamin K, as an antagonist to warfarin, increases the difficulty in returning the PT to a therapeutic level. As with all human-derived blood products, the risk of transmission of infectious agents through infusion of FFP must be weighed against the benefits of treatment.

The treatment of rodenticide poisoning is more of a problem. Because of the long half-life of these agents, prolonged therapy with vitamin K is often necessary. Concomitant administration of barbiturates has been suggested to shorten the time course (secondary to inducement of the hepatic microsomal enzyme system). Patients must be watched closely over a period of months for any recurrent bleeding symptoms. Actively bleeding patients should receive FFP.

In both warfarin toxicity and rodenticide poisoning, the efficacy of treatment should be evaluated with frequent monitoring of the PT.

ACQUIRED FACTOR INHIBITORS

20. What is a factor inhibitor?

Factor inhibitors are acquired circulating anticoagulants—typically antibodies that inhibit the function of a specific coagulation protein. Usually inhibitors occur in patients with congenital factor deficiencies after exposure to factor concentrates or FFP. However, inhibitors may also occur in patients with no history of factor deficiency. This chapter addresses only the latter situation (no prior history of factor deficiencies).

21. In the acquired setting, what are the different types of inhibitors?

Two types of inhibitors are identified in patients with no history of congenital factor deficiency:

1. Antibodies that specifically inhibit or neutralize the functional activity of a coagulant protein. Usually these antibodies are of the IgG class but occasionally IgM and IgA inhibitors are reported in the literature.

2. Paraprotein (monoclonal immunoglobulin or immunoglobulin fragment) produced in such diseases as multiple myeloma, Waldenstrom's macroglobulinemia, and some cases of lymphoma. By virtue of their nature and high plasma concentration, these paraproteins tend to bind nonspecifically to anything circulating in the plasma. Formation of noncovalent paraprotein/coagulation protein complexes interferes with the function of the latter.

22. Against which coagulation factors have specific inhibitors been identified?
Acquired inhibitors (antibodies) to factors VIII and V are among the most common. Inhibitors to the von Willebrand factor (VWF) have been reported in many patients with no history of hereditary disease. Inhibitors of factor I (fibrinogen), factor II (prothrombin), factor VII, factor X, and factor XI have been reported but are exceedingly rare. In nonhemophiliacs, inhibitors of factor IX are also extremely rare.

23. What are the clinical conditions associated with spontaneous coagulation factor inhibitors?
Spontaneous factor inhibitors arise in a number of different clinical settings:

Rheumatoid arthritis	Various dermatologic diseases (e.g., psoriasis,
Regional enteritis	pemphigus vulgaris, erythema multiforme,
Systemic lupus erythematosus	exfoliative dermatitis)
Myasthenia gravis	Infections
Scleroderma	Drug therapy (e.g., penicillins, sulfa drugs,
Pregnancy and the immediate	chloramphenicol, aminoglycoside antibiotics,
postpartum period	phenothiazines, phenytoin, arsenicals)
Hematologic and nonhematologic	Advancing age
malignancies	

Elderly patients account for a large fraction of those with no associated disease.

24. How do patients with acquired inhibitors clinically present?
Patients with acquired factor inhibitors usually present with bleeding symptoms ranging from soft-tissue hematomas to life-threatening intracranial hemorrhages. Factor inhibitor should be included in the differential diagnosis for patients with bleeding symptoms who have no previous history of bleeding. The diagnosis of a factor inhibitor, especially a factor VIII inhibitor, represents a possible life-threatening medical condition that requires close patient follow-up along with rapid intervention at any signs of hemorrhage.

25. What is the natural history of a factor inhibitor?
Because factor VIII inhibitors are the most common, they are the best studied of all acquired coagulation factor inhibitors. Approximately 12–40% of patients with factor VIII inhibitor die from hemorrhage. Patients with inhibitors for 1 year or longer have a greater likelihood of dying from bleeding complications. Without treatment, acquired factor VIII inhibitors may spontaneously remit in postpartum patients and in patients with no underlying conditions.

Factor V inhibitors are the second most common acquired antibody inhibitor. Bleeding problems are more variable than with factor VIII inhibitors. Factor V inhibitors have a high rate of spontaneous remission.

Antibody inhibitors to fibrinogen (factor I) are rare. However, paraprotein inhibitors to fibrin clot polymerization are more common. The clinical severity of the bleeding diathesis parallels the course of the underlying disease, with higher circulating levels of paraprotein predisposing to bleeding problems. Most patients with paraproteinemias do not develop hemorrhagic problems; significant bleeding is more commonly associated with IgM or IgA dysproteinemias.

Inhibitors to VWF are rare, but antibody inhibitors arising in patients with no underlying condition typically remit spontaneously. Paraprotein inhibitors to VWF can occur; bleeding problems respond to treatment of the underlying disease state.

Acquired factor XI inhibitors are also rare but deserve mention because some case reports suggest that they are not associated with hemorrhage but with an increased incidence of thrombosis.

The remainder of reported factor inhibitors are rare, and the natural course of the disease process is not well delineated.

26. How are acquired factor inhibitors diagnosed in the clinical laboratory?
Depending on which specific factor is inhibited, the aPTT, PT, or both may be prolonged
(see figure with question 4). Studies mixing aPTT and/or PT with normal plasma show
no significant correction. Specific factor assays can demonstrate the presence of an
inhibitor.

27. How are inhibitors quantitated?
The most common method in the United States is a Bethesda titer. By definition, an
inhibitor plasma that contains 1 Bethesda unit of antibody per milliliter will neutralize 50%
of factor activity in an equal volume of pooled normal plasma after incubation of the
mixture at 37° C for 2 hours. In other words, 1 Bethesda unit results in the inactivation of
50% of factor activity in a sample; 2 Bethesda units result in the inactivation of 75% of
factor activity; 3 Bethesda units result in the inactivation of 87.5% of factor activity, and
so on. Quantitation of acquired factor VIII inhibitors presents a special problem. Acquired
factor VIII inhibitors may show complex kinetics in their reactions with factor VIII. As a
result, it is quite possible for a patient to have a high-titer inhibitor, measurable levels of
factor VIII, and at the same time serious bleeding. Bethesda titers in such patients should
be viewed as estimates of inhibitor potency.

28. How are inhibitors treated?
Treatment for factor VIII inhibitors is tailored for the severity of bleeding and the potency
of the inhibitor. Minor soft-tissue bleeds may respond to conservative measures such as
immobilization or compression of the affected area. Minor or moderate bleeding with a
low-titer inhibitor (<5 Bethesda units) may respond to desmopressin (DDAVP). Severe
bleeding requires more aggressive intervention. Depending on the potency of the inhibitor
and the kinetics of its reaction with factor VIII, it may be possible to override it with transfusions of factor concentrate. Severe bleeding in a patient with an inhibitor titer less than
5 Bethesda units may respond to an initial bolus of 50–100 U/kg of factor VIII, followed
by a drip of 1000 U/hr. High-titer (>10–20 Bethesda units) inhibitors usually do not respond
well to treatment with high doses of human factor VIII concentrates. In an emergent
situation, however, it is worthwhile to try infusions of human factor VIII. Factor VIII
inhibitors show a significant degree of species specificity, and purified concentrate of
porcine factor VIII has been used successfully to treat bleeding with high-titer inhibitors.
It is important to obtain a Bethesda titer against porcine factor VIII before treatment.
    If no clinical response is obtained with either human or porcine factor VIII, several
other options exist. Prothrombin complex concentrates (PCC) or factor IX concentrates
contain a mixture of the vitamin K–dependent coagulation factors and possess factor VIII–
bypassing activity. Unfortunately, the use of PCC is not without risks, including scattered
reports of DIC and thromboembolic phenomena. A new product, recombinant human
factor VIIa concentrate, also possesses factor VIII–bypassing activity. At the present time,
experience with recombinant factor VIIa is limited. Other treatment modalities are
designed to lower inhibitor titers. Plasmapheresis with plasma exchange, plasmapheresis
with staphylococcus A columns to absorb the antibody inhibitor, immunosuppressive
therapy, and intravenous immunoglobulin have been used with some success. In many
cases, infusions of factor VIII combined with one or more of the preceding therapies has
been successful in treating refractory bleeding problems.
    The treatment of factor V inhibitors usually is less problematic than that of factor VIII
inhibitors. Many patients with factor V inhibitors do not exhibit bleeding symptoms, and
the rate of spontaneous remission is high. Bleeding symptoms in patients with acquired
factor V inhibitor have been successfully treated with FFP infusions, immunosuppressive
therapy, and/or platelet transfusions. Platelets contain approximately 20% of the whole
blood factor V. The use of platelet transfusions, however, is not without drawbacks. It is
possible to sensitize the recipient to platelet and HLA antigens. Once sensitized, the patient
may become refractory to further use of platelet transfusions.

The treatment of paraprotein inhibitors usually is aimed at the underlying disease. In acute bleeding problems, plasmapheresis with plasma exchange has been used successfully to lower the level of the circulating paraprotein.

29. What is the lupus anticoagulant? What is its significance?
The term lupus anticoagulant refers to a group of antiphospholipid antibodies that act to inhibit in vitro clot-based coagulation assays. The name lupus anticoagulant is a misnomer. The term was originally coined as descriptive, because the first patients had systemic lupus erythematosus (SLE) with bleeding symptoms. Since these first reports, it has become apparent that lupus anticoagulants usually are not associated with bleeding unless concomitant hemostatic abnormalities are present. In addition, many patients with the lupus anticoagulant do not have SLE.

A very small subset of patients with SLE and the lupus anticoagulant present with hypoprothrombinemia (low levels of factor II) and bleeding symptoms. These patients apparently have an antibody that clears factor II from the circulation.

The lupus anticoagulant is one of the most common causes of an isolated, prolonged aPTT. In recent years it has become apparent that the lupus anticoagulant is more frequently associated with thrombosis and the hypercoagulable state. Further information on the lupus anticoagulant is found in chapter 22.

MISCELLANEOUS

30. List two major mechanisms that result in acquired factor deficiencies in the patient with trauma.
 1. Dilutional coagulopathy resulting from large infusions of stored bank blood, packed red blood cells, or crystalloid solutions
 2. DIC (reviewed in chapter 16)

31. How is dilutional coagulopathy treated?
Dilutional coagulopathy is treated with transfusions of FFP. A rule of thumb is to provide one unit of FFP for every 5 units of whole bank blood or packed red blood cells. This approximation should be modified in the face of any complicating clinical conditions. In addition, actively bleeding patients with platelet counts <50,000/mm^3 or fibrinogen levels <75–100 mg/dl necessitate transfusion of platelet concentrates and cryoprecipitate, respectively.

32. Which factor deficiency has been associated with primary systemic amyloidosis? How is it treated?
Isolated acquired deficiency of factor X, which has been described in a number of patients with amyloidosis, is due to specific adsorption of factor X to amyloid fibrils. Transfusions of factor concentrate are not effective treatment. Treatment must be directed at the underlying disease.

BIBLIOGRAPHY

1. Galloway B: The laboratory response to the trauma patient. Trauma Q 3:63–69, 1987.
2. Hultin MB: Acquired inhibitors in malignant and nonmalignant disease. Am J Med 91(suppl 5A):95–135, 1991.
3. Kemkes-Matthes B, Bleyl H, Matthes KJ: Coagulation activation in liver diseases. Thromb Res 64:253–261, 1991.
4. Kunkel LA: Acquired circulating anticoagulants. Hematol Oncol Clin North Am 6:1341–1357, 1992.
5. Mammen EF: Coagulation abnormalities in liver disease. Hematol Oncol Clin North Am 6:1287–1299, 1992.
6. Martinez J, Palascak JE, Kwasniak D: Abnormal sialic acid content of the dysfibrinogenemia associated with liver disease. J Clin Invest 61:535–538, 1978.

7. Routh CR, Triplett DA, Murphy MJ, et al: Superwarfarin ingestion and detection. Am J Hematol 36:50–54, 1991.
8. Suttie JW: Recent advances in hepatic vitamin K metabolism and function. Hepatology 7:367–376, 1987.

22. THE HYPERCOAGULABLE STATE

Richard A. Marlar, Ph.D.

1. What is the hypercoagulable state?

The hypercoagulable state (sometimes called the prethrombotic state) is a catchall phrase for a group of poorly defined abnormalities associated with clinical laboratory tests (decreased protein C, antithrombin III, or plasminogen, and/or thrombocytosis) or clinical conditions (malignancy, pregnancy, or the postoperative state) that puts the patient at an increased risk for developing thromboembolic complications (deep venous thrombosis, pulmonary embolus, arterial thrombosis, myocardial infarction, stroke).[1,2,10] Also included are patients with recurrent thrombosis who have no recognizable predisposing factor(s).

2. Discuss the causes of the hypercoagulable state.

Currently, there is a growing list of primary and secondary causes of the hypercoagulable state, including both inherited abnormalities (hereditary thrombotic disease) and acquired abnormalities. The acquired conditions are usually secondary to some underlying clinical condition or disease process. When several acquired or inherited abnormalities occur simultaneously, the chance of developing thrombosis is enhanced. The underlying mechanisms of the hypercoagulable state are due to either excessive initiation of the hemostatic systems and/or loss of the regulatory systems (hypofibrinolysis).

3. Are the pathophysiologic bases for the acquired hypercoagulable states known?

Unfortunately, the mechanisms for activation of the coagulation system, loss of regulatory systems, or for hypofibrinolysis are unknown in the majority of acquired cases. Physiologic phenomena (pregnancy and the postpartum period) as well as pathologic abnormalities (atherosclerosis, malignancy, nephrotic syndrome, myeloproliferative disorders) are associated with hypercoagulability. Iatrogenic or drug interaction complications (prosthetic devices, oral contraceptives or estrogen therapy) also contribute to the induction of the hypercoagulable state.[2] It appears that multiple mechanisms must be aberrant to induce the hypercoagulable state in many of these disorders. Currently, a number of new laboratory tests (prothrombin fragment 1 and 2 [F_{1+2}] and thrombin-antithrombin complex [T-AT]) are being used to confirm the clinical suspicion of a hypercoagulable state and in some cases to diagnose a prethrombotic condition prior to clinical complications.[2] Unfortunately, the potential diagnostic advantage of many of these new tests has not as yet been fully demonstrated to provide a significant predictive value.

4. What aspects of the hemostatic mechanism are involved in the hypercoagulable state?

All mechanisms of hemostasis appear to be involved in the hypercoagulable state. The platelet and/or the endothelial cell plays a role in acquired abnormalities (thrombocytosis or vascular injury). To date, only the coagulation and fibrinolytic systems have been shown to be involved in hereditary thrombotic disease. For the coagulation system, only regulatory mechanisms are associated with hereditary thrombotic disease, whereas in the fibrinolytic system, the primary pathway components (plasminogen and tissue plasminogen activator (tPA)) are the major factors.[5] The endothelial cell is currently a "black box" with respect to the regulation of hemostasis and the hypercoagulable state. A considerable amount of work still needs to be completed to determine the role of this important pivotal component of the hemostatic system.

5. Discuss the concept of risk factors as they are associated with the hypercoagulable state.
A hypercoagulable **risk factor** is defined as any condition (acquired or inherited) that causes the patient to have a greater than normal chance for developing thrombosis.[2,8] The acquired factors can be due to acute or chronic conditions and may involve environmental, physiologic, or pathologic factors. The combination of factors and the severity necessary to cause thrombosis are currently unknown. A partial list of suspected acquired factors that, when dovetailed with the inherited abnormalities, increase the risk of thrombotic complications are provided in the table below. The concept of the risk factor in the hypercoagulable state is analogous to risk factors in heart disease.

Acquired Risk Factors for Hypercoagulability

PHYSIOLOGIC	PATHOLOGIC	ENVIRONMENTAL	IATROGENIC
Pregnancy	Malignancy	Smoking	Surgery
Postpartum	Liver disease	Stress	Postsurgical
Venous stasis	DIC	Heat	Oral contraceptive
	Lupus anticoagulant		drugs
	Vascular injury		Other drugs
	Inherited abnormalities		

6. How are risk factors important in causing thrombosis?
Hypercoagulable risk factors, both acquired and inherited, appear to magnify the potential for developing thrombosis synergistically.[2] The more risk factors that a patient develops, the greater the chance of thromboembolic complications. For example, if the only risk factor is inherited protein C deficiency, then the likelihood of thrombosis appears to be low. However, if several underlying acquired risk factors are present, such as pregnancy, vascular injury, and inflammation, then the risk of thrombosis is increased with each additional factor. Currently, the majority of risk factors and their importance in the development of the hypercoagulable state are unknown.

7. What is hereditary thrombotic disease?
Hereditary thrombotic disease (HTD), or thrombophilia, represents a group of abnormalities in which a patient has recurrent thrombotic complications and a positive family history of thrombosis because of a genetic defect(s) associated with coagulation, fibrinolysis, or their regulatory systems.[2,3,9] The first such deficiency, antithrombin III, was diagnosed in the early 1960s. Since then, several other deficiencies have been described and much has been learned about the hereditary nature of HTD. At least eight inherited abnormalities have been confirmed and several more are now suspected of causing HTD.[3,8] It should be noted that about 65–70% of the causes of HTD are still unknown.

Primary Hereditary Factors Associated with Hypercoagulability

FACTOR	PERCENT*
Known	
Antithrombin III deficiency	3
Protein C deficiency	10
Protein S deficiency	12
Plasminogen deficiency	1
Dysfibrinogenemia	1
tPA deficiency	1
PAI-1 excess	2
Heparin cofactor II	1

Table continued on following page.

Primary Hereditary Factors Associated with Hypercoagulability (Continued)

FACTOR
Suspected
Factor XII deficiency (homozygous)
Thrombomodulin
Tissue factor pathway inhibitor
Endothelial cell
Platelet

* The percent is the relative ocurrence of each disorder. About 70% of the cases of hereditary thrombotic disease have no known genetic cause (not found as yet).

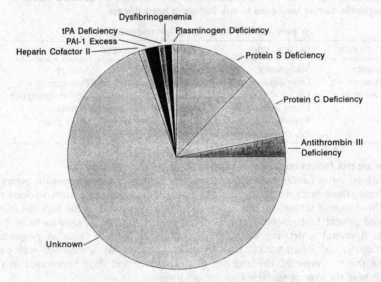

Primary hereditary factors associated with HTD

8. Describe the most common inherited deficiencies.

The prevalence (in percentage of families with HTD) for each deficiency is shown in the table and chart in question 7. To date, there is excellent evidence that a number of coagulation regulatory factors (protein C, protein S, and antithrombin III) and fibrinolytic factors (plasminogen, tPA) are inherited causes of HTD.[3,9,11] The most common known deficiencies appear to be protein C and protein S. There is a large percentage (65–70%) of individuals with apparent HTD in which the inherited cause has not been established. This large group may represent deficiencies associated with the suspected factors or as yet unrecognized abnormalities (endothelial cell functional defects).

9. How is HTD tansmitted?

The genetics associated with all of the known HTD causes are autosomal, usually with complete penetrance in the heterozygote.[3,9] However, there has been some heterozygous deficiencies with incomplete penetrance in which thrombotic complications are not present.

10. Describe a classic case of a patient with HTD.

A 34-year-old woman presented with deep venous thrombosis (DVT) involving the left lower extremity without a precipitating cause. History revealed a previous DVT after her first pregnancy. Her mother also had a "clotting problem" and died (probably of a pulmonary embolus) at the age of 37 after multiple hospitalizations and treatment with "blood thinners." The patient's brother had died 5 years previously of a massive pulmonary embolus.

The majority (approximately 90–95%) of patients with HTD usually present with venous thrombosis.[9] Arterial thrombosis is rarely reported. Venous thrombosis in unique vessels (mesenteric, hepatic, splenic) and thrombotic stroke in HTD may be more common based on the recognition of its hereditary nature by surgeons, neurologists, and general internists. The thromboembolic complication may occur spontaneously or may be related to some underlying event (risk factor), such as the postoperative state, trauma, or pregnancy.[9] Most patients with HTD have their first thrombotic episode between the ages of 18 and 40, with about 80–90% having had a clot by the age of 45. Symptoms usually do not manifest until after puberty (age 15).[9] The majority of patients have had multiple episodes of thrombosis and a positive family history. Currently, individuals in the age range of 18–45 years are usually evaluated for a hypercoagulable state or HTD after their firs episode of thrombosis.

A patient with thrombosis should be evaluated for a personal and family history ot clotting episodes and other acquired causes of hypercoagulability ruled out before an expensive work-up for HTD is initiated.[3,9]

In the case presented above, the patient and other family members tested were found to have protein S deficiency and were treated accordingly.

11. What is the lupus anticoagulant?
The lupus anticoagulant (LA) is an autoimmune disorder in which autoantibodies against phospholipid membranes develop. LA manifests in vitro with a prolongation of coagulation tests but paradoxically in vivo causes thrombosis in approximately 30% of the patients.[6,13] Therefore, LA is a hypercoagulable disorder.[6] The LA interferes with either coagulation regulatory mechanisms or perturbation of the endothelial cells to cause thromboembolic complications. The term "lupus anticoagulant" is a true misnomer. The term *lupus* was applied because this abnormality was first described in patients with systemic lupus erythematosus. The name "anticoagulant" comes from the laboratory artifact of prolonged coagulation tests, activated partial thromboplastin time (aPTT).[12] The LA is not exclusive to patients with systemic lupus erythematosus, but is found in a variety of other situations (viral infections, antibiotic and phenothiazine usage, and in otherwise normal individuals). The diagnosis of LA is based almost solely on a prolonged aPTT with no other cause (heparin or factor deficiency). But this disorder is not necessarily benign, with 30% of the patients developing thrombosis.

12. What are the laboratory diagnostic criteria for LA?
The laboratory diagnostic criteria for LA are not well defined.[12] If a patient has a prolonged aPTT (and heparin contamination has been ruled out), the next assay should be aPTT mixing studies. A patient with the LA will have only partial correction. A factor deficiency will have complete correction to the normal range. If the mixing studies suggest the presence of a LA, further more sensitive confirmatory tests such as dilute Russell viper's venom test (dRVVT) or platelet neutralization procedure (PNP) must be performed.[12] In conjunction with the coagulation tests, the patient's serum should be assayed for anticardiolipin antibodies. The presence of either anticardiolipin antibodies or a positive confirmatory test (dRVVT or PNP) in conjunction with the prolonged aPTT is the basis for the diagnosis of LA.[12]

13. How is LA treated?
The treatment of LA is controversial and can be difficult. Patients with diagnosed LA bu no underlying thrombotic complications should not be treated. Patients who develop venous thrombosis should be treated in the standard fashion as recommended for venous thrombosis. Monitoring heparinization may be difficult because of the initially prolonged aPTT. Heparin therapy should be monitored by a heparin assay or thrombin time. Individuals presenting with arterial thrombosis should be treated with aspirin and/or oral anticoagulant therapy. If the hypercoagulable state is difficult to control, prednisone may be used in conjunction with the other anticoagulant therapy.

14. How are protein C and protein S involved in the regulation of hemostasis?
Protein C and protein S are the two central components of a major *anti*thrombotic regulatory mechanism (both anticoagulant and profibrinolytic properties).[4,9] Protein C and protein S are vitamin K–dependent proteins similar to factors VII, IX, and X and prothrombin. The protein C/protein S mechanism involves numerous plasma factors, the platelet, and the endothelial cell. Protein C is activated by thrombin bound to an endothelial cell cofactor, thrombomodulin. Activated protein C, a serine protease, complexes in the presence of calcium ions with protein S either on an activated platelet surface or the endothelial cell surface. This complex rapidly inactivates factors Va and VIIIa to inhibit the coagulation system. The mechanism by which the protein C system works in fibrinolysis is not well understood.

15. Which fibrinolytic components affect the regulation of thrombosis?
The fibrinolytic system is analogous to and as complex as the coagulation system, involving a number of factors in plasma and the endothelial cell. It consists of two distinct initiating pathways, a common pathway, and a variety of regulatory mechanisms.[2,5] Plasminogen, the central enzyme of fibrinolysis, will increase the risk of thrombosis if hereditary deficiency is present. Abnormalities associated with the major activator of plasminogen in vivo, tPA, and its release from the endothelial cell are factors that affect the dissolution of a clot, increasing the risk of thrombosis. Finally, excessive levels of plasminogen activator inhibitor type 1 (PAI-1), the major regulator of tPA, have been shown to be increased in some patients with a history of thrombosis. The mechanisms by which the last two factors are regulated are unknown but are risk factors for thrombosis. Although not definitively proved, abnormalities of the other components of the fibrinolytic system, such as urokinase, may also increase the risk of thrombosis. Finally, the endothelial cell, a pivotal component of the fibrinolytic system, may be a significant culprit of the hypercoagulable state.

16. When is the optimal time to perform a work-up for a patient in whom HTD is suspected?
The best time for a definitive diagnosis of HTD is when the patient is asymptomatic and off all anticoagulation medication.[3,9] However, the majority of patients develop thrombosis prior to being worked up or are on long-term anticoagulation. For cost containment and to avoid the chance of obtaining erroneous results, laboratory evaluation should *not* be performed (1) during the early post-thrombotic periods, (2) when the patient is symptomatic, or (3) when the patient is on heparin or coumadin. Testing during these times may mask true results due to consumption or assay artifact. If evaluation is made during these times, hen only a tentative diagnosis can be assigned.[9] The confirmation of a hereditary abnormality can be made only after two abnormal values are obtained in the patient during an asymptomatic-nontreated state and similar values are identified in two other family members. The laboratory abnormalities must cosegregate with the thrombotic complications. When all criteria are met, then the patient and family can be labeled with a hereditary deficiency. If only the patient can be evaluated, a tentative diagnosis should be established.

17. What factors should be tested in patients with suspected HTD?
The best way to evaluate a patient with hypercoagulability due to HTD is to assay in a series of stages starting with the most common deficiencies.[9] Acquired causes of hypercoagulability must be ruled out before starting any testing. The most common acquired abnormality is the lupus anticoagulant. It must be remembered that the etiology of the hypercoaguability will be found in only about 30% of cases. The remaining 70% will remain undiagnosed and will eventually be assigned when research testing demonstrates the deficiencies and the relative importance.

The collection and preparation of blood or serum for subsequent testing is crucial. The blood collection must be from a nontraumatic blood draw and the sample prepared as rapidly as possible. The sample should be platelet free ($<10,000/\mu l$) and then rapidly frozen for subsequent testing.

Stages of a Work-Up for HTD

Stage 0 Rule out acquired causes of hypercoagulability Lupus anticoagulant	**Stage 3** tPA PAI-1 Venous occlusion test
Stage 1 Antithrombin III Protein C Protein S	**Stage 4** Tissue factor pathway inhibitor Heparin cofactor II
Stage 2 Plasminogen Dysfibrinogenemia	**Stage 5** Potentially new factors (research)

18. How are results interpreted for diagnosis of HTD?

The diagnosis of HTD can be complicated by a number of causes (underlying disease, acquired abnormalities, laboratory artifact). Interpretation must always be made with caution.[2,3,9] All acquired causes of abnormal coagulation values (e.g., liver disease, DIC, thrombosis, malignancy) must be eliminated prior to evaluation. A definitive diagnosis should never be made in a patient who is anticoagulated or has acquired abnormalities. If all known acquired causes of an abnormal value are eliminated and a hereditary basis is still suspected, confirmation of the abnormal value must be made on a second sample and in family studies. Cosegregation of thrombosis and the deficiency must be confirmed. If the patient is the only family member who can be tested, then only a tentative diagnosis should be assigned. The controversy associated with testing family members is discussed under Controversies.

19. What is the treatment for HTD?

The treatment should address the type of thrombotic event and the site of thrombosis rather than the deficiency.[7] In general, for DVT and pulmonary embolus, the first thrombotic event should be treated with heparin followed by 3–6 months of oral anticoagulant therapy. The second event is also treated with heparin followed by 6–12 months of oral anticoagulant therapy. The third and subsequent events are usually treated with lifelong oral anticoagulant therapy. In rare cases of protein C or protein S deficiency, the complication of warfarin-induced skin necrosis has been observed when large loading doses of warfarin are used without concurrent heparin.[9] All treatment regimens are highly individual and must be adjusted to the location, type, and past history of thrombosis.[7]

Patients at increased risk for thrombosis (e.g., surgery, pregnancy) with a known deficiency or past history of thrombosis should be treated prophylactically.[2,7,9] However, some evidence suggests that the risks of anticoagulation may outweigh the benefits of prophylactic treatment. The bottom line with respect to prophylactic treatment is that it must be considered on an individual basis.

CONTROVERSIES

20. Should family members of patients with HTD undergo a work-up?

A significant debate is occurring as to whether asymptomatic family members should undergo a work-up when HTD has been diagnosed in a symptomatic member.

For:

A diagnosis of a deficiency state in an asymptomatic family member can pinpoint the potential increased thrombtic risk to each family member. He or she can then be educated about the deficiency and thrombotic signs. Additionally, it will help in genetic counseling and family planning.

Against:
The asymptomatic family member is subsequently labeled for life with a deficiency even though he or she remains asymptomatic. Insurance companies may not insure a patient with this preexisting condition.

The consensus at this time is to perform a work-up for family members because it offers the opportunity to educate family members, to eliminate acquired risk factors, and to assess the individual's risk of thrombosis.

21. Should unaffected deficient members of a family with a history of thrombosis be treated prophylactically?
Prophylactic treatment of asymptomatic members with HTD is controversial. A number of physicians currently treat asymptomatic patients with known deficiencies with prophylactic heparin when they are undergoing increased-risk procedures (surgery). The routine daily prophylactic treatment of an asymptomatic family member is usually not recommended because of inherent risks of long-term oral anticoagulation. This approach is highly individualized, with the physician and patient making the final decision. As guidelines, families with only DVT and pulmonary embolu are probably not at sufficient risk to treat a patient prophylactically except when undergoing surgery. However, if there has been significant large vessel, unique site of thrombosis, or stroke affecting the family, then prophylactic treatment might be considered.

BIBLIOGRAPHY

1. Ansell JE: Hypercoagulability: A conceptual and diagnostic approach. Am Heart J 114:910, 1987.
2. Bauer KA: Pathobiology of the hypercoagulable state: Clinical features, laboratory evaluation, and management. In Hoffman R, Banz E, Shathel S, et al (eds): Hematology: Basic Principles and Practice. New York, Churchill Livingstone, 1991, pp 1415–1430..
3. Comp PC: Hereditary disorders predisposing to thrombosis. Prog Hemost Thromb 8:71, 1986.
4. Esmon CT: The regulation of natural anticoagulant pathways. Science 235:1348, 1987.
5. Francis CW, Marder VJ: Physiologic regulation and pathologic disorders of fibrinolysis. In Coleman RW, Hirsh J, Marder VJ, Salzman EW (eds): Hemostasis and Thrombosis: Basic Principles and Clinical Practice, 2nd ed. Philadelphia, J.B. Lippincott, 1987, p 358.
6. Gastineau DA, Kazmier FJ, Nichols WL, Bowie EJW: Lupus anticoagulant: An analysis of the clinical and laboratory features of 219 cases. Am J Hematol 19:265, 1986.
7. Hirsh J, Dalen JE, Deykin D, Poller L: Oral anticoagulants: Mechanism of action, clinical effectiveness, and optimal therapeutic range. Chest 102:312S, 1992.
8. Mammen EF, Fujii Y: Hypercoagulable states. Lab Med 20:611, 1989.
9. Marlar RA, Mastovich S: Hereditary protein C deficiency: A review of the genetics, clinical presentation, diagnosis and treatment. Blood Coag Fibrinolysis 1:319–330, 1990.
10. Schafer AI: The hypercoagulable states. Ann Intern Med 102:814, 1985.
11. Thaler E, Lechner K: Antithrombin III deficiency. Clin Haematol 10:369, 1981.
12. Triplett DA: Laboratory diagnosis of lupus anticoagulants. Semin Thromb Hemost 16:190, 1990.
13. Triplett DA, Brandt JT: Lupus anticoagulant: Misnomer, paradox, riddle epiphenomenon. Hematol Pathol 2:121, 1988.

23. NEUTROPENIA

Russell C. Tolley, M.D.

1. What is the definition of neutropenia?
Neutropenia is a neutrophilic granulocyte count—or absolute neutrophil count (ANC)—of less than 1500/mm^3. The ANC is calculated by multiplying the total white blood cell (WBC) count by the percentage of band neutrophils and segmented neutrophils:

$$\text{ANC} = \text{WBC count} \times (\% \text{ bands} + \% \text{ segmented neutrophils}) \times 0.01$$

Neutrophil counts of less than $2000/\text{mm}^3$ are uncommon, but some normal individuals of Yemenite Jew or African descent may have counts as low as $1000/\text{mm}^3$ with no apparent disease.

2. What is the risk of infection with neutropenia?

Generally speaking, the lower the neutrophil count, the higher the risk of infection. In studies of bone marrow transplantation, the risk of infection rises dramatically when the ANC falls below $500/\text{mm}^3$. However, the risk of infection also varies with the nature of the primary disease process and the duration of neutropenia. Usually, neutropenia from marrow hypoplasia (due to chemotherapy, aplastic anemia, or other causes of marrow failure) has the greatest risk for infection. Neutropenia associated with a cellular marrow (chronic idiopathic neutropenia in adults, chronic benign neutropenia of infancy, or hypersplenism) usually has less risk of infection.

3. How do infections in acute and chronic neutropenia differ?

In acute neutropenia, *Staphylococcus aureus, Pseudomonas aeruginosa, Escherichia coli,* and *Klebsiella* sp. are common causes of infection, which often presents as sepsis. Patients with severe chronic neutropenia and autoimmune neutropenia, however, have recurrent sinusitis, stomatitis, gingivitis, and perirectal infections but usually do not become septic.

4. How are neutropenias classified?

Like anemias, neutropenias can be classified into categories of (1) decreased production, (2) sequestration from the circulating pool to marginated or tissue pools, (3) increased destruction or utilization, or (4) a combination of the above. Because techniques of measurement are cumbersome and not easily available, most authors divide the neutropenias into two categories: acquired or intrinsic.

5. What are the causes of acquired neutropenia?

Drug-induced neutropenia
Marrow-infiltrating disorders
Benign familial neutropenia
Chronic idiopathic neutropenia
Isoimmune neutropenia
Increased margination of WBCs
Infection with human immunodeficiency virus (HIV)

Postinfectious neutropenia
Nutritional deficiencies
Chronic benign neutropenia of childhood
Autoimmune neutropenia
Metabolic diseases
Immunologic abnormalities

Chronic acquired neutropenias also can be subdivided into those with splenomegaly (Felty's syndrome, congestive splenomegaly, Gaucher's disease, sarcoidosis, and other infectious diseases) and those without splenomegaly (chronic idiopathic neutropenia, benign familial neutropenia, and chronic benign neutropenia of childhood).

6. How do drugs cause neutropenia? Which agents cause neutropenia most often?

A history of chemotherapy is easily obtained, but many other therapeutic agents may cause neutropenia. The mechanism can involve direct marrow destruction (as with many chemotherapy agents), immune-mediated damage to neutrophil precursors in the bone marrow, or peripheral destruction or clearance of neutrophils. Fortunately, most drug-related neutropenias are due to dose-dependent suppression of bone marrow. After the offending agent is stopped, return of the neutrophil count to normal usually occurs within a few days, preceded by monocytosis (as in the recovery of the neutrophil count after chemotherapy). On rare occasions, chloramphenicol may cause a dose-independent aplastic anemia. The drugs that most commonly cause neutropenia include:

Phenothiazines (chlorpromazine, promazine)
Antithyroid agents (propylthiouracil, methimazole)
Ethanol
Antibiotics (chloramphenicol, semisynthetic penicillins, sulfonamides)
Meprobamate (tranquilizer)
Nonsteroidal anti-inflammatory drugs
Antiepileptics (carbamazepine, phenytoin)
Analgesics (salicylates, dipyrone, aminopyrine)

7. What are the common causes of postinfectious neutropenia?
Neutropenia can be seen after **viral infections**, a common cause in children. Viral diseases such as hepatitis A and B, influenza, Kawasaki disease, measles, rubella, and varicella have been implicated; the neutropenia can last for weeks. HIV infection, usually in later stages, can cause neutropenia in both adults and children and is usually associated with a hypercellular marrow. **Nonviral agents**, such as staphylococcus, mycobacterium tuberculosis, and rickettsiae, also can cause neutropenia. Brucellosis and tularemia have been associated with low neutrophil counts, and any cause of sepsis can be associated with a severe neutropenia. Increased utilization and margination probably account for low neutrophil counts in the case of sepsis. A low neutrophil count in streptococcal pneumonia is a poor prognostic sign. The mainstay of therapy is treatment of the underlying infection.

8. What are the characteristic findings in neutropenia associated with HIV infection?
Neutropenia is seen in more than 70% of patients with acquired immunodeficiency syndrome (AIDS) and is usually associated with a hypercellular marrow and a late myeloid arrest in the WBC precursors. Both hypersplenism and antineutrophil antibodies can be found in many patients.

9. What is benign familial leukopenia? What ethnic populations are usually involved?
Benign familial leukopenia is characterized by a mild neutropenia (2100–2600/mm³) with no increased risk of infection. This disorder is seen in several ethnic groups, including Yemenite Jews, West Indians, and people of African descent. The bone marrow biopsy appears normal; this finding represents a genetic variation in the regulation of the circulating neutrophil counts.

10. What is seen on the peripheral blood smear in individuals with neutropenia due to a bone marrow-infiltrating process?
If the bone marrow is infiltrated with either infection or metastatic cancer, other findings from the physical examination and history often lead to a diagnosis. In many patients, however, the peripheral smear shows a myelophthisic picture, with an increase in percentages of immature cell forms from all lines (reticulocytes, nucleated red cells, myeloid precursors, and giant platelets). This condition is sometimes indicative of a marrow infiltrated with metastatic carcinoma or, more rarely, an infectious agent such as mycobacterium.

11. Lack of which vitamins can cause neutropenia?
Vitamin B12 or folate deficiency can cause neutropenia with or without anemia. The bone marrow biopsy shows megaloblastic changes with ineffective myelopoiesis. Neutropenia and anemia associated with a megaloblastic bone marrow have been seen in the DIDMOAD syndrome (diabetes insipidus, diabetes mellitus, optic atrophy, deafness). In this syndrome hematologic abnormalities have been responsive to thiamine.

12. Deficiency of which heavy metal can cause isolated neutropenia?
Nutritional deficiency of copper and inherited deficiency of transcobalamin II have been known to cause ineffective myelopoiesis, megaloblastic changes in the marrow, and neutropenia.

13. What are the characteristics of chronic benign neutropenia of infancy and childhood?
Chronic benign neutropenia of childhood is a "chronic state of mature neutrophil depletion with a compensatory increase in immature granulocytes in the bone marrow analogous to erythroid hyperplasia in hemolytic anemia."[8] This disease occurs in the first 3 years of life, with 90% of cases occurring before the age of 14 months. Infection is a common presenting symptom, but the relationship is unclear because infections in this age group are common. Neutrophil counts are characteristically normal at birth, yet less than $500/mm^3$ at presentation. The majority of patients have detectable antineutrophil IgG antibodies that react with neutrophils, suggesting an immune mechanism. Immunosuppressive therapy is effective. Most of the infections are easily treated during the neutropenia, and some infants still can mount a neutrophil response. Although an unusual patient remains neutropenic into the adult years, 95% recover by 4 years of age. The bone marrow is normo- or hypercellular. High-dose intravenous gamma globulin, steroids, and granulocyte colony-stimulating factor (G-CSF) can be effective in raising the neutrophil count but are rarely indicated because of the usually benign nature of this disorder. Effective and expedient treatment of infections is the mainstay of therapy. Care must be taken not to confuse this diagnosis with more severe causes of neutropenia in infancy.

14. What is chronic idiopathic neutropenia?
Along with benign familial neutropenia and chronic benign neutropenia of childhood, chronic idiopathic neutropenia is a chronic neutropenia not usually associated with splenomegaly. The diagnosis is applied to neutropenias that do not fit into other categories. Age of onset is quite variable, and neutrophil counts are usually between 200 and $500/mm^3$. A normal to increased number of immature granulocytes can be found in the bone marrow (suggesting arrested maturation). Antineutrophil antibodies are usually absent, G-CSF concentrations are usually normal, and cytogenetic analysis of the marrow is normal. A neutrophil response to stimuli can still be seen, and the clinical course is often mild.

15. What is the treatment for chronic idiopathic neutropenia?
Splenectomy, corticosteroids, and cytotoxic agents have been used successfully in treating chronic idiopathic neutropenia. Recently filgrastim (G-CSF) has been used successfully to raise the leukocyte count. Treatment should be reserved for patients with significant recurrent infections because the clinical course of the disease may be mild.

16. What are the immune causes of neutropenia?
Even though immune mechanisms are implicated in cases of neutropenia that have been called idiopathic, a few causes of immune neutropenia are well established. Isoimmune neutropenia occurs in newborn infants when antibodies are transferred from the mother to the infant. Autoimmune neutropenia due to neutrophil-associated antibodies can occur at any time, from childhood to old age. Immunologic abnormalities such as hyper- or hypogammaglobulinemia, T-cell defects, and natural killer-cell abnormalities, as well as other autoimmune diseases, can cause neutropenia in childhood. Patients usually present with frequent infections and hepatosplenomegaly. Many have a family history of neutropenia. Severe cases have been treated with allogeneic bone marrow transplantation.

T-gamma lymphocytosis is a disorder in which clonal proliferation of lymphocytes is associated with a normocellular marrow, maturational arrest in neutrophils, and peripheral neutropenia. Although the course of this disease may be benign, some individuals have been successfully treated with gammaglobulin.

17. What is the treatment for isoimmune neutropenia in newborns?
Isoimmune neutropenia in newborns is identical in pathogenesis to Rh hemolytic disease: prenatal sensitization to neutrophil antigens with subsequent IgG antibodies that cross the placental barrier to the newborn. The disorder occurs in 0.2% of births. The newborn may be asymptomatic or present with sepsis. Antineutrophil antibodies are usually detected in

both the infant's and mother's serum. Bone marrow biopsy performed on the infant is
normocellular and displays a late maturational arrest. Neutropenia usually resolves in
12–15 weeks, although on rare occasions it lasts as long as 6 months. Appropriate antibiotics are the usual treatment; intravenous gamma globulin also has been used successfully.

18. What are the causes of autoimmune neutropenia?

Autoimmune neutropenia can be (1) isolated (i.e., the only hematologic abnormality),
(2) secondary to other autoimmune diseases such as rheumatoid arthritis or systemic lupus
erythematosus, or (3) related to immune mechanisms triggered by infections or drugs. The
neutropenia is moderate to severe, with hypercellular marrow and late myeloid maturational
arrest. Hepatosplenomegaly is seen in about half the patients, and presentation can be at
any age. Neutropenia can be associated with a concurrent idiopathic thrombocytopenia
purpura (ITP) or hemolytic anemia. Various antineutrophil antibodies of the IgG or IgM
type may be detected, and, as in some cases of chronic idiopathic neutropenia, immune
complexes have been found. Patients with rheumatoid arthritis, neutropenia, and splenomegaly have Felty's syndrome, a complex autoimmune disorder. Methotrexate treatment
sometimes decreases the levels of antineutrophil antibody and concurrently increases the
neutrophil count. Other patients with a severe autoimmune neutropenia (ANC <500/mm³)
and recurrent infections can be treated with intravenous gamma globulin or steroids.
Cytotoxic therapy has been used in other immune neutropenias as well as in rheumatoid
arthritis. Splenectomy provides no lasting benefit.

19. Which metabolic diseases are associated with neutropenia?

Neutropenia has been seen in patients with ketoacidosis and hyperglycemia, hyperglycinuria,
orotic aciduria, methylmalonic aciduria, and glycogen storage disease type Ib. Hypothyroidism may cause neutropenia. Treatment focuses on the underlying disease whenever possible.

20. What are the causes of neutrophil margination? Is it related to the adult respiratory distress syndrome (ARDS)?

Complement activation clearly can cause acute and chronic neutropenia due to increased
adherence and aggregation in endothelia. Etiologies such as hemodialysis, membrane
oxygenators, severe burns, and transfusion reactions have been implicated. Paroxysmal
nocturnal hemoglobinuria also generates complement-mediated neutrophil destruction.
Lung dysfunction and pulmonary infiltrates have been seen in some patients, suggesting
that the neutrophil may play a role in the pathogenesis of ARDS. This theory, however, has
not been proved.

21. What is hypersplenism? How is it treated?

Splenomegaly from any cause can produce neutropenia, usually in association with mild
thrombocytopenia and anemia. Splenic sequestration and increased peripheral utilization
are proposed mechanisms. Predisposition to infection is variable, although usually it is not
severe enough to cause symptoms. Splenectomy increases the blood counts but should be
reserved for patients with recurrent severe infections.   -

22. What are the intrinsic causes of neutropenia?

Dyskeratosis congenita is an X-linked disorder characterized by integument abnormalities
in association with mild neutropenia or, in some cases, pancytopenia. The bone marrow is
hypocellular. Kostmann syndrome (infantile agranulocytosis) is an inherited disorder that
presents in infancy with recurrent severe infections and neutropenia. Bone marrow
examination reveals myeloid hypocellularity with an arrest at the promyelocyte stage. Bone
marrow culture reveals G-CSF-dependent colony growth. This previously fatal disorder
responds well to G-CSF in vivo. Shwachman-Diamond-Oski syndrome presents in the first
decade of life with neutropenia, metaphyseal dysplasia, and pancreatic insufficiency. Severe,
sometimes fatal, infections occur in over half the patients. Chediak-Higashi syndrome is the

rare inherited syndrome of oculocutaneous albinism, progressive neurologic impairment, and giant granules in many cells, including neutrophils. Severe neutropenia is also seen. The syndrome of agranulocytosis, lymphoid hypoplasia, and thymic dysplasia is known as reticular dysgenesis. The bone marrow is hypoplastic with few myeloid precursors, and all patients die in infancy unless treated with a bone marrow transplant. Cyclic neutropenia is a dominantly inherited disorder of variable expression with neutropenia that recurs about every 15–35 days. The course of the disease tends to be benign, although recurrent infections can be severe and may cause death. Age of presentation is variable, and the marrow is hypoplastic during episodes of neutropenia. Furthermore, isolated neutropenia can be seen in other states of marrow failure, such as refractory anemia, aplastic anemia, and Fanconi's anemia.

23. What is the work-up for neutropenia?
If the patient is without symptoms, physical findings, or historical data that merit further evaluation, clinical observation is the best approach. This is especially true if the patient has a recent history of a viral infection or discontinues a medicine known to cause neutropenia. Complete blood counts must be done twice weekly for 6 weeks if cyclic neutropenia is suspected. In children, the most common causes of isolated neutropenia are benign, and isolated neutropenia is rarely the presentation of malignancy at any age. If thrombocytopenia or anemia is present, if the patient presents with infection, or if the neutropenia persists, bone marrow aspiration and biopsy should be performed. Serum immunologic evaluation, assessment of levels of antineutrophil antibody, and a work-up for collagen vascular disease may then be merited.

24. How is neutropenia managed?
Management of infection is of major concern in the neutropenic patient. Many of the inflammatory signs of infection may not be present because of the inability to mount a neutrophil response. Therefore, the combination of fever and neutropenia usually requires immediate use of broad-spectrum antibiotics. The organisms that cause infection are usually from the gastrointestinal tract and the skin, and therapy should be aimed at gram-negative as well as gram-positive organisms. Intravenous gammaglobulin and steroids have had limited usefulness in some instances of immune-related neutropenia, and both G-CSF and allogeneic bone marrow transplantation have been used successfully in certain cases of severe chronic neutropenia.

BIBLIOGRAPHY

1. Coates T, Baehner R: Leukocytosis and leukopenia. In Hoffman R, Benz EJ, Shattil SJ, et al (eds): Hematology: Basic Principles and Practice. New York, Churchill Livingstone, 1991.
2. Dale DC, Guerry D, Wewerka JR, et al: Chronic neutropenia. Medicine 58:128, 1979.
3. Fronteira M, Myers AM: Peripheral blood and bone marrow abnormalities in the acquired immunodeficiency syndrome. West J Med 147:157, 1987.
4. Hammond WP, Price TH, Souza LM, Dale DC: Treatment of cyclic neutropenia with granulocyte colony-stimulating factor. N Engl J Med 320:1306, 1989.
5. Heimpel H: Drug-induced agranulocytosis. Med Toxicol Adverse Drug Exp 3:449, 1988.
6. Kyle RA: Natural history of chronic idiopathic neutropenia. N Engl J Med 302:908, 1980.
7. Wright DG, et al: Human cyclic neutropenia: Clinical review and long-term follow-up of patients. Medicine 60:1, 1980.
8. Zeulzer WW, Bajoghli M: Chronic granulocytopenia in childhood. Blood 23:359, 1964.

24. MYELODYSPLASTIC SYNDROMES

Jeanette Mladenovic, M.D.

1. Name the components of the triad that suggest the clinical diagnosis of myelodysplastic syndrome (MDS).

The hematologic constellation of a chronic refractory cytopenia, a bone marrow with increased cellularity, and dysmyelopoietic abnormalities in bone marrow precursors is sufficient to presume the clinical disorder of MDS.

2. Which categories of diseases are included in MDS? What are the diagnostic criteria for each subgroup?

There is a widely accepted classification of MDS proposed by the FAB (French-American-British) group, paralleling the classification of leukemias. The classification is based on morphologic criteria that include the numbers of myeloblasts and ring sideroblasts in the marrow, the numbers of circulating blasts and monocytes in the blood, and the presence or absence of Auer rods. The five types of MDS along with their distinguishing diagnostic criteria are listed below.

Myelodysplastic Syndromes

	PERIPHERAL BLOOD		BONE MARROW	
	% CIRCULATING BLASTS	% MONOCYTES	% BLASTS	% RING SIDEROBLASTS
Refractory anemia (RA)	<1	Not increased	<5	<15
Refractory anemia with ring sideroblasts (RAS)	<1	Not increased	<5	>15
Chronic myelomonocytic leukemia (CMML)	<5	>10^9/L	≥20	Insignificant
Refractory anemia excess blasts (RAEB)	<5	Not increased	5–20	Insignificant
Refractory anemia with excess blasts in transformation (RAEB-T)	≤5	Not increased	20–30 and/or Auer rods	Insignificant

As can be seen from the above table, the myelodysplastic syndromes consist of five separate entities, many of which have overlapping characteristics that can be distinguished by the predominant blood and marrow characteristics. The importance of this classification can be seen in patient prognosis, indications for therapy, and therapeutic outcomes.

3. Why is the term "myelodysplastic syndrome" misleading?

The term might lead one to believe that the bone marrow is simply abnormal but not neoplastic in nature. This is not the case. The bone marrow in MDS represents the clonal proliferation of an abnormal stem cell. Thus, although a megaloblastic marrow due to B12 deficiency might be considered dysmyelopoietic in descriptive terms, it is not a clonal abnormality of the stem cell representing conversion to neoplasia. Older terms for MDS such as "preleukemia" might in fact be more appropriate. Today, however, these groups of entities are most commonly called MDS.

4. Describe the clinical presentation of a patient with MDS.
The clinical presentation of MDS has no specific features. The most common presentation is that of an elderly man with fatigue, weakness, and exertional dyspnea, often related to anemia. Most patients present asymptomatically with an abnormality noted in their routine peripheral blood count. Splenomegaly and hepatomegaly are seen in only 5–10% of patients. A small number of patients may present with infection related to neutropenia or hemorrhage secondary to thrombocytopenia. Occasionally, MDS may manifest itself with a unique clinical syndrome. For instance, arthralgias may be the initial complaint in some patients. Rare clinical entities such as diabetes insipidus, acute neutrophilic dermatosis (Sweet's disease) or a serositis syndrome resembling systemic lupus erythematosus may present concurrently with MDS.

5. How frequently are various cytopenias found in MDS?
The most frequent presentation is anemia, which is found in >85% of patients. This anemia is characterized by hypoproliferation, with an increase in the mean cell volume. There may be acquired hemoglobinopathies (hemoglobin H disease) or enzyme deficiencies (pyruvate kinase) complicating this anemia.

Neutropenia is often accompanied by a monocytosis, which is present in about half the patients with this diagnosis. Thrombocytopenia is found in about 25% of patients at the time of diagnosis, but mild thrombocytosis may also occur. The abnormality in platelets may be accompanied by abnormal platelet function, leading to prolonged bleeding and abnormal in vitro aggregation responses. Often patients have lymphocyte abnormalities such as lymphopenia with decreased numbers of natural killer cells and/or helper lymphocytes.

6. What are the peripheral blood smear clues to the diagnosis of MDS?
Because this is a disorder of the myeloid stem cell, there may be abnormalities in all three cell lines on the peripheral blood smear. In addition to abnormalities noted in the differential criteria (percentage of circulating blasts and monocytosis), there may be several other findings that suggest a myelodysplastic abnormality. The red blood cells themselves may be macrocytic or may consist of a second population of cells that are hypochromic and coarsely stippled. There may be a number of misshapen cells with nucleated red blood cells, basophilic stippling, and Heinz bodies. Immature white blood cells that usually do not circulate in the peripheral blood may be evident. The nuclear anomaly of Pelger-Huët is frequently seen with bilobed or even ring-shaped nuclei. Cytoplasmic granules may be decreased or absent. The platelets may be abnormal in appearance in addition to their abnormal numbers. There may be large platelets, poorly granulated platelets, or circulating fragments of megakaryocytes. In summary, abnormalities in more than one cell line are highly suggestive of the diagnosis of MDS, especially in the absence of peripheral circulating blasts.

7. Characterize the marrow abnormalities of MDS.
Marrow cellularity is usually increased but occasionally may be normal or hypoplastic. When there appears to be decreased cellularity, there are still islands of abnormal appearing cells, which are often atypical megakaryocytes. The erythroid series is usually hyperplastic with megaloblasts and apparent nuclear cytoplasmic maturation abnormalities. There are nuclear fragments in stippled erythroblasts with poorly hemoglobinized cells. On staining for iron with Prussian blue, an increase in macrophage iron is usually found. More importantly, however, there is an increased number of erythroblasts that contain siderosomes (cytoplastic ferritin-containing vacuoles), such that these cells are referred to as abnormal sideroblasts. On occasion, these sideroblasts have mitochondrial iron aggregated around the nucleus in a ring shape (thus ringed sideroblast). Ring sideroblasts are most common in acquired refractory sideroblastic anemia. Granulocytic hyperplasia also is frequently observed. Abnormalities of the granulocytes similar to those in the peripheral smear consist

of hypogranulation, Pelger-Huët anomalies and increased numbers of blasts and other early white cells precursors. Megakaryocytes are usually present or increased with micro-megakaryocytes often present.

8. What are the most common cytogenic abnormalities seen in MDS? How do they influence prognosis?

Up to 50% of patients with MDS may have chromosomal abnormalities. Most often these abnormalities consist of chromosomal losses or gains such as 5q−, 7−, and 8+ abnormalities. None of these abnormalities is unique for classes or subgroups of MDS. The specific structural abnormalities of acute nonlymphocytic leukemia are less common in MDS. In MDS, virtually every chromosome has been affected. In general, the more complex and the greater numbers of cells that show evidence of chromosomal cytogenic abnormalities, the worse the prognosis. This is true with the exception of the 5q− syndrome associated with refractory anemia, which usually predicts a good prognosis.

9. What do we know of the pathogenesis of MDS?

As noted previously, MDS is a group of clonal disorders. How clonal abnormalities result in cytopenias in MDS is not clear. Although it is commonly held that MDS results from ineffective hematopoiesis with intramedullary destruction of precursors, data to support this hypothesis have not been clearly demonstrated. It may be that failure of differentiation due to abnormal progenitors or hematopoietic growth factors is important in the observed phenotype. This hypothesis has arisen from abnormalities of hematopoietic in vitro colony growth. The molecular bases of abnormalities in MDS remain to be determined. A number of target genes have been shown to have mutations (ras, c-fms), but these have been inconsistent and likely represent only one clue to the puzzle of abnormal myeloproliferation in this disease.

10. Which factors predispose to the development of MDS?

Usually MDS arises without specific or apparent cause. However, patients with MDS have a greater than expected exposure to benzene. Likewise, cancer treatment, especially with alkylating agents and radiation therapy, is an important factor in the predisposition to MDS. These patients have an overall risk of about 10% in 10 years for the development of MDS with transition to acute nonlymphocytic leukemia. On rare occasions, aplastic anemia and paroxysmal hemoglobinuria will evolve into MDS.

11. Characterize and distinguish primary from secondary MDS.

Although phenotypically these syndromes appear similar, they differ in several aspects. Therapy-related MDS occurs at a variable age depending on the antecedent exposure to chemotherapy. Although abnormalities in the blood are similar, the bone marrow may more often be hypocellular in secondary MDS. The course is often more rapid, and the presentation more commonly that of myelodysplastic syndrome in transition to acute nonlymphocytic leukemia in secondary MDS. It is unclear whether some diseases, in addition to chemotherapy, predispose to MDS (such as multiple myeloma, Hodgkin's disease, other lymphomas, and polycythemia vera). Most patients with therapy-related MDS have clonal chromosomal abnormalities, and three-fourths of these patients will have more than one chromosomal abnormality at presentation. Often these syndromes follow a more aggressive course and appear to respond to therapy less well.

12. How common is leukemic transformation in MDS?

Overall, with the recognition of earlier disease as MDS, only about 20% of patients undergo leukemic transformation of their disease. This incidence varies with respect to the FAB category. Refractory anemia with ring sideroblasts shows the lowest leukemic transformation (5%), whereas refractory anemia with excessive blasts in transformation undergoes true leukemic transformation up to 50% of the time. Refractory anemia (10%), refractory anemia with excessive blasts (23%), and chronic myelomonocytic leukemia (20%) are in the intermediate range.

13. What is the cause of death in patients with MDS that does not evolve into acute leukemia?

Mortality from infection or hemorrhage occurs in about 25% of patients. Because this is a disease of the elderly, death from other entities is likely in many patients who have had MDS for years. Iron overload may occur in patients who undergo frequent transfusions. The clinical appearance of hemochromatosis is more frequent in patients who are HLAA3+, suggesting that sideroblastic anemia and transfusion therapy in combination with a genetic predisposition result in hemochromatosis.

14. An elderly woman with refractory macrocytic anemia and splenomegaly is likely to have which MDS?

This patient likely has the 5q– syndrome. This entity is seen in elderly women who present with refractory macrocytic anemia and who often have a long and uneventful course other than the occasional need for transfusion. These patients have splenomegaly (up to 50%) with platelets that are normal or increased in number. The region of the break point of the 5q chromosome contains genes for major hematopoietic growth factors, including interleukins 3,4,5, macrophage colony-stimulating factor (M-CSF), granulocyte-macrophage colony-stimulating factor (GM-CSF), and the proto-oncogene c-*fms*, which is the M-CSF receptor. However, how the abnormality in this chromosomal area relates to the clinical presentation of MDS remains to be discovered.

15. A patient with MDS asks if he will need to quit his job in the next year. How should he be answered?

It is important to determine the clinical subclass of MDS that the patient has, because varying overall prognoses coupled to prognostic factors delineate the expected natural history. The best prognosis is usually for refractory anemia and refractory anemia with ring sideroblasts, with the worst prognosis being for refractory anemia with excessive blasts and refractory anemia with excessive blasts with transformation, whereas chronic myelomonocytic leukemia is intermediate (22 months). A simple scoring system consists of assigning 1 point to each of the following: bone marrow blasts >5%, platelets <100,000, neutrophils <2.5 or >16, and hemoglobin <10 gm (total possible score 4). The total score correlates with length of survival: ≤1 = 62 months; 2 or 3 = 22 months; 4 = 8.5 months. Thus, taking into account the natural history of the patient's disease, you as a physician and the patient may decide the patient's own desires with respect to the immediate and long-term course of action.

16. Who should be treated for MDS?

Many patients require only supportive therapy (transfusions) and treatment of infectious complications for their disease. Treatment is required in those patients whose disease evolves into acute nonlymphocytic leukemia and who elect treatment. To consider cure, treatment must be aimed at eradication of the abnormal clone.

Alternatively, the availability of recombinant human hematopoietic growth factors has been effective in improving cytopenias in some patients. For instance, erythropoietin has led to an increase in hemoglobin concentration in approximately one-fifth of anemic patients regardless of their erythropoietin levels. Occasionally, G-CSF or GM-CSF may transiently improve the white blood cell count. Likewise, it is possible that recombinant IL-3 may result in short-term hematopoietic improvement. Because of the current cost of recombinant growth factors and the limited improvement in outcome, they should be used on experimental protocol or only sparingly in these patients.

Another approach is the use of nontoxic differentiation agents in clinical trials. However, both retinoic acid and 1-25-dehydroxyvitamin D3 have resulted in only minimal responses in MDS. Alpha interferon likewise should be used sparingly. Standard therapy with glucocorticoids and danazol may transiently improve counts in a limited number of patients. In short, these palliative measures do not change the long-term outcome of this disease.

17. How has chemotherapy fared in MDS?
Low-dose chemotherapy or conventional chemotherapy has proved ineffective in changing the overall survival. However, the use of intensive chemotherapy coupled with bone marrow transplantation on some occasions may be appropriate. These aggressive approaches should be considered in young patients who have undergone leukemic transformation. Therapy-related MDS does not preclude utilization of this approach. Since up to 40% of patients may die during aggressive chemotherapy, the overall intention to treat must consider this high possibility of mortality.

BIBLIOGRAPHY

1. Besa EC: Myelodysplastic syndromes. Med Clin North Am 76:599–617, 1992.
2. Doll DC, List AF (eds): Myelodysplastic syndromes. Semin Oncol 10:1, 1992.
3. Greenberg PL: In vitro marrow culture studies in the myelodysplastic syndromes. Semin Oncol 19:34, 1992.
4. Griffin JD (ed): Myelodysplastic syndromes. Clin Haematol 15:909, 1986.
5. Heim S: Cytogenetic findings in primary and secondary MDS. Leuk Res 16:43, 1992.
6. Kantarjian HM, et al: Treatment of therapy-related leukemia and myelodysplastic syndrome. Hematol Oncol Clinic North Am 7:81–107, 1993.
7. Liu E, et al: Mutations of the Kirsten-*ras* proto-oncogene in human preleukaemia. Nature 330:186, 1987.
8. Mathew P, Tefferi A, Dewald GW, et al: The 5q⁻ syndrome: A single institution study of 43 consecutive patients. Blood 81:1040–1045, 1993.
9. Nowell PC: Chromosome abnormalities in myelodysplastic syndromes. Semin Oncol 19:25, 1992.
10. Tricot G, et al: Prognostic factors in the myelodysplastic syndromes: Importance of initial data on peripheral blood counts, bone marrow cytology, trephine biopsy and chromosomal analysis. Leuk Res 16:109, 1992.
11. Vallespi T, et al: Myelodysplastic syndromes: A study of 101 cases according to the FAB classification. Br J Haematol 61:83, 1985.

25. HYPEREOSINOPHILIC SYNDROMES

Russell C. Tolley, M.D.

1. What is an eosinophil? How does it function?
Eosinophils develop in the bone marrow like neutrophils and have characteristic red-staining granules that contain a unique peroxidase. By secreting the contents of the granules in the vicinity of large parasites such as *Schistosoma mansoni,* they inflict damage to the cell wall of the organisms. The blood pool of eosinophils is relatively small compared with the number of eosinophils in tissues.

2. What is eosinophilia?
The absolute level of eosinophils can be obtained by multiplying the percent of eosinophils on the differential by the white blood cell (WBC) count:

$$\text{absolute eosinophil count} = \text{WBC} \times \% \text{ eosinophils} \times 0.01$$

Normal levels do not exceed $350/\text{mm}^3$; levels above $1000/\text{mm}^3$ direct attention to the causes of eosinophilia.

3. Does the eosinophil count vary during the day?
Yes. The number is lowest in the afternoon and highest in the morning.

4. Which growth factors stimulate the production of eosinophils? Where are the genes for these growth factors located?
The most specific growth factor is interleukin-5 (IL-5), a cytokine found in the serum of patients with parasitic infections. In mice it has been shown to increase specifically the production of eosinophils. Granulocyte/macrophage-colony stimulating factor (GM-CSF) and IL-3 are also known to increase production of eosinophils but not specifically. Of interest, all three of these genes are located on the long arm of chromosome 5 and within very close proximity to each other.

5. What are some of the secondary causes of eosinophilia?
Allergic states, including hayfever, asthma, and drug reactions, which are associated with elevated serum levels of IgE
Parasitic diseases
Vasculitides, including Wegener's granulomatosis, Churg-Strauss syndrome, and a number of pulmonary infiltrative disorders
Malignancies such as Hodgkin's disease, non-Hodgkin's lymphoma, and, more rarely, carcinoma, which may also cause acute myeloblastic leukemia, myeloproliferative disorders, and myelodysplastic states with eosinophilic differentiation
Collagen vascular diseases and autoimmune disorders, including rheumatoid arthritis, dermatomyositis, and periarteritis nodosa, which may be confirmed through serologic tests (serum complement levels, antinuclear antibodies) or tissue biopsy

6. Is there a way to remember the causes of eosinophilia?
The acronym NAACP is useful:
  N   Neoplasm
  A   Allergies
  A   Asthma
  C   Collagen vascular diseases
  P   Parasites
Obviously, this acronym does not identify every possible cause, but it does include the more common causes.

7. Which parasitic diseases cause eosinophilia?
Schistosomiasis is a major source of infection outside the United States and a common cause of eosinophilia. Filariasis, trichinosis, hookworm and Ascaris infection, visceral larva migrans, and strongyloidiasis also can cause marked eosinophilia.

8. What are the most common causes of eosinophilia in the United States?
Allergic and hypersensitivity reactions are the most common underlying causes of eosinophilia in adults. Visceral larva migrans due to *Toxocara canis* also is common in children.

9. How does a child get visceral larva migrans?
This disorder results when children eat dirt infected with eggs   odes, whose natural host is the dog *(Toxocara canis)* or cat *(Toxocara cati).* The larvae then migrate through the gastrointestinal tract to tissues, causing an illness characterized by fever, intense eosinophilia, wheezing, pneumonitis, and hepatosplenomegaly. If reinfection is prevented, the disorder may be self-limiting.

10. Name some commonly used drugs that cause eosinophilia.
Sulfonamides, iodides, nitrofurantoin, phenytoin, and aspirin may cause elevated eosinophil counts.

11. What is the hypereosinophilic syndrome (HES)? How is it treated?
Idiopathic HES is a primary disorder of unknown etiology, also known as Loffler's syndrome, eosinophilic leukemia, and disseminated eosinophilic collagen disease. It is associated with serious morbidity and mortality; some past reviews of untreated patients show a 3-year survival rate of only 12% and a median survival of 9 months. HES is characterized by white blood cell counts between 15,000 and 150,000/mm^3, marked eosinophilia on differential with up to 70% eosinophils, and increased eosinophils and eosinophil precursors on marrow examination. Fever, anemia, and hepatosplenomegaly also are commonly seen. Prominent cardiac findings, including emboli from mural thrombi, abnormal EKGs, congestive heart failure, murmurs, and left ventricular hypertrophy, may be observed, along with pulmonary abnormalities and neurologic dysfunction. Many patients succumb to a progressive endomyocardial fibroelastosis. The etiology is thought to be eosinophilic infiltration of tissues with resultant tissue damage. Therapy consists of decreasing the eosinophilia with either corticosteroids or hydroxyurea. With the advent of corticosteroid and cytotoxic therapy for HES, 5-year survival rates of 70–90% have been reported.

12. How is the diagnosis of HES made?
Patients with no underlying disorder known to cause eosinophilia and with persistence of eosinophilia for 6 months in association with underlying organ dysfunction that is otherwise unexplained fall into the category of HES. Of interest, the male predominance is 9:1.

13. What pulmonary disorders are associated with hypereosinophilia?
As mentioned above, parasitic infections and HES can produce pulmonary infiltrates and eosinophilia. Fungi such as coccidioides or bronchopulmonary aspergillosis, a disorder of asthmatic patients, may cause hypereosinophilia. Bronchopulmonary aspergillosis tends to produce segmental and central pulmonary infiltrates, with eosinophils in the sputum as well. Coccidioides presents with fever, pulmonary infiltrates, arthralgias, and erythema nodosum. Hypersensitivity reactions to molds in grain dust (farmer's lung), allergic granulomatosis (vasculitis with features of polyarteritis nodosa and pulmonary infiltrates), and sarcoidosis (suggested by hilar adenopathy on roentgenogram) are associated with eosinophilia.

Chronic eosinophilic pneumonia is a debilitating illness of unknown etiology with fever, weight loss, and characteristic peripheral lung infiltrates on roentgenogram. Asthmatic symptoms and eosinophilia in the blood and/or sputum are present. The lung infiltrates promptly disappear with corticosteroid treatment.

14. Can eosinophilia be inherited?
Yes. This eosinophilia is generally a mild, rare disorder that is usually associated with an autosomal dominant pattern and a benign clinical course.

15. What causes the damage in patients with eosinophilia?
Damage results both from the mass effect of eosinophilic infiltration of tissue and from proteins liberated when eosinophils degranulate. The most important protein released appears to be major basic protein (MBP), which is toxic to cells. MBP can be demonstrated in sputum of patients with asthma or in serum of patients with eosinophilia.

16. What are Charcot-Leyden crystals?
These characteristic crystals are found both in the cytoplasm of eosinophils and in the extracellular environment when degranulation occurs. They are thought to contain lysophospholipase and to be inert once they are formed.

17. What is the relationship between eosinophilia and leukemia?
The association between eosinophilia and leukemia is unclear. In fact, the existence of a true eosinophilic leukemia is debated. In some cases, eosinophilia associated with leukemia is a poor prognostic factor, as in acute lymphocytic leukemia with eosinophilia and a t(5,14)

(q13;q32) transformation. Alternatively, eosinophilia in patients with acute myelomonocytic leukemia and an inversion of chromosome 16 carries a favorable prognosis.

18. What is eosinophilia-myalgia syndrome (EMS)?
EMS was first identified in 1989. Patients presented with a variety of symptoms, but all patients have myalgias and most have eosinophilia. EMS can be debilitating, with ultimate development of scle odermalike skin lesions and peripheral neuropathies. Eosinophil counts are modestly elevated but have been as high as 36,000/dl. EMS bears a striking resemblance to toxic oil syndrome as well as other hypereosinophilic syndromes.

19. What causes EMS?
The exact cause is still unknown. The greatest association appears to be with the identification of a novel amino acid consisting of two L-tryptophan molecules. This compound was created in the manufacturing process of L-tryptophan but only at selected manufacturing sites. Some individuals who develop EMS demonstrate abnormal tryptophan metabolism. It may be that both impurities in the manufacturing process and abnormal metabolism are required for development of the syndrome.

BIBLIOGRAPHY

1. Dvorak AM, Letourneau L, Login GR, et al: Ultrastructural localization of the Charcot-Leyden crystal protein (lysophospholipase) to a distinct crystalloid-free granule population in mature human eosinophils. Blood 72:150, 1988.
2. Fausci AS, Harley JB, Roberts WC, et al: The idiopathic hypereosinophilic syndrome: Clinical, pathophysiologic, and therapeutic considerations. Ann Intern Med 97:78, 1982.
3. Frigas E, Loegering DA, Solley GO, et al: Elevated levels of the eosinophil granule major basic protein in the sputum of patients with bronchial asthma. Mayo Clin Proc 56:345, 1981.
4. Gabig TE: Hypereosinophilic syndromes. In Hoffman R, Berz E, et al (eds): Hematology: Basic Principles and Practice. New York, Churchill Livingstone, 1991, pp 567–571.
5. Larson RA, Williams SF, Le Beau MM, et al: Acute myelomonocytic leukemia with abnormal eosinophils and inv(16) or t(16;16) has a favorable prognosis. Blood 68:1242, 1986.
6. Naiman JL, Oski FA, Allen FH, Diamond LK: Hereditary eosinophilia: Report of a family and review of the literature. Am J Hum Genet 16:195, 1964.
7. Olsen EGJ, Spry CJF: The pathogenesis of Loffler's endomyocardial disease, and its relationship to endomyocardial fibrosis. Prog Cardiol 8:281, 1979.
8. Parrillo JE, Fauci AS, Wolff SM: Therapy of the hypereosinophilic syndrome. Ann Intern Med 89:167, 1978.
9. Varga J, Uitto J, Jimenez SA: The cause and pathogenesis of the eosinophilia-myalgia syndrome. Ann Intern Med 116:140, 1992.
10. Weller PF: The immunobiology of eosinophils. N Engl J Med 324:110, 1991.

26. ANEMIA AND IDIOPATHIC THROMBOCYTOPENIC PURPURA

George Rajan, M.D., Miho Toi, M.D., and Adam M. Myers, M.D.

ANEMIA

1. How common is anemia in acquired immunodeficiency syndrome (AIDS)?
Anemia is common in patients with human immunodeficiency virus (HIV) infection and becomes more common with disease progression. In asymptomatic HIV infection, anemia is seen in 10% to 20% of patients. In patients with full-blown AIDS with opportunistic infections, anemia is seen in 70% to 90% of cases.

2. What causes anemia in AIDS?

All three classic mechanisms of anemia can contribute to the development of anemia in patients with AIDS: (1) decreased bone marrow production, (2) increased peripheral destruction, and (3) blood loss. Direct invasion by HIV of bone marrow cells results in ineffective hematopoiesis and/or problems of cell egress from the marrow. Additionally, dysregulation of the host immune system leads to increased peripheral destruction and/or inhibition of hematopoiesis. Secondary complications of AIDS such as infections and malignancies, and their treatments, also contribute.

3. What abnormalities would you anticipate in the peripheral blood smear in the anemic patient with AIDS?

Anemia in HIV infection is typically normochromic and normocytic with a mild degree of anisocytosis and poikilocytosis. Red blood cell (RBC) macrocytosis also is commonly seen, especially when the patient is being treated with drugs such as azidothymidine (AZT), dapsone, and sulfamethoxazole-trimethoprim. The reticulocyte count is low or normal, suggesting depressed erythropoiesis as the predominant mechanism of anemia.

Frequently, there is evidence of early RBC release in the form of polychromasia. Enlarged left-shifted hyposegmented neutrophils, large vacuolated monocytes, and large granular lymphocytes also may be seen. The presence of schistocytes suggests a concomitant microangiopathic process like disseminated intravascular coagulation (DIC) or thrombotic thrombocytopenic purpura (TTP).

4. What do iron studies show in a patient with HIV-related anemia?

Results of iron studies resemble those of anemia of chronic disease. Hypoferremia with decreased iron reutilization but with increased iron stores is typical. Hence, one sees low serum iron and binding capacity and an elevated serum ferritin. Iron stores may especially be increased when the patient is transfusion dependent.

5. When should a serum B12 estimation be ordered in a patient with anemia and HIV infection?

B12 levels are lower than normal in as many as 25% of patients with AIDS probably because of a gastropathy. Characteristically, these low B12 levels occur in the absence of neutrophilic hypersegmentation, RBC macrocytosis, and megaloblastic changes in bone marrow. Although this reduction is not clinically significant and often not associated with complications, it may increase the hematologic toxicity of AZT.

6. How often does hemolysis occur in patients with HIV infection?

Anti-red blood cell antibodies produce a positive direct Coombs test in approximately 20% of patients with AIDS. In a study with the use of the direct antiglobulin test (DAT) for immunoglobulin G (IgG), IgM, and anti-C3b, 85% of patients with AIDS, 68% of patients with AIDS-related complex (ARC) and 46% of healthy homosexuals were Coombs positive. Yet, it must be emphasized that clinically significant hemolysis is rare.

7. Bone marrow examination in a patient with AIDS shows what characteristics?

Characteristically, the marrow cellularity is normocellular to hypercellular even in the presence of peripheral cytopenias. The erythroid precursors are decreased and frequently dysplastic, with the myeloid to erythroid ratio ranging from 2:1 to 5:1 (which is high). Megakaryocytes are either adequate or increased and lymphoid aggregates are occasionally present. There also is a tendency toward increased reticulin formation, which may account for the many "dry taps" when marrow aspirations are performed in patients with AIDS.

8. What does significantly depressed hematopoiesis out of proportion to other cell lines suggest?

It suggests *Mycobacterium avium-intracellulare* infection, which is more likely to occur when CD4 cell counts are low.

9. Are there any other associations between infections and anemia?
Parvovirus B19 should be added to the list of pathogens that can contribute to anemia in persons with HIV infection. This also is particularly true if the anemia is severe and/or if there is red blood cell aplasia on bone marrow biopsy.

10. How is anemia in HIV infection treated?
Treatment is generally aimed at the underlying cause, which may include antiretroviral measures, treating opportunistic infections and malignancies, replacing deficient substrates, discontinuing myelosuppressive drugs, and treating coexistent hemolysis or blood loss. Often, repeated transfusions may be required to maintain the patient's hematocrit.

11. When should erythropoietin be used to treat anemia in AIDS?
Erythropoietin (EPO) is a glycoprotein hormone produced by the kidney that directs the development and maintenance of the red blood cell mass. Typically, a patient with AIDS has a blunted response to anemia compared with healthy persons, but patients taking AZT may have unusually high levels of EPO. Studies have shown that patients with endogenous EPO levels <500 mg/ml had a significant reduction in their transfusion requirement and an improvement in overall quality of life after exogenous EPO was administered. With higher (>500 mg/ml) baseline levels of EPO, no benefit is seen with exogenous administration of EPO.

IDIOPATHIC THROMBOCYTOPENIC PURPURA (ITP)

12. How common is thrombocytopenia in HIV-infected persons?
Thrombocytopenia occurs in 3–8% of HIV-seropositive individuals, whereas the incidence is 30–45% of HIV-infected individuals with fully developed AIDS. Thrombocytopenia occurs in HIV-infected patients regardless of the risk group to which they belong (e.g., homosexual men, intravenous drug abusers, and hemophiliacs). It also occurs in all age groups.

In HIV-seropositive patients with hemophilia, ITP is the most frequently observed HIV-related condition. Among the hemophilic HIV-positive population, the cumulative 10-year incidence of thrombocytopenia was found to be 43% in adults and 27% in children.

13. How do thrombocytopenic HIV-infected patients usually present?
Thrombocytopenia itself may occur as a part of the acute viral syndrome with initial HIV infection. One-third of thrombocytopenic HIV-infected patients present with easy bruising, petechiae, or bleeding. Other hematologic abnormalities also are found in 60% of these individuals (e.g., neutropenia with or without anemia). Spontaneous significant clinical bleeding usually does not occur.

14. Define thrombocytopenia.
Thrombocytopenia is a platelet count of <150,000/μl. HIV-infected persons with ITP usually have a moderate presentation with platelet counts between 40,000 and 60,000/μl. Occasionally, platelet counts of <10,000/μl are seen.

15. What are the mechanisms of thrombocytopenia in AIDS?
   1. Increased peripheral destruction of platelets
   2. Decreased production as a result of bone marrow failure

16. How can these two problems be distinguished?
Increased destruction of platelets can be documented by kinetic studies using homologous platelets labeled with chromium. These studies have demonstrated reduced platelet survival and increased splenic sequestration, which is similar to what is found in ITP without HIV infection. In clinical practice, however, this study is rarely necessary. Elevated

platelet-associated immunoglobulins (often higher than those with chronic ITP) are frequently seen. Indirect tests for antiplatelet antibodies also are usually positive. Circulating immune complexes are found in two-thirds of HIV-infected patients. If these tests are positive, it suggests that there is an increased peripheral destruction of platelets.

17. Isn't the bone marrow biopsy the "gold standard" in the diagnosis of ITP?

A bone marrow biopsy should be considered if the etiology of the thrombocytopenia from the above tests is still not clear. The bone marrow biopsy in patients with HIV infection is typically hypercellular with normal or increased numbers of megakaryocytes. Dysmegakaryocytopoiesis may be found occasionally. Hypercellular bone marrow from HIV infection may be a result of "HIV marrow"—failure of production and/or egress of cells rather than a reflection of an increased marrow effort to make platelets. This HIV marrow can suggest that a peripheral destructive process is operative when the process actually may be impaired production. However, if patients are taking medications that are potentially toxic to bone marrow (i.e., trimethoprim-sulfamethoxazole, AZT), a bone marrow biopsy will help assess for this toxicity. Drug toxicity may be evidenced by the presence of vacuolation of erythroid precursors and/or marrow hyperplasia.

18. What is the immunologic cause of thrombocytopenia in HIV-infected persons?

1. Platelet autoantibodies in HIV-infected persons with or without thrombocytopenia are found. These antibodies react with a 25-kilodalton (kd) antigen found on normal platelets but not on other blood cells. Conventional platelet-reactive autoantibodies of the type seen in chronic ITP also are found.

2. Nonspecific deposition of immune complexes on the surface of platelets with subsequent clearance of opsonized platelets may also occur. This hypothesis is supported by the finding of anti-HIV antibodies and the absence of detectable HIV antigens in these immune complexes. Platelets are, in effect, innocent bystanders. Circulating platelet-associated immune complexes may be made of anti-F(ab')$_2$ antibodies complexed with the F(ab')$_2$ portion of normal IgG. Some of these complexes are found to contain anti-HIV antibodies bound to anti–anti-HIV antibodies (anti-idiotypic antibodies). This finding suggests a link between HIV infection and the host's immune response in the etiology of thrombocytopenia.

19. What is the cause of ineffectiveness of bone marrow production in HIV-infected persons?

The direct effect of HIV infection of megakaryocytes may contribute to thrombocytopenia. The presence of viral RNA has been found in the platelets of thrombocytopenic HIV-infected individuals by in situ hybridization. Dysplastic changes of megakaryocytes have also been observed in the bone marrow of HIV-infected individuals. Affected megakaryocytes may not be able to compensate for platelet destruction.

20. When should ITP be treated?

In 11–32% of patients with thrombocytopenia, the disease regresses spontaneously without therapy. Treatment is probably not indicated in patients with thrombocytopenia and no clinical significant bleeding or need for emergency surgery. Those with ITP should not be treated on the basis of the platelet counts alone.

21. When should patients with ITP be transfused?

Traditionally, the threshold for platelet transfusion in asymptomatic patients (for prophylaxis) has been 20,000/μl. There is no clear evidence of an increased bleeding risk with platelet counts <20,000/μl. However, a rapid fall in the platelet count or concomitant fever may increase this bleeding risk. Some reports suggest an increased hemorrhage with platelet counts <1,000/μl. This 20,000/μl guideline was based on studies done on patients with leukemia, not with ITP. The value of platelet transfusion in patients with ITP has not been adequately studied. If a patient is symptomatic, a trial platelet transfusion may be given followed by a platelet count 1 hour later. A patient with increased destruction will not respond appropriately to transfused platelets and there will be little increase in the platelet count. A patient with bone marrow failure should respond with an increased platelet count after the transfusion (approximately 10,000 platelets/μl increase per transfused unit). Platelet transfusion also may be considered when an invasive procedure is planned (i.e., tooth extraction, bronchoscopy, colonoscopy). Tooth extraction is the ultimate test for hemostasis, and careful preprocedural evaluation is needed. It is here where the role for intravenous immunoglobulin (IV IgG) is more clear (see below).

22. What drug therapies should be considered in thrombocytopenic patients?
AZT should be tried first when thrombocytopenia is not clinically significant. AZT has been found to increase platelet levels within 2 weeks of initiation of therapy. The effect of AZT on thrombocytopenic patients may be explained by the mechanism described above (see question 19).

Intravenous (IV) IgG is transiently effective in most patients. IV IgG can be used prior to elective surgery or when a more immediate response is clinically indicated (i.e., acute hemorrhage). The doses commonly used are either 1 gm/kg for 1 day or 2–3 consecutive days or 400 mg/kg for 5 consecutive days. The use of IV IgG is limited by the transient effects, high cost, and the usual need for hospitalization.

Adrenal glucocorticoids have a 70–90% response rate. When conventional doses of corticosteroids are given, they are relatively well tolerated. Prednisone, 80 mg/day, in a divided dose should begin to raise platelet counts in 3–5 days, but few patients maintain their response when the steroids are discontinued.

Danazol has been reported to have some efficacy and can spare the use of adrenal glucocorticoids. However, long-term remission on danazol alone has not been established. Danazol has been used in patients with ITP without HIV infection with a slightly better response rate than in HIV-infected patients with ITP. Danazol is an attenuated androgen with mild virilizing effects. The commonly used dose is 300–800 mg daily. Response is usually seen within 2 months, but it may take up to 6 months with lower doses. Danazol is generally well tolerated. Other side effects include fluid retention, persistent nausea, and hepatitis.

Splenectomy has a 75% response rate. Owing to the infectious complications, splenectomy should be performed only for persistence of profound symptomatic thrombocytopenia either steroid dependent or unresponsive to treatment. Antipneumococcal vaccination must be provided ideally 10–14 days prior to splenectomy.

Alpha-interferon (alpha-IFN) given in low doses (3 million units three times weekly) has been tried in a few cases and found to be effective. Alpha-IFN may provide antiretroviral action and thus may be beneficial to the HIV-infected thrombocytopenic patients.

In one study,[19] anti-rhesus antibodies (Anti-Rh$_0$(D) immunoglobulin) injected into Rh+(D+) patients was found to be effective in 9 of 14 patients.

23. Are there any risks of treatment in thrombocytopenic HIV-infected patients?
HIV-infected persons are already immunocompromised and they often have other coexisting opportunistic infections. The use of glucocorticoids and danazol depresses macrophage and lymphocyte function in these persons already at risk. Severe infections complicating immunosuppressive treatments have been reported. Steroids should be avoided in hepatitis B surface antigen carriers. The possible contribution of immunosuppressive therapy to the development of AIDS is unclear. Long-term use of steroids should be avoided because of these and other significant side effects.

24. Why don't individuals with ITP have significant bleeding?
Thrombocytopenia is fairly well tolerated in HIV-infected patients with ITP. It appears that there are two factors contributing to the low incidence of significant bleeding. One is the better quality of the platelet present in ITP. The circulating platelets are relatively young owing to increased production and early release, and young platelets function more efficiently. This is different from thrombocytopenia caused by underproduction as a result

of bone marrow failure in which bleeding may be life threatening (i.e.; hypoplasia due to AZT toxicity). Another reason is that platelet factor 3 (PF_3) is released when platelets are destroyed. PF_3 presence in increased amounts accelerates the intrinsic clotting pathway. This will, in turn, offset the risk of significant bleeding.

25. Does the presence of ITP predict the clinical course of HIV illness?
The process of thrombocytopenia is not a prognostic factor in HIV-seropositive persons. However, earlier studies reported that the frequency of thrombocytopenia was inversely correlated with the CD4+ lymphocyte counts. The incidence of thrombocytopenia was found to be 2.9% with CD4 cells >700/μl and 10.8% with CD4 cells <250/μl.

BIBLIOGRAPHY

ANEMIA

1. Aboulafia DM, Mitsuyasu RT: Hematologic abnormalities in AIDS. Oncol Clin North Am 5:195, 1991.
2. Groopman JE, Faber D: Hematopoietic growth factors in AIDS. Semin Oncol 19:608, 1992.
3. de Mayolo JA, Temple JD: Pure red cell aplasia due to parvovirus B19 infection in a man with HIV infection. South Med J 83:1480, 1990.
4. Donahue RE, Johnson MM, Zon Li, et al: Suppression of in-vitro hematopoesis following human immunodeficiency virus infection. Nature 326:200, 1987.
5. Henry DH, Beall GN, Benson CA, et al: Recombinant human erythropoietin in the treatment of anemia associated with human immunodeficiency virus (HIV) infection and Zidovudine therapy: Overview of four clinical trials. Ann Intern Med 117:739, 1992.
6. Herbert V: B12 deficiency in AIDS. JAMA 260:2837, 1988.
7. Fischl M, Galpin JE, Levine JD, et al: Recombinant human erythropoietin for patients with AIDS treated with Zidovudine. N Engl J Med 322:1448, 1990.
8. Telen MJ, Robert KB, Barlett JA: HIV associated autoimmune hemolytic anemia: Report of a case and review of the literature. J AIDS 3:933, 1990.
9. Zon Li, Groopman JE: Hematological manifestations of the human immunodeficiency virus (HIV). Semin Hematol 25:208–218, 1988.

ITP

10. Abrams DI, Kiprov DD, Goedert JJ, et al: Antibodies to human T-lymphotropic virus type III and development of the acquired immunodeficiency syndrome in homosexual men presenting with immune thrombocytopenia. Ann Intern Med 104:47–50, 1986.
11. Bel-Ali Z, Dufour V, Najean Y: Platelet kinetics in human immunodeficiency virus induced thrombocytopenia. Am J Hematol 26:299–304, 1987.
12. Bettaieb A, Fromont P, Louache F, et al: Presence of cross-reactive antibody between human immunodeficiency virus (HIV) and platelet glycoproteins in HIV-related immune thrombocytopenic purpura. Blood 80:162–169, 1992.
13. Beutler E: Platelet transfusions: The 20,000/μL trigger. Blood 81:1411–1413, 1993.
14. Eyster ME, Rabkin CS, Hilgartner MW, et al: Human immunodeficiency virus-related conditions in children and adults with hemophilia: Rates, relationship to CD4 counts, and predictive value. Blood 81(3):828–834, 1993.
15. Gaydos LA, Freireich EJ, Mantel N: The qualitative relation between platelet count and hemorrhage in patients with acute leukemia. N Engl J Med 266:905–909, 1962.
16. Karpatkin S: Immunologic thrombocytopenic purpura in HIV-seropositive homosexuals, narcotic addicts and hemophiliacs. Semin Hematol 25(3):219–229, 1988.
17. Louache F, Bettaieb A, Henri A, et al: Infection of megakaryocytes by human immunodeficiency virus in seropositive patients with immune thrombocytopenic purpura. Blood 78(7):1697–1705, 1991.
18. Northfelt DW, Kaplan LD, Abrams DI: Continuous, low dose therapy with Interferon-A for human immunodeficiency virus (HIV)–related immune thrombocytopenic purpura. Am J Hematol 38:238–239, 1991.
19. Oksenhendler E, Bierling P, Brossard Y, et al: Anti-RH immunoglobulin therapy for human immunodeficiency virus–related immune thrombocytopenic purpura. Blood 71(5):1499–1502, 1988.
20. Oksenhendler E, Bierling P, Farcet JP, et al: Response to therapy in 37 patients with HIV-related thrombocytopenic purpura. Br J Haematol 66:491–495, 1987.

III. Malignant Hematology

27. ACUTE LEUKEMIA: CLASSIFICATION AND LABORATORY EVALUATION

Mitchell A. Bitter, M.D.

1. What are the findings in the complete blood count (CBC) and leukocyte differential in patients with acute leukemia (AL)?

AL is typically associated with cytopenias in the CBC, and blasts in the peripheral blood film. The most constant findings are anemia and thrombocytopenia. Thrombocytopenia is seen in over 90% of cases, with severe thrombocytopenia ($<50 \times 10^9/L$) in more than half. In about half of patients, the WBC will be normal or low, and the absolute neutrophil count is low in over half of cases.

Peripheral blood blasts are usually identified in acute myelogenous leukemia (AML) but are variable in number. Oftentimes, blasts are not identified in the 100-cell count but may be seen if the blood film is scanned at low power.

2. What information is needed from the laboratory before therapy is initiated in the patient with suspected AL?

When a patient with suspected AL is evaluated, hematopathologists and hematologists must address three questions. In order of importance:

1. Is it really AL?
2. Is it AML or acute lymphoblastic leukemia (ALL)?
3. How should the leukemia (AML or ALL) be subclassified?

The importance of the first question is self-evident. Because therapy differs significantly in AML and ALL, the second question is clinically important (see chapter 28). The modalities used to make this distinction are addressed below.

Once a firm diagnosis of AML or ALL has been rendered, subclassification (see below) is undertaken to provide prognostic information, and in some circumstances it will influence the choice of a therapeutic regimen.

3. Which benign conditions are sometimes mistaken for AL in the bone marrow? In the blood film?

It should be stated at the outset that the diagnosis of AL is **not** based primarily on examination of the blood film. Rather a diagnosis of AL should be rendered only after examination of the bone marrow. Both a bone core biopsy and aspirate should be obtained.

In a well-processed specimen, the diagnosis of AL is generally not difficult. Occasionally, benign disorders may be difficult to distinguish from AL. The best examples are (1) florid megaloblastic anemia (may be confused with erythroleukemia); (2) suppressed bone marrows with superimposed infections (e.g., in the alcoholic with pneumonia).

In the peripheral blood film, myelophthisic anemias (anemias due to marrow infiltration), including disseminated tuberculosis or fungal infection, may show a picture of cytopenias and immature mononuclear cells. However, in these disorders, blasts are not generally prominent.

The inexperienced morphologist may have difficulty distinguishing reactive lympho-cytoses, such as in mononucleosis syndromes, from AL. The morphologic findings that help distinguish blasts and reactive blasts are listed and illustrated below.

AL is almost always associated with thrombocytopenia, which is severe ($<50 \times 10^9/L$) in $>50\%$ of cases. Although thrombocytopenia is common in mononucleosis syndromes, it is usually mild. A diagnosis of AL should be reconsidered in the face of a normal or near normal platelet count.

Morphologic Features of Reactive Lymphs and Blasts

	BLAST	REACTIVE LYMPH
Size	Large	Large
Nuclear/cytoplasmic ratio	Higher	Lower
Nucleoli	May be prominent	May be prominent
Chromatin	Fine	Clumped

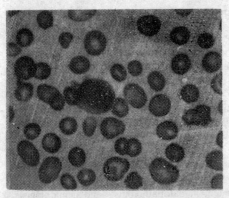

Myeloblast. Myeloblasts are generally two to four times the size of the red blood cells. Their chromatin is finely granular, and one to three nucleoli are often seen. The nuclear to cyto-plasmic volume ratio is generally high (relatively little cytoplasm is seen). Granules or Auer rods may be present in the cytoplasm (not shown). (See also Figure 7, Color Plates.)

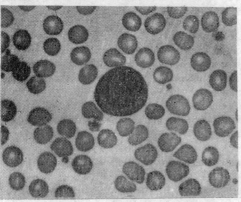

Reactive lymph. Like the myeloblast, the reactive lymph may be a large cell, and a nucleolus may be seen (not shown). Gran-ules may even be present in the cytoplasm (not shown). The reactive lymph is dis-tinguished from the blast by its coarser chromatin (note the clumped chromatin) and its somewhat lower nuclear to cyto-plasmic ratio. (See also Figure 5, Color Plates.)

4. How is AML distinguished from ALL?

As discussed above, after a definitive diagnosis of AL is made, the choice of a therapeutic regimen depends on whether the leukemia is ALL or AML. The two most important modalities used to distinguish AML from ALL are morphologic examination and cyto-chemistry. These are low cost and may be rapidly performed. In difficult cases, more costly and time-consuming studies may be required.

In about 80–90% of cases, the distinction between AML and ALL can be readily made by the experienced morphologist. Morphologic differences between myeloblasts and lymphoblasts are listed and illustrated below. However, in some cases, morphologic distinction is difficult or impossible. Furthermore, even the experienced morphologist is occasionally surprised when a case that was thought to be AML turns out to be ALL and vice versa. Therefore, at a minimum, myeloperoxidase or Sudan black B stains, which are positive in blasts of AML, should be performed to confirm the morphologic impression in any new AL. These stains are rapid and can be performed within an hour, if need be, either on blood (if blasts are present) or marrow aspirate. Other modalities useful in difficult cases and that are performed regularly in some institutions include the following:

1. Immunophenotyping by flow cytometry or immunocytochemistry for lymphoid and myeloid antigens.

2. Detection of terminal deoxynucleotidyl transferase (TdT), a nuclear protein seen in >95% of ALL and 15% of AML.

3. Cytogenetics, which show different abnormalities in AML versus ALL.

4. Immunoglobulin and T-cell receptor gene rearrangement studies.

The results of cytogenetic and gene rearrangement studies are generally not back in time to influence initial therapy.

Features of Myeloblasts and Lymphoblasts

	MYELOBLAST	LYMPHOBLAST
Size	Large	Smaller
Amount of cytoplasm	More	Less
Nucleoli	Conspicuous	Often inconspicuous
Granules	Frequent, fine	Uncommon, coarse
Auer rods	Observed in 50%	Absent
Myeloperoxidase	Positive	Negative

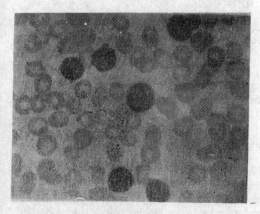

Lymphoblasts. As compared with the myeloblast, lymphoblasts are smaller (cell size one and a half to three times that of the red blood cells). They have inconspicuous nucleoli, coarser chromatin, and scant cytoplasm.

5. How is ALL subclassified?

After a diagnosis of AL is made, and it is determined to be ALL (see question 11 for AML subclassification), the disorder is subclassified in a number of ways. Subclassification provides prognostic information and may be used to stratify patients to receive different therapeutic regimens. Classification is based on:

1. Clinical parameters such as age, blood counts, and performance status (see chapter 28)

2. Morphology of the blasts

3. Immunophenotype of the blasts

4. Pattern of cytogenetic abnormalities

6. Is morphologic classification of ALL prognostically significant?
ALL is classified into three subtypes (L1, L2, and L3) based on the morphology of the blasts. This is known as the French-American-British (FAB) System of Classification. In adults, the great majority of ALLs are L1 and L2. This distinction (L1 versus L2) has, at best, minor prognostic significance. A small number of cases (~3-5%) are L3. These patients have a disorder that overlaps with Burkitt's lymphoma, and although they represent an uncommon subtype, they are important to distinguish for therapeutic purposes.

7. Is immunologic classification clinically significant?
In myeloid cells, lineage (i.e., neutrophil versus eosinophil) and stage of maturation (i.e., blast versus promyelocyte) can often be determined based on morphology. This is not true for lymphocytes. You cannot generally tell a T cell from a B cell based on morphology, and only gross stages of maturation are morphologically distinguishable—lymphoblast versus lymphocyte. Therefore, lineage and stage of maturation are determined based on the reactivity of the malignant population with a number of antibodies to cell surface constituents either using flow cytometry or immunocytochemistry.

ALL is subclassified into a number of immunologic categories. An abbreviated listing is given below. In univariate analyses, these groups differ in prognosis. However, immunologic phenotype is sometimes correlated with other prognostic factors. For instance, patients with T-cell ALL often have a high WBC, which is associated with poorer prognosis. Immature B-lineage ALL in the elderly is often associated with the t(9;22) (Philadelphia chromosome), which portends a dismal outlook (see below). Therefore, in multivariate analyses, the prognostic importance of immunologic classification is lessened.

Immunologic Classification of ALL

SUBTYPE	MAJOR MARKERS	FREQUENCY (%)
B-precursor (common ALL)	TdT+, CD19+, CD10+	75
T-ALL	TdT+, CD7+	20
B-ALL	CD19+, SIg+	5

TdT = terminal deoxynucleotidyl transferase; SIg = monoclonal surface immunoglobulin.

8. What are the clinical and laboratory features of T-cell ALL?
Patients with T-ALL are often teens or young adults with a male predominance. In more than 50%, the leukemic population in the thymus forms a mediastinal mass. Patients tend to have high WBC, often over $50 \times 10^9/L$.

9. For prognosis and therapeutic decision making, what is the most important cytogenetic abnormality in ALL?
By far the most important cytogenetic abnormality in adult ALL is the t(9;22) (Philadelphia chromosome). This reciprocal translocation between the long arms of chromosomes 9 and 22 bring together the *abl* proto-oncogene (9q34) and the *bcr* gene (22q11). A fusion gene is formed that encodes a protein with high tyrosine kinase activity, which is important in leukemogenesis.

This translocation is most strongly associated with chronic myelogenous leukemia in which it is observed in 95% of patients. However, it is also present in 20-30% of adults with ALL, and over half of all ALL in the elderly may be associated with the t(9;22). The presence of this translocation may identify patients with little chance (0-20%) of long-term remission after conventional ALL chemotherapy. The t(9;22) is associated with immature B-lineage in most cases. This association may account for the poorer prognosis of immature B-lineage ALL, as compared with T-cell ALL, which has been observed in some studies of adult ALL. This clinically important genetic rearrangement may be detected by molecular genetic methods in addition to traditional cytogenetics.

10. Overall, which clinical and laboratory findings are most important in determining prognosis in ALL?

Because ALL is most commonly seen in children, more is known about prognostic factors in children than in adults. Although a number of factors bear on prognosis, the most important in children are age, WBC, cytogenetics, and response to initial chemotherapy. In adults, WBC, cytogenetics, and response to chemotherapy are important, as are factors relating to the ability of the patient to withstand induction chemotherapy such as age and performance status.

11. How is AML subclassified?

Like ALL, AML is subclassified based on: (1) clinical parameters, (2) morphology, and (3) cytogenetics. Immunologic subclassification is less important than in ALL. Marker studies are most useful in identifying minimally differentiated AML (M0) and myeloid lineages that do not express myeloperoxidase such as acute megakaryoblastic leukemias (M7).

12. Is morphologic classification of AML clinically important?

AML is subclassified morphologically into the eight types listed below. This is the FAB System of Classification of AML. These subtypes have some clinical differences such as the propensity of monoblastic leukemia (M5) to infiltrate tissues; however, with the exception of one subtype—acute promyelocytic leukemia (APL, M3), treatment is generally the same for all FAB subtypes.

Classification of AML

M0	AML with minimal differentiation
M1	AML without maturation
M2	AML with maturation
M3	Acute promyelocytic leukemia
M4	Acute myelomonocytic leukemia
M5	Acute monocytic leukemia
M6	Acute erythroleukemia
M7	Acute megakaryoblastic leukemia

It is critical to diagnose APL correctly and to differentiate it from other subtypes of AML. APL accounts for about 10% of patients with AML. Approximately 70% of these patients have laboratory evidence of disseminated intravascular coagulation (DIC) at the time of presentation, which is often exacerbated by the initiation of conventional chemotherapy.

In the past, these patients had a high mortality rate during induction chemotherapy; however, patients who survived induction chemotherapy had an excellent chance of long-term disease free survival. Recently, it has been shown that patients respond well to all-*trans*-retinoic acid, which may induce a complete remission in most patients with far less toxicity than conventional chemotherapy. Future investigation regarding this treatment will combine all-*trans*-retinoic acid with conventional combination chemotherapy.

13. What do the abnormal promyelocytes in APL look like?

As will be discussed below, APL is associated with a particular chromosomal translocation. However, because of the prolonged turnaround time of cytogenetic studies, the diagnosis of APL is generally a morphologic one, with cytochemistry and immunologic markers serving as useful adjuncts.

In the most common form of APL, Wright-stained smears of the leukemic cells show lobated or kidney-shaped nuclei with the cytoplasm stuffed with scarlet-staining granules. Auer rods are prominent and many may be seen in a single cell. About 25% of APL cases are more difficult to recognize because the granules are below the limit of resolution of the light microscope. Therefore, the cells often appear agranular. These "microgranular" APLs must be recognized by their nuclear features alone. Many of these cases are misdiagnosed as other forms of AML. Patients with microgranular APL have the same problems with DIC as do patients with the more common form of APL, and they respond well to all-*trans*-retinoic acid.

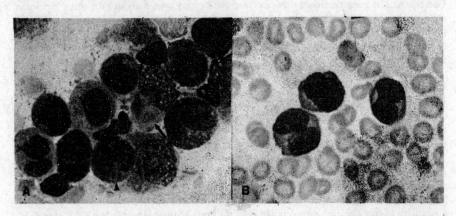

A, Hypergranular acute promyelocytic leukemia (M3). The arrowhead indicates an abnormal promyelocyte showing the typical bilobed nucleus. The arrow shows a degenerating cell with numerous Auer rods in its cytoplasm. *B*, Microgranular acute promyelocytic leukemia (M3V). Like the hypergranular promyelocytes depicted in *A*, these cells from a patient with the microgranular variant of APL show the typical bilobed nuclei. However, the heavy cytoplasmic granulation observed in the hypergranular form is not observed in the microgranular variant. These cases are easily mistaken for monocytic leukemia by the inexperienced morphologist. (See also Figure 8, Color Plates.)

14. Which cytogenetic abnormalities in AML are favorable and which are unfavorable?

Cytogenetic abnormalities are detected in about 80% of cases of AML. Several of them are correlated with clinical findings and prognosis. Three cytogenetic abnormalities have been considered by many to be prognostically favorable. The t(15;17) is specific for APL and, in some centers, all or nearly all patients with APL have had this abnormality. The clinical findings of APL are discussed above and in chapter 28. The t(8;21) and certain abnormalities of chromosome 16, including a pericentric inversion (the inv[16]), have been considered to be favorable. These patients have had extremely high rates of complete remission (>90%); however, remissions may not be particularly durable (in contrast to the t([15;17]). In some studies, but not in others, patients with the inv(16) have had an extremely high incidence of central nervous system relapse.

Many studies have shown that deletions involving the long arms of chromosomes 5 and 7 are associated with therapy-related AML (t-AML). In some studies, 60–80% of t-AMLs are associated with these abnormalities. T-AML and deletions involving the long arms of chromosomes 5 and 7 are considered to auger a poor prognosis.

BIBLIOGRAPHY

1. Bitter MA, LeBeau MM, Rowley JD, et al: Associations between morphology, karyotype and clinical features in myeloid leukemias. Hum Pathol 18:211–255, 1987.
2. Borowitz MJ: Acute lymphoblastic leukemia. In Knowles DM (ed): Neoplastic Hematopathology. Baltimore, Williams & Wilkins, 1992, pp 1295–1314.
3. Cheson BD, Cassileth PA, Head DR, et al: Report of the National Cancer Institute-sponsored workshop in definitions of diagnosis and response in acute myeloid leukemia. J Clin Oncol 8:813–819, 1990.
4. Glass JP, Van Tassel P, Keathing MJ, et al: Central nervous system complications of a newly recognized subtype of leukemia: AMML with a pericentric inversion of chromosome 16. Neurology 37:639–644, 1987.
5. Larson RA, Williams SF, LeBeau MM, et al: Acute myelomonocytic leukemia with abnormal eosinophils and inv(16) or t(16;16) has a favorable prognosis. Blood 68:1242–1249, 1986.

6. Lestingi TM, Hooberman AL: Philadelphia chromosome-positive acute lymphoblastic leukemia. Hematol Oncol Clin North Am 7:161–175, 1993.
7. Litz CE, Brunning RD: Acute myeloid leukemias. In Knowles DM (ed): Neoplastic Hematopathology. Baltimore, Williams & Wilkins, 1992, pp 1315–1349.
8. Samuels BL, Larson RA, LeBeau MM, et al: Specific chromosomal abnormalities in acute nonlymphocytic leukemia correlate with drug susceptibility in vivo. Leukemia 2:79–83, 1988.
9. Schiffer CA, Lee EJ, Tomiyasu T, et al: Prognostic impact of cytogenetic abnormalities in patients with de novo acute nonlymphocytic leukemia. Blood 73:263–270, 1989.
10. Walters R, Kantarjian HM, Keating MJ, et al: The importance of cytogenetic studies in adult lymphocytic leukemia. Am J Med 89:579–587, 1990.
11. Warrell RP, Frankel SR, Miller WH, et al: Differentiation therapy of acute promyelocytic leukemia with tretinoin (all-*trans*-retinoic acid). N Engl J Med 324:1385–1393, 1991.

28. ACUTE MYELOGENOUS AND LYMPHOCYTIC LEUKEMIA

Nicholas J. DiBella, M.D.

1. Describe the laboratory features that would make one suspect that a patient has acute leukemia.

White count is elevated in over half of patients; however, approximately 15% will have a normal white blood count and 33% of patients will present with neutropenia. The presence of blasts in the peripheral smear is noted in 85%. Over 80% of patients will also have anemia and thrombocytopenia. Thus, the absence of anemia or thrombocytopenia typically militates against a diagnosis of acute leukemia.

2. What is the differential diagnosis of pancytopenia or isolated neutropenia?

Aplastic anemia, bone marrow replacement with other hematologic malignancies, including lymphoma, myelofibrosis, myelodysplastic syndromes, hypersplenism, immune cytopenia such as associated with lupus, HIV infections, or drug toxicity; megaloblastic anemias to include vitamin B12 or folate deficiency and hypersplenism.

3. The French-American-British (FAB) classification lists eight different subtypes of acute myelocytic leukemia. Give at least three of these subtypes.

Acute myeloblastic leukemia with minimal differentiation	M0
Acute myeloblastic leukemia without maturation	M1
Acute myeloblastic leukemia with maturation	M2
Hypergranular acute promyelocytic leukemia	M3
Acute myelomonocytic leukemia	M4
Acute monocytic leukemia	M5
Erythroleukemia	M6
Acute megakaryoblastic leukemia	M7

4. Name clinical features that distinguish acute monocytic leukemia from the other subtypes.

There is more frequent involvement of the gums, skin, and central nervous system.

5. If the pathologist reports that the bone marrow stain for myeloperoxidase and Sudan black stain are positive, which kind of acute leukemia should be suspected—acute myelocytic leukemia (AML) or acute lymphocytic leukemia (ALL)?

AML. To summarize, AML is Sudan black positive and myeloperoxidase positive. ALL is negative for these two stains but can be positive for periodic acid–Schiff (PAS).

6. Do patients with AML usually require prophylactic central nervous system (CNS) therapy?
No. Patients with AML rarely develop meningeal leukemia compared with patients with ALL.

7. Is granulocyte colony-stimulating factor (G-CSF) contraindicated in patients with ALL?
No. There is no risk of stimulating the blasts with G-CSF. G-CSF presumably stimulates only granulocytic blasts and not lymphoblasts. There is still some controversy as to whether it is contraindicated in AML.

8. Is disseminated intravascular coagulation (DIC) associated with acute promyelocytic leukemia (M3)?
Yes, presumably because the granules contained in promyelocytes when released can trigger the coagulation cascade, that is, they are thrombogenic.

9. Should allopurinol be started prior to therapy in patients with both AML and ALL?
Yes. Hyperuricemia can occur in either form of acute leukemia but may be more common in ALL owing to rapid lysis of blasts that can result in renal insufficiency without adequate hydration and allopurinol therapy.

10. What is the overall cure rate in AML?
Although the complete remission rate is quite high, one must distinguish complete remission rate from cure rate. If the leukemia recurs in the first five years despite an initial complete remission, then the chance for cure diminishes accordingly. In general, the chance for a cure in AML is between 15 and 30% as opposed to an initial complete remission rate of 65–80% in most adults under the age of 60 years.

11. Which two chemotherapeutic drugs are most often used in the treatment of AML?
Cytosine arabinoside (ARA-C) and daunorubicin.

12. Which drugs are typically used in the treatment of ALL?
The most commonly used drugs include vincristine, prednisone, daunorubicin, intrathecal methotrexate, and L-asparaginase; maintenance therapy usually includes 6-mercaptopurine and methotrexate.

13. What factors predispose to so-called tumor lysis syndrome?
- High white blood cell count
- Hyperuricemia
- Elevated LDH
- Impaired renal function
- Sepsis
- Dehydration

14. Describe the leukostasis syndrome. How is it managed?
Patients with an exceptionally high white blood cell (WBC) count (generally >100,000) may develop a syndrome resulting from blasts aggregating in the capillaries. The most common manifestations are cardiopulmonary with acute respiratory insufficiency and a pulmonary edema or pneumonia-type picture; central nervous system (CNS) manifestations, including headache and possibly progressing to a strokelike syndrome. This is considered a medical emergency and requires rapid reduction of the WBCs, including leukapheresis, chemotherapy, or CNS radiation. For reasons that are not entirely clear, this syndrome is primarily seen in AML, ALL, and chronic myelogenous leukemia (CML) but rarely in chronic lymphocytic leukemia (CLL).

15. What is a chloroma?
It is an unusual tumor composed of granulocytic malignant cells as is seen in AML; chloroma refers to the green color of the cut surface of these tumors due to the high level of myeloperoxidase. Chloromas sometimes develop prior to the diagnosis of AML or CML.

16. List the poor risk factors in ALL.
- Increasing age after 10 years
- WBC count >15,000
- Male sex
- Presence of the Philadelphia chromosome
- Leukemic involvement of CNS
- L3 morphology

17. What is the cure rate in childhood ALL and adult ALL?
In children, the complete remission rate is generally in excess of 90% and the cure rate at 5 years is at least 50%; patients who complete 2.5–3 years of maintenance therapy without relapse have a >80% chance of cure rate. In adults, one could expect at least a 25% disease-free survival and with some more aggressive regimens, 35–40% 5-year survival.

18. When should human leukocyte antigen (HLA) typing be performed and in which types of acute leukemia?
HLA typing should be performed in patients with either ALL or AML at the time of diagnosis if adequate lymphocytes are present in the peripheral blood and the patient is under the age of 50 years. HLA typing is primarily performed in preparation for possible bone marrow transplantation.

19. Define the following forms of bone marrow transplantation: syngeneic, allogeneic, and autologous.
   Syngeneic refers to bone marrow derived from an identical twin; allogeneic refers to a nonidentical donor who is otherwise HLA compatible; and autologous refers to the patient's own bone marrow.

20. When should bone marrow transplantation be considered in adult ALL or adult AML? What are the results?
Bone marrow transplantation generally should be considered at the time of the first relapse or the second remission in either ALL or AML; some data suggest that transplantation during the first remission may improve the cure rate, but this has not been proved. The results with first relapse or second remission are approximately 25–30% long-term cure rate for both AML and ALL. The value of autologous bone marrow transplantation is not proven.

21. What are potential sites of relapse in ALL?
The CNS, testes, or bone marrow. The primary reason relapse can occur in the CNS and testes is presumably because chemotherapy does not achieve very high concentrations in these tissues and, therefore, the leukemia has the chance to grow in these sites. Prophylaxis of the testes is not generally performed because of the sterilizing potential and the lack of obvious efficacy in improving the cure rate.

22. Should management of patients with neutropenia (<500 absolute neutrophil count) include reverse isolation?
No. There is no proof that reverse isolation decreases the risk of infection.

23. Does the use of prophylactic systemic antibiotics decrease the risk of infection in neutropenia?
No. There is no evidence that their use decreases the risk of infection.

24. When a patient with neutropenia has a fever, should systemic antibiotics be administered even though there is no obvious source of infection?
Yes. Once a patient is neutropenic, urgency is appropriate in starting antibiotics rather than waiting for the cultures to come back positive; the sooner antibiotics are initiated, the better chance of reversing an episode of sepsis or other serious infection.

25. Are there dietary limitations in a patient with neutropenia?
Yes. Patients should not receive fresh fruit or vegetables that may be a source of bacterial contamination.

26. In patients with leukemia, should further chemotherapy be avoided until the neutropenia resolves?
No. Patients need to be treated based on the presence of leukemia in the bone marrow, not based on peripheral neutropenia.

27. How should leukemic involvement of the CNS be managed?
Typically, it is managed by using intrathecal chemotherapy via lumbar puncture or preferably using an Ommaya reservoir; drugs used include cytosine arabinoside or methotrexate. These drugs are administered usually twice a week until the CNS has cleared; if a systemic complete remission is achieved; then monthly thereafter. Hydrocortisone and radiation therapy may also be added.

28. What factors predispose to renal failure in acute leukemia?

Hyperuricemia	Intravenous x-ray contrast material
Sepsis	Renal infiltration by leukemia
Drug toxicity (e.g., aminoglycosides)	

BIBLIOGRAPHY

1. Bennett JM, Catovsky D, Daniel M, et al: Proposed revised criteria for the classification of acute myeloid leukemia. Ann Intern Med 103:626–629, 1985.
2. Cheson BD, Cassileth PA, Head DR, et al: Report on the National Cancer Institute Sponsored Workshop on Definitions of Diagnosis and Response to Acute Myeloid Leukemia. J Clin Oncol 8:813–819, 1990.
3. Cuttner J, Meyer R, Ambinder EP, Young T-H: Hyperleukocytosis in adult leukemia. In Bloomfield CD (ed): Chronic and Acute Leukemias in Adults. The Hague, Martinus Nijhoff, 1985, pp 263–282.
4. Yates J, Glidewell O, Wiernik P, et al: Cytosine arabinoside with daunorubicin or adriamycin for therapy of acute myelocytic leukemia: A CALGB study. Blood 60:454–462, 1982.
5. Clarkson B, Ellis S, Little C, et al: Acute lymphoblastic leukemia in adults. Semin Oncol 12:160–179, 1985.
6. Cohen LF, Balow JE, Magrath IT, et al: Acute tumor lysis syndrome: A review of 37 patients with Burkitt's lymphoma. Am J Med 68:486–491, 1980.
7. Hoelzer D, Thiel E, Loffler H, et al: Prognostic factors in a multicenter study for treatment of acute lymphoblastic leukemias in adults. Blood 71:123–131, 1988.
8. Omura G, Raney M: Longterm survival of adult acute lymphoblastic leukemia: Follow-up of a Southeastern Cancer Study Group Trial. J Clin Oncol 3:1053–1058, 1985.

---

29. CHRONIC LYMPHOCYTIC LEUKEMIA

Robert S. Kantor, M.D.

---

1. Define chronic lymphocytic leukemia.
Chronic lymphocytic leukemia (CLL) is a malignant proliferation of small lymphocytes that tend to accumulate in the bone marrow, peripheral blood, lymph nodes, spleen, and liver. CLL is an indolent disease with a natural history usually measured in years.

2. Which type of lymphocyte is malignant in CLL?
Although a rare form of T-cell CLL exists, nearly all cases arise from relatively well-differentiated B lymphocytes. Note that some investigators use the term "chronic lymphocytic leukemia" to refer to the general category of indolent lymphocytic leukemias, of which there are several (see question 14). In this chapter, CLL refers specifically to B-cell chronic lymphocytic leukemia.

3. How common is CLL?
CLL is the most common type of leukemia, accounting for 30% of all cases. The incidence is 3.9 and 2.0 per 100,000 in men and women, respectively. Ninety percent of patients are over age 50, although rare cases in children do occur.

4. What is the etiology of CLL?
The etiology of CLL is unknown. Although a direct mode of inheritance has not been established, first-degree relatives of patients with CLL carry a three times normal risk of developing CLL or other lymphoid malignancies. Neither radiation nor retroviruses have been implicated as a cause of CLL.

5. Discuss the common symptoms of CLL.
Approximately 25% of patients are asymptomatic and diagnosed as a result of routine clinical or laboratory examination. Those who are symptomatic commonly present with nonspecific complaints such as fatigue and malaise even in the absence of anemia. Specific symptoms such as early satiety or bleeding and bruising can be attributed to splenomegaly and thrombocytopenia, respectively. Occasionally, patients present with infection or have noted lymph node enlargement.

6. What is the significance of fever in patients with CLL?
In the absence of infection, fever is rare in CLL, whereas fever is a common constitutional symptom in other lymphoid neoplasms.

7. Describe the physical findings in CLL.
Lymphadenopathy is present in 80% of patients. Cervical, supraclavicular, and axillary nodes are most commonly involved. The lymph nodes are usually mobile, nontender, and have a rubbery feel. The spleen is enlarged 50–70% of the time and hepatomegaly is present in <50% of patients. Petechiae and bruising are uncommon. Rarely, massive lymphadenopathy may produce extremity lymphedema and biliary, renal, or upper airway obstruction.

8. What are the peripheral blood findings in CLL?
Lymphocytosis is universal, and the absolute lymphocyte count usually exceeds $15 \times 10^9/L$ at the time of diagnosis. Granulocytopenia, anemia, and thrombocytopenia are common. The peripheral blood smear reveals an abundance of relatively normal-appearing small lymphocytes. (See Figure 10, Color Plates.)

9. What is a "smudge cell"?
CLL lymphocytes tend to rupture during preparation of the peripheral smear. These ruptured forms have a distinct appearance known as smudge cells. (See Figure 10, Color Plates.) The presence of smudge cells should always raise the suspicion for CLL.

10. Describe the bone marrow in CLL.
The marrow is always involved. Either focal or diffuse infiltration can be seen on core biopsies. The extent of marrow infiltration directly correlates with prognosis.

11. It is known that patients with CLL are predisposed to infection. What are the immunologic defects associated with CLL?
Granulocytopenia due to marrow infiltration is almost always present. Hypogammaglobulinemia is present 75% of the time, the degree of which directly correlates with clinical stage and risk of infection. Functional abnormalities in B cells and T cells can be demonstrated in virtually all patients.

12. Why do anemia and thrombocytopenia occur in CLL?
The primary reason is disruption of normal marrow hematopoiesis by the infiltrating lymphocytes. Splenomegaly, when present, causes sequestration of normal blood cells.

Autoimmune hemolytic anemia or autoimmune thrombocytopenia may develop and can be particularly troublesome.

13. How is the diagnosis of CLL made?
The history, physical examination, peripheral blood counts, and lymphocyte morphology are usually all that are required to diagnose CLL in the clinical setting. Published criteria for the diagnosis of CLL require peripheral blood lymphocytosis along with either evidence of marrow infiltration or the documentation of B-cell markers (usually by flow cytometry) on the peripheral blood lymphocytes. The bone marrow biopsy and peripheral blood B-cell markers need only be studied when the diagnosis is uncertain or in a research setting.

14. What is the differential diagnosis of CLL?
There are several indolent lymphocytic malignancies related to CLL. These include prolymphocytic leukemia, Waldenström's macroglobulinemia, leukemic phase of lymphomas, hairy cell leukemia, T-cell CLL, adult T-cell leukemia, large granulocytic leukemia, and cutaneous T-cell lymphoma.

Small lymphocytic lymphoma (diffuse, well-differentiated lymphoma) is often diagnosed on lymph node biopsies obtained from patients with CLL. This type of lymphoma is histologically identical to CLL. The distinction between these two entities simply depends on whether or not peripheral blood involvement is present.

15. How is CLL distinguished from these related disorders?
Clinical and morphologic findings are usually sufficient. However, the diagnosis can be confirmed by determining the immunologic phenotype of the malignant lymphocytes using flow cytometry analysis. (See chapter 31, questions 16 and 17, for a discussion of flow cytometry.) Flow cytometry uses monoclonal antibodies to identify cell surface antigens that are unique to an individual type of lymphocyte (e.g., normal cell, CLL cell, T-helper cell).

16. What are the flow cytometry findings in CLL?
A B-cell phenotype is documented by the presence of the cell surface antigens termed CD19, CD20, and CD21. The antigen called CD5 is normally found only on T lymphocytes. However, the diagnosis of CLL is confirmed when CD5 is paradoxically expressed on the same cells that express the above B-cell markers. Flow cytometry has significantly increased our understanding of lymphoid malignancies and is now widely available.

17. What is the natural history of CLL?
The natural history can be determined by the clinical stages of the disease. Patients may be assigned a stage based on the clinical findings and blood counts. A bone marrow biopsy is not necessary to determine the clinical stage. Clinical stage correlates well with expected survival. The Rai and Binet staging systems are commonly encountered.

Rai Staging System for Chronic Lymphocytic Leukemia

STAGE	FINDINGS	MEDIAN SURVIVAL (MONTHS)
0	Lymphocytosis ($>15 \times 10^9/L$)	>150
I	Lymphocytosis plus lymphadenopathy	100
II	Lymphocytosis plus splenomegaly	70
III	Lymphocytosis plus anemia (Hgb $<11/g/dL$)	19
IV	Lymphocytosis plus thrombocytopenia (platelet $<100 \times 10^9/L$)	19

In stages II–IV, lymphadenopathy may be present or absent; in stages III–IV, splenomegaly may be present or absent. Anemia and thrombocytopenia due to an autoimmune syndrome should not be used to determine stage.

18. Are there any other prognostic factors in CLL?
Yes. Other factors that adversely influence survival include disease progression, extensive or diffuse marrow infiltration, a rapid lymphocyte doubling time, and the presence of chromosomal abnormalities on karyotype analysis. The degree of peripheral lymphocytosis does not correlate well with prognosis.

19. At what white blood cell count should treatment be initiated?
This is a trick question. The absolute white blood cell count alone never influences treatment decisions. The white blood cell count can reach very high levels (e.g., >500 × 10^9/L), in asymptomatic patients.

20. If that is true, then when should patients be treated?
As with other indolent lymphoid malignancies (e.g., hairy cell leukemia, low-grade lymphoma), treatment is indicated only when symptoms occur. It has been clearly established that treatment of asymptomatic patients with these disorders does not result in improved survival compared with those treated later when symptoms occur. Asymptomatic patients who are treated are exposed to unnecessary risks of chemotherapy.

Specific indications for treatment include infection, symptomatic or unsightly lymphadenopathy, and symptomatic splenomegaly, anemia, or thrombocytopenia. Constitutional symptoms, such as fatigue and malaise, occasionally necessitate treatment. Hemolytic anemia and immune thrombocytopenia are exceptions, as these disorders require therapy whether or not symptoms occur.

21. What is the optimal treatment for CLL?
Optimal treatment has not yet been defined. Several treatments can control the disease; however, remissions, whether complete or partial, are usually short lived. Alkylating agents such as chlorambucil (Leukeran) or cyclophosphamide (Cytoxan) are typically administered with or without prednisone as initial therapy. Combination chemotherapy is tried next. Recently, the nucleoside analogues fludarabine (Fludara) and 2-chlorodeoxyadenosine (Leustatin or 2-CdA) have been shown to be highly effective even in patients refractory to combination chemotherapy.

22. How effective are the alkylating agents?
About 60% of patients improve with chlorambucil or cyclophosphamide (either agent alone or with prednisone. Ten percent of these responses are complete (disappearance of all measurable disease) and the remaining 50% of responses are partial.

23. What can be done when CLL is resistant to alkylating agents?
Combination chemotherapy such as cyclophosphamide, vincristine (Oncovin), and prednisone (COP regimen) or doxorubicin (Adriamycin) plus COP (CHOP regimen) result in transient improvement about 50% of the time with very few complete responses.

24. What is the role of the nucleoside analogues?
Fludarabine and 2-CdA interfere with adenosine metabolism leading to intracellular accumulation of toxic metabolites and resultant cell death. These drugs each produce complete response rates of 15% and partial response rates of 50% in patients resistant to standard chemotherapy. These drugs are significantly less toxic than standard chemotherapeutic agents. Both drugs are presently under investigation in previously untreated patients and for use in combination with alkylating agents.

25. Are there any other effective therapies for CLL?
Yes. Radiation is useful for localized symptomatic lymphadenopathy. Biologic treatments such as interferon and interleukin may have activity and are being investigated.

26. What is the cause of death in patients with CLL?
Because CLL is generally a disease of the elderly, 30% die of unrelated causes. Fifty percent die of infection, 15% from complications of therapy, and the remainder from hemorrhage, hemolysis, or vital organ infiltration.

27. Can CLL be cured?
A rare patient under the age of 50 may be cured with high-dose chemotherapy plus radiation therapy, followed by HLA-matched, sibling donor, bone marrow transplantation. However, even though long disease-free intervals are often achieved with standard therapy, CLL is not considered to be a curable disease. It remains to be seen whether the use of fludarabine or 2-CdA as early or initial treatment or in combination with standard therapies can improve the long-term prognosis. Regardless, it is apparent that the natural history of CLL may be significantly improved by these new agents.

BIBLIOGRAPHY

1. Foon KA, Rai KR, Gale RP: Chronic lymphocytic leukemia: New insights into biology and therapy. Ann Intern Med 113:525, 1990.
2. Foon KA, Todd RF: Immunologic classification of leukemia and lymphoma. Blood 68:1, 1986.
3. Keating MJ, Kantarjian H, Talpaz M, et al: Fludarabine: A new agent with major activity against chronic lymphocytic leukemia. Blood 74:19, 1989.
4. Lee RG, Bithell TC, Foerster J, et al (eds): Wintrobe's Clinical Hematology. Philadelphia, Lea & Febiger, 1993.
5. Piro LD, Carrera CJ, Beutler E, Carson DA: 2-Chlorodeoxyadenosine: An effective new agent for the treatment of chronic lymphocytic leukemia. Blood 72:1069, 1990.
6. Rai KR, Sawitsky A, Cronkite EP, et al: Clinical staging of chronic lymphocytic leukemia. Blood 46:219, 1975.
7. Tefferi A, Phyliky RL: A clinical update on chronic lymphocytic leukemia. I. Diagnosis and prognosis. Mayo Clin Proc 67:349, 1992.
8. Tefferi A, Phyliky RL: A clinical update on chronic lymphocytic leukemia. II. Critical analysis of current chemotherapeutic modalities. Mayo Clin Proc 67:457, 1992.
9. Williams WJ, Beutler E, Erslev AJ, Lichtman MA (eds): Hematology. New York, McGraw-Hill, 1990.

30. CHRONIC MYELOGENOUS LEUKEMIA

Michael T. Parra, M.D.

1. What is chronic myelogenous leukemia (CML)?
CML, one of the myeloproliferative disorders, is characterized by the clonal proliferation of an early stem cell. This generally results in an elevated number of granulocytes, but erythroid and megakaryocytic cells also may be elevated. Clinical distinction of CML from the other myeloproliferative disorders (essential thrombocytosis, polycythemia vera, and myeloid metaplasia) is often difficult. CML can be distinguished cytogenetically by identification of the Philadelphia chromosome in the leukemic cells.

2. What is the Philadelphia chromosome?
The Philadelphia chromosome results from a balanced translocation of material between chromosomes 9 and 22, t(9:22) (q34; q11). This translocation transposes a protooncogene called c-*abl* from its normal location on chromosome 9 to a new location on chromosome 22 that is called the breakpoint cluster region, *bcr*. The result is creation of a new

fusion gene, *bcr/abl*. The protein product of this fusion gene functions as a tyrosine kinase, similarly to c-*abl* but with increased enzymatic activity. This translocation can be demonstrated, with various molecular techniques, in >95% of individuals diagnosed with CML.

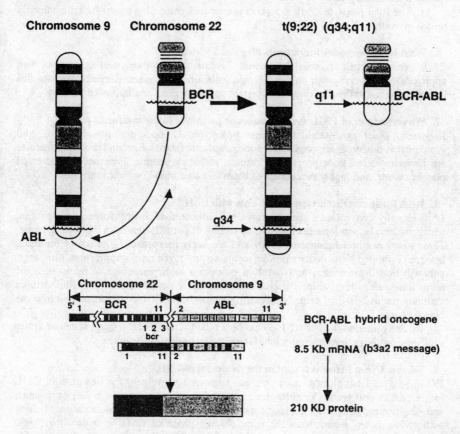

The Philadelphia chromosome in CML and associated molecular abnormalities. (From Kantarjian HM, Deisseroth A, Kurzrock R, et al: Chronic myelogenous leukemia: A concise update. Blood 82:691–703, 1993, with permission.)

3. Does the *bcr/abl* gene cause CML?

Yes. This gene has been placed into bone marrow cells and injected into irradiated mice. The cells then repopulate the killed bone marrow of the mice, which develop clinical disorders consistent with CML. This important finding suggests not only that the *bcr/abl* gene causes CML, but also that it is the only genetic event necessary for the development of CML.

4. What is the typical clinical presentation of CML?

The clinical presentation of CML is varied. Presentation can occur as young as 15 years or as old as 80 years. About 40% of all patients are asymptomatic at the time of diagnosis. In 20% of patients hepatosplenomegaly is present, and an additional 54% present with only splenomegaly. Approximately 50% of all patients present with anemia (hemoglobin <12gm/dl), and approximately 60% of all patients present with white blood cell counts >100,000/dl. (See Figure 9, Color Plates.) Occasionally significant weight loss, fever, chills, anorexia, and fatigue also may be associated with the disease.

5. What are the three phases of CML?

1. The **indolent** or **chronic phase** of CML generally lasts about 3 years.
2. The **accelerated phase** lasts for 1–1½ years. Treatment in this phase can result in return to a chronic phase.
3. The **final phase** of CML is a short accelerated phase (3–6 months) that commonly results in death.

6. What is the prognosis for patients diagnosed with CML?

CML generally runs its course in about 7 years. In the past, median survival was approximately 3 years, with only 20% of patients alive at 5 years. Recently, survival has improved because of earlier diagnosis, better supportive care, and improved therapy.

7. Which features of CML assist in assessing prognosis in the individual patient?

In general, older age, weight loss, hepatosplenomegaly, poor performance status, and symptoms at diagnosis are considered poor prognostic factors. Certain laboratory features are also considered poor prognostic features, including anemia, increased or decreased platelet counts, and higher percentage of blasts in either blood or bone marrow.

8. What is the current therapy for patients with CML?

Until recently conventional therapy for CML consisted of hydroxyurea and busulfan, which produce hematologic remission in up to 80% of patients treated in the chronic phase. These drugs can be administered orally and are fairly inexpensive. The use of busulfan, however, is limited by its toxicity profile, including prolonged myelosuppression. Moreover, although both hydroxyurea and busulfan produce a high percentage of remissions, the remissions are not durable. Patients demonstrate a persistence of the Philadelphia chromosome in >90% of cells. Neither drug alters the inevitable transformation into the blastic phase.

Recently interferon alpha (INF-α) has been used to treat CML; this agent demonstrates similar hematologic response rates and far greater cytogenetic responses.

9. What is INF-α? How is it used in the treatment of CML?

INF-α, derived from human leukocytes, has been used actively for the treatment of CML for the past several years. Complete hematologic response rates are seen in 70% of patients, and 40% achieve complete cytogenetic remission. The median survival of patients treated with INF-α–based regimens in the early chronic phase of CML is approximately 60 months. Long-term reports at this time indicate that 25% of patients maintain a durable cytogenetic remission. These data suggest the superiority of INF-α over conventional therapy, as measured by cytogenetic response and survival.

10. What are the toxicities of INF-α?

INF-α is associated with both early and late toxicity. Early toxicities, characterized by a flulike illness, are generally self-limiting as tachyphylaxis develops within 1–2 weeks. Symptoms can be managed by (1) treating with Tylenol, (2) administering doses at bedtime, (3) starting therapy at 50% of the target dose, and (4) substituting hydroxyurea for INF-α therapy until the white cell count can be decreased to <20,000/dl.

Late effects of INF-α therapy include fatigue, weight loss, neurologic toxicity, and immune-mediated toxicity. These symptoms result in discontinuation of therapy in a significant number of patients.

11. Is splenectomy indicated in the treatment of CML?

Generally not. Studies have demonstrated no survival advantage for patients who undergo splenectomy. Splenectomy may be considered, however, for symptomatic relief (when splenomegaly is massive) or when hypersplenism limits therapy (e.g., anemia or thrombocytopenia requiring dose reduction of drugs).

12. What is the role of bone marrow transplantation in treatment of CML?

Of patients treated with allogenic bone marrow transplantation, 38% are disease-free at 5 years. Because CML runs its course in about 7 years, bone marrow transplantation may offer hope for an otherwise incurable disease. The therapy, however, is risky. Depending on the age of the patient, it can be associated with a mortality rate up to 25%.

13. When should bone marrow transplantation be considered for patients with CML?

This is a controversial subject. Allogenic bone marrow transplantation is a highly toxic therapy but may offer cure. In general, younger patients in the early chronic phase who have a matching related donor will do better and should be offered bone marrow transplantation. Because of the associated morbidity and mortality, patients who do not have a related donor, who are older (>55 years), or who are in the later phases of CML should be treated first with alpha interferon.

BIBLIOGRAPHY

1. Alimena G, et al: Interferon alpha 2B as therapy for the Philadelphia chromosome positive chronic myelogenous leukemia. Blood 72:642, 1988.
2. Canellos GT: Chronic granulocytic leukemia. Med Clin North Am 60:1001, 1988.
3. Cervantes F, Rozman C: A multi-variant analysis of prognostic factors in chronic myeloid leukemia. Blood 60:1298, 1982.
4. Golde DW, Champlin RE: Chronic myelogenous leukemia: Recent advances. Blood 65:1039, 1985.
5. Goldman JM, et al: Bone marrow transplantation for patients with chronic myeloid leukemia. N Engl J Med 314:202, 1986.
6. Kantarjian HM, et al: Characteristics of accelerated disease in chronic myelogenous leukemia. Cancer 61:1441, 1988.
7. Kantarjian HM, et al: Chronic myelogenous leukemia: A multi-variant analysis of the associations of patient characteristics and therapy with survival. Blood 66:1326, 1985.
8. Kantarjian HM, Deisseroth A, Kurzrock R, et al: Chronic myelogenous leukemia: A concise update. Blood 82:691, 1993.
9. Kluin-Nelenans JC, et al: CML treated by interferon alpha 2B vs. hydroxyurea alone. Blood 80:385A, 1992.
10. Rowley JD: A new consistent chromosomal abnormality in chronic myelocytic leukemia identified by quinacrine, *floricine*, and Giemsa staining. Nature 243:290, 1973.
11. Silver R: Chronic myeloid leukemia: Perspective of the clinical and biological issues of the chronic phase. Hematol Oncol Clin North Am 4:319, 1990.
12. Snyder DS, et al: Treatment of chronic myelogenous leukemia with bone marrow transplantation. Bone Marrow Transplant 4:535, 1990.
13. Sokal JE, et al: Prognostic discrimination: Good risk chronic granulocytic leukemia. Blood 63:789, 1984.

31. HAIRY CELL LEUKEMIA

Robert S. Kantor, M.D.

1. What is hairy cell leukemia (HCL)?

HCL is a malignant disorder of well-differentiated B lymphocytes. HCL is a chronic leukemia whose cell of origin is similar to that of chronic lymphocytic leukemia (CLL); however, the clinical presentation of HCL is quite distinct. HCL was first described in 1958 and was then referred to as leukemic reticuloendotheliosis.

2. Name the three most characteristic features of HCL.
1. Pancytopenia
2. Bone marrow infiltration
3. Splenomegaly

3. Who gets HCL?
HCL is generally a disease of elderly men, although it has been reported in persons in their early 20s. The median age of onset is 50 years and 75% of patients are men.

4. How important is HCL?
HCL is a rare disease. Only 600 cases per year are diagnosed in this country, accounting for 2% of adult leukemia. HCL is quite important though, as research into this rare disorder has broadened our understanding of immunology and led to the development of effective new drugs that are useful in HCL and other lymphoproliferative disorders.

5. What causes HCL?
The etiology of HCL is unknown. Radiation exposure has been associated with HCL, but this remains controversial. There have been isolated familial occurrences; one involved three siblings, all with the HLA A1, B7 haplotype. The retrovirus HTLV-II has been implicated in two atypical cases of T-cell HCL.

6. Why is the disease called "hairy" cell leukemia?
The hairy cell is like no other cell encountered in the peripheral blood and is usually easy to recognize on a Wright-stained smear. (See Figure 11, Color Plates.) Hairy cells are mononuclear with abundant pale cytoplasm. Cytoplasmic projections (pseudopods or microvilli) give the cells their hairy appearance.

7. Describe the clinical features of HCL.
The presenting symptoms of HCL are directly attributable to the cytopenias and splenomegaly.

Clinical Features of HCL

CLINICAL FINDINGS	INCIDENCE (%)
Weakness, fatigue	80
Fever, night sweats	20
Early satiety, weight loss	25
Infection	20–30
Hemorrhage, bruising	20–30
Abdominal pain	20–30
Lymphadenopathy	0–5
Petechiae, ecchymoses	20–30
Hepatomegaly	15
Splenomegaly	90

Note that although most infections in patients with HCL are produced by typical gram-positive cocci and gram-negative rods, there does seem to be a predisposition to atypical mycobacterial infections such as *Mycobacterium avium-intracellulare.*

8. How are these findings different from CLL?
Actually, almost any of the signs and symptoms listed in the above table can be seen in CLL. However, lymphadenopathy almost always accompanies such findings in CLL but is rarely (<5%) encountered in HCL.

9. Why is the term hairy cell leukemia a misnomer?

Only 10–15% of patients with HCL are actually leukemic (WBC count >10 × 10⁹/L). The majority of patients are leukopenic. The laboratory findings are described below.

Laboratory Features of HCL

LABORATORY FINDINGS	INCIDENCE (%)
Leukocytosis	10–15
Leukopenia	65
Granulocytopenia	75
Monocytopenia	90
Anemia	80
Thrombocytopenia	80
Pancytopenia	50
Hairy cells visible on blood smear	85
Elevated liver function tests	10
Monoclonal paraprotein	1–3

10. What are the typical bone marrow features of HCL?

First, a "dry tap" is often encountered on attempting to aspirate the marrow because of fibrosis, which can be demonstrated by silver reticulin staining of the core biopsy. Second, the hairy cells have a "fried egg" appearance because of a halo of clear cytoplasm around the nuclei and distinct cellular borders. The marrow can be either focally or diffusely infiltrated.

11. Describe the TRAP stain. How is it important?

Tartrate-resistant acid phosphatase (TRAP) staining is extremely useful in distinguishing HCL from other similar disorders. Incubation of normal lymphocytes and those of other hematologic disorders with tartrate renders these cells unstainable for acid phosphatase. Hairy cells are resistant to tartrate inhibition (owing to acid phosphatase isoenzyme 5) and readily take up acid phosphatase stain. TRAP activity, once thought to be pathognomonic for HCL, is now known to be rarely present in other lymphoproliferative disorders and thus somewhat limits the usefulness of this test.

12. Name three causes of the pancytopenia often seen in HCL.

1. Disruption of marrow hematopoiesis by HCL infiltration
2. Splenic sequestration of circulating blood cells
3. Dilutional effect of increased plasma volume (which accompanies splenomegaly)

13. How is the diagnosis of HCL made?

The history, examination, and laboratory findings are extremely important. The diagnosis is confirmed by morphologic identification of hairy cells in the blood, marrow, or spleen. TRAP staining, electron microscopy, and flow cytometry (see below) help distinguish HCL from other lymphoproliferative diseases.

14. What is the differential diagnosis of HCL?

Hairy cells are not found in any other disorder. Atypical forms of HCL do exist and must not be confused with other related disorders. The differential diagnosis includes CLL, prolymphocytic leukemia, large granular lymphocytic leukemia, splenic lymphoma with villous lymphocytosis, monocytoid B-cell lymphoma, and the malignant histiocytic syndromes.

15. How is HCL separated from these disorders?

Usually morphology alone is enough. TRAP staining can help, but recall that this is not entirely specific. Electron microscopy is helpful to identify the cytoplasmic projections but is expensive and not available outside major centers. Flow cytometry analysis of circulating or marrow lymphocytes is the most specific, cost-effective test available.

16. What is flow cytometry?
Lymphocytes express cell-specific surface antigens that can be readily identified with fluorescent-labeled monoclonal antibodies (MoAbs). Each type of lymphocyte (e.g., hairy cell, normal cell, CLL cell) expresses a unique set of cellular antigens, thus allowing MoAb identification. A flow cytometer passes individual MoAb-labeled cells through a column where fluorescence is quantified, thus immunologically identifying each individual cell.

17. Why is flow cytometry so important?
Flow cytometry has significantly increased our understanding of HCL and related disorders by generating a complete, reproducible immunologic profile of each such disease. This technique is now available in most major medical centers. When the cellular antigens termed CD11c, CD22, CD25, and B-Ly7 are identified by flow cytometry, the diagnosis of HCL is ensured.

18. Define the natural history of untreated HCL.
Ten percent of patients will have a benign course and never require therapy. Most patients, however, develop progressive pancytopenia and splenomegaly, thus requiring intervention. The median survival for untreated patients is about 5 years.

19. When is treatment for HCL required?
Generally, patients are observed until infection or symptomatic cytopenias or splenomegaly occur.

20. How is HCL treated?
The treatment of HCL has dramatically changed during the last several years. Splenectomy, once the mainstay of therapy, is now virtually contraindicated because of the availability of several highly effective new drug therapies. Treatment options include splenectomy, recombinant human interferon alpha (IFN-α), and the two nucleoside analogues deoxycoformycin (DCF) or 2-chlorodeoxyadenosine (2-CdA). Chemotherapy, hormones, steroids, and radiation are rarely effective.

21. What can splenectomy accomplish?
Splenectomy improves blood counts in 98% of cases owing to removal of splenic sequestration and reduction in plasma volume. However, most patients develop progressive pancytopenia within 1 year on account of progressive marrow disease. Splenectomy is associated with significant perioperative morbidity and a long-term risk of recurrent pyogenic infection. Pneumococcal vaccination should be administerd to all patients who are under consideration for splenectomy.

22. Is interferon alpha effective?
Yes. About 70% of patients improve, but complete responses (normal blood counts, <5% hairy cells in the marrow, and no splenomegaly) are rare. IFN-α is administered subcutaneously for 1 year. Toxicity is significant, and most patients relapse within 1 to 2 years after stopping therapy. Subsequent courses usually lead to drug resistance.

23. How effective are the nucleoside analogues?
Very. These new drugs interfere with adenosine metabolism, leading to intracellular accumulation of toxic metabolites and resultant cell death.

Deoxycoformycin (DCF, Pentostatin) induces complete responses in about 60% of patients and partial improvement in 25%. Most of the complete responses are long lasting. DCF is administered intravenously every other week for 3–6 months. It is highly immunosuppressive with serious infections observed in about one-third of those treated.

2-Chlorodeoxyadenosine (2-CdA, Leustatin) induces complete responses in 90% with the remainder experiencing near-complete responses. These remissions (whether complete or partial) are long lasting, with only a rare patient resistant to therapy or relapsing. 2-CdA is administered via a single 7-day infusion. The only toxicity is culture-negative fever in about 40% of patients.

24. Can HCL be cured?
The initial results with DCF and 2-CdA do suggest a curative potential for HCL. Both drugs have produced complete remissions lasting up to 8 years at the time of this writing. Over 300 patients have now been treated with 2-CdA. Of the 90% complete responders, only about 1% have relapsed. Only time will tell if these long-term remissions will translate into cures. Regardless, it is apparent that the natural history of HCL has been significantly improved by these new therapeutic modalities.

BIBLIOGRAPHY

1. Alexander SD, Spiers TD, Moore D, et al: Remissions in hairy-cell leukemia with pentostatin (2'-deoxycoformycin). N Engl J Med 316:825, 1987.
2. Bouroncle BA, Wiseman BK, Doan CA: Leukemic reticuloendotheliosis. Blood 13:609, 1958.
3. Foon KA, Todd RF: Immunologic classification of leukemia and lymphoma. Blood 68:1, 1986.
4. Golomb HM, Fefer A, Golde DW, et al: Update of a multi-institutional study of 195 patients with hairy cell leukemia treated with interferon alfa-2b. Proc Am Soc Clin Oncol 6:215, 1990.
5. Lee RG, Bithell TC, Foerster J, et al (eds): Wintrobe's Clinical Hematology. Philadelphia, Lea & Febiger, 1993.
6. Piro LD, Carrera CJ, Carson DA, Beutler E: Lasting remissions in hairy cell leukemia induced by a single infusion of 2-chlorodeoxyadenosine. N Engl J Med 322:1117, 1990.
7. Saven A, Piro LD: Treatment of hairy cell leukemia. Blood 79:1111, 1992.
8. Williams WJ, Beutler E, Erslev AJ, Lichtman MA (eds): Hematology. New York, McGraw-Hill, 1990.

32. NON-HODGKIN'S LYMPHOMA: CLASSIFICATION AND PATHOLOGY

Mitchell A. Bitter, M.D.

1. In a patient with several enlarged lymph nodes, which lymph node should be biopsied?
As a general rule, the largest lymph node should be chosen for biopsy. It is always a temptation to biopsy a smaller, superficial node if it is more easily accessible. However, in some cases, the smaller node may not show diagnostic findings and thereby delay diagnosis or even result in an erroneous diagnosis. A common fallacy holds that inguinal lymph nodes should not be biopsied because they may show nonspecific, confusing, histologic changes that may obscure the correct diagnosis. However, if an inguinal node is the largest node, and it does not predate the patient's illness, it should be chosen for biopsy.

2. What kind of lymph node biopsy should be performed? How should a tissue specimen be handled before it gets to the laboratory if lymphoma is suspected?
Unless a lymph node is massive and cannot be removed in toto for technical reasons, all lymph node biopsies should be excisional (rather than incisional). The tissue should be delivered without delay to the pathology department without fixation. If the tissue is placed in fixative, microbiologic cultures and special studies such as molecular genetic tests and cytogenetics cannot be performed. Furthermore, immunologic marker studies are severely limited.

3. What is the purpose of lymphoma classification?
In the clinical setting, lymphoma classification is based on the observation that the morphologic features of a lymphoma are useful in predicting (although imperfectly) the clinical behavior and response to therapy of a lymphoma. Lymphoma subtype is factored into a number of clinical decisions including: Should the lymphoma be treated at all? If so, should it be treated for cure or should treatment be palliative? What is the regimen most likely to be effective? What is the patient's overall prognosis?

4. What is the Working Formulation?
A number of systems of lymphoma classification are used in clinical practice. Each system uses different terminology, which has led to great confusion among clinicians and pathologists. In 1982, the Working Formulation was proposed. It was based on a National Cancer Institute (NCI) study of over 1,000 cases of lymphoma. It was put forth as a system that could be used to "translate" the terminology of one classification system into another to facilitate evaluation of the results of clinical trials. The Working Formulation was not intended to supplant the classification systems already in use. However, over the years, that is exactly what happened. The Working Formulation has become the most widely used system of lymphoma classification in the United States and Canada.

The Working Formulation divides lymphomas into three broad categories: low, intermediate, and high grade. However, many clinicians consider two broad categories of lymphomas: indolent lymphomas, those which are not generally curable; and aggressive lymphomas, which may be treated for cure. As a generalization, the low-grade lymphomas of the Working Formulation roughly correspond to the former and the intermediate and high grade lymphomas roughly correspond to the latter.

Working Formulation (Simplified)

GRADE	% IN ADULTS
Low	
Diffuse, small lymphocytic	4
Follicular, predominantly small cleaved cell	23
Follicular, mixed small cleaved and large cell	8
Intermediate	
Follicular, predominantly large cell	4
Diffuse, small cleaved cell	7
Diffuse, mixed small and large cell	7
Diffuse, large cell	20
High	
Large cell immunoblastic	8
Lymphoblastic	4
Small noncleaved	5
Miscellaneous	10

5. How reproducible is the morphologic classification of lymphoma?
Many clinicians are surprised to learn of the poor reproducibility of some aspects of lymphoma classification even among expert hematopathologists. It has been shown that hematopathologists reproducibly recognize follicular versus diffuse architecture (approximately 90% reproducibility). Unfortunately, reproducibility of the specific lymphoma subtype is poor. In one study, among expert hematopathologists, interobserver agreement ranged from 21–65% depending on the observers and the classification system. Moreover, some expert hematopathologists agreed with themselves only slightly more than half (range for different experts 53–93%) of the time!

Placing this information into perspective, how certain can the oncologist be of the histologic classification of a lymphoma rendered by the pathologist? Obviously, this depends on the pathologist. However, in general, pathologists are good at making the most important histologic distinction in terms of therapeutic decisions—low grade versus intermediate or high grade. Other major distinctions that influence choice of a therapeutic regimen, for instance, distinction between lymphoblastic versus small noncleaved cell lymphoma, are reproducible by expert hematopathologists, especially if immunologic marker studies are available. However, some distinctions are poorly reproducible; for instance, is a follicular lymphoma small cleaved cell type or mixed small cleaved and large cell type? Fortunately, most of these poorly reproducible distinctions are less important in clinical decision-making.

In general, lymphoma diagnosis and classification are best made by pathologists with a great deal of experience in the field. However, it is important to remember that many distinctions are irreproducible even among expert hematopathologists. Therefore, if a local pathologist calls a given case a follicular small cleaved cell lymphoma, and the national "expert" calls it a follicular mixed small cleaved and large cell lymphoma, do not assume that the local pathologist is "wrong" and the expert is "right."

6. What is immunophenotyping?

Immunologic marker studies are widely used to characterize malignant lymphomas. These studies may be performed using flow cytometry or by immunohistochemistry. The former technology utilizes a semiautomated instrument that rapidly measures up to three fluorescence signals (up to three antibodies) on a large number of cells and correlates these measurements with other parameters, including cell size.

The technique of immunohistochemistry demonstrates the binding of antibodies to the lymphoma cells on microscope slides and allows the pathologist visually to correlate the pattern of antibody staining with the histology and cytology of the lymphoma. Either technique may be used to characterize a lymphoma, and each has relative advantages and disadvantages.[5,8]

7. What clinically useful information is derived from immunologic marker studies of lymphomas?

In some institutions, comprehensive and costly panels of antibodies are used to characterize every new case of malignant lymphoma. These studies can be useful in helping to answer a number of clinically important questions.

1. **Is a malignant tumor a lymphoma or a poorly differentiated carcinoma?** In some cases, it may be difficult or impossible to determine if a tumor is a lymphoma or a carcinoma by microscopic examination alone. In such cases, antibodies that recognize lymphoid cells (such as CD45) and epithelial cells (such as cytokeratin) may be very useful.

2. **Is an atypical lymphoid proliferation malignant or is it an unusual reactive lesion?** In difficult cases, the demonstration of clonality (for instance, the abnormal cells all express kappa light chain rather than the normal mixture of both kappa- and lambda-positive cells) indicates a given proliferation is malignant rather than reactive. Lymphoma cells may also fail to express antigens present on normal B or T cells or express combinations of antigens not observed in normal cells.

3. **How should the lymphoma be classified?** Because many of the morphologic subtypes of non-Hodgkin's lymphoma in the Working Formulation have characteristic immunophenotypic profiles, immunophenotyping can be useful as an adjunct to morphology to improve the accuracy and reproducibility of morphologic classification. For instance, in a difficult case, if the immunophenotype is consistent with the proposed morphologic diagnosis, that diagnosis can be rendered with greater confidence. Alternatively, if the immunophenotype is inconsistent with the tentative morphologic diagnosis, that diagnosis should be reconsidered. Immunophenotyping may also be used to subclassify a lymphoma within a given histologic group. For instance, is a large cell lymphoma of T or B lineage? The possible significance of this distinction is addressed below.

8. Is it clinically important whether a large cell lymphoma has a T- or B-cell phenotype?
At present, this issue is not resolved. Early studies indicated that this distinction did not influence patient outcome. More recently, some studies have suggested that immunophenotype in large-cell lymphoma is important. Some groups report shorter disease-free survival in T-cell diffuse large-cell lymphoma when compared with patients with B-cell lymphomas showing similar histology.[2] More definitive information awaits the results of large-scale prospective studies which are underway.

Other immunophenotypic information has been reported by some to influence prognosis in large cell lymphoma. Lack of expression by the lymphoma cells of major histocompatibility complex (MHC) class I and class II antigens has been reported to be associated with shortened survival. Data correlating the percentage of proliferating cells (as determined by staining with the proliferation-associated marker Ki-67) with clinical outcome in large-cell lymphoma have yielded conflicting results.

9. What are immunoglobulin and T-cell gene rearrangement studies?
These studies, which employ the techniques of molecular biology, have been introduced into clinical diagnosis over the last decade.[6]

Early in maturation, lymphoid cells rearrange their immunoglobulin (B cells) and T-cell receptor genes (T cells). This process allows the cells to generate enough different antigen recognition molecules to be able to respond to all of the antigens that will be encountered during a lifetime.

Each cell reconfigures its antigen recognition genes in a slightly different way. Therefore, the size and electrophoretic mobility of rearranged antigen receptor genes will differ for each cell after restriction endonuclease digestion. In addition, the mobility of each will differ from the unrearranged antigen receptor genes of nonlymphoid cells. The mobility of the unrearranged genes is termed **germline**. Because the mobility of each rearranged DNA fragment differs, no distinct bands, other than germline (contributed in part by nonlymphoid cells in the sample), are seen in Southern blots.

Lymphomas are derived from neoplastic transformation and proliferation of a single cell, which occur after the cell has rearranged its antigen receptor genes. All of its progeny have identical antigen receptor gene configurations and therefore identical electrophoretic mobility. This clone is seen as a new distinct band (other than germline) after electrophoresis. Current methodology can detect rearranged bands contributed by as few as 2% to 5% clonal cells.

10. How are immunoglobulin and T-cell gene rearrangement studies used in lymphoma diagnosis?
In clinical practice, immunoglobulin and T-cell receptor gene rearrangement studies are used (1) to assess clonality and thereby help to determine if a given proliferation is malignant and (2) to assign lineage. A prominent rearranged band (a strong band in a position other than germline) indicates a significant clone is present and supports a diagnosis of non-Hodgkin's lymphoma. Faint rearranged bands contributed by small populations of clonal cells need to be interpreted individually in conjunction with clinical and other laboratory information to determine the clinical significance and biologic potential of the clone.

Immunoglobulin and T-cell rearrangement studies may be helpful in uncommon cases where immunophenotypic studies are unable to assign lineage (T versus B). The presence of clonal immunoglobulin gene rearrangement without T-cell receptor rearrangement supports B lineage and clonal T-cell receptor rearrangement without immunoglobulin rearrangement supports T lineage.

11. What are the most important cytogenetic abnormalities in non-Hodgkin's lymphoma (NHL)?
Three cytogenetic abnormalities are strongly associated with particular types of NHL. The most common recurring translocation in NHL is the t(14;18) (reciprocal translocation

between chromosomes 14 and 18), which is seen in approximately 80% of follicular lymphomas and 20% of diffuse large-cell lymphomas. Several groups have investigated the prognostic significance of the t(14;18) in diffuse large-cell lymphoma. Although some groups report a lower rate of complete remission or shorter disease-free survival, other studies have failed to confirm these results.

The t(8;14) is strongly associated with small noncleaved cell lymphoma, including Burkitt's lymphoma. It may also be seen in large-cell and large-cell immunoblastic lymphomas, particularly in HIV-infected patients.

Although not entirely specific, the t(11;14) is strongly associated with a relatively newly recognized form of malignant lymphoma that has several names, including centrocytic lymphoma, mantle cell lymphoma, and intermediately differentiated lymphocytic lymphoma. Most examples of this lymphoma are intermediate grade. They are generally classified as diffuse, small cleaved cell lymphomas using the Working Formulation.

12. What are the most important molecular genetic rearrangements in NHL?

The three cytogenetic abnormalities described above result in genetic rearrangements involving specific genes. Not only are these rearrangements critical in lymphomagenesis, but molecular genetic tests that identify these abnormalities may be used for diagnosis and for rare tumor cell detection in a variety of specimens.

The t(14;18) brings the *BCL-2* (B-cell leukemia/lymphoma-2) gene (18q21) under the regulatory influence of the immunoglobulin (Ig) heavy chain gene (14q32), resulting in overproduction of the *BCL-2* protein in tumor cells. Polymerase chain reaction (PCR)–based tests have been shown to be useful in detecting lymphoma in the bone marrow of these patients, particularly after therapy. The t(8;14) causes inappropriate expression of the *myc* proto-oncogene (8q24), and the t(11;14) results in disregulation of the *BCL-1* gene (11q13).

13. In NHL, what information is more important in determining therapy, histologic classification (grade) or stage? In Hodgkin's disease?

In part because of the unpredictability of spread in NHL, it is generally treated with chemotherapy. The choice of chemotherapeutic regimen depends to a large extent on the histologic subtype (grade) of the lymphoma. Therefore, in NHL, grade is more important than stage.

Because Hodgkin's disease generally spreads in a predictable fashion from one node group to the next, nonbulky localized disease in adults can be treated with radiotherapy. Advanced-stage disease is treated with chemotherapy. The chemotherapeutic regimens used in these patients is not dependent on the histologic subtype of Hodgkin's disease. Moreover, stage for stage, survival in advanced-stage disease is probably similar for all histologic subtypes. Therefore, in Hodgkin's disease, tumor stage is more important than grade in determining therapy.

BIBLIOGRAPHY

1. Berard CW, Bloomfield C, Bonadonna G, et al: Classification of non-Hodgkin's lymphomas. Reproducibility of major classification systems. Cancer 55:91–95, 1985.
2. Grogan TM, Miller TP: New biologic markers in non-Hodgkin's lymphomas. Hematol Oncol Clin North Am 5:925–933, 1991.
3. Hardy R, Horning SJ: Molecular biologic studies in the clinical evaluation of non-Hodgkin's lymphoma. Hematol Oncol Clin North Am 5:891–900, 1991.
4. LeBeau MM: Chromosomal abnormalities in non-Hodgkin's lymphomas. Semin Oncol 17:20–29, 1990.
5. Sheibani K: Immunohistochemical analysis of lymphoid tissue. In Knowles DM (ed): Neoplastic Hematopathology. Baltimore, Williams & Wilkins, 1992, pp 197–213.
6. Sklar J: Antigen receptor genes: Structure, function, and techniques for analysis of their rearrangements. In Knowles DM (ed): Neoplastic Hematopathology. Baltimore, Williams & Wilkins, 1992, pp 215–244.

7. The non-Hodgkin's lymphoma pathologic classification project. National Cancer Institute sponsored study of classification of non-Hodgkin's lymphomas. Cancer 49:2112–2135, 1982.
8. Willman CL: Flow cytometric analysis of hematologic specimens. In Knowles DM (ed): Neoplastic Hematopathology. Baltimore, Williams & Wilkins, 1992, pp 169–195.

33. LOW-GRADE AND HIGH-GRADE NON-HODGKIN'S LYMPHOMAS

David S. Hanson, M.D.

1. What are the usual tests obtained in staging a patient who has been diagnosed with malignant lymphoma by adequate excisional biopsy?
Staging generally involves a careful history and physical examination with attention to such symptoms as weight loss, fevers, night sweats, and pruritus. The physical examination must pay careful attention to all lymph node areas, including the throat, neck, supraclavicular region, axilla, epitrochlear lymph nodes, and inguinal region, as well as a careful abdominal examination. Laboratory evaluation generally includes a complete blood count with erythrocyte sedimentation rate and evaluation of hepatic function that must include a serum alkaline phosphatase. It is generally important to determine the adequacy of renal function as well. Radiographic studies often include chest radiograph, abdominal/pelvic computed tomographic (CT) scanning and may also involve further more aggressive radiographic evaluation as dictated by symptoms. Such investigation may include further abdominal evaluation with sonography, radionuclide bone scanning, or plain radiographs if there is evidence of bony involvement and further CT scanning, which may include evaluation of the chest in patients with equivocal chest radiographs or head or other neural magnetic resonance imaging (MRI) for patients with neurologic symptoms or signs. In addition, bilateral bone marrow biopsies with aspiration provide important information in the staging of patients with lymphoma.

2. Why is the staging of a lymphoma important?
Treatment decisions are often based on the stage of disease at presentation. For example, patients with early-stage low-grade lymphomas can be successfully treated with radiation therapy, whereas patients with advanced-stage low-grade lymphomas are much more apt to be managed when symptomatic with chemotherapy. Early-stage high-grade lymphomas can be treated with a combination of radiation therapy coupled with a brief course of multi-agent combination chemotherapy, whereas patients with more advanced intermediate- and high-grade lymphomas are treated with combination chemotherapy alone. Patients with intermediate- or high-grade lymphomas who have demonstrable bone marrow involvement are at much greater risk of central nervous system involvement, which requires futher treatment in addition to the combination chemotherapy usually employed.

3. How are the staging procedures used to determine the clinical stage of non-Hodgkin's lymphoma?
Staging non-Hodgkin's lymphoma parallels the Ann Arbor Staging Classification for Hodgkin's disease:
　　Stage I: involvement of a single lymph node region or single extralymphatic organ.
　　Stage II: involvement of two or more lymph node regions or extralymphatic sites on the same side of the diaphragm.
　　Stage III: involvement of lymph node regions or extralymphatic organs or sites on both sides of the diaphragm.

Stage IV: diffuse or disseminated involvement of more than one extralymphatic organ with or without associated lymph node involvement. In addition, involvement of the bone marrow confers stage IV designation.

The National Cancer Institute has modified the staging scheme for lymphomas based on the Ann Arbor classification. For low-grade lymphomas, the National Cancer Institute modified staging schema denotes:

Stage I: localized disease that roughly parallels Ann Arbor stages I and II.

Stage II: disseminated disease paralleling Ann Arbor stages III and IV.

Intermediate and high-grade lymphomas are grouped into three stages by the National Cancer Institute modified staging schema:

Stage I: localized nodal or extranodal disease and is roughly equivalent to Ann Arbor stage I disease.

Stage II: two or more nodal sites of disease or localized extranodal involvement plus draining nodes with none of the following characteristics present: Karnofsky performance status <70, "B" symptoms, any mass greater than 10 cm in diameter, serum lactate dehydrogenase (LDH) >500 international units or three or more extranodal sites of disease.

Stage III: stage II plus any of the poor prognostic features mentioned above.

4. Which lymphoma is the solid tumor equivalent of chronic lymphocytic leukemia (CLL)?
Small lymphocytic lymphoma, composed of well-diffferentiated small lymphocytes, represents the solid tumor equivalent of CLL. In most instances, small lymphocytic lymphoma will progress to CLL.

5. What is the most common kind of follicular lymphoma?
Small cleaved cell lymphoma is by far the most common type of follicular lymphoma. (See Figure 13, Color Plates.)

6. Is there a circulating phase of follicular small cleaved cell lymphoma?
Follicular small cleaved cell lymphoma is far less likely to be associated with lymphoid cells circulating in the peripheral blood than small lymphocytic lymphoma. However, on occasion, circulating cells will be found in the peripheral blood. (See Figure 12, Color Plates.) These cells appear different from the usual cells seen in chronic lymphocytic leukemia in that the nuclei exhibit clefts or notches (so-called buttock cells). Although this disease entity has been referred to as lymphosarcoma cell leukemia, this term has fallen out of favor because it has been used to describe a variety of malignant lymphomas with a circulating phase that can vary widely in their clinical behavior.

7. Which low-grade lymphomas have the greatest biologic potential to require treatment within 12 months of diagnosis?
Of the low-grade lymphomas, follicular mixed, small cleaved cell and large-cell lymphoma is clinically the most aggressive. This is probably because of the presence of the large-cell component, whose role is likely replicative, in contradistinction to the small-cell component, which likely contributes more to the multiple organ involvement seen in low-grade lymphomas.

8. What is the median survival for a patient diagnosed with low-grade lymphoma?
In general, persons with a low-grade lymphoma have a median survival of about 6 years. This underscores the fact that although most of the low-grade lymphomas are treatable (that is, patients will respond to chemotherapy), this treatment results only in palliation and not in long-term cure of the underlying disease.

9. Discuss criteria used to treat patients with low-grade lymphomas.
Because low-grade lymphomas may grow slowly, treatment is often not indicated at the time of diagnosis. In fact, patients with low-grade lymphomas may not require therapy for up to several years following their diagnosis. However, when patients are debilitated by "B" symptoms or have symptomatic lymphadenopathy or cytopenias, they are often times

treated with palliative radiation therapy, palliative chemotherapy, and on occasion both. Although treatment is often associated with symptomatic and clinical improvement, there is little proof that treatment actually affects survival.

10. What is the most common shared clinical characteristic of the intermediate- and high-grade lymphomas?
These diseases are grouped because ot their tendency to disseminate and grow rapidly. Their prognosis is unfavorable unless moder:n intensive multiagent chemotherapy or chemotherapy combined with radiation therapy induces a sustained complete remission. In contradistinction to the low-grade lymphomas, if a complete remission is achieved and sustained for a period beyond 2 years, the likelihood of being cured from these intermediate- or high-grade lymphomas is high.

11. What factors are associated with a poor prognosis in intermediate/high-grade lymphoma?
Tumor bulk appears to be a very important prognostic factor. Whether this tumor bulk is related to stage or bulk of disease, patients with advanced-grade or bulky disease have a poorer prognosis than patients who present with early-stage, low-bulk disease. In addition, elevation of serum LDH may also be associated with a poor prognosis.

12. How are patients with localized intermediate/high-grade lymphoma generally treated?
Patients with early stage intermediate/high–grade lymphoma (excluding lymphoblastic lymphoma, Burkitt's lymphoma, adult T-cell leukemia lymphoma, and human immunodeficiency virus [HIV]-associated lymphoma) can generally be treated with a combination of multiagent chemotherapy and involved-field radiation therapy. In general, these are a highly selected group of patients with non-bulky (<10 cm) stage IA and IIA disease. Nearly all these patients will achieve a complete remission, and the vast majority will be free of disease at 2 years.

13. How are patients with advanced intermediate/high–grade non-Hodgkin's lymphoma generally treated?
In general, these patients (except those with lymphoblastic lymphoma, Burkitt's lymphoma, adult T-cell leukemia/lymphoma, and HIV-associated lymphoma) are treated with multiagent combination chemotherapy. The most common of these regimens is CHOP (Cytoxan cyclophosphamide], hydroxydaunorubicin [Adriamycin], Oncovin [vincristine], and prednisone). In general, four full-dose cycles of chemotherapy are given on schedule (every 3 weeks). The patient is then completely restaged. Patients who have a complete response after four cycles of combination chemotherapy have the highest likelihood of being maintained in complete remission. All such patients are given at least an additional two cycles of chemotherapy. Further maintenance therapy is of no demonstrated value.

14. What characteristics at presentation increase the risk of central nervous system (CNS) involvement in patients with intermediate/high–grade lymphoma?
Patients with bone marrow involvement are statistically at higher risk of CNS involvement. In addition, patients with primary paranasal sinus disease and possibly testicular disease may also be at increased risk of CNS involvement. In many of these patients, CNS prophylaxis may be indicated as a component of primary therapy. Patients at risk for CNS involvement should have an evaluation for CNS involvement at the time of staging. This evaluation generally includes a lumbar puncture with routine chemistries and cell counts, as well as cytologic evaluation of the spinal fluid.

15. What is Burkitt's lymphoma?
Burkitt's lymphoma is a specific, aggressive subtype of small noncleaved cell high-grade no. -Hodgkin's lymphoma. (See Figure 14, Color Plates.) Endemic, or African, Burkitt's

lymphoma is associated with the Epstein-Barr virus (EBV) and the t(8;14), chromosomal translocation is very often demonstrated. The most common sites of involvement are the jaw and the orbit. Prolonged survival can occur with treatment with cyclophosphamide. A sporadic form of Burkitt's lymphoma occurs in the United States and throughout the world. It is rarely associated with the EBV, although the chromosomal translocation t(8;14) is very often demonstrated. In contradistinction to African Burkitt's lymphoma, the abdomen, gastrointestinal tract, and bone marrow are most often involved and therapy requires multiple-agent combination chemotherapy, including CNS prophylaxis.

16. Which high-grade lymphoma pathologically resembles an acute leukemia?
Lymphoblastic lymphoma pathologically resembles acute lymphocytic leukemia, particularly when diagnosed early by examination of bone marrow and peripheral blood. These patients commonly present with mediastinal masses. These masses can cause significant clincal difficulty, including superior vena cava syndrome, and pericardial effusions and tamponade, as well as pleural effusions. This is primarily a disease of adolescent and young males.

17. Which high-grade lymphoma is most strongly associated with a viral etiology?
Adult T-cell lymphoma/leukemia is probably caused by the HTLV-I virus. Though this disease was initially described in Japan, it is also endemic in the Caribbean. Patients present with fairly classic clinical constellation of lymphadenopathy, organomegaly, hypercalcemia, bone involvement, and CNS involvement. Response to treatment to date has been poor, with death occurring within a year of diagnosis.

18. What are the clinical characteristics of acquired immunodeficiency syndrome (AIDS)– related lymphomas?
AIDS-related or HIV-related lymphomas are usually high-grade B-cell malignancies of the small noncleaved cell type or the large-cell immunoblastic type. In addition to involvement of multiple lymph node sites, these lymphomas frequently involve extranodal sites such as the gastrointestinal tract, bone, and CNS. Although patients do respond to treatment with multiagent chemotherapy, their treatment is complicated by relatively significant cytopenias. In general, patients whose only manifestation of AIDS is lymphoma are the best candidates for therapy.

19. Are there other immunodeficiency states associated with the development of lymphoma?
Patients with congenital immunodeficiencies such as agammaglobulinemia, Wiskott-Aldrich syndrome, or ataxia telangiectasia have an inordinately high risk of the development of lymphoma. Similarly, patients with autoimmune disease such as rheumatoid arthritis, systemic lupus erythematosus, Hashimoto's thyroiditis, and Sjögren's syndrome are at increased risk of developing non-Hodgkin's lymphoma. Finally, patients who are iatrogenically immunosuppressed (such as organ transplant recipients) are at increased risk for non-Hodgkin's lymphoma. Interestingly, patients who can tolerate tapering of their immunosuppressive regimen may experience spontaneous resolution of their lymphoma, although this approach as a singular treatment is rare.

20. What is the most common form of solitary extranodal lymphoma?
Primary gastrointestinal lymphoma is the most common form of solitary extranodal lymphoma and presents in two clinical ways. The **Mediterranean type** commonly presents in the second decade of life, is a disease that generally involves the proximal jejunum and duodenum, and may be associated with alpha heavy chain disease. These patients commonly present with symptoms of diarrhea and malabsorption. Response to treatment is relatively poor. In contradistinction, the so-called **Western type** of primary gastrointestinal lymphoma presents later in life, most commonly in the fourth or later decades. The stomach is the most commonly involved organ, although this disease can present in the small bowel or colon as well. Diarrhrea and/or malabsorptive symptoms are uncommon. However, this

form of disease is much more likely to be associated with gastrointestinal bleeding and hepatosplenomegaly. Five-year survival after treatment, which may include surgery, is approximately 40%.

21. Discuss the characteristics of primary CNS lymphoma.
Primary CNS lymphoma is almost always of B-cell origin and high histologic grade. Lesions are primarily parenchymal, and multiple lesions in 30–40% of cases. In addition, the leptomeninges may be involved in up to 30% of cases at diagnosis and at a much higher frequency when patients are taken to autopsy. This disease entity is associated with both congenital and acquired immune deficiency, as well as advanced age. Patients generally present with neurologic changes or headaches. Diagnosis requires either stereotactic biopsy or formal surgical exploration, as the majority of these patients will not have associated systemic lymphoma.

22. What is Richter's transformation?
It is the development of diffuse large-cell lymphoma in a patient with a history of chronic lymphocytic leukemia or other low-grade well-differentiated lymphoid neoplasm. This large-cell lymphoma is clinically and histologically more aggressive than the usual large-cell lymphoma and as a consequence has a poor prognosis.

BIBLIOGRAPHY

1. Blayney DW, et al: The human T-cell leukemia/lymphoma virus associated with American adult T-cell leukemia/lymphoma. Blood 62:401, 1983.
2. Coleman CN, et al: Treatment of lymphoblastic lymphoma in adults. J Clin Oncol 4:1628, 1986.
3. Connors JM, et al: Brief chemotherapy and involved field radiation therapy for limited stage aggressive lymphoma. Ann Intern Med 107:25, 1987.
4. Fisher RI, et al: Comparison of a standard regimen (CHOP) with three intensive chemotherapy regimens for advanced, non-Hodgkin's lymphoma. N Engl J Med 328:1002, 1993.
5. Korsmeyer SJ: Immunoglobulin and T-cell receptor genes reveal the clonality, lineage and translocation lymphoid neoplasms In DeVita VT Jr, Hellman S, Rosenberg SA (eds): Important Advances in Oncology 1987. Philadelphia, J.B. Lippincott, 1987, pp 3–15.
6. Magrath IT, et al: An effective therapy for both undifferentiated (including Burkitt's) lymphomas and lymphoblastic lymphomas in children and young adults. Blood 63:1102, 1984.
7. National Cancer Institute sponsored study of classifications of non-Hodgkin's lymphomas. Summary and description of a working formulation for clinical usage. Cancer 49:2112, 1982.
8. Rosenberg SA: Karnofsky Memorial Lecture. The low-grade non-Hodgkin's lymphomas: Challenges and opportunities. J Clin Oncol 3:299, 1985.
9. Yunis JJ, et al: Distinctive chromosomal abnormalities in histologic subtypes of non-Hodgkin's lymphoma. N Engl J Med 307:1231, 1982.

34. CUTANEOUS LYMPHOMAS

Jill Lacy, M.D.

1. Primary lymphomas of the skin comprise a heterogeneous group of tumors. What are the three major categories of cutaneous lymphomas?
1. The mycosis fungoides (MF)/Sézary syndrome complex (also more recently referred to as cutaneous T-cell lymphoma, CTCL): a low-grade T-cell lymphoma comprising predominantly small lymphocytes that display the immunophenotype of mature "helper" (CD4⁺) lymphocytes.

2. T-cell lymphomas comprising large cells, described as anaplastic, large cell, immunoblastic, or pleomorphic: These "peripheral T-cell lymphomas" often express an aberrant immunophenotype with loss of pan–T-cell antigens.

3. B-cell lymphomas that display the spectrum of histopathologies encountered in nodal lymphomas.

2. What is the natural history of CTCL?
CTCL is an indolent low-grade lymphoma, and most patients afflicted with this disease survive years if not decades. However, the overwhelming majority of patients cannot be cured, and thus many patients ultimately die of complications related to their lymphoma.

3. How do patients with CTCL typically present?
Prior to a definitive diagnosis of CTCL, most patients give a history of years of an intermittent pruritic eczematous skin disorder often misdiagnosed as eczema or other benign processes. This phase is referred to as the premycotic phase. As the disease progresses, eczematous lesions evolve into erythematous, indurated plaques, described as the plaque phase, at which time a definitive pathologic diagnosis on skin biopsy is usually possible. The majority of patients (70%) are diagnosed in the plaque phase.

4. Discuss some of the pathologic features that characterize CTCL.
CTCL is an epidermotropic tumor. Characteristic pathologic features include a bandlike infiltrate of atypical lymphoid cells in the upper dermis. Pautrier's abscess, a small collection of atypical lymphoid cells within the epidermis, is an important histologic feature that helps confirm the diagnosis.

5. Describe the evolution and spread of CTCL.
Typically, plaque lesions increase in number and size to involve an increasing percentage of the body surface area. The plaques also increase in thickness evolving into nodules or tumors that often ulcerate and become secondarily infected. As the disease progresses, lymph node involvement occurs, and overt visceral dissemination is present in the majority of patients in the terminal stages of the disease. Although any visceral site may be involved with CTCL, common sites include bone marrow, liver, lung, and spleen.

6. Give the two major causes of death in patients with CTCL.
1. Progressive lymphoma, frequently after transformation to an intermediate- or high-grade T-cell malignancy
2. Infection secondary to breakdown of the normal skin barrier

7. The staging system recently adopted for CTCL is a modified TNM system based on the extent and nature of skin involvement (T), nodal involvement (N), visceral metastases (M), and blood involvement (B). Describe the categories of skin involvement.

T1: limited plaques (plaques involving less than 10% of the body surface area)

T2: generalized plaques
T3: cutaneous tumors
T4: generalized erythroderma

8. What is the importance of staging in CTCL?
Stage is a predictor of prognosis and influences treatment-related decisions. Over 90% of patients with stage I disease are alive at 5 years. In contrast, less than 50% of patients with stage IV disease survive 2 years. With respect to treatment, patients with disease limited to the skin can usually be managed with a variety of topical therapies, whereas patients with visceral involvement may require systemic chemotherapy.

9. Define the Sézary syndrome.
The Sézary syndrome is a variant of CTCL in which patients present with or develop diffuse erythema of the skin (generalized erythroderma) in association with the presence of

circulating malignant T cells, or Sézary cells (>10%) in the peripheral blood. Intense pruritus is characteristic of the generalized erythroderma and often results in severe excoriations and ulcerations. Approximately 15% of patients with CTCL actually present with the Sézary syndrome.

10. What is the general approach to the treatment of patients with CTCL?
Because the major manifestations of CTCL are confined to the skin until the late stages of the disease, the approach to treatment of this disease has been the utilization of a variety of topical treatments to control cutaneous symptoms. The use of systemic chemotherapy in early-stage disease has not been shown to affect outcome and, thus, is not routinely used in initial management of CTCL.

11. What is an appropriate staging work-up in patients diagnosed with CTCL?
The initial staging evaluation should include a thorough physical examination, with special attention directed to assessing the extent of skin involvement and the presence of palpable lymph nodes. The peripheral blood should be examined carefully for the presence of circulating Sézary cells and a chest radiograph obtained. Routine staging computed tomographic (CT) scans, bone marrow biopsies, and liver biopsies are not necessary unless signs and symptoms suggest visceral involvement.

12. Describe the topical therapies that are effective in the treatment of CTCL.
   1. **Radiation therapy:** Because CTCL is exquisitely radiosensitive, radiation therapy is an effective treatment modality for control of cutaneous disease. Two types of radiation therapy are used. Electron beam radiation delivers a superficial dose of radiation and can be used to treat the total skin surface. Toxicities are limited to the skin (e.g., erythema, desquamation, hair loss, damaged sweat glands) and usually subside after completion of therapy. Electron beam therapy is highly effective treatment for superficial cutaneous disease; the overall response rate to "total skin" electron beam therapy is nearly 100% (including complete and partial responders), with >90% of patients with limited plaque involvement attaining complete remission. Traditional orthovoltage radiation is used to treat small fields ("spot" radiation) to control specific symptomatic tumors or thick plaques requiring more penetrating radiation.
   2. **Topical chemotherapy:** The topical application of nitrogen mustard is effective therapy for patients with plaque-stage disease. Treatment is applied to the entire skin until disease clearance (often 6–12 months), followed by maintenance therapy for one to two years. Toxicities include hypersensitivity reactions and secondary skin cancers with long-term usage.
   3. **PUVA (psoralin ultraviolet A) photochemotherapy:** This involves exposure to long-wave UVA light after oral ingestion of methoxypsoralen, a photosensitizing drug that covalently binds DNA and causes cell death after activation by UVA light. Treatment is given three times weekly until disease clearance is achieved, followed by a tapering maintenance regimen. As with other topical therapies, results are best in patients without tumors or thick plaques. Acute toxicities include pruritus and "sunburn"; the major long-term complication is the development of secondary skin cancers.

13. What is photophoresis and what is its role in the treatment of CTCL?
This is an experimental form of therapy that involves the administration of oral methoxypsoralen followed by extracorporeal circulation of the blood with exposure of leukocytes to long-wave UVA light prior to reinfusion. This therapy is most effective in patients with erythroderma and/or the Sézary syndrome.

14. What is the role of systemic chemotherapy in the treatment of CTCL?
Although systemic chemotherapy results in objective responses in approximately two-thirds of patients with CTCL, it is not curative. Furthermore, the addition of systemic chemotherapy

to topical therapies does not improve the efficacy of topical therapy alone. Thus, the role of systemic chemotherapy is limited to palliation of symptoms that cannot be controlled with topical therapy. Patients with advanced cutaneous disease, symptomatic nodal or visceral involvement, or the Sézary syndrome can derive palliation from a variety of single agents or combinations of drugs, including alkylating agents, methotrexate, etoposide, doxorubicin, prednisone, bleomycin, cis-platinum, and fludarabine. In addition, multidrug chemotherapy regimens are appropriate in the setting of transformation to a high-grade T-cell lymphoma.

15. Is interferon effective in the treatment of CTCL?
Yes. Interferon has good activity against CTCL, including disease refractory to other therapies. The combination of PUVA with interferon is highly effective in preliminary studies and is a promising new treatment strategy.

16. List some of the recent novel systemic therapies that have been used in the treatment of CTCL.

Retinoids	Antithymocyte globulin	High-dose thymidine
Cyclosporine	Monoclonal antibodies	

17. How do the B- and T-cell lymphomas of the skin, excluding mycosis fungoides, usually present?
Patients with non–mycosis fungoides cutaneous lymphoma usually present with skin nodules, tumors, or plaques that are reddish or violaceous in color.

18. Is the approach to the work-up and management of non–mycosis fungoides lymphomas of the skin any different from that of extracutaneous lymphomas?
No. Although the non–mycosis fungoides cutaneous lymphomas comprise a heterogeneous group of tumors, they are best managed by utilizing the same principles that guide the management of typical extracutaneous non-Hodgkin's lymphoma. Thus, these patients should have an adequate biopsy to confirm the diagnosis, with immunophenotyping, if possible, and a complete staging evaluation, with a body CT scan and bone marrow biopsies. The appropriate treatment modality (radiation, chemotherapy, or both) is dictated by the pathologic subtype and grade, as well as the stage. Thus, a patient with an intermediate-grade diffuse large-cell lymphoma of the skin should be treated with multidrug chemotherapy. In contrast, a patient with a low-grade follicular small cleaved cell lymphoma restricted to the skin (stage I) should be treated with involved field radiation therapy.

BIBLIOGRAPHY

1. Abel EA, Deneau DG, Rafber EM, et al: PUVA treatment of erythrodermic and plaque-type mycosis fungoides. J Am Acad Dermatol 4:423, 1981.
2. Abel EA, Sendagorta E, Hoppe RT, Hu CH: PUVA treatment of erythrodermic and plaque-type mycosis fungoides: 10-year follow-up study. Arch Dermatol 123:897, 1987.
3. Abel EA, Wood GS, Hoppe RT: Mycosis fungoides: Clinical and histologic features, staging, evaluation, and approach to treatment. CA Cancer J Clin 43:93, 1993.
4. Axelrod PI, Lorber B, Vonderheid EC: Infections complicating mycosis fungoides and Sézary syndrome. JAMA 267:1354, 1992.
5. Bunn PA, Ihde DC, Foon KA: The role of recombinant interferon alpha-2a in the therapy of cutaneous T-cell lymphoma. Cancer 57:1689, 1986.
6. Bunn PA Jr, Lamberg SI: Report of the committee on staging and classification of cutaneous T-cell lymphoma. Cancer Treat Rep 63:725, 1979.
7. Edelson RL: Cutaneous T cell lymphoma: Mycosis fungoides, Sézary syndrome, and other variants. J Am Acad Dermatol 2:89, 1980.
8. Edelson R, Berger C, Gasparro R, et al: Treatment of cutaneous T-cell lymphoma by extracorporeal photochemotherapy: Preliminary results. N Engl J Med 316:297, 1987.

9. Hoppe RT, Abel EA, Deneau DG, Price NM: Mycosis fungoides: Management with topical nitrogen mustard. J Clin Oncol 5:1796, 1987.
10. Hoppe RT, Cox RS, Fuk ZY, et al: Electron beam therapy in the treatment of mycosis fungoides: The Stanford experience. Cancer Treat Rep 63:691, 1979.
11. Kaye FJ, Bunn PA, Steinberg SM, et al: A randomized trial comparing combination electron-beam radiation and chemotherapy with topical therapy in the initial treatment of mycosis fungoides. N Engl J Med 321:1784, 1989.
12. Lambert WC: Premycotic eruptions. Dermatol Clin 3:647, 1985.
13. Van Vloten WA, De Vroome H, Noordijk EM: Total skin electron beam irradiation for cutaneous T cell lymphoma (mycosis fungoides). Br J Dermatol 112:697, 1985.
14. Wieselthier JS, Koh HK: Sézary syndrome: Diagnosis, prognosis, and critical review of treatment options. J Am Acad Dermatol 22:381, 1990.
15. Wood GS, Burke JS, Horning S, et al: The immunologic and clinicopathologic heterogeneity of cutaneous lymphomas other than mycosis fungoides. Blood 62:464, 1983.

35. MULTIPLE MYELOMA AND MACROGLOBULINEMIAS

Madeline J. White, M.D.

1. What is multiple myeloma (MM)?

MM is an uncontrolled malignant proliferation of plasma cells. In almost all cases, these cells make an excess amount of monoclonal immunoglobulin (IgG, IgA, IgD, IgE) or kappa (κ) or lambda (λ) light chains.

2. Where in the normal development of the B cell does the malignant transformation occur?

Heavy (H) and light (L) chain variable regions are identical, which indicates that the malignant transformation has occurred before the plasma cell stage in the pre-B cell population or even earlier. Some investigators hypothesize that myeloma is initiated at the hematopoietic stem cell level, because myeloid dysplasia with myeloma may be seen and multiple hematopoietic lineage-associated antigens may be present on the malignant cells (early B-cell, T-cell, natural killer cell, myeloid, erythroid, and megakaryocytic markers).

3. In what population is myeloma commonly seen?

The incidence of myeloma rises with age. The mean age at diagnosis is 65 years. Onset before age 40 is very uncommon. Men are affected more frequently than women. Afro-Americans have a higher incidence than whites.

4. What are some potential risk factors for myeloma?

The cause for myeloma is unknown, but potential risk factors include radiation exposure and occupational exposures (e.g., farming, use of pesticides, benzene, organic solvents).

5. Which cytokine is considered the major growth factor for myeloma?

Interleukin-6 (IL-6) is the major myeloma growth factor. It may serve as a differentiating agent, moving pre-myeloma cells into mature plasma cells. IL-6 causes C-reactive protein to rise. This protein can be used as a marker for IL-6 levels.

6. When plasma cell tumors arise, describe the pattern of distribution that can be seen.

Usually, myeloma presents as multiple lytic tumors in the bone or as a diffuse plasmacytosis in the bone marrow with a osteoporotic picture (10% to 30%). Rarely (3%), osteosclerotic lesions can be seen. This is called multiple myeloma (MM). Single plasmacytomas can occur in the bone and usually represent an earlier presentation of MM. This is called solitary myeloma (5%). Localized extramedullary plasmacytomas can appear in non-myeloid tissue, especially upper airways, without bone marrow involvement. Median survivals for solitary myeloma and extramedullary plasmacytomas are longer than for MM.

7. How do plasma cell tumors cause disease?

In addition to the effects of the myeloma proteins, plasma cell neoplasms cause disease from local tumor growth and from the effects of secreted factors such as osteoclast-activating factor (a combination of IL-6, IL-1β and TNF-β). Bone pain, fractures, hypercalcemia, and nerve compression can occur. Local marrow suppression and/or replacement can lead to severe anemia. Other cytokines can suppress normal immunoglobulin production, leading to infections.

8. What types of infections are common in myeloma?

Because normal immunoglobulin synthesis is depressed in myeloma, humoral immunity is impaired. Patients are susceptible to infections, especially bacterial types. *Streptococcus pneumoniae* and *Staphylococcus aureus* are frequent pathogens. Gram-negative organisms invade as well. Cellular immunity is better preserved, although some T-cell function is impaired.

9. What are some dysfunctions caused by the secretion of large amounts of the myeloma (M) proteins in the circulation?

The proteins can cause increased plasma volume, can displace plasma water causing pseudohyponatremia, and can accumulate and/or aggregate leading to hyperviscosity. Decreased anion gap can occur as chloride and bicarbonate are retained to balance the protein's net positive charge. M proteins can coat platelets and interfere with their function. Rarely, M proteins have antibody activity and react against common antigens (red blood cell [RBC] polysaccharides, bacterial polysaccharides, myelin-associated glycoprotein, actin, tubulin, nuclear components, insulin, lipoproteins, and immunoglobulins). Proteins that bind to coagulation factors can enhance bleeding tendencies. Cold sensitivity can occur if M proteins precipitate as cryoglobulins at ambient temperatures. As amyloid and nonamyloid L chains, M proteins can deposit in cardiac, nerve, and renal tissues, causing dysfunction.

10. Describe some specific problems caused by deposition of the M proteins in the kidney.

About 50% of patients with myeloma show evidence of renal dysfunction caused by M proteins.

Renal tubular dysfunction: L chains that are filtered, reabsorbed, and catabolized are damaging to tubular cells. You can see defects in proximal and distal tubular function (nephrogenic diabetes insipidus, impaired acidification and concentration, distal renal tubular acidosis). In some patients, adult Fanconi's syndrome develops as the tubules lose the ability to reabsorb amino acids, glucose, and phosphate.

Myeloma kidney: With L chain excretion and decreased glomerular filtration rate, intratubular L chain concentration increases, leading to cast formation, especially in the distal tubules. Acute and chronic interstitial inflammation ensues. Renal failure develops more commonly in those excreting λ chains than those excreting κ chains.

Amyloid kidney and L chain deposition disease: Nonamyloid L chains and amyloid can be deposited in the kidney along tubular basement membrane, glomeruli, blood vessels, or interstitium. Tubular casts are not prominent. Deposits in the glomeruli cause nephrotic syndrome. If urine protein electrophoresis (UPEP) shows a tubular pattern (major L chain and minor albumin peaks), myeloma cast nephropathy is likely. If UPEP shows glomerular pattern (albumin $\geq$ L chain), amyloid or L chain deposition is found.

11. Besides these problems, what other kinds of renal disease can occur in patients with myeloma?
Plasma cell infiltration, urinary tract infection, hypercalcemia, uric acid nephropathy, dehydration, nephrotoxic antibiotics, contrast nephropathy, and cryoglobulins can damage renal function.

12. Discuss some symptoms, signs, or laboratory tests that should prompt you to think of myeloma.
Kyle and others list unexplained weakness or fatigue, back pain, osteoporosis, osteolytic lesions, recurrent infections, anemia, increased erythrocyte sedimentation rate, hypercalcemia, renal insufficiency, Bence Jones proteinuria, increased total protein, decreased anion gap, and hyponatremia. It would be in the differential diagnosis of sensorimotor neuropathy, nephrotic syndrome, carpal tunnel syndrome, refractory congestive heart failure, orthostatic hypotension, and malabsorption.

13. What is the most common immunoglobulin type found in myeloma?
IgG monoclonal proteins are found in about 55% of myelomas. IgA is the next most common type. IgD and IgE are uncommon. Light chain–only myeloma occurs in about 20% of cases. Biclonal production can occur (0.5–2.5%), the most common combination being IgG and IgA (33%). Rarely, no monoclonal protein is found in serum or urine. These plasma cells cannot produce the protein or cannot secrete the protein extracellularly.

14. Can the serum protein electrophoresis (SPEP) miss the M protein spike?
If the spike is very small, it can be obscured by the normal immunoglobulins. Immunoelectrophoresis should identify the monoclonal band. If only L chains are produced, they do not accumulate in the serum unless there is severe renal failure. SPEP may only show hypogammaglobulinemia. A 24-hour urine protein electrophoresis must be done to find the L chains.

15. In addition to a serum protein electrophoresis, what tests are needed to diagnose and stage myeloma?
• Urine protein electrophoresis. Remember urine dipsticks are insensitive for L chains.
• Quantitative immunoglobulins.
• Immunoelectrophoresis.
• Skeletal survey (skull, cervical, thoracic, and lumbar spine, pelvis, arms and forearms, thighs, and legs).
• Bone marrow aspirate and biopsy.
• Complete blood count, serum calcium, serum creatinine, serum uric acid, serum lactate dehydrogenase (LDH), and serum β_2-microglobulin.

16. Once these tests have been done, what criteria are used for diagnosis?
Here are criteria adapted from DeVita's text[7] to diagnose active MM in symptomatic patients.
Major Criteria
1. Plasmacytoma on tissue biopsy.
2. Bone marrow plasmacytosis with >30% plasma cells.
3. Monoclonal globulin spike on serum electrophoresis exceeding 3.5 gm/dl for G peaks or 2.0 gm/dl for A peaks. Greater than or equal to 1.0 gm/24 hours of kappa or lambda light chain excretion on urine electrophoresis in the absence of amyloidosis.
Minor Criteria
1. Bone marrow plasmacytosis 10% to 30%.
2. Monoclonal globulin spike present but less than the levels defined above.
3. Lytic bone lesions.
4. Normal IgM <50 mg/dl, IgA <100 mg/dl, or IgG <600 mg/dl.
The diagnosis of myeloma requires *a minimum of* one major criterion plus 1 minor criterion *or* three minor criteria that must include criteria nos. 1 and 2.

17. How do these tests help in staging myeloma?

Many groups use the Durie-Salmon[12] staging system that looks at indicators of tumor volume. High tumor mass is confirmed when any of the following are present:
1. Hemoglobin <8.5 gm/dl.
2. Corrected calcium >12 mg/dl.
3. Extensive skeletal destruction and major fractures.
4. IgG spike >7 gm/dl, IgA peak >5 gm/dl, or urine L chains >12 gm/24 hours.

Low tumor mass is indicated when all of the following are present:
1. Hemoglobin >10 gm/dl
2. Normal calcium
3. Normal bones on radiography or solitary bone plasmacytoma only
4. IgG spike <5 gm/dl, IgA spike <3 gm/dl, or urine L chains <4 gm/24 hours.

Intermediate tumor mass falls in between.

These groups are subclassified depending on renal function: A—serum creatine <2 mg/100 ml; B—serum creatinine ≥2 mg/100 ml.

More recently, high β_2-microglobulin (>6 mg/L), LDH >300, chromosomal abnormalities, and plasma cell labeling index (LI) add to the list of poor prognostic features.

18. Why do myeloma bone lesions fail to show up on bone scan?

Cytokines from the myeloma cells inhibit bone formation. Osteoblast activity is suppressed and no radionuclide is taken up. Plain radiographs can be negative in 20% of cases. Computed tomography (CT) and magnetic resonance imaging (MRI) can detect myelomatous involvement where radiographs are negative.

19. List some clues that help distinguish myeloma from metastatic carcinoma involving th vertebra.

Weinstein[19] summarizes that a collapsed vertebra but preservation of the pedicles can be seen in myeloma. The disc is usually intact. A paraspinous mass is frequently present.

20. Name other variants of multiple myeloma.

Smoldering multiple myeloma has an M protein >3 gm/dl and more than 10% plasma cells in the bone marrow but causes no anemia, renal insufficiency, or bone lesions. Osteosclerotic myeloma can be part of the POEMS syndrome (polyneuropathy, organomegaly, endocrinopathy, M protein, and skin changes). The hematocrit is normal or high. Hypercalcemia and renal insufficiency are rare.

21. When and how do you treat myeloma?

If patients are asymptomatic and have no anemia, bone lesions, or renal compromise, treatment may be postponed until the disease progresses. The standard treatment is a combination of melphalan and prednisone. This may be very toxic if the patient has renal failure. Combination chemotherapy using three to five drugs is sometimes initiated in younger patients with aggressive disease to get a higher response rate. Multidrug therapy has not yet been shown to improve survival. Vincristine, dexamethasone, and doxorubicin (Adriamycin) (VAD) or dexamethasone alone have activity as salvage therapy. Some centers are offering autologous bone marrow transplant to patients <70 years of age with any stage of the disease or allogeneic transplant to patients <55 years of age with poor prognostic features at diagnosis as well as with relapse, progression, or refractory disease. Interferon may play a role in maintaining remission once it is induced. Radiation therapy is useful for local painful lesions.

22. Compare Waldenström's macroglobulinemia (WM) to MM.

WM is a low-grade lymphoid malignancy. It is one seventh as common as MM. In the bone marrow, WM appears as a proliferation of small, basophilic lymphocytes (plasmacytoid lymphocytes). Mast cells are increased. The M protein produced is an IgM monoclonal protein that circulates as a pentamer. The lympocytic proliferation causes hepatosplenomegaly in about 38% of patients with adenopathy in about 30%. Bone pain is rare. Lytic lesions are seen in <10%. Renal failure is not common, but sensorimotor neuropathy can be a prominent feature.

23. What are common symptoms in WM?
Fatigue, weakness, and bleeding are common presenting symptoms. As the disease progresses, severe anemia, constitutional symptoms (night sweats, weight loss), hyperviscosity, organomegaly, and adenopathy may force treatment.

24. How do M proteins cause hyperviscosity?
The amount of M protein alone, in relation to the plasma fluid, can cause increased viscosity and sluggish blood flow. Proteins that tend to polymerize or aggregate can increase viscosity at a lower level of protein. IgM circulates as a pentamer and IgA as a dimer. A subtype of IgG, IgG3, tends to aggregate. Although most patients will be symptomatic at viscosities >4 centipoise (nl <1.8), the correlation is not perfect.

25. If hyperviscosity is present, what do you expect to find on history and physical examination?
Chronic nasal bleeding, oozing from gums, and at times gastrointestinal bleeding occur. Patients describe blurring and loss of vision. Fundi show flame hemorrhages, sausagelike segmentation of retinal veins, and papilledema. Impaired circulation in the nervous system is manifested as dizziness, headache, vertigo, nystagmus, hearing loss, ataxia, paresthesias, diplopia, somnolence, and even coma. Congestive heart failure can occur.

26. What features of IgM hyperviscosity allow plasmapheresis to be effective?
IgM pentamers are distributed predominantly in the intravascular space (76%). This is in contrast to the distribution of IgG (45%) and IgA (42%). For IgM, there is no large extravascular pool to replace the plasma pool once the pheresis pulls out the M protein. Chemotherapy should be used to decrease new protein production.

27. Because chronic lymphatic leukemia (CLL) also can have an IgM spike, how can you distinguish WM from CLL?
Compared with CLL, WM will have a larger M spike, usually >3 gm/dl. The bone marrow will show "plasmacytoid" lymphocytes and increased mast cells. No lymphocytosis is present.

BIBLIOGRAPHY

1. Alexanian R, Dimopoulos M, Delasalle K, Barlogie B: Primary dexamethasone treatment of multiple myeloma. Blood 80:887, 1992.
2. Barlogie B (ed): Multiple myeloma. Hematol Oncol Clin North Am 6:211, 1992.
3. Barlogie B, Alexanian R, Jagannath S: Plasma cell dyscrasias. JAMA 268:2946, 1992.
4. Barlogie B, Epstein J, Selvanayagam P, Alexanian R: Plasma cell myeloma—New biological insights and advances in therapy. Blood 73:865, 1989.
5. Barlogie B, Gale RP: Multiple myeloma and chronic lymphatic leukemia: Parallels and contrasts. Am J Med 93:443, 1992.
6. Cavo M, Galieni P, Zuffa E, et al: Prognostic variables and clinical staging in multiple myeloma. Blood 74:1774, 1989.
7. DeVita VT, Hellman S, Rosenberg SA (eds): Cancer: Principles and Practices of Oncology. Philadelphia, J.B. Lippincott, 1989.
8. Dimopoulos MA, Barlogie B, Smith LS, Alexanian R: High serum lactate dehydrogenase level as a marker for drug resistance and short survival in multiple myeloma. Ann Intern Med 115:931, 1991.
9. Dimopoulos MA, Goldstein J, Fuller L, et al: Curability of solitary bone plasmacytoma. J Clin Oncol 10:587, 1992.
10. Dimopoulos MA, Kantarjian H, Estey E, et al: Treatment of Waldenström macroglobulinemia with 2-chlorodeoxyadenosine. Ann Intern Med 118:195, 1993.

11. Dimopoulos MA, Moulopoulos A, Smith T, et al: Risk of disease progression in asymptomatic multiple myeloma. Am J Med 94:57, 1993.
12. Durie BGM, Salmon SE: A clinical staging system for multiple myeloma. Cancer 36:842, 1975.
13. Greipp PR: Advances in the diagnosis and management of myeloma. Semin Hematol 29(Suppl 2):24, 1992.
14. Hoffman R, Benz EJ, Shattel SJ, et al (eds): Hematology: Basic Principles and Practice. New York, Churchill Livingstone, 1991.
15. Lee GR, Bithell TC, Foerster J, et al (eds): Wintrobe's Clinical Hematology. Philadelphia, Lea & Febiger, 1993.
16. Mandelli F, Avvisati G, Amadori S, et al: Maintenance treatment with recombinant interferon alpha-2b in patients with multiple myeloma responding to conventional induction chemotherapy. N Engl J Med 322:1430, 1990.
17. Miralles GD, O'Fallon JR, Talley NJ: Plasma-cell dyscrasia with polyneuropathy: The spectrum of POEMS syndrome. N Engl J Med 327:1919, 1992.
18. Redmond B, Pyzdrowski KL, Elson MK, et al: Brief report: Hypoglycemia due to a monoclonal insulin-binding antibody in multiple myeloma. N Engl J Med 326:994, 1992.
19. Weinstein RS: Bone involvement in multiple myeloma. Am J Med 93:591, 1992.
20. Williams WJ, Beutler E, Erslev AJ, Lechtman MA (eds): Hematology. New York, McGraw-Hill, 1990.

36. HODGKIN'S DISEASE

George Mathai, M.D., and William A. Robinson, M.D., Ph.D.

1. Who gets Hodgkin's disease?

Although Hodgkin's disease may occur at any age, the classic bimodal age distribution shows one peak at 20–29 years (mainly of the nodular sclerosis [NS] histology) and a second peak at 60 years or older (mainly of the lymphocyte-depleted [LD] histology). Despite male predominance in children under age 10 years, the sex distribution becomes nearly equal at the two age peaks. In the United States, Caucasians account for more than 90% of all cases. The disease is also associated with small family size, high standard of living, and high level of maternal education.

2. What cells are found in biopsies of patients with Hodgkin's disease?

Reed-Sternberg (RS) cells
RS cell precursors
Host inflammatory cells
Cells appearing in response to cytokines liberated by RS cells

3. What is the Reed-Sternberg cell?

Reed-Sternberg (RS) cells are giant cells with two or more nuclear lobes and huge eosinophilic, inclusionlike nucleoli. The classic RS cell has a symmetrical, mirror-image nucleus that creates the "owl-eye" appearance. (See Figure 15, Color Plates.)

Variants or precursors of RS cells can also be identified. The lacunar cell, a small variant of the RS cell, is seen in nodular sclerosis histology. The popcorn-cell variants may be seen in lymphocyte-predominance histology, and a sarcomatous RS variant is seen in lymphocyte-depletion Hodgkin's disease.

RS cells and variants, which have the phenotype of activated lymphoid cells, express antigens Ki-1 (CD30), Leu-M1 (CD15), HLA-DR, Tac (CD25), and T9 (transferrin receptor). Leukocyte common antigen (LCA or CD45), which is absent in most cases of Hodgkin's disease, helps to distinguish Hodgkin's disease from non-Hodgkin's lymphoma (NHL).

4. Are Reed-Sternberg cells found only in Hodgkin's disease?
No. RS cells have been seen rarely in other types of cancer (e.g., breast and lung cancer, melanoma); they also have been seen in certain inflammatory states (e.g., myositis, infectious mononucleosis). RS cells are diagnostic for Hodgkin's disease only in the proper histologic setting.

5. Describe the four histologic types of Hodgkin's disease.
The original classification by Lukes et al. of the histopathology of Hodgkin's disease has been revised according to the Rye classification:
   1. **Nodular sclerosis** (NS), the most frequent histologic type in the United States, is associated with a good prognosis. Hematoxylin and eosin (H&E) stains show eosinophilic collagen bands of varying width surrounding blue lymphoid nodules. (See Figure 16, Color Plates.) Some cells may seem to be sitting within a cleared area. These lacunar variants of the RS cell are an artifact of cell fixation. NS has been subdivided into grades I and II. Grade II, which shows areas of lymphocytic depletion or numerous pleomorphic RS giant cells, has a worse prognosis than grade I.
   2. In **lymphocyte-predominant** (LP) Hodgkin's disease the affected tissue consists primarily of small lymphocytes and benign epithelioid histiocytes. Diagnostic RS cells are rare. RS cell variants with large folded, twisted, or multilobar nuclei and small nucleoli are called popcorn cells. Two subtypes, nodular and diffuse, are seen. Nodular Hodgkin's disease may sometimes progress to lymphocytic depletion or large-cell NHL.
   3. **Lymphocyte depletion**, as the name suggests, is characterized by depletion of lymphocytes and frequently by focal necrosis. This variant may be associated with a febrile wasting syndrome, presenting often with subdiaphragmatic involvement and bone-marrow infiltration.
   4. **Mixed cellularity** is the second most common type. RS cells are frequent, along with reactive histiocytes, eosinophils, neutrophils, plasma cells, small lymphocytes, and small foci of necrosis. There is usually focal or partial involvement of lymph nodes.

6. What causes Hodgkin's disease?
The cause is unknown. Investigators have long argued that Hodgkin's disease may not even be a malignancy. The clustering of childhood cases and cases within families suggests an infectious etiology. A viral etiology has been proposed, and DNA of the Epstein-Barr virus (EBV) has been demonstrated in RS cells of some patients with Hodgkin's disease. Subsequent studies have disputed these theories.

Although chromosomal translocations are common in NHL and are thought to play a role in pathogenesis, no consistent chromosomal abnormalities (except hyperdiploid RS cells) can be demonstrated in Hodgkin's disease.

7. How does the clinical presentation of Hodgkin's disease differ from that of non-Hodgkin's lymphoma?
Hodgkin's disease commonly presents as cervical adenopathy, which may remain isolated or spread to contiguous lymph-node groups. NHL does not present with this characteristic contiguous spread. Generalized lymphadenopathy is a rare presentation for Hodgkin's disease but is commonly seen in low-grade NHL.

When found above the diaphragm, Hodgkin's disease is often limited to the supradiaphragmatic area. If identified below the diaphragm, the disease is more often widely disseminated. Similar statements are **not** true for NHL.

Hodgkin's disease can present in the adolescent or young adult as a large mediastinal mass. High-grade histologies of NHL may have similar presentations.

Bulky abdominal adenopathy or involvement of Waldeyer's ring suggests NHL rather than Hodgkin's disease.

8. What signs or symptoms may suggest the diagnosis of Hodgkin's disease?
Often patients with Hodgkin's disease complain of generalized pruritus. They also may describe lymph node pain with alcohol ingestion and generally are anergic. Thus, they do not respond to normal skin antigens such as mumps and candida; if previously positive for tuberculosis, they are now negative.

9. What are B symptoms in the staging of Hodgkin's disease?
B symptoms, which are specific and prognostic, include:
Unexplained fever of 101°F (38.5°C) or higher
Drenching night sweats
Loss of more than 10% of body weight in the previous 6 months

10. Describe the staging classification and the staging evaluation of a patient with Hodgkin's disease.
The Ann Arbor staging classification for Hodgkin's disease recognizes both a clinical and a pathologic stage. Stages are determined according to the number of lymph node regions (not sites) involved and whether the disease affects one or both sides of the diaphragm. The designation E denotes a direct extranodal extension of lymph node disease that potentially can be encompassed in a radiation portal.

Ann Arbor Staging Classification for Hodgkin's Disease*

STAGE	FEATURES
I	Involvement of a single lymph node region (I) or a single extralymphatic organ or site (I_E)
II	Involvement of 2 or more lymph node regions on the same side of the diaphragm (II), or 1 or more lymph node regions with an extralymphatic site (II_E)
III	Involvement of lymph node regions on both sides of the diaphragm (III), possibly with an extralymphatic organ or site (III_E), the spleen (III_S), or both (III_{SE})
IV	Diffuse or disseminated involvement of 1 or more extralymphatic organs (identified by symbols), with or without associated lymph node involvement

* All stages are subclassified as A (asymptomatic) or B (fever, sweats, and loss of more than 10% of body weight).

Clinical staging evaluation proceeds as in the table below.

Recommended Steps for Staging Evaluation of Patients with Hodgkin's Disease

History and examination
  B symptoms: weight loss >10%
    during previous 6 months,
    documented fever, night sweats
  Detailed physical examination
Radiology
  Plain chest radiograph
  Computed tomography (CT) of
    thorax, abdomen, and pelvis
Hematology
  Full blood count
  Erythrocyte sedimentation rate
  Bone marrow biopsy, bilateral

Biochemistry
  Tests of liver function
  Albumin, lactate dehydrogenase (LDH),
    calcium
Under special circumstances
  Ultrasound scanning
  Magnetic resonance imaging
  Bipedal lymphangiogram
Other imaging techniques
  Isotope scanning
  Gallium
  Technetium
  MUGA (multiple-gated acquisition
    blood-pool scan)

In 1989 an international multidisciplinary committee modified the Ann Arbor staging classification. This modification, called the Cotswold recommendations, gave due importance to computed tomography scans and other imaging modalities in defining extent of disease.

Cotswold Staging Classification

STAGE	FEATURES
I	Involvement of a single lymph node region or lymphoid structure (e.g., spleen, thymus, Waldeyer's ring)

II	Involvement of 2 or more lymph node regions on the same side of the diaphragm
	    The mediastinum is a single site; hilar lymph nodes are lateralized.
	    The number of anatomic sites should be indicated by a subscript (e.g., II_3)

III	Involvement of lymph node regions or structures on both sides of the diaphragm
	    III_1: with or without splenic hilar, celiac, or portal nodes
	    III_2: with paraaortic, iliac, mesenteric nodes

IV	Involvement of extranodal site(s) beyond that designated E
	    A: No symptoms
	    B: Fever, drenching sweats, weight loss
	    X: Bulky disease
	        $>1/3$ widening of mediastinum
	        >10 cm maximal dimension of nodal mass
	    E: Involvement of a single extranodal site, contiguous or proximal to known nodal site
	    CS: Clinical stage
	    PS: Pathologic stage

11. What are the current views regarding staging laparotomy?

Occult Hodgkin's disease is discovered at laparotomy in at least 25% of patients with only supradiaphragmatic disease on clinical evaluation. The controversy about staging laparotomy can be eased by the philosophy that laparotomy should be avoided unless the findings will change treatment significantly.

Staging laparotomy is required:
For patients with clinical stage I, II, and IIIA disease when radiation therapy alone is being considered. Such patients will benefit from combined modality treatment if extensive splenic (>4 nodules) or periaortic nodes are found at laparotomy.

Staging laparotomy is not required:
1. For patients with clear clnical stage IIIB or IV disease who are scheduled for chemotherapy.
2. For patients with a bulky mediastinal mass ($>1/3$ the diameter of the chest), who benefit most from combined modality treatment.
3. For patients with isolated high cervical or nonbulky mediastinal involvement and lymphocyte-predominant or nodular sclerosing Hodgkin's disease, who may be managed by subtotal nodal radiation alone.

12. What are the treatment modalities available for Hodgkin's disease? What are the current recommendations?

The three treatment modalities available for Hodgkin's disease are radiation therapy, combination chemotherapy, and combined modality treatment (radiation and chemotherapy). The current recommendations for the various stages are as follows:
1. **Stages IA/IIA**—subtotal nodal radiation
2. **Stages IB/IIB**—combination chemotherapy

3. **Stage IIIA**—combination chemotherapy alone. Patients with minimal laparotomy-defined stage IIIA disease may be treated with subtotal or total nodal radiation.

4. **Bulky mediastinal disease**—combined modality treatment

5. **Stages IIIB/IV**—combination chemotherapy

13. Describe the three different fields of radiation used in Hodgkin's disease.

1. **Subtotal nodal or lymphoid radiation** consisting of mantle and spade fields is commonly used for stages IA, IIA, and pathologic stage IIB.

2. **Total nodal or lymphoid radiation** consisting of mantle and inverted-Y fields is used for stages IIB and IIIA.

3. **Involved field radiation** is only for sites of known disease and is commonly used in combination with chemotherapy.

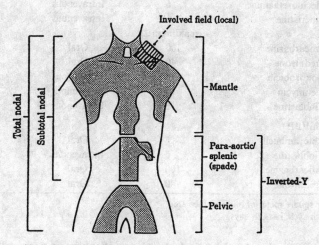

Radiation fields used in Hodgkin's disease.

14. Is the chemotherapy used in Hodgkin's disease the same regardless of stage?

The choice of chemotherapy should be individualized to the patient and stage of disease. Patients who desire to preserve fertility should avoid MOPP (the combination of nitrogen mustard, Oncovin, prednisone, and procarbazine) (see table below). Patients receiving combined modality therapy for bulky mediastinal disease should avoid ABVD (the combination of Adriamycin, bleomycin, vinblastine, and dacarbazine) (see table below) because of the added pulmonary and cardiac toxicity of radiation when combined with bleomycin and Adriamycin.

Newer studies are attempting to identify even less toxic regimens of combination chemotherapy to be used with involved field radiation for lower-stage (I and II) disease.

Common Chemotherapeutic Regimens Used in Hodgkin's Disease .

REGIMEN	RECOMMENDED DOSE* (mg/m²)	ROUTE	CYCLE DAYS†
1. MOPP			
Mechlorethamine	6	Intravenous	1 and 8
Vincristine	1.4	Intravenous	1 and 8
Procarbazine	100	Oral	1–14
Prednisone	40	Oral	1–14

Table continued on following page.

Common Chemotherapeutic Regimens Used in Hodgkin's Disease (Continued)

REGIMEN	RECOMMENDED DOSE* (mg/m²)	ROUTE	CYCLE DAYS†
2. ABVD			
Doxorubicin	25	Intravenous	1 and 15
Bleomycin	10	Intravenous	1 and 15
Vinblastine	6	Intravenous	1 and 15
Dacarbazine	375	Intravenous	1 and 15
3. MOPP–ABVD in alternating monthly cycles	As for MOPP and ABVD above		
4. MOPP-ABV hybrid			
Mechlorethamine	6	Intravenous	1
Vincristine	1.4 (maximum 2)	Intravenous	1
Procarbazine	100	Oral	1–7
Prednisone	40	Oral	1–14
Doxorubicin	35	Intravenous	8
Bleomycin	10	Intravenous	8
Vinblastine	6	Intravenous	8
5. ChlVPP			
Chlorambucil	6	Oral	1–14
Vinblastine	6	Intravenous	1 and 8
Procarbazine	100	Oral	1–14
Prednisone	40	Oral	1–14

* Per square meter of body surface area.
† Each cycle lasts 28 days.

15. What can be done for the patient who relapses after primary treatment?

ᶠ the primary treatment is radiation therapy, the patient should receive combination
hemotherapy. Of patients salvaged with chemotherapy after radiation therapy, 50% can
ᵇe cured.

If the patient relapses after combination chemotherapy, the interval from treatment to
relapse should be considered. Some investigators argue that patients who relapse more than
1 year after treatment did not receive dose-intensive therapy. These patients may be treated
with the same regimen that they initially received. Patients who relapse less than 1 year after
treatment should be considered to have aggressive disease and receive a regimen of drugs
different (non–cross-resistant) from the initial regimen.

16. When should a bone marrow transplant be considered in the treatment of Hodgkin's disease?

Autologous bone marrow transplantation has been used as salvage therapy for individuals
with relapsed Hodgkin's disease. Long-term responses are seen in 20–40% of patients. This
form of therapy may be considered in patients who relapse early (<1 year) after primary
therapy. Studies are under way to identify high-risk patients who may benefit from therapy
during their first remission.

17. How can one tell when a patient is cured of Hodgkin's disease?

ᵢndividuals who are disease-free for more than 10 years after therapy may be considered
cuᵣed.

18. Which individuals have the highest rate of relapse?
Relapse cannot be predicted accurately in Hodgkin's disease. Poor prognostic factors, however, have been identified. Tumor bulk and stage appear to be the most important prognostic factors. Of interest, the presence of a residual radiographic abnormality is not associated with a greater relapse rate. The presence of B symptoms (generally signifying greater tumor burden) is a poor prognostic factor. Low hematocrit and high lactate dehydrogenase (LDH) also have been associated with a higher rate of relapse. The histopathology has been suggested to have prognostic significance but should **not** guide the choice of therapy.

19. Is Hodgkin's disease an AIDS-defining illness?
No. Although it is the most common non–AIDS-defining cancer, the prevalence may be secondary to the high incidence of Hodgkin's disease in the group of individuals acquiring the AIDS virus (young adults).

20. What are the complications of therapy for Hodgkin's disease?
The common complications after therapy for Hodgkin's disease are as follows:
1. **Hypothyroidism** is seen in 10–20% of patients treated with mantle radiation therapy (see figure on p. 151) and correctable by replacement therapy.
2. **Sterility** is seen in women after pelvic radiation. MOPP chemotherapy causes sterility in men.
3. **Pneumonitis** is seen after mantle radiation.
4. **Cardiac toxicity** (a higher incidence of pericardial disease) is seen when both Adriamycin-based chemotherapy and radiation are given.
5. **Aseptic necrosis of femoral heads** is associated with prednisone in MOPP chemotherapy.
6. **Secondary neoplasms**
   (1) Acute nonlymphocytic leukemia occurs 3–10 years after treatment in 2–10% of patients treated with a combination of MOPP chemotherapy and radiation. The 12-year estimate of leukemia development after treatment is 1.3% for chemotherapy alone, 10.2% for radiation plus MOPP chemotherapy, 0% for radiation plus ABVD chemotherapy, and 4.8% for radiation plus other regimens.
   (2) NHL may develop, usually with high grade B-cell tumors.
   (3) Epithelial tumors and sarcomas are also known to develop in patients treated for Hodgkin's disease.
7. **Neurologic complications** may include neuropathy after vincristine therapy and myelopathy after radiotherapy.

21. Describe the appropriate follow-up of patients after completion of treatment.
Most relapses occur within the first 3–4 years after therapy. Treated individuals should be followed every 2 months for the first 2 years, then every 3 months for the next 2 years, and then every 6 months. Appropriate procedures during follow-up include:

Appropriate Follow-up of Patients

History and physical examination at each visit
Complete blood count with sedimentation rate at each visit
Chemistry panel every 6 months for 4 years
Chest radiograph yearly for 10 years
Computed tomography scans of involved areas yearly for 4 years
Thyroid function tests yearly
Sterility testing before and after treatment if desired by the patient

BIBLIOGRAPHY

1. Anderson J, Canellos GP: MOPP vs. ABVD vs. MOPP alternating with ABVD in advanced Hodgkin's disease [abstract]. Proceedings of the International Conference on Malignant Lymphomas, Lugano, Switzerland, 1990.
2. Armitage JO: Bone marrow transplantation in the treatment of patients with lymphoma. Blood 73:1749, 1989.
3. Brain MC, Carbone PP: Current Therapy in Hematology/Oncology, 4th ed. Philadelphia, B.C. Decker, 1992.
4. Hoffman R, Benz EJ, Shattil SJ, et al: Hematology: Basic Principles and Practice. New York, Churchill Livingstone, 1991.
5. Hoppe RT: The contemporary management of Hodgkin disease. Radiology 169:297, 1988.
6. Longo DL, Young RC, Wesley M, et al: Twenty years of MOPP chemotherapy for Hodgkin's disease. J Clin Oncol 4:1295, 1986.
7. Santaro A, Bonfante V, Bonadonna G: Salvage chemotherapy with ABVD in MOPP-resistant Hodgkin's disease. Ann Intern Med 96:139, 1982.
8. Santaro A, Viviani SS, Valagussa P, et al: CCNU, etoposide, prednimustine (CEP) in refractory Hodgkin's disease. Semin Oncol 13:23, 1986.
9. Urba WJ, Longo DL: Hodgkin's disease. N Engl J Med 326:678, 1992.
10. Williams SF, Farah R, Golomb HM: Hodgkin's disease. Hematol Oncol Clin North Am 3: 1989.

IV. General Care of the Cancer Patient

37. CARCINOGENESIS

George E. Moore, M.D., Ph.D.

1. How is carcinogenesis defined?
The alteration of normal cells into malignant cells is almost always a multistage evolution of genetic and epigenic alterations that eventuate in cells that escape the normal growth constraints of the host.

2. What are the stages of carcinogenesis?
The multistage process[6,7,8,11,13] may include the following:
1. Mutation/activation of a cell may involve unconstrained factors of growth, advantageous metabolic patterns, oncogenes, inactivated suppressor gene functions, and autonomy from cell-cell controls.
2. Selective clonal growth—usually from single cell with a new growth advantage which permits further mutations.
3. Selection of additional "malignant features" allows progression from benign hyperplasia to autonomous neoplastic growth.
4. Multiple clonal cancers developing from mutations with varying mosaics of genetic and functional activities develop even more autonomy from dependence on hormones and other host factors.
5. Additional changes promote invasion and autonomy of metastases—first of clumps of cells and then even single cells.
Note: The birth of single malignant cells is probably very common, a daily occurrence, but their sustained growth is rare. Suppressive interaction with defensive host factors occurs at all levels. Indeed the regression of established malignancies as well as precancerous lesions has been authenticated.
The stages outlined above are not necessarily distinct and each stage probably includes multiple alterations of antigenicity, regulatory enzymes, inappropriate expression of growth factors and other centers of genome activation.

3. What are the classes of carcinogens?

Physical agents	Vital agents	Rarely, chronic
Chemical compounds	Foreign body reactions	inflammation

Carcinogens may also be divided into:

Inherited genetic defects	Foreign body reactants—asbestos fibers
Social agents such as tobacco and alcohol	Chronic inflammation such as ulcerative colitis
Occupational exposures such as the benzenes	Iatrogenic agents such as cancer chemotherapeutic drugs, radiation,
Radiation from many sources	and estrogens given to pregnant
Contaminants of the food chain such as aflatoxin B	women that caused vaginal cancers in their daughters

4. What are major examples of inherited susceptibilities to cancer?

Li-Fraumeni syndrome—cancers of multiple organs
Xeroderma pigmentosa—cancers of the skin and melanoma
Familial polyposis coli
Familial retinoblastosis or Cowden's syndrome—cancer of the breast
   and other organs
DiGeorge syndrome—leukemia.

Note: Some of these traits increase reactivity to environmental agents, whereas others reflect rather specific lack of host defenses. Some are single gene defects, whereas most involve multiple activator and suppressor genes and a sequence of genetic changes.

Note: Carcinogenesis must be considered as an alteration of the "normal" rate of "spontaneous" mutations that rarely produce cancerous cells and that may escape host surveillance. The implication that unusually high mutation rates of selected DNA sequences may reflect a genetic trait is important.[19]

5. In addition to chimney sweep's cancer, what are other historical causes and noncauses of cancers?

There were and continue to be many "causes" of cancers with and without known biologic rationale. There were "cancer houses," which were kept vacant or burned. Many different microorganisms, various soil conditions and water supplies, water contaminants, and dietary substances such as smoked fish, raw fish, and spices have also been thought to cause cancers.

Thyroid tumors developed in the trout of certain streams; a problem that was immediately solved by the addition of iodine to the water—an observation of direct relevance to humans.

The observation of nasal cancers in snuff users was made centuries ago.

Women who pointed their paint brushes dipped in uranium salts by twirling them between their lips and then painted the numbers on watches developed horrible carcinomas and sarcomas of the mouth and jaws (1915 to 1925). Pioneers in the use of radiation developed skin cancers and leukemias (1907 to 1945).

The uranium miners in the Schneeberg area of Saxony in Europe had increased lung "disorders." Ironically, the minerals were not mined for their radioactivity but for the beautiful colors they imported to glass.

Presently, there is a fear of radiation from radon seepage from the ground and into homes and schools which is greatly exaggerated.

Many years ago, cancer of the urinary bladder was associated with infestation by the trematode *Schistosoma haematobium*.

6. How are carcinogens identified?

Most human carcinogens such as tobacco and vinyl chloride have been identified first by clinical observation.

Most carcinogens are mutagens and therefore fruit flies *(Drosophila)*, molds *(Neurospora)*, bacteria, round worms, and a variety of experimental animals have been used as test subjects. Cultured human and rodent cells have been very useful in studies of carcinogenesis but are less applicable for screening purposes. Various routes of delivery and extended application of the substances to animals may be required. For example, topical applications, ingestion, injections, and the exposure of pregnant animals at various doses are necessary.

The complexity of such assays can be imagined when one considers that some carcinogens are metabolites, others require growth-promoting agents, and specific exposures may be limited to specific cells of specific species at specific ages with and without additional "promoting" agents.

The Ames test is an assay of mutagenesis of bacteria. It is a valuable screen but is limited in direct significance for human carcinogenesis.

7. Do we know any causes of frequent human cancers?

The search for specific causes is not simple, as demonstrated by our absolute failure to identify the cause(s) of the pandemic of gastric cancer during the middle of the 20th century.

Even the evident causation of lung cancer by cigarette smoking was not clarified until 1950. Carcinogens have been identified in smoke, and there are excellent studies of the progressive histologic and cytologic changes in the bronchial epithelium of smokers.

The association of skin cancer with sunlight and ionizing radiation has been known for many years. The susceptibility of thyroid and hemopoietic cells to radiation-induced carcinogenesis has been authenticated.

8. What are some of the animate causes of cancers?

These include viruses such as the Epstein-Barr virus and the papillomaviruses, and indirectly parasitic infestations such as schistosomiasis, and perhaps infection with *Helicobacter pylori*, which induces chronic gastritis.

Viruses such as SV-40 are used to immortalize cells in the laboratory, but they seem unable to complete the evolution of carcinogenesis without the aid of additional stimuli. From a historical view, mention should be made of the discovery of sarcoma virus by Roux (1911), papillomavirus by Shope (1933), mouse mammary virus by Bittner (1936), leukemia virus by Gross (1951), polyomavirus by Stewart (1957), and many others in both plants and animals.

As molecular assays become available, the detection of many more viral sequences at various stages of carcinogenesis in humans seems reasonable.

9. Discuss the iatrogenic causes of cancers.

There is a risk of cancer, although low, from diagnostic and therapeutic radiation, from many chemotherapeutic agents such as the alkylating agents and other antimetabolites, hormones such as estrogens, growth hormone (which causes leukemia), and even the implantation of iron-dextran. Any intensely biologically active medication must be suspect. For example, the antibiotic metronidazole apparently causes lung adenomas in mice, azidothymidine (AZT) is carcinogenic in rodents, and tamoxifen, which is being used as preventative of breast cancer, causes hepatocellular cancers in rodents and rarely uterine carcinomas in humans.

A dramatic example of medical carcinogenesis was the use of diethylstilbestrol for threatened abortion in many thousands of women and whose daughters subsequently developed carcinomas of the vagina and exocervic from ages 7 to 28.[18]

Radioactive thorium dioxide (Thorotrast) provided excellent angiograms but also caused a variety of malignancies.[4]

Foreign bodies such as the metallic replacements of joints and struts for fractured bones and the various meshes have not been shown to be carcinogenic in humans, in contrast to rodents.[14]

A separate indirect category of carcinogenesis includes the immunosuppressive agents required for organ transplants.[16]

10. What are the effects of immunosuppression on carcinogenesis?

An exception to the long precancerous period—10 to over 30 years—is the rapid progression of cancers in those patients with acquired immunodeficiency syndrome (AIDS), probably those with malaria, and those immunosuppressed by medication.[16] Explosive cancerous growth occurs. Reversal of the immunosuppression may cause regression of the cancers—a confirmation of the importance of normal regulatory controls.

11. Explain the Delany Clause.

This infamous legislation in 1958 declared that anything added to our food chain that caused cancer in animals under any circumstances must be excluded—the theory of **zero tolerance.**

Unfortunately, many experimental animals are very susceptible to carcinogens that may in massive doses cause cancers, but these assays are not always relevant to humans.[2,12]

Controversies rage as to the optimal method(s) of testing and the species used for assays. Even the definition of "carcinogen" is inexact. From a practical standpoint, animal testing is limited to mice and rats. Confounding issues are the age at which the exposure is begun, the route and length of applications, dosage that is often at a maximal tolerated level, nutrition, and sex of the animals. The functional activities of host organs must be considered as well as the burden of "normal" viruses and bacteria in the test animal.

Indeed, the roles of the carcinogenist, the Food and Drug Administration (FDA), and the Environmental Protection Agency (EPA) regulators are not happy ones. The tortured saga of cyclamate, an artificial sweetener, began in 1970 with the report of bladder cancers in rats. It was removed from the market during a general hysteria and by political pressures unrelieved by science.

12. Are the recent claims of carcinogenicity associated with "natural" foodstuffs reasonable?
It is estimated that 99.9% of carcinogens in our foods are of natural origin.[2] These natural carcinogenic substances include mold toxins such as aflatoxins, certain bracken ferns, cycasin from the cycad nut, mushrooms (pyrrolizidine alkaloids), safroles (formerly used to flavor root beer), and even molecules in coffee. A popular drink in South America, "mate," which is a hot infusion of the leaves of the *Ilex* tree, has been implicated in cancers of the pharynx and esophagus.

Health food stores continue to advertise untested concoctions and vitamins as cancer preventatives and some even for treatment such as the latest craze—shark cartilage. Carcinogens have been isolated from both herbal medicines and teas.

In brief, it is impossible to avoid all carcinogens but fortunately most are of only experimental interest rather than significant dangers to humans. Undoubtedly, additional natural and synthetic carcinogens will be identified and will evoke terrifying headlines and rarely some will require preventive action.

13. Do cancers develop at sites of chronic inflammation? Are they associated with some chronic diseases?
Yes to both. Ulcerative colitis, usually after 10 years, is associated with colon cancer. Most cancers of the gallbladder are found with cholelithiasis. Chronic ulcers of the leg from stasis, old burn sites (Marjolin's ulcer), and persistent sinus tracts may evolve into cancers. The recent implication of a bacterial infection with gastritis and gastric cancer is interesting.[4]

In contrast to rodents, humans rarely ever have malignant reactions to foreign bodies. Asbestosis is an exception, and there is some evidence that other fibers such as glass wool and wood splinters may be dangerous. Controversies concerning the actual dangers of asbestos to humans are tainted by social and political imagery and biases.

Lung cancer or, more accurately, bronchial carcinomas result in part from the continuous cellular injury and repair plus exposure to the carcinogens in cigarette smoke. Cigarette smoke is the single greatest preventable carcinogenic threat.

Asiatic people who smoke "cigars" with the smoldering end within the mouth develop oral cancers as, of course, do chewers of betel nut concoctions and tobacco.

The development of skin cancers in Kashmiris at the abdominal site burned by the heated kangri bowl held against it for warmth was reported by missionary brothers in 1900.[9]

As a personal note from a surgeon oncologist, the emotional diatribes about the dangers of asbestos have departed from any and all scientific data. There has not been the predicted disastrous epidemic of asbestos-related deaths.[15] In Colorado, there has been no increase in mesothelioma deaths, which remain at about seven per year. The billions of dollars spent in removing asbestos from public buildings such as schools has benefited a new industry and countless lawyers at the expense of education.

Trauma is commonly blamed by patients for the development of cancers ("A baseball hit my breast")—these claims are legal rather than biologic. However, rarely trauma and the regeneration of tissues associated with it may aid in indirectly promoting carcinogenesis, as has been demonstrated experimentally.[5]

14. What are the intervals between exposure to a carcinogen and the development of cancer?
A number of years are required for carcinogenesis in the human. For example, asbestos-related cancers in nonsmokers rarely develop in less than 15 years and more often become evident in 25 to 40 years. Multiple exposures to ionizing radiation may eventuate in skin cancers and leukemia after only a few years, whereas malignancies of connective tissue cells and adenocarcinomas may take 15–30 years to develop. Smoking-induced cancers often require 15 or more years of exposure. **Note:** Cessation of exposure usually partially decreases the risk of malignancy.

Just as in experimental animals, youthful exposures are more dangerous and the carcinogenic interval is shorter.

15. Discuss the roles of oncogenes and suppressor genes in carcinogenesis.
These families of regulator genes[19]—oncogenes are positive growth regulators and suppressor genes are negative regulators—are subject to genetic segregation, deletion, mutation, and alterations of expression.

About 100 oncogenes and 6 or 7 suppressor genes have been identified. Both can be carried, activated, or inactivated by viruses or viral proteins and both may be altered by mutation, mutational amplification, expression out of sequence, and activation/suppression by translocation to an abnormal chromosomal site.

16. What are examples of oncogenes and suppressor genes in human malignancies?
In Burkitt's lymphoma, the *myc* oncogene is frequently translocated from chromosome 8 to 14. In many neuroblastomas, one of the many *myc* oncogenes is highly amplified. Mutational forms of the K-*ras* oncogene are present in cancers of the colon, bladder, bronchi, and pancreas. Translocations may expose or form critical hybrid transcripts with oncogenes. The famous Philadelphia chromosome is an altered chromosome 22 and brings into juxtaposition the important *bcr* gene and the c-*abl* proto-oncogene from chromosome 9.

The complexity involved in sorting out similar translocations, deletions, mutations, suppressors, and activations taking place on multiple chromosomes during *multiple sequential* stages of carcinogenesis numbs the mind.

The first suppressor genes identified were the *Rb* gene, whose deletion from chromosome 13 is associated with retinoblastoma, and the *p53* gene on chromosome 17. Alteration or deletion of *p53* has been detected in nearly 50% of certain human tumors.

Remember, our knowledge of the interactions of these genes is primitive and the exact roles are probably much more complicated than reflected by initial studies, but there is no doubt of their role in human carcinogenesis and the subsequent evolution of malignancies.

17. Are there preventive carcinogenic dietary patterns?
In my opinion, there is no conclusive evidence of carcinogenesis directly attributable to eating habits except obesity, which may accelerate aging of tissues and cells—a lessening of good health. Most information is derived from epidemiologic studies. Obesity has been related to breast cancer, a lack of fiber or stool bulk with colon cancer, the ingestion of hot liquids with carcinoma of the pharynx and esophagus, and the excessive use of grilled and smoked meat and fish with gastric cancer.

Experimental data suggest various antioxidants may negate or inhibit stage progression of many carcinogens—even asbestos—in experimental animals. Unfortunately, the toxicity of acceptable agents for human use has been excessive. There is a great popular interest in vitamins C and E as preventatives.

Rather nebulous epidemiologic studies have suggested a reduced risk of colon cancer in persons taking aspirin regularly. There are supporting observations of both human and animal tumor inhibition with nonsteroidal anti-inflammatory drugs.

Agents that cause cellular differentiation and maturation have been effective in experimental animals and may have clinical usefulness in the future.

In brief, lifestyle and dietary patterns that will slow aging are probably helpful but unproven preventatives.

18. How can we escape exposure to carcinogens?

You can't—even vegetables and fruits touted for optimal diets contain carcinogens that would be banned if used as artificial food flavorings! One should minimize exposure to ultraviolet light and ionizing radiation, especially persons with sensitive skin such as those with blonde and red hair, blue eyes, and freckles.

Those with familial risks require identification and regularly scheduled diagnostic procedures such as mammography, colonoscopy, and the inspection of dermal abnormalities.

In the future, some of the genetic factors will be identified and perhaps eliminated by genetic engineering.

19. Why haven't epidemiologic studies of human carcinogenesis been more successful?

Carcinogenesis is complex and may extend over many years and may progress in only a tiny percentage of the persons at risk. Simple small correlations that are spewed out from interview studies and manipulative computer analyses are often erroneous. Indeed, the most common epidemiologic study of cancer causation is one denying a prior report.

"Causes" of cancers have many confounders: genetic factors, different target organ/cells, age, sex, pregnancy, multiple carcinogens, multiple "promoting" agents, infectious agents, dosage- and time-related/multiple exposures, and specific alterations of systemic and local immunities, some of which are associated with aging.

The list of spurious results is endless: EMF (electromagnetic fields), radio phones, radar, Alar, caffeine, hair coloring, food additives, and many "capitalistic products," such as cotton clothing, "new car odor," and many "occupational exposures." (Hobbies are rarely studied.)

Assertions of carcinogenesis are subject to emotional, political, and legislative interpretations, which in turn are affected/driven by scientific uncertainties, selective polemics, ambitions, and seemingly last of all valid biologic data.

Actually, most if not all human carcinogens were first identified by personal observations. The confirmation of these observations by epidemiologic studies has been very important.

Environmental factors other than tobacco and ultraviolet light probably cause <10% of malignancies but 90% of the headlines.

Exposures to infectious agents, environmental factors, and other diverse health factors will always evolve and change over the years, which further minimizes the ability of epidemiologic studies to detect causative agents.

BIBLIOGRAPHY

1. Acheson ED, Hadfield EH, MacBeth RG: Carcinoma of the nasal cavity and accessory sinuses in woodworkers. Lancet 1:311–312, 1967.
2. Ames BN, Gold LS: Too many rodent carcinogens: Mitogenesis increases mutagenesis. Science 249:970–971; 250:970–971, 1990.
3. Anderson M, Storm HH: Cancer incidence among Danish Thorotrast-exposed patients. J Natl Cancer Inst 84:1318–1325, 1992.
4. Bock FG, Moore GE: Carcinogenic activity of cigarette—Smoke condensate. I. Effect of trauma and remote X-irradiation. J Natl Cancer Inst 22:401, 1959.
5. Discoveries and Opportunities in Cancer Research: Cancer Research 51:#18 supplement 5015–5086, 1991.
6. Carcinogenesis. These 532 abstracts provide an excellent introduction to current research. Proc Am Assoc Cancer Res 34:99–187, 1993.
7. Druker BJ, Mamon HJ, Roberts TM: Oncogenes, growth factors, and signal transduction. N Engl J Med 321:1383–1391, 1989.
8. Neve EF, Neve A: Kangri-burn cancer. Br Med J 2:1255–1256, 1923.

9. Feinstein AR, Horwitz RI, Spitzer WO, Battista RN: Coffee and pancreatic cancer: The problems of etiological science and epidemiologic case-control research. JAMA 246:957–961, 1981.
10. Harris CC: Chemical and physical carcinogenesis: Advances and perspectives for the 1990s. Cancer Res (Suppl 51):5023–5044, 1991.
11. Hay A: Testing times for the tests. Nature 350:555–556, 1991.
12. Koeffler HP, McCormick F, Denny C: Molecular mechanisms of cancer. West J Med 155:505–513, 1991.
13. Moore GE, Palmer QN: Money causes cancer, ban it. JAMA 238:397, 1977.
14. Mossman BT, Bignon J, Corn M, et al: Asbestos: Scientific developments and implications for public policy. Science 247:294–301, 1990.
15. Penn I: Depressed immunity and the development of cancer. Clin Exp Immunol 46:459–474, 1981.
16. Stone R: News and comments. Science 254:928–931, 1991.
17. Ulfelder H: The stilbestrol-adenosis-carcinoma syndromes. Cancer 38:426–431, 1976.
18. Vogt PK: Cancer genes. West J Med 158:273–278, 1993.
19. Yurij Ionov M, Peinado S, Malkhosyan D, et al: Ubiquitous somatic mutations in simple repeated sequences reveal a new mechanism for colonic carcinogenesis. Nature 363:558–561, 1993.

38. THE USE OF MOLECULAR DIAGNOSTICS IN MALIGNANCY

Vincent L. Wilson, Ph.D.

1. Why use molecular genetics if cytogenetic analysis is available?

In relevant cases, the molecular genetic tests are generally more rapid and precise. Cytogenetics can only detect deletions and other mutations that span approximately 1 million bases in size. Molecular genetics can detect mutations as small as a single base substitution. Therefore, molecular genetics will more readily detect a diagnostic mutation in the retinoblastoma gene than cytogenetics. Diagnostic and cancer-predisposing mutations are not generally detectable without molecular genetic approaches. Molecular techniques also enable the detection of minimal residual disease, because clonal markers of cancer cells, such as chromosomal translocations and gene rearrangements, are detectable when present at a level of only one cancer cell in a million. However, molecular genetics will see only the tree, specific branch, or leaf and not the forest. Cytogenetics may provide the detection of other relevant chromosomal changes that are prognostic to the specific cancer.

2. What are the four categories of molecular genetic testing services?

1. **Predisposition to cancer.** A number of genes (e.g., *RB, p53, APC, WTl, NFl*) have been found to have the capacity to carry heritable mutations. These inherited mutations are usually present in all tissues and cells of the body and predispose the individual to cancer. In some cases, such as in multiple endocrine neoplasia (MEN) types 1 and 2b, the specific predisposing gene has not been identified. However, in these cases, the genomic loci is known and the inheritance of the offending allele and thus the presence or absence of cancer predisposition can be determined by linkage analysis. The gene for MEN 2a has just recently been identified.[4]

2. **Amplification of specific genes.** Cells normally contain two copies (alleles) of each gene. However, cancer cells often lose some genes and/or amplify other genes. The increase in the number of copies (generally referred to as gene copy number) and/or the amplified transcription or expression of a few genes has been correlated with poor prognosis in selective cancers (e.g., N-*myc* in neuroblastoma and HER2/*neu* in breast cancer).[1,10]

3. **Markers of clonality.** Most malignancies are clonal in that they arose from a single cell and therefore all of the tumor cells contain the same genetic errors. Any molecular

diagnostic marker can be considered a marker of clonality. However, not all moelcular changes found in the cancer cells will necessarily be in each and every cell of the tumor. The Philadelphia (Ph') chromosomal translocation, also known as a *bcr-abl* gene rearrangement, is a diagnostic marker of clonality, whereas a specific immunoglobulin gene rearrangement may be present in only a subclone of the lymphoma under study.[13]

4. DNA fingerprinting for transplantation. Using molecular probes and other polymorphic markers, an individual's DNA can be fingerprinted. DNA fingerprinting and/or markers of clonality can be used to monitor the outgrowth of the donor cells (and the cancer cells) in bone marrow transplant recipients. DNA typing of HLA phenotypes for the identification of acceptable matches of donors and recipients also falls under this category.

3. What is the difference between a genetic marker and a gene?
A genetic marker has no biologic function. A gene may carry a cancer-causing mutation, but the genetic marker allows the offending mutation or gene to be identified. A marker may be a DNA sequence or gene used as a probe or DNA sequences used as primers for the polymerase chain reaction (PCR) amplification of a specified loci. Thus, a genetic marker may identify a specific mutation or a polymorphic site in an individual's DNA.

4. When is a genetic error considered a germline mutation?
A genetic error is considered germline and heritable when it is present in all cells (normal as well as tumor) of the body. Most cancer associated mutations are somatic in origin and are only found in the tumor. However, when a tumor-associated mutation also is identified in normal adjacent tissue and/or in the DNA isolated from peripheral circulating leukocytes, then it is germline. Such a germline error could have been inherited from a carrier parent or it could be a new mutation arising in the gametes or the resultant conceptus.

5. Is the sibling of a patient with unilateral retinoblastoma at risk for cancer?
Yes. The parents of a retinoblastoma-affected child have approximately a 6% risk of another child with retinoblastoma. This value has been empirically determined.[16] However, if the retinoblastoma mutation can be identified and it is a germline error (predisposing mutation), then the inheritance of this lesion by a sibling can be determined. The risk of the occurrence of a retinoblastoma tumor is approximately 90% in a newborn child who is known to carry a predisposing lesion. This is because the penetrance of a retinoblastoma-predisposing mutation is approximately 90%. Only about 10% of retinoblastoma cases are the result of the inheritance of a predisposing lesion from an affected or asymptomatic carrier parent. However, 30–40% of patients with retinoblastoma carry a heritable mutation (including the 10% who inherited the predisposing mutation from a parent). The majority of these cases are new mutations.

6. Should a patient with retinoblastoma with a germline mutation receive radiation or chemotherapy?
Depending on the clinical evaluation of the patient with retinoblastoma, radiation and/or chemotherapy may be required to treat the disease. However, individuals who carry germline cancer-predisposing mutations are at a higher risk of cancer. The exposure of predisposed patients to other DNA-damaging and carcinogenic agents (e.g., radiation and almost all chemotherapeutic agents) will increase the probability of a second primary tumor. In a patient with retinoblastoma, a second primary tumor may occur in the uninvolved retina, the unaffected eye, bone, or numerous soft tissue localities.

7. Can the diagnostic mutation in retinoblastoma always be found?
Finding the diagnostic mutation can be a laborious and expensive proposition. Only about 15% of these mutations are large enough (deletions and rearrangements) to be seen by standard molecular biology techniques, and only about 5% are large enough to be seen by cytogenetic methods. Approximately 85% of these cancer causing mutations are single

point mutations, which are generally the result of a base substitution. These point mutations occur almost anywhere within the retinoblastoma (RB) gene. No "hot spots" for mutation have been found in this gene. Since the RB gene contains approximately 4.5 kilobases (kb) of coding sequences distributed in 27 exons that are spread over a 200 kb of DNA sequences, finding a point mutation can be a tedious job. When the risk of retinoblastoma in a sibling or other relative is in question, linkage analysis is the best approach. However, advances in technology may enable the rapid sequencing of large genes and genomic DNA regions to be performed more rapidly and cheaply in the near future.

8. How can the individual members of an FAP (familial adenomatous polyposis) family who are predisposed to cancer be identified?

As in the above case of retinoblastoma, sequencing the entire gene (adenomatosis polyposis coli [APC] in FAP cases) in question is generally beyond the realm of most DNA diagnostic laboratories. An alternative to direct sequencing is the use of linkage analysis. Linkage analysis is the use of genetic markers that are polymorphic in the human population and are closely linked to the disease gene under study. Polymorphic markers in the APC gene and surrounding genomic DNA region enable the identification of which allele (disease gene or normal gene) was inherited from each parent. These procedures require that the family under study contain two or more affected family members, so that the disease allele can be identified with specific patterns discerned by polymorphic markers. Linkage analysis also requires that the family be "informative," such that the inheritance of different alleles can be followed by differences in the polymorphic marker patterns. For instance, if all of the polymorphic markers used provide the same patterns in both parents, then the inheritance of the disease allele cannot be determined in their offspring and the family is said to be "uninformative." Fortunately, very few families are uninformative, as new genetic markers are being found that have higher frequencies of polymorphism within the human population.

9. What other tumor suppressor genes are involved in human cancer?

A tumor suppressor gene is, by definition, a gene that allows cancer to develop when the gene or its protein product is absent or nonfunctional. The RB gene is the prototype human tumor suppressor gene. However, owing to the exponential advances being made in the molecular etiology of human cancer, tumor suppressor genes are being identified at a rapid rate. At present, other tumor suppressor genes that have been characterized include $p53$, $WT1$, $NF1$, APC, $PTPase$, and $NM23$, which is a putative metastatic suppressor gene.[2,7] Other tumor suppressor genes will probably be found in regions involved in the inheritance of MEN types 1 and 2b, as well as other familial forms of cancer.

Owing to the intimate involvement of tumor suppressor genes in normal cellular functions and controls (i.e., both the RB and the $p53$ gene are important to cell cycle regulation), tumor suppressor genes are extremely important in human cancer. The second most common genetic error that has been observed in human cancer is a mutation in the $p53$ gene. Unfortunately, this also means that the number of target loci that need to be surveyed for mutations in tumor DNA specimens may be large, albeit some of these tumor suppressor genes may be found not to be involved in certain cancers.[7]

10. What does it mean when a cancer patient's tumor specimen was found to express the MDR1 gene?

When the multidrug resistance gene (MDR1) is highly expressed in the tumor cells, then these cells are generally resistant to a large number of chemotherapeutic drugs. However, treatment regimens generally include more than one agent and the tumor may not be resistant to one or more of the drugs in the combination. Additional agents that can inactivate the MDR1 protein are also under study in clinical trials. Molecular techniques enable the level of expression of a given gene to be determined by quantitating the amount of gene specific mRNA present in the tumor cells. Such information may be especially valuable in selective cases in which the first choice of treatment fails to reduce the tumor burden.[3]

11. What value is the determination of N-*myc* gene copy number in neuroblastoma cases?
The number of copies of the N-*myc* gene has been found to be an independent indicator of prognosis in neuroblastoma. The presence of greater than 10 copies of N-*myc* suggests a poor prognosis, whereas less than three copies is an indicator of a good prognosis. However, this is only one of several independent prognostic factors that must be considered in each case of neuroblastoma.[10]

The function of the N-*myc* gene is unknown, but it has been identified as a proto-oncogene with the potential to become activated and involved in the development of human cancer. Increased expression of this gene may be important to the aggressiveness of neuroblastoma. However, it has been the increase in N-*myc* gene copy number that correlates with poor prognosis.

12. What does T- and B-cell gene rearrangements tell us about a specific lymphoma case?
Molecular genetic methods have now been added to immunologic methods in the analysis of tumor specimens for specific rearrangements in the antigen receptor genes of T- and B-lymphoid cells. Tumor cell–specific rearrangements of the V, D, and J segments of the immunoglobulin (B cells) and the T-cell receptor (TCR) (T cells) genes can be identified by Southern blotting and probing and/or by polymerase chain reaction (PCR) techniques. In general, it has been thought that if a tumor cell–specific rearrangement of the immunoglobulin genes is found that the lymphoma is of B-cell origin and of T-cell origin if a rearrangement is found in the TCR genes. Although this is still valuable information, one must be careful in the interpretation of the molecular results. Often many different antigen gene rearrangements occur in lymphoid tumor cells such that more than one may be identified by PCR techniques. Only one of these will truly be clonal, whereas the others may involve subpopulations of the tumor cells. Unfortunately, a TCR gene rearrangement may be occasionally found in a B-cell tumor (or an immunoglobulin gene rearrangement in a T-cell tumor) owing to this apparent lack of genetic stability in the tumor cells. Thus, the determination of gene rearrangements in more than one location (both immunoglobulin and TCR genes) is important to the identification of clonal markers and the cell type of origin for the tumor.[13]

13. Do all cases of chronic myelogenous leukemia (CML) carry Ph′ chromosomal translocations [t(9;22)(q34;q11)]?
Greater than 98% of all CML cases have a major *bcr* (M-*bcr*) gene rearrangement (*bcr-abl* translocation) whether or not cytogenetics can detect a Ph′ chromosome. When a leukemia case is suspected to be CML, then molecular techniques are more accurate and efficient in detecting the *bcr-abl* translocations, especially if there is a submicroscopic DNA translocation present. Most often, suspected CML cases that do not contain a M-*bcr* gene rearrangement can be reclassified as a myeloproliferative disorder. However, a few CML cases (<2%) have been reported that do not contain a M-*bcr* rearrangement, although the disease course of these few cases may be different from the M-*bcr* rearrangement–positive CML. The classification of CML based on the presence of a M-*bcr* rearrangement or on the clinical picture remains a controversial subject. Note, however, that the presence of a Ph′ chromosome is **not** diagnostic of CML (see question 14).

14. Is the sequence location of the breakpoint in a Ph′ chromosomal translocation of diagnostic importance?
The *bcr-abl* gene translocations occur in two regions of the *bcr* gene, the major (M-*bcr*) and the minor (m-*bcr*) regions. The *bcr* gene rearrangements that involve the minor region also present with a Ph′ chromosome. Only M-*bcr* rearrangements are found in CML cases. However, acute lymphoblastic leukemia (ALL) cases can have a *bcr* gene rearrangement in either the M-*bcr* and the m-*bcr* regions, although not all ALL cases carry a *bcr* gene rearrangement. A few rare cases of AML also have a m-*bcr* rearrangement. Thus, a CML case that presents in blast crisis and has a Ph′ chromosome could be misdiagnosed based

on cytogenetics data alone. Rearrangements of m-*bcr* can only be detected with molecular techniques, and PCR is the most common and efficient method of testing. Thus, the presence of a Ph′ chromosome is not by itself diagnostic of CML.

15. Can the progression or status of leukemia be monitored even during remission?

Owing to the sensitivity of molecular genetic techniques such as PCR, the detection of tumor cells during the course of therapy can be followed in patients. For example, chromosomal translocations (such as the *bcr-abl* translocation) can be detected by PCR techniques when the level of tumor cells in the peripherally circulating blood is only one cell in a million. Thus, minimal residual disease can be detected when the disease is in remission. This can be performed in any patient in whom a tumor cell marker has been defined by PCR techniques. Therefore, the course of leukemic disease can be followed when specific gene rearrangements or other translocations (e.g., t[1;19], t[14;18], etc.) are present.

16. Why should DNA analysis be performed in bone marrow transplant cases?

Bone marrow transplants have become more common in recent years in the management of malignancies. The standard serologic techniques for typing donor versus patient cells have limitations in their ability to separately classify cross-reactive subtypes. HLA typing at the DNA level enables the expansion of the surface antigen (serologic) subtypes into many more subgroups. Thus, better patient-donor matches can be found using DNA HLA typing leading to improved patient recovery and prognosis. However, the DNA typing cannot replace the serologic procedures at present and is used as supplementally distinguishing information. DNA typing will undoubtedly begin to dominate the bone marrow and other organ typing in future years as we learn more about the human genome and human genes.

CONTROVERSIES

17. Discuss the use of *HER*-2/*neu* gene amplification data as a prognostic factor in breast and ovarian cancer.

Correlation between increased expression of the *neu* oncogene (also called the *HER*-2 or *erb*B-2 gene) and the long-term survival (>5 years) of individuals diagnosed with breast or ovarian carcinomas have been published by a few investigators. These results have been controversial, as several papers have been published showing that the study of other patient populations did not find this correlation. However, the data boil down to statistics and are highly dependent on the classification and staging of the disease. Although the statistics appear to be firm and the correlation may end up being accurate, how this information will be used in the clinical management of the disease is still under consideration.[1]

BIBLIOGRAPHY

1. Anderson TJ: C-erbB-2 oncogene in breast cancer: The right target or a decoy? Hum Pathol 23:971–972, 1992.
2. Boyd JA, Barrett JC: Tumor suppressor genes: Possible functions in the negative regulation of cell proliferation. Mol Carcinog 3.325–329, 1990.
3. Chabner BA, Wilson W: Reversal of multidrug resistance. J Clin Oncol 9:4–6, 1991.
4. Donis-Keller H, Dou S, Chi D, et al: Mutations in the RET proto-oncogene are associated with MEN 2A and FMTC. Hum Mol Genet 2:851–856, 1993.
5. Fearon ER, Vogelstein B: A genetic model for colorectal tumorigenesis. Cell 61:759–767, 1990.
6. Haber DA, Buckler AJ, Glaser T, et al: An internal deletion within an 11p13 zinc finger gene contributes to the development of Wilms' tumor. Cell 61:1257–1269, 1990.
7. Harris CC, Hollstein M: Clinical implications of the p53 tumor-suppressor gene. N Engl J Med 329:1318–1327, 1993.
8. Kinzler KW, Nilbert MC, Vogelstein B, et al: Identification of a gene located at chromosome 5q21 that is mutated in colorectal cancers. Science 251:1366–1370, 1991.
9. Lion T, Izraeli S, Henn T, et al: Monitoring of residual disease in chronic myelogenous leukemia by quantitative polymerase chain reaction. Leukemia 6:495–499, 1992.

10. Look T, Hayes FA, Shuster JJ, et al: Clinical relevance of tumor cell ploidy and N-myc gene amplification in childhood neuroblastoma: A pediatric oncology group study. J Clin Oncol 9:581–591, 1991.
11. Malkin D, Li FP, Strong LC, et al: Germ line p53 mutations in a familial syndrome of breast cancer, sarcoma, and other neoplasms. Science 250:1233–1238, 1990.
12. Marshall CJ: Tumor suppressor genes. Cell 64:313–326, 1991.
13. Sklar J, Weiss LM: Applications of antigen receptor gene rearrangements to the diagnosis and characterization of lymphoid neoplasms. Annu Rev Med 39:315–334, 1988.
14. Srivastava S, Zou Z, Pirollo K, et al: Germline transmission of a mutated p53 gene in a cancer-prone family with Li-Fraumeni syndrome. Nature 348:747–749, 1990.
15. Wiggs J, Nordenskjold M, Yandell D, et al: Prediction of the risk of hereditary retinoblastoma, using DNA polymorphisms within the retinoblastoma gene. N Engl J Med 318:151–157, 1988.
16. Wiggs JL, Dryja TP: Predicting the risk of hereditary retinoblastoma. Am J Ophthalmol 106:346–351, 1988.
17. Yandell DW, Campbell TA, Dayton SH, et al: Oncogenic point mutations in the human retinoblastoma gene: Their application to genetic counseling. N Engl J Med 321:1689–1695, 1989.

39. HEREDITARY MALIGNANCIES

Henry T. Lynch, M.D., and Jane F. Lynch, B.S.N.

1. What is meant by the terms "familial" and "hereditary" cancer?

"Familial" is a rather imprecise term that expresses an increased risk for cancer based on a clustering of cancers in a family. The term was first used by investigators in the 1920s to the 1950s when assessing the family histories of patients with cancers of the breast, stomach, and colon and comparing these site-specific cancers with the family histories of controls who lacked one of these site-specific cancers. These studies showed that the first-degree relatives of such patients would have a two- to threefold increased risk for this same site-specific cancer when compared with the controls. The familial concept did not take into consideration age of onset or the possible integral association of other forms of cancer. The concept is useful because a patient, for example, with a first-degree relative with cancer of the breast and possibly no other information available on the family history would, because of the two- to threefold increased risk for breast cancer, be a candidate for more intensive surveillance. It is always desirable to search for evidence that could be consonant with a hereditary etiology.

Hereditary cancer, on the other hand, implies a mendelian inherited predisposition to cancer. This may involve cancer of a specific anatomic site, such as breast cancer, or it could involve breast cancer in association with other cancer types, such as ovarian cancer in the hereditary breast-ovarian cancer syndrome. In hereditary cancer, one would expect to see a pattern of segregation of the cancer(s) within the family in accord with the particular hereditary cancer syndrome of concern and its mendelian inheritance pattern, either autosomal dominant, autosomal recessive, or X-linked. Recent work in cytogenetics, gene linkage, and molecular genetics has provided highly specific findings that confirm the hereditary etiology in certain hereditary cancer syndromes.

2. In compiling a family history of cancer, how extensively should the physician pursue this matter?

Ideally, the family history should be compiled through what is referred to as the modified nuclear pedigree. This involves a detailed description of the cancer history in the patient's first-degree relatives, including mother and father, siblings, and progeny, and in second-degree relatives, especially both sets of grandparents, aunts, and uncles. By extending the history to older second-degree relatives, one will be dealing with persons who more than likely have passed through the highest cancer risk age and, thus, will be more genetically informative than the patient's siblings and progeny. The history should include cancer of *all* anatomic sites and any premonitory stigmata such as the presence of café au lait spots or neurofibromas in von Recklinghausen's neurofibromatosis (NF-1) or multiple atypical moles, as in the familial atypical multiple mole melanoma (FAMMM) syndrome. It is always important to pursue the history through the paternal as well as the maternal lineage, because even in sex-limited tumors such as the breast, ovary, or endometrium, cancer-free males may be obligate gene carriers.

3. What are the cardinal features that characterize hereditary forms of cancer?
Hereditary forms of cancer are characterized by a cancer phenotype that has the following features: (1) early age of cancer onset, although the range in age of onset may be quite variable within and between families; (2) multiple primary cancers with specific combinations such as colon and endometrium in Lynch syndrome II or the breast and ovary in the hereditary breast-ovarian cancer syndrome; (3) premonitory physical stigmata, or biomarkers of genotypic susceptibility, or both in certain syndromes (e.g., the mentioned, multiple atypical moles in the FAMMM syndrome); (4) distinctive pathologic features such as medullary thyroid carcinoma in multiple endocrine neoplasia type II and type III; and, finally, (5) mendelian patterns of tumor transmission. However, it must be appreciated that not all of these features apply when considering any specific patient or family, because there may be marked variation in expression of any of these phenotypic features of hereditary cancer's natural history. Nevertheless, these cardinal features are sufficiently pervasive as to assist the clinician effectively in identifying hereditary cancer-prone families.

4. What is meant by Knudson's "two-hit" hypothesis for the explanation of cancer etiology?
In 1971, Dr. Alfred G. Knudson, Jr. proposed what is now known as the "two-hit" or two-mutation model for carcinogenesis. This was based on studies of patients with retinoblastoma wherein he proposed that those with the hereditary form of the disease harbored a germ-line mutation and required a second "hit," which was a postconceptional somatic mutation. Sporadic cases, on the other hand, lack the germline mutation and thereby require two somatic mutations for retinoblastoma to occur. The two-hit model explained the earlier age of onset and the excess of bilaterality in the hereditary form of retinoblastoma when compared with its sporadic variant. The sporadic variant requires two somatic "hits," a fact that partially explains its later age of onset and the decrease in bilateral cancer occurrences.

5. How important is age of the patient at onset of cancer as a predictor of genetic etiology?
The fraction of cancer that is believed to be genetically induced is substantially greater in patients below age 40. Age at onset of cancer is particularly important in several of the major cancer sites of public health importance, particularly breast, colon, and ovary. For example, it is estimated that as many as 50% of patients with any of these cancers with onset below age 40 will have family histories consonant with a hereditary cancer syndrome. The likelihood of such cancer-affected patients having a genetic etiology appears to increase in direct proportion to the *decrease* in the age at onset of that cancer. In patients with strikingly early age of cancer onset, in the absence of a positive family history, a new germline mutation may have occurred in one of the patient's parents. Other explanations for a negative family history, yet potential genetic etiology, may be important. These include death of key relatives at early ages from causes other than cancer, lack of accurate data about cause of death, or reduced penetrance of the deleterious gene.

6. Is hereditary breast cancer a single syndrome, or are there multiple hereditary breast cancer-prone disorders?
Hereditary breast cancer is exceedingly heterogeneous and involves a variety of differing syndromes, each of which appears to show an autosomal dominant mode of genetic transmission. These disorders include site-specific breast cancer; the hereditary breast-ovarian cancer syndrome; families showing breast cancer clustering very early in life, often

in the mid 20s and early 30s, referred to as the extraordinarily early–onset breast cancer syndrome; hereditary breast cancer in association with gastrointestinal tract cancers; the Li-Fraumeni (SBLA) syndrome (discussed subsequently); and breast cancer in association with multiple trichilemmomas and thyroid cancer in Cowden's syndrome.

7. What is the tumor spectrum that characterizes the Li-Fraumeni (SBLA) syndrome?
The acronym SBLA was coined by Lynch et al.[4] to explain the syndrome's tumor spectrum, also referred to—more popularly—as the Li-Fraumeni syndrome. The "S" stands for sarcoma; the "B" for breast cancer and brain tumors; the "L" for carcinoma of the lung and larynx, leukemia, and lymphoma; and the "A" for adrenocortical carcinoma. This is an exceedingly complex disorder that is most likely due to the pleiotropic effects of a p53 germline mutation, and that appears to be responsible for a litany of cancer types in this disorder. Early age of onset and multiple primary cancer, as in most forms of hereditary cancers, also are characteristics of this disease. Other tumors that appear to be integral to SBLA syndrome include neuroblastoma, Wilms' tumor, and pancreatic carcinoma. Undoubtedly, as data on more families are accrued and extended, with meticulous attention to cancer of *all* anatomic sites, and with correlation of molecular genetic studies of newly identified germline (p53) mutations, knowledge about its full tumor complement will increase.

8. Is hereditary colorectal cancer a single disease or is it heterogeneous with multiple genotypes?
Hereditary colorectal cancer is exceedingly heterogeneous. It includes the following seven syndromes:
   1. Familial adenomatous polyposis coli (FAP), which accounts for about 0.4% of all colorectal cancer
   2. Hereditary juvenile polyposis coli, which is even more rare than FAP
   3. Hereditary flat adenoma syndrome (HFAS), the frequency of which is unknown
   4. Hereditary nonpolyposis colorectal cancer (HNPCC), also called Lynch syndromes I and II, which accounts for at least 6% of the total colorectal cancer burden
   5. Familial forms of ulcerative colitis and Crohn's disease, which are associated with increased susceptibility to colorectal cancer
   6. Peutz-Jegher syndrome
   7. Hereditary common adenomatous polyps and colon cancer, which are exceedingly prevalent.

9. How are the Lynch syndromes defined?
   Lynch syndrome I is an autosomal dominantly inherited predisposition to colorectal cancer (CRC) in the absence of florid colonic polyps that is characterized by early age of CRC onset (average age 45), an increased proclivity to CRC occurrence in the proximal colon (approximately 70%), and an excess of synchronous and metachronous CRC.
   Lynch syndrome II contains all of the aforementioned features of Lynch syndrome I with respect to the colon but in addition shows a highly significant excess of carcinomas of the endometrium, ovary, transitional cell carcinoma of the ureter and renal pelvis, adenocarcinoma of the small bowel and stomach, and hepatobiliary carcinoma.

10. Are there any premonitory stigmata or biomarkers of genotypic risk that can aid in the diagnosis of the Lynch syndromes?
The only premonitory stigmata for the Lynch syndromes are the cutaneous signs of the Muir-Torre syndrome; namely, sebaceous adenomas, sebaceous carcinomas, and multiple keratoacanthomas. However, these features have been identified in only a small subset of Lynch syndrome II kindreds. There have been no common identifiable biomarkers that show sufficient sensitivity and specificity to the Lynch syndromes phenotypes. However, certain striking clinical features warrant concern—cancers of the proximal colon, age younger than 40, occurrence in two or three primary relatives in the absence of multiple

colonic polyps, and/or one or more primary relatives with early (younger than age 45) onset endometrial carcinomas.

11. What are the surveillance and management indications for the Lynch syndromes?

The most important aspect of screening is education of the patient and his or her physician about the significance of the genetics and natural history of cancer in the Lynch syndromes. We initiate this education of our patients at high risk by the late teens. Because about 70% of CRCs occur proximal to the splenic flexure, with one third occurring in the cecum, we initiate colonoscopy at age 25 and repeat it every other year through age 35 and then annually thereafter. We recommend no less than subtotal colectomy for the first occurrence of CRC, because about 45% of patients will have a second primary cancer by 10 years after the initial CRC if only a limited resection is performed. In Lynch syndrome II, surveillance in women includes aspiration curettage of the uterus because of the risk for endometrial carcinoma. We are researching the use of pelvic probe ultrasound, Doppler color blood flow imaging, and CA-125 in screening for ovarian cancer. We initiate this screening at age 25 and repeat it annually. Should a woman develop CRC and should she have completed her family, we would offer prophylactic total abdominal hysterectomy and bilateral salpingo-oophorectomy.

12. Has the gene for the Lynch syndromes been identified?

The gene for the Lynch syndromes is believed to be located at a susceptibility locus on chromosome 2 (2p15-16).[8] The gene is now referred to as COCA 1.

13. What is the natural history and tumor spectrum of familial adenomatous polyposis (FAP)?

FAP is the paradigm for hereditary forms of cancer. The syndrome was first described in the 1880s and is characterized by the presence of multiple (in some cases thousands) of adenomatous colonic polyps. The polyps start at a very early age in the rectosigmoid area of the colon; therefore, rigid sigmoidoscopy can be used to establish the diagnosis. However, in spite of more than 100 years of experience with this syndrome, it has been shown that 59% of patients with FAP die of CRC.[2] The reason for this is clear. Physicians simply are not taking adequate family histories of their high-risk patients, and, in turn, they are not educating and/or extending surveillance to their patients and their patients' high-risk (first-degree) relatives. This is a pity and needs to be resolved.

The tumor spectrum in FAP has become extensive. The second most common cancer in FAP is periampullary carcinoma, and the third most common tumors are desmoids, often located intra-abdominally. Some desmoid tumors are believed to be initiated by surgery—occurring an average of 2 years following surgery. It has been estimated that 5% to 10% of patients with FAP, particularly those with Gardner's phenotypic variant (osteomas, epidermoid cysts, and supernumerary teeth) and other less frequently occurring phenotypic features will be at risk for desmoid tumors. Gardner's syndrome variant is thought to be located at the same APC (5q) locus as FAP and may represent a separate mutation in this large gene. Other cancers integral to FAP and its Gardner's variant include papillary thyroid carcinoma, brain tumors, sarcomas, cancers of the small bowel, stomach (particularly in FAP occurrences in Japan), hepatoblastoma, hepatobiliary carcinoma, and pancreatic carcinoma.

We initiate screening of first-degree relatives in FAP families by the age of 10 to 12 years. In addition to rigid sigmoidoscopy or flexible sigmoidoscopy, we recommend upper endoscopy because of the stated risk for periampullary carcinoma.

Recently, the gene for FAP has been cloned and is located on chromosome 5q (see subsequent discussions).

14. Ulcerative colitis and Crohn's disease have shown a significant association with cancer. Is there any evidence for familial aggregation of these inflammatory bowel disorders?

The etiopathogenesis of these inflammatory bowel diseases (IBD) remains elusive. Nevertheless, genetic factors may play an important role. Reports of familial clustering of

Crohn's disease (CD) and ulcerative colitis (UC) have been observed for many decades. Although HLA haplotypes have not been found to associate with the IBD trait, there is evidence that healthy relatives of affected individuals have functional or immunologic abnormalities, including increased intestinal permeability, complement dysfunction, or, in certain circumstances, the presence of autoantibodies in the serum.

Undoubtedly, environmental and psychologic factors and their interaction with host factor susceptibility are important. An autosomal dominant model for CD and UC has been suggested, as has polygenic inheritance.[7]

15. What are the molecular events involved in the genesis of hereditary and sporadic colorectal cancer?

Most investigators believe that the molecular substrate responsible for the critical events in carcinogenesis involve genes that regulate cell proliferation and differentiation. These are referred to as *oncogenes* (or activator genes) and *tumor suppressor genes*. Alteration in the expression or structure of these genes may give rise to the perturbations of cell growth, which is the linchpin in neoplasia. Studies of colorectal tumors has led to the discovery of three new tumor suppressor genes; namely APC (adenomatous polyposis coli), DCC (deleted in colon cancer), and p53.

Oncogenes are retroviral genes that are responsible for in vitro cell transformation. In normal human cells, these are referred to as proto-oncogenes, whereas in their activated form in human tumors, they are referred to as v-*onc*. Certain oncogenes appear to have a physiologic role in cell division and differentiation and are considered to be the target for mutagenesis in the neoplastic setting. Those oncogenes most frequently involved in colorectal tumors are c-Ki-*ras* and c-*myc*. Other oncogenes that are involved in large bowel tumors, although less frequently, are c-*src*, c-*myb*, and c-*erb*.

Tumor suppressor genes are a relatively small group whose main role is to inhibit cell proliferation and tumorigenicity. In FAP, it has been found that colon cancer in this hereditary cancer disorder is determined by point mutations in APC, which is inherited through the germline and is located on chromosome 5q21. The APC tumor suppressor gene is believed to lose its ability to suppress cell division by its loss or inactivation. Thus, it involves loss of both allelic forms of the gene either by chromosomal deletion or point mutation or, possibly, both events may occur. Because both alleles must be "lost" for cellular transformation to occur, tumor suppressor genes are considered to be recessive. In contrast to this recessive mode, oncogenes may act through alteration of a single allele, and this is sufficient to cause transformation. Other tumor suppressor genes, as mentioned above, are also involved in these processes.

Following the identification of the APC locus on chromosome 5q, deletions and point mutations were identified in another large gene referred to as MCC (mutated in colorectal cancer). As many as 55% of cancers have been shown to contain deletions involving MCC. MCC is not believed to be the gene responsible for FAP. Nevertheless, it is believed to be a common site for mutagenesis, and may therefore be another colorectal tumor suppressor gene. Finally, DCC, which is located on chromosome 18, is believed to be a candidate tumor suppressor gene. Herein deletions affecting the DCC locus have been found in 73% of cancers but only in about 11% of adenomas.

Much evidence has now been accumulated relevant to deletions on the short arm of chromosome 17 involving the p53 allele, which is believed to be a tumor suppressor gene. The p53 gene is considered to be the commonest genetic abnormality described to date in human cancer of many types, including colorectal cancer.

16. How can the multistage theory of carcinogenesis be applied to colorectal cancer?

Bert Vogelstein, M.D. of Johns Hopkins Medical School has pioneered the concept that multiple events are required in the genesis of colorectal cancer.[11] He has postulated that normal mucosa in the presence of a germline APC mutation in the FAP paradigm will lead to a hyperproliferative mucosa, which then will evolve to a small adenoma. In the presence of a K-*ras* mutation, this small adenoma will evolve to a large adenoma, and in the presence of the p53 mutation and a chromosome 18q deletion, a locally invasive carcinoma will arise. It is not fully clear what molecular events are responsible for a locally invasive carcinoma to emerge into a metastatic carcinoma.

In sporadic colorectal carcinoma, it is believed that normal mucosa will transform to a small adenoma through an APC mutation, an MCC mutation, a *ras* mutation, a chromosome 5q deletion, or a c-*myc* activation. The rest of the events involved in the FAP findings will then take place in the sporadic setting.

17. Is there a hereditary etiology for neuroendocrine tumors?
A variety of neuroendocrine tumors appear to have a hereditary etiology. Foremost of these are multiple endocrine neoplasia (MEN) type I, which involves parathyroid, pituitary, and pancreatic islet cell tumors. In addition, loss of heterozygosity at a site located on chromosome 11 may be present. MEN type IIa (or MEN II) involves a predisposition to medullary thyroid carcinoma and pheochromocytoma (which are often bilateral); MEN type IIb (or MEN III) is also referred to as the multiple mucosal neuroma syndrome. This disorder, in addition to the predisposition to medullary thyroid carcinoma and pheochromocytoma, shows multiple mucosal neuromata (dysplasias of neurocristic Schwann cells) and peripheral extensions of neurocristic ganglion cells, as well as a marfanoid habitus and abnormalities of intestinal neural plexuses, referred to as gangliomatosis of the bowel. The MEN syndromes are autosomal dominantly inherited.[1]

18. Is hereditary pheochromocytoma heterogeneous?
Pheochromocytoma, in addition to its integral association with MEN IIa and IIb, also occurs in von Recklinghausen's neurofibromatosis (NF-1 variety) and in von Hippel-Lindau disease. Each of these disorders has an autosomal dominant inheritance as may isolated pheochromocytoma.

19. What is the tumor spectrum in MEN I (Wermer's syndrome)? Where is the MEN I locus located?
Tumors of the parathyroid, anterior pituitary, and endocrine pancreas constitute the tumor spectrum in MEN I. Genetic-linkage studies of patients with MEN I and deletion findings in their tumors have enabled the mapping of the MEN I locus to chromosome 11q13.

20. Where is the gene located for MEN IIa and MEN IIb and hereditary site-specific medullary thyroid cancer?
The genes for MEN IIa and IIb, as well as for hereditary site-specific medullary thyroid carcinoma, are localized in the pericentromeric region of chromosome 10. The finding that each of these three clinically distinct familial cancer syndromes maps to the same chromosomal region suggests that all are allelic mutations at the same locus or that they represent a cluster of genes involved in the regulation of neuroendocrine tissue development.

21. Does pancreatic cancer show familial aggregation?
Two case-control studies have demonstrated a significant familial aggregation of pancreatic cancer. Studies of extended kindreds have also shown, albeit rarely, pancreatic cancer occurring through multiple generations in a pattern of transmission suggestive of an autosomal dominant inherited factor. Pancreatic cancer has also occasionally been shown to be integrally associated with hereditary pancreatitis, MEN I, Lynch syndrome II, von Hippel-Lindau syndrome, and a subset of the FAMMM syndrome, and it has been seen in ataxia-telangiectasia and in a single family with insulin-dependent diabetes mellitus.

22. What is the evidence for hereditary etiology in carcinoma of the stomach?
Gastric carcinoma has been identified in families with FAP, particularly from Japan, as well as in Lynch syndrome II kindreds. There have been family reports of site-specific

gastric cancer appearing through multiple generations, which is consistent with an autosomal dominant mode of inheritance. Gastric cancer has also been observed at extremely early ages in patients with ataxia-telangiectasia. There is also believed to be an association between pernicious anemia and stomach cancer. Gastric cancer is frequently associated with blood group A.

23. Does intraocular malignant melanoma show evidence of a genetic etiology?

There have been rare occurrences of families with intraocular malignant melanoma (IOM) occurring on a site-specific basis consonant with an autosomal dominantly inherited etiology. IOM has also been shown to be an integral finding in a subset of families with FAMMM syndrome.

In a survey of medical records of 45 patients with histologically diagnosed IOM at the University of Texas MD Anderson Hospital and Tumor Institute, a patient with IOM had a similarly affected sibling with histologically verified IOM. A second, unrelated family was referred during the course of the study wherein IOM was found through three generations.[3]

24. What is the evidence for the role of genetic factors in Hodgkin's disease and in non-Hodgkin's lymphoma?

Knowledge of the role of genetics in the etiology of Hodgkin's disease (HD) and non-Hodgkin's lymphoma (NHL) is limited. There have been occasional families with a remarkably increased occurrence of HD, NHL, or both. In one such family, NHL was histologically verified in a mother and in all five of her daughters.[5] One of the NHL-affected daughters had a daughter with HD. It was suggested that these hematogenous malignancies were autosomal dominantly inherited in this family. There also have been families with only HD, others with only NHL and, more rarely, families with both HD and NHL transmitted in a manner suggestive of this same mode. However, it must be emphasized that familial occurrences of lymphoma are relatively rare and, herein, the familial aggregation of NHL occurs less frequently than the familial aggregation of HD.

X-linked lymphoproliferative disease of Purtillo is a special example of NHL occurring at a markedly early age of onset and restricted to males, because the gene is located on the X chromosome. In SBLA syndrome, lymphoma is one of the integral forms of cancer and is transmitted in accord with an autosomal dominantly inherited factor.

Evidence linking genetics, immunology, and environmental factors in the etiology of lymphomas has been emerging during the past two decades. For example, immunologic anomalies and/or disorders in lymphomas have been shown to occur in the following mendelian inherited settings:

1. Several sex-linked recessive disorders, including Bruton's agammaglobulinemia, Wiskott-Aldrich syndrome, and the mentioned X-linked lymphoproliferative disorder of Purtillo

2. Autosomal recessively inherited traits, including ataxia-telangiectasia, Chédiak-Higashi syndrome, common variable immunodeficiency, Sjögren's syndrome, and familial microcephaly syndrome

Lymphoma has also been described in families prone to systemic lupus erythematosus, which is a disorder that may be familial in some cases.

25. What are cancer-associated genodermatoses? How many of these syndromes are known to exist?

A diagnosis of a cancer-associated genodermatosis implies that the disorder of concern harbors a specific form of cutaneous stigmata in association with cancer of the skin, brain, bone, or viscera and that it is mendelian inherited. At least 50 differing hereditary cancer-associated genodermatoses show autosomal dominant, autosomal recessive, and X-linked modes of inheritance. Therefore, one should be aware of the important dermatologic signs, because these stigmata may provide a beacon to a hereditary cancer syndrome diagnosis. Examples of cancer-associated genodermatoses include the following:

1. The already-mentioned FAMMM syndrome is characterized by the presence of multiple atypical moles and cutaneous malignant melanoma. Intraocular melanoma and/or pancreatic cancer may occur in a subset of FAMMM kindreds.

2. Multiple hamartoma syndrome (Cowden's syndrome) includes cutaneous lesions such as dome-shaped, flat-topped papules, verrucous lesions, punctate keratoderma of the palms, multiple angiomas and lipomas, gingival and palatal papules, as well as a scrotal tongue. These patients are at high risk for carcinoma of the breast, including bilateral occurrence. Papillary thyroid cancer also occurs in excess in this disorder.

3. Peutz-Jegher syndrome is characterized by multiple pigmented macular spots of the lips, buccal mucosa, conjunctiva, periorbital area, and digits. Affected patients also have multiple intestinal harmatomatous polyps that may contain adenomatous features and are predisposed, albeit weakly, to adenocarcinoma of the colon and small bowel (duodenum). Granulosa cell tumors of the ovaries also occur in this disease.

4. In xeroderma pigmentosum (XDP) affected patients have an exquisite cutaneous photosensitivity to sunlight. They have excessive freckling in sun-exposed areas of the skin in the first years of life, with early degeneration of the skin leading to freckling, telangiectasia, keratosis, papillomas, and eventually to carcinomas and melanomas. The eyes may also be affected with photophobia, lacrimation, and keratitis, with resulting opacities. DNA repair deficiency to ultraviolet light has shown extant heterogeneity in XDP by virtue of at least eight complementation groups based on their DNA repair phenotypes.

26. Where is the retinoblastoma gene located? Has it been cloned?

The retinoblastoma locus has been mapped to the chromosome region 13q14. Constitutional chromosome 13 deletions in retinoblastoma patients share a loss of this region, and tumor cells frequently share similar chromosome 13 deletions. The gene for retinoblastoma was cloned by Hen-Hwa Lee in 1987.

The retinoblastoma model is an important one in that this rare childhood cancer of the eye has provided evidence supporting the prevailing concept with regard to the unmasking of recessive mutations in carcinogenesis. Specifically, it is the loss or deletion of *both* genes in the genetic model (a germline mutation and somatic loss) that accounts for the early onset and bilateral nature of hereditary retinoblastoma, whereas in the sporadic model, both somatic gene losses occur resulting in unilateral retinoblastoma of later onset.

27. Do any other cancers occur in patients with retinoblastoma?

Patients with the hereditary form of retinoblastoma harbor an increased proclivity for other cancers, including brain tumors, carcinoma of the lung and breast, malignant melanoma, and especially osteogenic sarcoma.

28. What is the germline mutation responsible for the Li-Fraumeni (SBLA) syndrome?

Mutation of the p53 gene, located on the short arm of chromosome 17, has been identified in the Li-Fraumeni (SBLA) syndrome. This gene has now been cloned.[6]

29. At least two distinct forms of neurofibromatosis exist—NF-1 and NF-2. What is the difference between NF-1 and NF-2?

NF-1 is an autosomal dominant disorder that affects about 1 in 5000 people. It was previously called von Recklinghausen's disease or peripheral neurofibromatosis. However, the term NF-1 was adopted in 1987 to make a clear distinction between the two definite categories of neurofibromatosis.

NF-1 is characterized by the presence of multiple hyperpigmented macules known as café au lait spots; dermal, subcutaneous and plexiform neurofibromas; iris (Lisch) nodules; axillary freckling; and optic nerve gliomas. The gene for NF-1 is on the proximal long arm of chromosome 17 (17q11.2).

NF-2 had been previously called central neurofibromatosis or bilateral acoustic neurofibromatosis, as well as hereditary bilateral vestibular schwannoma syndrome. This autosomal dominant disorder affects about one in 50,000 individuals. It is characterized by bilateral acoustic neuromas, posterior subcapsular cataracts, meningiomas, trigeminal nerve tumors, schwannomas, spinal cord ependymomas, and dermal, subcutaneous, and plexiform neurofibromas. The gene for NF-2 is located on the distal long arm of chromosome 22.[9]

30. What is the tumor spectrum in von Hippel-Landau disease? Has it been linked to a tumor suppressor gene? If yes, please give the gene's location.
Von Hippel-Lindau disease (VHL) is a hereditary cancer syndrome (autosomal dominant) characterized by a predisposition to the development of retinal, cerebellar, and spinal hemangioblastomas. In addition, these high-risk patients have a markedly increased susceptibility to renal cell carcinoma and pheochromocytoma.

The gene for VHL has been mapped to chromosome 3p25-p26. Flanking markers have been identified and should lead to the cloning of this tumor suppressor gene. Once the gene is cloned, patients at increased risk will be more readily identifiable. Such an advance should then lead to marked improvement in the clinical management of families with VHL, in that the accuracy of presymptomatic diagnosis will be significantly advanced.

31. Is there an excess risk of cancer among the heterozygous carriers of the ataxia-telangiectasia gene?
Ataxia-telangiectasia (A-T) is an autosomal recessive disorder in which cancers develop in affected homozygotes at an enormous rate (approximately 100 times higher than in unaffected age-matched controls). Because A-T is inherited as an autosomal recessive disorder, one can predict that there will be many heterozygous individuals in the general population, and indeed they constitute about 1% of the general population.

Swift et al. showed that cancer rates were significantly higher in the relatives of patients with A-T as opposed to their spouses.[10] The estimated risk of cancer of all types among the heterozygotes as compared with noncarriers was 3.8 in men and 3.5 in women. When considering breast cancer in women, the relative risk was 5.1. Swift et al. concluded from this study that the A-T gene predisposed heterozygotes to cancer, particularly breast cancer in women.

BIBLIOGRAPHY

1. Anderson RJ, Lynch HT: Familial risk for neuroendocrine tumors. Curr Opin Oncol 5:75–84, 1993.
2. Arvanitis ML, Jagelman DG, Fazio VW, et al: Mortality in patients with familial adenomatous polyposis, Dis Colon Rectum 33:639–642, 1990.
3. Lynch HT, Anderson DE, Krush AJ, et al: Hereditary and intraocular malignant melanoma. Cancer 21:119–125, 1968.
4. Lynch HT, Mulcahy GM, Harris RE, et al: Genetic and pathologic findings in a kindred with hereditary sarcoma, breast cancer, brain tumors, leukemia, lung, laryngeal, and adrenal cortical carcinoma. Cancer 41:2055–2064, 1978.
5. Lynch HT, Marcus JN, Weisenberger D, et al: Genetic and immunopathologic findings in a lymphoma family. Br J Cancer 59:622–626, 1989.
6. Malkin D, Li FP, Strong LC, et al: Germ line p53 mutations in a familial syndrome of breast cancer, sarcomas, and other neoplasms. Science 250:1233, 1990.
7. McConnell RB: Genetic aspects of etiopathic inflammatory bowel disease. In Kirsner JB, Shorter RG (eds): Inflammatory Bowel Disease, 3rd ed. Philadelphia, Lea & Febiger, 1988, pp 87–95.
8. Peltomaki P, Aaltonen LA, Sistonen P, et al: Genetic mapping of a locus predisposing to human colorectal cancer. Science 260:810–819, 1993.
9. Roos KL, Dunn DW: Neurofibromatosis. CA 42:241–254, 1992.
10. Swift M, Morrell D, Massey R, et al: Incidence of cancer in 161 families affected by ataxia-telangiectasia. N Engl J Med 325:1831–1836, 1991.
11. Vogelstein B, Fearon ER, Hamilton SR, et al: Genetic alterations during colorectal tumor development. N Engl J Med 319:525–532, 1988.

40. CANCER SCREENING AND EARLY DETECTION

Mona Bernaiche Bedell, R.N., B.S.N., O.C.N.

1. When is cancer screening most beneficial?
Benefit is greatest when the disease is fairly common and early diagnosis and treatment result in a decline in cancer deaths.

2. What are important characteristics of a cancer screening test?
Ideally, a screening test or procedure should be simple and inexpensive to perform, safe and clinically acceptable to the patient, accurate (have high sensitivity and specificity), and most importantly result in an improved outcome.

3. Why isn't CA-125 used to screen for ovarian cancer?
Currently, studies do not support routine use of CA-125 to screen for ovarian cancer because of the cost and the relatively low incidence of ovarian cancer, and also because CA-125 levels are elevated in <50% of patients with early disease. Elevated levels of CA-125 can be found in benign conditions such as endometriosis, pregnancy, menses, pelvic inflammatory disease, uterine fibroids, and liver disease. Levels of CA-125 also can be elevated with cancers of the fallopian tube, lung, breast, pancreas, and colon.

4. Has a high-risk population for ovarian cancer been described?
There appears to be a genetic or familial association, although a specific gene has not been identified. Use of CA-125 is recommended for women with familial histories or symptoms of ovarian cancer.

5. Do data support annual screening with Papanicolaou (Pap) smears?
Randomized control trials were not conducted prior to widespread use of Pap smears, but a convincing body of evidence exists to support its benefit. Cervical cancer mortality has decreased more than 70% over the last 40 years because of use of Pap smears in screening.

6. Are we successful at screening all women for cervical cancer?
No. There is evidence that high-risk women in lower socioeconomic groups and the elderly are not adequately screened. The incidence of advanced disease at diagnosis remains high in these groups. Efforts must be made to target these women for screening.

7. Who is at risk for developing colorectal cancer?
High risk patients are those with:
1. Personal history:

    Sporadic colorectal adenomas   Breast, ovarian, or endometrial cancer
    Colorectal cancer   Radiation therapy
    Inflammatory bowel disease

2. Family history:

    Familial adenomatous polyposis   Hereditary nonpolyposis colorectal
    Gardner's syndrome   cancer syndromes
    Turcot's syndrome   Flat adenoma syndrome
    Oldfield's syndrome   Sporadic colorectal cancer
    Juvenile polyposis   Sporadic colorectal adenoma

8. Should there be special surveillance for those at high risk for colorectal cancer?
High-risk individuals should be identified for special surveillance. Screening for individuals with one affected first-degree relative should begin at ages 35 to 40 and include annual rectal examinations, annual occult blood testing, and flexible sigmoidoscopy every 3–5 years.

9. Will periodic fecal occult blood testing (FOBT) reduce overall mortality from colorectal cancer?
Current data do not suggest this. Clinical trials are now underway to assess the effectiveness of FOBT in reducing mortality from colon cancer. FOBT is positive in only 50–70% of patients with cancer. In addition, 20–30% of patients with adenomatous polyps, a precursor of colorectal cancer, will be identified.

10. What are the detection rates for colorectal cancer using digital rectal examination (DRE) and flexible sigmoidoscopy?
Approximately 10% of colon cancers will be identified by DRE, and 50% to 60% of cancers will be found by flexible sigmoidoscopy.

11. Who is at risk for breast cancer?
All women are at risk. Many risk factors have been identified, but over 75% of breast cancers are diagnosed in women without known risk factors. At very high risk are women with a personal history of breast cancer or family history of premenopausal and/or bilateral breast cancer in a mother or sister.

12. How effective is mammography in detecting breast cancer?
Mammography is effective in identifying 85% to 90% of all breast cancers. When mammography is combined with physical examination, mortality from breast cancer is reduced in women over 50 years of age.

13. Does a diagnosis of a benign breast condition increase a woman's risk for breast cancer?
There is little or no increased risk for cancer in women with most types of benign breast conditions. Risk is minimal for nonproliferative diseases and moderate for proliferative disease without atypia. Risk is highest for atypical hyperplasia, especially in premenopausal women and women with a family history of breast cancer.

14. Does the use of screening chest radiography and sputum cytology in smokers have an effect on survival?
No significant improvement in overall mortality from lung cancer has been demonstrated. Current screening methods have not been successful in detecting lung cancers in the earliest phases. Nearly two thirds of cases are metastatic at the time of diagnosis.

15. Are risks for lung cancer reduced for smokers who quit after years of smoking?
Yes. Future risks of death from lung cancer can be markedly reduced. Several years after quitting and gradually over 15 years, cancer risk approaches that of nonsmokers. Studies have shown that even a brief message from physicians will encourage about 5% of patients to quit smoking. Assuming this rate of success, over 2.5 million smokers will quit each year with this simple intervention.

16. Does early detection and treatment alter mortality associated with prostate cancer?
No. Early detection and treatment have never been shown to reduce mortality. Mortality rates have remained the same for over 30 years.

17. Which screening tests are currently used to detect prostate cancer?
Digital rectal examination has traditionally been the "gold standard" for screening, although its effectiveness is limited. The use of prostate-specific antigen and transrectal

sonography are currently being studied for use in screening and early detection in asymptomatic men. None of these screening tests has been proved to reduce mortality.

CONTROVERSIES

18. Is breast self-examination (BSE) effective in early detection of breast cancer?
Recommendations vary for and against its use and the role it plays in early detection of breast cancer.
For:
BSE is simple, easy to perform, noninvasive, and a low-cost examination that could potentially result in early detection of breast cancer. Its greatest value may be for women in areas in which there is limited access to physical examination and mammography. Greater awareness could result in earlier detection of breast cancer.
Against:
The evidence is inconclusive that BSE reduces breast cancer mortality. Searching monthly for breast cancer may cause unnecessary fear and anxiety for some women. In other women, BSE may promote a false sense of security. Often when lesions become palpable to patients, they may be larger and more advanced.

19. What would be the effect of early diagnosis of prostate cancer?
Controversy exists over the issue of screening and what impact it would have.
For:
There is optimism that newer screening techniques will detect early prostate cancer where the potential for cure is high.
Against:
Screening may increase the detection rate of clinically insignificant prostate cancers. Once detected, many men would be subjected to unnecessary morbidity from screening tests and morbidity and mortality from treatment. Prostate cancer remains latent in the majority of men and never causes clinically apparent disease.

BIBLIOGRAPHY

1. American Cancer Society: Cancer Facts and Figures. New York, American Cancer Society, 199
2. Battista N, Grover SA: Early detection of cancer: An overview. Ann Rev Public Health 9:21, 1988.
3. Cole P, Morrison AS: Basic issues in population screening for cancer. J Natl Cancer Inst 64:5, 1980.
4. Creasman WT, DiSaia PJ: Screening in ovarian cancer. Am J Obstet Gynecol 165:7, 1991.
5. Gerber GS, Chodak GW: Routine screening for cancer of the prostate. J Natl Cancer Inst 83:329, 1991.
6. Hayward RA, Shapiro MF, Freeman HE, Corey CR: Who gets screened for cervical and breast cancer? Results from a new national survey. Arch Intern Med 148:1177, 1988.
7. Hulka BS: Cancer screening: Degrees of proof and practical application. Cancer 62:1176, 1988.
8. Joseph AM, Byrd JC: Smoking cessation in practice. Prim Care 16:83, 1989.
9. London SJ, Connoly JL, Schnitt SJ, Colditz GA: A prospective study of benign breast disease and the risk of breast cancer. JAMA 267:941, 1992.
10. Ransohoff DF, Lang CA: Screening for colorectal cancer. N Engl J Med 325:37, 1991.
11. Roetzheim RG, Herold AH: Prostate cancer screening. Prim Care 19:637, 1992.
12. Seidman HS, Stellman SD, Mushinski MH: A different perspective on breast cancer risk factors: Some implications of non-attributable risk. CA 32:3, 1982.
13. Smart RS, Chu KC, Conley VL, et al: Cancer screening and early detection. In Holland JF, Frei E, Bast RC, et al (eds): Cancer Medicine. Philadelphia, Lea & Febiger, 1993. pp 408–409.
14. Winawer SJ, Schottenfeld D, Flehinger BJ: Colorectal cancer screening. J Natl Cancer Inst 83:242, 1991.

41. CANCER PREVENTION

Richard F. Bakemeier, M.D., and Dennis J. Ahnen, M.D.

1. What is meant by the term primary prevention?

Carcinogenesis of most (if not all) tissues is thought to be a multistage process that results from exposure of a genetically susceptible host to a cancer-inducing environment. Primary prevention attempts to modify factors that are either intrinsic to the host or extrinsic within the environment. Primary preventive measures (smoking cessation, dietary modification, micronutrient supplements) may act at any stage of carcinogenesis (initiation, promotion, progression) before the appearance of histologically recognizable cancer.

2. What is meant by the term secondary prevention?

Secondary prevention attempts to identify and treat premalignant or early malignant lesions to prevent progression and death from cancer. Secondary preventive measures (screening mammography, Pap smears, sigmoidoscopy, prostate specific antigen) may be applied to populations at different relative risks. In general, the higher the risk of a given population, the more successful the screening program will be and the more intense the secondary prevention effort should be (e.g., sigmoidoscopy for average-risk populations but colonoscopy for first-degree relatives of patients with the hereditary nonpolyposis colorectal cancer syndrome).

3. What is meant by the term chemoprevention?

Chemoprevention is the use of specific quantities of a chemically defined compound to prevent the development of a premalignant or malignant lesion or to cause regression of a premalignant lesion. For example, Sulindac has been proposed as a chemopreventive agent to prevent the development of colonic adenomas and to cause regression of established adenomas in patients with familial adenomatous polyposis.

4. What are the clinically relevant differences between a chemoprevention trial and a dietary prevention trial?

In the United States a chemoprevention trial is much simpler to implement and to evaluate than a dietary intervention trial. Giving (or taking) a pill is easier than teaching someone to change daily dietary intake (or trying to change your own). Monitoring compliance to a specific supplement (pill counts, serum levels) is much simpler than monitoring compliance with a significant dietary modification (food frequency questionnaires, stool fiber content).

5. List six general dietary principles designed to decrease cancer risk and publicized by the American Cancer Society.

1. Avoid obesity. Increased caloric intake appears to enhance tumor growth in certain animal models. Exercise appears to be inversely related to the incidence of certain cancers in humans and may involve expenditure of dietary calories.

2. Decrease total fat intake. Epidemiologic and animal studies suggest a direct relationship between fat intake and the incidence of breast, colon, and prostate cancers (see below).

3. Include a variety of vegetables and fruits in the daily diet to provide fiber, vitamins, and chemical agents that demonstrate cancer preventive qualities in experimental models.

4. Eat more high-fiber foods, such as whole grain cereals, vegetables, and fruits. Insoluble fiber decreases the transit time of the fecal stream and thereby can be expected to reduce the contact between carcinogens and the intestinal mucosal cells. High-fiber foods also bind carcinogens and influence the composition of bile acids in ways favorable to cancer prevention.

5. Limit consumption of alcoholic beverages. Increased alcohol intake has been associated with cancers of the oral cavity, esophagus, liver, and breast.

6. Limit consumption of smoked and nitrite-cured foods. Smoking may create carcinogenic agents in foods. Nitrites may lead to the formation of highly carcinogenic nitrosamines from proteins in the acidic milieu of the stomach.

6. What relation does dietary fat have to cancer formation?

Epidemiologic evidence relating estimated fat intake among the populations of various countries to age-adjusted deaths from breast, colon, or prostate cancer indicates a linear correlation between the two. In general, nations, such as the United States, with high estimated fat intake have high death rates from these cancers, whereas nations with low estimated fat intake, such as Thailand, have low death rates. Animal experiments controlling the amount of dietary fat support a role for dietary fat in cancer promotion, as in spontaneous mouse mammary tumors and carcinogen-induced rat mammary tumors. Other human studies, particularly with breast cancer, have shown variable relationships between reported dietary fat intakes and incidence of breast cancer (see question 12).

7. What evidence relates vitamin A and carotenoids to cancer prevention?

Epidemiologic studies indicate that patients with lung cancer, even early in the clinical course and apparently well-nourished, have lower serum levels of retinol (animal vitamin A) and beta-carotene than controls. (Beta-carotene consists essentially of two molecules of vitamin A, which can be split and made available when needed). Dietary surveys have demonstrated that individuals with the highest intakes of beta-carotene (found in carrots, squash, and spinach) also have the lowest incidence of certain cancers. Vitamin A is essential for normal growth and development, and it is particularly involved in differentiation and maturation of epithelial cells. The precise mechanisms involved in a protective effect of vitamin A have not been defined, but evidence indicates a role in the modulation of protein kinase-C, a receptor for certain tumor-promoting agents. Derivatives of vitamin A and beta-carotene, as well as these micronutrients themselves, are undergoing chemoprevention trials involving patients at high risk for the occurrence or recurrence of tumors of the aerodigestive tract (see below).

8. What evidence relates vitamin C to cancer prevention?

The epidemiologic evidence for a role of vitamin C in cancer prevention is impressive for cancers of the stomach, esophagus, oral cavity, and pancreas. Some evidence suggests a significant protective effect for breast cancer. The striking decrease in the incidence of gastric cancer in the United States over the past half-century has been attributed at least in part to the greater availability of citrus fruits throughout the year, with an associated increase in dietary vitamin C and its antioxidant effects. (A decrease in nitrite-preserved foods, concomitant with increased availability of refrigeration, also has been implicated.) Antioxidants, including also vitamin E and beta-carotene, may have important anticancer effects by protecting cells from damage caused by free radicals.

9. What are cruciferous vegetables? Why do they appear relevant to cancer prevention?

Cruciferous vegetables include broccoli, cauliflower, and brussels sprouts, whose stems share certain structural features indicated by the reference to a cross in their collective name. Epidemiologic studies have related dietary intake of such vegetables to decreased incidence of certain cancers. Recent evidence has demonstrated at least four classes of chemicals found in cruciferous vegetables that inhibit experimental tumors in animals or in vitro by various mechanisms. One of these agents is an isothiocyanate compound that induces detoxification enzymes (glutathione transferase, quinone reductase) in liver cells. Another agent, an indole, alters estrogen metabolism, resulting in metabolites that act as antiestrogens and compete with estrogens that have cancer-enhancing properties. A third chemical is a selenium-containing compound that appears to inhibit tumor promotion. Vegetables may also contain potentially carcinogenic chemicals in addition to cancer-preventing chemicals, leading to the general principle that a desirable diet has a broad variety of vegetables, with none consumed in great excess.

10. What is the suggested relationship between garlic and cancer?
Epidemiologic studies in China and Italy suggest that garlic in the diet may be associated with a reduced risk of gastric cancer. Laboratory experiments using in vitro and in vivo tumor models have suggested possible mechanisms for tumor prevention; inhibition of tumor promotion by garlic extracts seems likely.

11. What nutritional preventive or chemopreventive agents have been proved effective?
None has been rigorously proved effective. Dietary recommendations (low intake of fat, high intake of fruits and vegetables, high intake of fiber) can be made based on strong epidemiologic and animal data, but they have not been proved effective by formal clinical evaluation (such trials are underway). In the population of Lixuian, China, which has a very low intake of several micronutrients, dietary supplementation with various micronutrients (beta-carotene, selenium, vitamin E, retinol, zinc) has been shown to induce a modest decrease in total deaths from cancer (9%) and in deaths from stomach cancer (21%). Whether this type of intervention would be of any benefit in populations with a typical Western diet is not known. In certain high-risk groups, chemoregression of premalignant lesions has been induced by chemopreventive agents (retinol in patients with actinic keratoses, Sulindac in adenomas in patients with adenomatous polyposis coli). Numerous clinical chemoprevention trials are ongoing to evaluate the efficacy of several agents. Because of the design considerations discussed in question 14, most ongoing trials are conducted in high risk groups.

12. What dietary manipulations are under investigation in the National Cancer Institute's Women's Health Initiative?
Half the women in the Women's Health Initiative will continue their usual diet, generally including about 40% of calories from fat. The other half will have a diet in which approximately 20% of calories come from fat. Complex carbohydrates, fiber-containing foods, fruits, and vegetables will thereby be increased in the diet of the second group to provide adequate caloric intake. The 75,000 or so subjects will also be randomized to either a placebo or a combination of calcium carbonate and vitamin D3 supplementation. These two groups of women will be followed for at least 9 years, with particular attention to incidence of breast and colon cancer and bone fractures that reflect incidence of osteoporosis. (A nondietary portion of the Women's Health Initiative involves randomization to either estrogen, estrogen plus progestogen, or placebo.)

13. What are the characteristics of an ideal chemopreventive agent?
An ideal chemopreventive agent would be highly effective, nontoxic, free (or inexpensive), easy to administer, easy to comply with, and widely available. No agent is likely to meet all of these criteria, but they need to be kept in mind in the design of clinical trials. Development of highly effective interventions should become increasingly simplified as the genetic and biochemical events responsible for the early stages of carcinogenesis are defined. The short-term and long-term toxicities (phase I trials) of these agents will need to be carefully evaluated prior to phase II or III trials. Agents known to have significant toxicity (Sulindac), high cost (finasteride), limited availability (Taxol), or cumbersome administration requirements (octreotide) are not as attractive for large-scale clinical trials as an ideal compound would be.

14. What are the differences in study design between cancer chemopreventive and cancer chemotherapeutic trials?
1. Chemopreventive trials are larger, more complex, and more delicate than chemotherapeutic trials because chemopreventive agents are intended for use by large numbers of people, most of whom will never develop cancer. As a result, no significant toxicity is acceptable for a chemopreventive agent.

2. Phase I chemotherapeutic trials are designed to define the maximal dose that does not cause life-threatening toxicity. In contrast, the goal of a phase I chemopreventive trial is to define the maximal nontoxic dose of the compound.

3. Phase II chemotherapeutic trials are designed to determine if one or more of the tolerated doses of the agent causes objective regression of a cancer. In contrast, phase II chemoprevention trials are designed to determine if one or more nontoxic doses of an agent have a biologic effect on the relevant tissue (inhibition of prostaglandin synthesis or regression of adenomas in the colon by Sulindac, for example).

4. Phase III chemotherapeutic trials are controlled studies designed to determine the treatment efficacy of an agent and usually can be completed with hundreds of patients followed from a few months to a few years. In contrast, a phase III chemopreventive trial is designed to determine if an agent can prevent the occurrence of a premalignant or a malignant lesion.

5. Chemopreventive trials with incidence of cancer as the endpoint in average-risk populations typically require thousands of patients to be followed for as long as decades (the tamoxifen trial is designed to follow 50,000 women for 10 years; the finasteride trial plans to enroll 18,000 patients and follow them for 7 years). Because such large trials are very expensive, strong epidemiologic data, consistent animal data, and favorable phase I and II clinical trials are required to justify a phase III chemopreventive trial. Identification of high-risk populations and reliable intermediate endpoints can simplify such trials substantially.

15. What is meant by the terms intermediate endpoint and biomarker?
An intermediate endpoint is a feature of one or more of the early stages of carcinogenesis that may be used as a surrogate endpoint (in place of cancer itself) for a primary prevention trial. Intermediate endpoints can be histologic (adenomas in the colon, dysplasia in the lung or cervix), genetic (K-*ras* or p53 mutation), or biologic (proliferative rate of a tissue). The term biomarker is often used to describe intermediate endpoints but can also be used to describe features that establish the biologic effect of an agent on relevant tissue, regardless of whether the feature is intrinsic to the process of carcinogenesis. For example, inhibition of prostaglandin synthesis can be used as a biomarker of the effects of Sulindac on the colon without knowing whether inhibition of prostaglandin synthesis is essential for any chemopreventive effect(s) of the agent.

BIBLIOGRAPHY

1. Bal DG, Foerster SB: Dietary strategies for cancer prevention. Cancer 72:1005–1010, 1993.
2. Byers T: Dietary trends in the United States. Relevance to cancer prevention. Cancer 72:1015–1018, 1993.
3. Chlebowski RT, Butler J, Nelson A, Lillington L: Breast cancer chemoprevention. Tamoxifen: Current issues and future prospective. Cancer 72:1032–1037, 1993.
4. Correa P: Vitamins and cancer prevention. Cancer Epidemiol Biomarkers Prev 1:241–243, 1993.
5. Dorant E, van den Brandt PA, Goldbohm RA, et al: Garlic and its significance for the prevention of cancer in humans: A critical view. Br J Cancer 67:424–429, 1993.
6. Dwyer JT: Diet and nutritional strategies for cancer risk reduction. Focus on the 21st century. Cancer 72:1024–1031, 1993.
7. Greenwald P, Kramer B, Weed D: Expanding horizons in breast and prostate cancer prevention and early detection. The 1992 Samuel C. Harvey Lecture. J Cancer Educ 8:91–107, 1993.
8. Howe GR, Hirohata T, Hislop G, et al: Dietary factors and risk of breast cancer: Combined analysis of 12 case-control studies. J Natl Cancer Inst 82:561–569, 1990.
9. Laboyle D, Fucher D, Vielh P, et al: Sulindac causes regression of rectal polyps in familial adenomatous polyposis. Gastroenterology 101:635–639, 1991.
10. Lippman SM, Benner SE, Hong WK: Chemoprevention. Strategies for the control of cancer. Cancer 72:984–990, 1993.
11. Suh O, Mettlin C, Petrelli NJ: Aspirin use, cancer, and polyps of the large bowel. Cancer 72:1171–1177, 1993.
12. Zhang Y, Talalay P, Cho C-G, Posner GH: A major inducer of anticarcinogenic protective enzymes from broccoli: Isolation and elucidation of structure. Proc Natl Acad Sci USA 89:2399–2403, 1992.

42. CANCER CHEMOTHERAPY: PREVENTION AND MANAGEMENT OF COMMON TOXICITIES

Amy W. Valley, Pharm.D., BCPS, and Laura L. Boehnke, Pharm.D.

1. Why is toxicity a major problem in cancer chemotherapy?

The drugs used in cancer chemotherapy are unique in that they have a very narrow therapeutic window. The dosage needed for antitumor effect is not much different from the dosage that causes potentially lethal toxicity. Because many of these toxicities are irreversible or life-threatening once they occur, emphasis should be placed on prevention. The table below summarizes the major toxicities of the most commonly used antineoplastic agents.

Major Toxicities of Commonly Used Antineoplastic Agents

GENERIC NAME (BRAND NAME)	TOXICITIES
Bleomycin (Blenoxane)	Pulmonary toxicity*, fevers, hypersensitivity reactions, dermatologic toxicity (mucositis, desquamation)
Carboplatin (Paraplatin)	Myelosuppression*, moderate to severe nausea and vomiting
Cisplatin (Platinol)	Nephrotoxicity*, very severe nausea and vomiting, neurotoxicity*
Cyclophosphamide (Cytoxan) Ifosfamide (Ifex)	Myelosuppression*, hemorrhagic cystitis (Ifosfamide*), moderate to severe nausea and vomiting, SIADH
Cytarabine, Ara-C (Cytosar-U)	Myelosuppression*, mucositis, severe nausea and vomiting[†], neurotoxicity[†], conjunctivitis[†]
Dacarbazine (DTIC)	Severe nausea and vomiting, myelosuppression*, flulike symptoms, phlebitis
Daunorubicin (Cerubidine) Doxorubicin (Adriamycin)	Myelosuppression*, cardiotoxicity*, moderate to severe nausea and vomiting, complete alopecia, vesicants
Etoposide, VP-16 (Vepesid)	Myelosuppression*, hypotension with rapid infusion
5-Fluorouracil (Adrucil, others)	Myelosuppression*, mucositis*, diarrhea*, phlebitis
Methotrexate (Mexate, others)	Myelosuppression*, mucositis*, nephrotoxicity[†], photosensitivity
Mitoxantrone (Novantrone)	Myelosuppression*, moderate nausea and vomiting, cardiotoxicity
Nitrogen mustard (mechlorethamine, Mustargen)	Myelosuppression*, severe nausea and vomiting
Vincristine (Oncovin) Vinblastine (Velban)	Neurotoxicity (vincristine*), vesicant, SIADH, myelosuppression (vinblastine* only)

* = Dose-limiting side effect(s).
[†] = With high-dose regimens.
SIADH = syndrome of inappropriate secretion of antidiuretic hormone.

MYELOSUPPRESSION

2. Do all chemotherapy drugs cause myelosuppression?

In cancer chemotherapy, the dose-limiting side effect (DLSE) is defined as the toxicity that determines the maximal tolerated dose. Although myelosuppression is a common DLSE of the antineoplastic agents, a few agents do not produce this effect, such as bleomycin and vincristine. Patient-specific factors also significantly influence the risk for bone marrow toxicity. Empirical dosage reductions of myelosuppressive agents are often made for the first chemotherapy treatment in patients with low baseline white blood cell or platelet counts, diminished bone marrow reserve from previous chemotherapy or radiation therapy, tumor involvement of bone marrow, and impaired capability for drug elimination. The last factor is related to the pharmacokinetic profile of the myelosuppressive agent. For example, if a marrow toxic drug depends upon renal excretion for elimination, the patient with impaired renal function will have higher drug levels and be at increased risk for myelosuppression. When myelosuppressive drugs are used in combination chemotherapy regimens, the dosages are less than when the drugs are used as single agents to prevent additive toxicity.

3. When should patients be monitored for chemotherapy-induced myelosuppression?
The bone marrow is a common site of toxicity because many chemotherapy agents targe rapidly dividing cells, including committed blood cell precursors. Direct stem cell damage is not common, but when it does occur, it is usually related to use of the alkylating agents. Myelosuppression does not usually occur immediately after chemotherapy administration. Blood components that have already been produced by the bone marrow must be consumed before the effect is realized. White blood cells (WBCs), especially granulocyte precursors, are usually affected to the most significant degree because of their short lifespan (6-12 hours). Platelets (5-10 day lifespan) are also affected, but usually to a lesser degree than white blood cells. Erythrocytes have the longest lifespan (120 days) and are affected to the least degree. Usual nadirs (lowest blood cell counts) after chemotherapy occur at 7-14 days, with recovery by 21-28 days. Patients should have a complete blood count (CBC) with differential performed 1-2 weeks after chemotherapy to assess marrow toxicity. Exceptions to this time frame include the nitrosoureas and mitomycin C, which produce more prolonged patterns of nadir (4-6 weeks) and recovery (6-8 weeks). Planned courses of chemotherapy may be delayed while waiting for blood counts to recover. For safe resumption of chemotherapy, a WBC count $\geq 3000/mm^3$ or absolute neutrophil count (ANC) $\geq 1500/mm^3$ and platelet count $\geq 100,000/mm^3$ are usually required. The ANC may be calculated by multiplying the percentage of neutrophils (segmented + banded neutrophils) by the total WBC count.

4. What is the most appropriate management for patients who experience myelosuppression?
Marrow suppression is an expected phenomenon in leukemic patients receiving induction chemotherapy. In contrast, myelosuppression is an undesirable side effect in patients receiving chemotherapy for treatment of other malignancies. Most patients with solid tumors do not experience clinically significant myelosuppression after standard-dose chemotherapy. If neutropenia or thrombocytopenia occurs, doses of the myelosuppressive drug(s) may be reduced on subsequent cycles. Another alternative for patients who experience significant neutropenia (ANC $<500/mm^3$) is the use of the colony-stimulating factors (CSFs). Granulocyte-CSF (G-CSF) and granulocyte-macrophage CSF (GM-CSF) may be used to maintain full doses of chemotherapy and to prevent recurrence of neutropenia. In this setting, the CSFs are started the day after chemotherapy concludes and are continued throughout the period of neutropenic risk (7-14 days). CSFs are covered in more detail in another chapter. The use of CSFs in the treatment of established neutropenia is more controversial. To date, no preponderance of data supports routine clinical use of these costly drugs in uncomplicated neutropenia. Patients with neutropenic fever should receive prompt empirical treatment with broad-spectrum antibiotics. The management c ͨ infections in immunocompromised patients is covered in another chapter.

Unfortunately, no CSFs currently available can prevent or treat thrombocytopenia. Epoetin alfa (erythropoietin) has recently been approved for the management of chronic cancer-related anemia. Significant anemia (hematocrit $<25\%$) and thrombocytopenia (platelet counts $<20,000/mm^3$) are managed with transfusions of blood products. Patients receiving myelosuppressive chemotherapy must be counseled about signs and symptoms of infection and bleeding and instructed to seek prompt medical attention if they experience such effects.

GASTROINTESTINAL TOXICITY

5. How common are nausea and vomiting with chemotherapy?
An estimated 1–10% of cancer patients refuse or prematurely discontinue chemotherapy because of nausea and vomiting (N/V). In addition, the complications of uncontrolled N/V can delay scheduled courses of chemotherapy and significantly impair the patient's quality of life. These complications include anorexia, malnutrition, dehydration, electrolyte and acid-base imbalance, gastrointestinal mucosal tears, wound dehiscence, aspiration pneumonia, and the development of anticipatory N/V. The reported incidence of chemotherapy-induced N/V varies markedly and depends on several factors:

1. **Emetogenic potential** of the chemotherapy agent(s). Not all chemotherapy agents cause N/V. This factor is the most important determinant of risk.

2. **Dosage** of the chemotherapy agent. For example, high-dose cytarabine often produces severe N/V, whereas low-dose cytarabine is associated with a low incidence.

3. **Method of administration.** For example, doxorubicin given as a rapid intravenous bolus is associated with a moderately high incidence of N/V, but when given as a continuous intravenous infusion over 24 hours the incidence is mild.

4. **Patient-specific factors.** Previous N/V experience with chemotherapy influences the outcome with subsequent treatment regimens. Patients with a history of heavy alcohol use (>5 mixed drinks per day) have a decreased incidence of N/V.

5. **Use of antineoplastic agents in combination regimens.** Many combination regimens are associated with additive or synergistic N/V.

Relative Emetogenic Potential of Antineoplastic Drugs

HIGH (>90%)	MODERATELY HIGH (60–90%)	MODERATE (30–60%)	MODERATELY LOW (10–30%)	LOW (<10%)
Cisplatin	Carmustine (BCNU)	Doxorubicin	5-Fluorouracil	Vincristine
Dacarbazine (DTIC)	Cyclophosphamide	Daunorubicin	Cytarabine[†]	Chlorambucil
Mechlorethamine	Dactinomycin	Mitomycin C	Bleomycin	Tamoxifen
Streptozocin	Carboplatin		Methotrexate	
Cytarabine*	Ifosfamide		Etoposide (VP-16)	

* High-dose therapy (>500 mg/m²)
† Low-dose therapy (<500 mg/m²)
Adapted from Durivage HJ, Burnhan NL: Prevention and management of toxicities associated with antineoplastic drugs. J Pharm Pract 4:27–48, 1991.

6. How is the most appropriate antiemetic regimen selected?
Several antiemetics are available and selection depends on desired potency, adverse effects, patient-specific factors, and cost, as described below. In general, all antiemetic regimens are most effective when given to **prevent** N/V. The antiemetic regimen should be started before chemotherapy administration and should be continued around the clock throughout the period of N/V risk. For most chemotherapy drugs, the period of N/V risk is 24–36 hours; there are, however, exceptions. Cisplatin, for example, is associated with a delayed phase of N/V at 48–72 hours after the drug is administered. Antiemetic coverage should be provided on a regular schedule throughout this time period (3 days after cisplatin). N/V control should always be reassessed before each chemotherapy treatment.

1. **Potency.** Using the information presented in the table above and in question 5, the risk for N/V can be estimated for the chemotherapy regimen that is to be given. Some

antiemetics are effective only against mild to moderate emetogens, while others are effective against even the most emetogenic antineoplastics. The more "potent" antiemetics are not used routinely for all chemotherapy regimens because of adverse effects and/or cost. In general, combination antiemetic therapy is indicated for patients receiving moderately to highly emetogenic regimens of chemotherapy.

2. **Adverse effects.** Antagonism of dopamine receptors in the chemoreceptor trigger zone (CTZ) is the mechanism of action for many of the currently available antiemetic agents (e.g., phenothiazines, butyrophenones, metoclopramide). Unfortunately, the antidopamine effects may also lead to extrapyramidal side effects such as dystonic reactions, pseudo-parkinsonism, and akathisia. Other antiemetics, such as the serotonin antagonists, lack these side effects (see table below).

3. **Patient-specific factors.** For example, patients with anticipatory N/V may benefit from the anxiolytic and amnestic effects of benzodiazepines. Patients <30 years of age are at higher risk for extrapyramidal side effects.

4. **Cost.** Although highly effective, the use of serotonin antagonists is limited by high cost.

Comparison of Antiemetic Agents

CLASS GENERIC (BRAND)	POTENCY*	ADVERSE EFFECTS	COST	COMMENTS
Phenothiazines Prochlorperazine (Compazine) Thiethylperazine (Torecan)	Mild to moderate	Mild sedation, anticholinergic effects, EPS	+	Side effects minimal, multiple routes of administration (PO/IV/IM/PR)
Butyrophenones Haloperidol (Haldol) Droperidol (Inapsine)	Mild to moderate	Mild sedation, EPS	+	Low doses effective, less EPS than with antipsychotic doses
Benzodiazepines Lorazepam (Ativan)	Mild	Sedation, amnesia, respiratory depression (uncommon)	+	Anxiolytic effects useful in some patients, used to prevent/treat anticipatory N/V
Cannabinoids Dronabinol (Marinol)	Mild to moderate	Sedation, anticholinergic effects, euphoria/dysphoria	++	Appetite stimulation useful side effect
Corticosteroids Dexamethasone (Decadron) Methylprednisolone (Solu-Medrol)	Moderate to severe	Short-term effects: insomnia, agitation, mild euphoria, perirectal burning w/IV use	+	Not for long-term use due to side effects
Metoclopramide (Reglan)	Severe	Sedation, EPS (premedicate with Benadryl), diarrhea	++	Against severe emetogens, must use doses of 1–3 mg/kg and combine with corticosteroids
Serotonin Antagonists Ondansetron (Zofran) Granisetron (Kytrel)†	Severe	Mild headache, constipation	+++	Combine with corticosteroids against severe emetogens

*Expressed as efficacy against antineoplastic agents of mild, moderate, or severe emetogenic potential.
† Investigational agent soon to be marketed.
EPS = extrapyramidal side effects such as pseudo-parkinsonism, dystonias, and akathisia; PO = orally; IV = intravenously; IM = intramuscularly; PR = rectally.

7. How should mucositis in the patient receiving chemotherapy be prevented and treated?
The gastrointestinal (GI) mucosa is composed of epithelial cells with a high mitotic index and rapid turnover rate, making it a common site of chemotherapy-induced toxicity. The subsequent inflammation, or mucositis, can lead to painful ulcerations, local infection, and inability to eat, drink, and swallow. The disruption of the GI mucosal barrier may also provide an avenue for systemic microbial invasion. The time course for development and resolution of mucositis often parallels the time course for neutropenia. Agents most commonly associated with mucositis include 5-fluorouracil (5-FU) and methotrexate. The most effective means of preventing mucositis is good oral hygiene. Patients at high risk for this toxicity should be evaluated by a dentist before chemotherapy and instructed to rinse their mouth frequently with baking soda and salt water or chlorhexidine (Peridex) rinses after chemotherapy. For patients receiving 5-FU treatment, the use of ice (oral cryotherapy) may decrease the risk for mucositis. Once mucositis has developed, treatment is mainly supportive, including use of topical or systemic analgesics and oral hygiene (including the rinses described above). Severe cases may require intravenous hydration. Local infections due to *Candida* species and herpes simplex viruses are common in these patients. Suspicious lesions should be cultured and appropriate antifungal and/or antiviral treatment instituted. Antifungal therapy may be delivered topically for mild infections (thrush), using clotrimazole (Mycelex) troches or nystatin (Nilstat, others) oral suspension. For more severe oral or esophageal fungal infections, systemic treatment with oral ketoconazole (Nizoral) or fluconazole (Diflucan) is indicated.

Mucosal damage can occur at any point along the entire length of the GI tract. In the lower portion of the GI tract, the damage can be manifested as diarrhea (mild to life-threatening in nature) and abdominal pain. Support with intravenous fluids and electrolyte supplementation should be initiated promptly in severe cases. Once infectious causes have been ruled out, diarrhea can be treated safely with antispasmodics, like Lomotil or loperamide (Immodium). Recently, the somatostatin-analog octreotide has been used successfully to treat severe cases of 5-FU–induced diarrhea.

8. What treatment strategies can be used to enhance appetite in the patient with cancer?
The complications of cancer cachexia are a common cause of death in patients with cancer. In this patient population, malnutrition appears to result from a combination of decreased caloric intake and increased metabolic requirements caused by the tumor. The most common causes of decreased intake include anorexia, chronic nausea, alterations of taste or smell, pain, dysphagia, and depression. Several measures have been employed to increase appetite in these patients. Clinical studies have shown that megestrol acetate (Megace), a progestational agent, stimulates appetite and produces weight gain in patients with cancer, as well as patients with AIDS. The initial starting dose is 160 mg/day in divided doses. If no response occurs within 1–2 weeks, the dosage can be titrated upward to a maximum of 800 mg/day. Because megestrol acetate is quite expensive, the drug should be discontinued if no benefit is seen. Other drugs used for appetite stimulation include the cannabinoid dronabinol (Marinol), corticosteroids, cyproheptadine (Periactin), and medroxyprogesterone acetate (Provera). For patients who experience loss of appetite due to a feeling of persistent abdominal fullness or GI obstruction, metoclopramide (Reglan) may be beneficial. Patients with anorexia due to pain or depression should receive specific treatment of these disorders. Improvement of caloric intake, however, does not address the problem of metabolic alterations caused by the tumor. Consequently, not all patients benefit from these interventions, especially if they are initiated after cancer cachexia is in the advanced stages.

COMMON ORGAN-SPECIFIC TOXICITIES

9. How can cisplatin-induced nephrotoxicity be prevented?
During the early clinical trials of cisplatin, nephrotoxicity emerged as the dose-limiting side effect. Further experience with the drug has revealed that nephrotoxicity can usually

be prevented or minimized with adequate hydration. Like other heavy metals, cisplatin concentrates in the kidneys, where it can cause necrosis of the proximal and distal tubules. The effects are both dose-related and cumulative. Increases in blood urea nitrogen (BUN) and serum creatinine are evident 1-2 weeks after cisplatin administration and usually reverse within 1-2 weeks in time for the next treatment. With repeated courses, however, the nephrotoxicity may worsen or become irreversible. Patients with preexisting renal dysfunction or patients receiving other nephrotoxic drugs are at highest risk for toxicity.

Cisplatin nephrotoxicity may be prevented by vigorous hydration before, during, and after drug administration. Various regimens have been employed successfully. The common factors of these regimens include use of a chloride-containing intravenous hydration solution (0.9% normal saline or dextrose 5%/0.9% normal saline), and maintenance of adequate urine output ($\geq$100 ml/hr). The chloride solution is important to maintain the intrarenal cisplatin in its most nontoxic form. Maintenance of adequate urine output may require use of diuretics like mannitol or furosemide (Lasix). The renal damage also leads to decreased tubular reabsorption of electrolytes. Patients receiving cisplatin require frequent magnesium and potassium supplementations. Adequate antiemetics for control of delayed emesis must be provided (see questions 5 and 6). Dehydration from uncontrolled emesis increases the risk for significant nephrotoxicity. Before each treatment, patients should have their BUN, serum creatinine, and electrolytes reevaluated. Several strategies for further prevention of cisplatin nephrotoxicity are under investigation, including the development of less toxic analogs and use of chemoprotectants such as ethiofos (WR-2721). Carboplatin, a cisplatin analog with minimal nephrotoxicity, is an alternative to cisplatin for some tumor types.

10. The chronic dose-limiting side effect of doxorubicin is cardiotoxicity. At what total cumulative dose should doxorubicin be discontinued?

The cardiac toxicity of doxorubicin (Adriamycin) is most commonly manifested as congestive heart failure (CHF), which may progress to cardiomyopathy. The etiology of the cardiac damage is believed to be formation of free oxygen radicals, induced by doxorubicin-iron complexes. Mortality from this toxicity is as high as 60%. The risk for development of cardiotoxicity depends on several factors. The most important is a total cumulative dosage of 450-550 mg/m^2, when the doxorubicin has been administered as an intravenous bolus every 3-4 weeks. The incidence of CHF below a cumulative dose of 450-550 mg/m^2 is only 0.1-0.2%. However, the incidence increases to 30% for cumulative doses exceeding 550 mg/m^2. Administration of the drug on a weekly basis or as a continuous infusion may safely permit higher cumulative doses, presumably because of lower peak doxorubicin concentrations in the heart. Other risk factors for doxorubicin cardiotoxicity include age (young children or the elderly), preexisting cardiac disease, concomitant treatment with other cardiotoxic agents, and prior mediastinal irradiation. Although cumulative dosage determines risk, actual cardiac function determines whether treatment should be discontinued. A baseline left ventricular ejection fraction (LVEF) is usually evaluated before administration of doxorubicin and monitored throughout treatment. If the LVEF decreases by 10% and the value is <50%, doxorubicin therapy is discontinued. Although analogs of doxorubicin (e.g., mitoxantrone [Novantrone], idarubicin [Idamycin]) have less cardiotoxicity than doxorubicin, some degree of cardiotoxicity is associated with their use. Future cardioprotective agents, like the iron chelator ICRF-187 (ADR-529), may prevent or minimize this side effect. Once cardiotoxicity occurs, the clinical management is the same as for any other type of CHF or cardiomyopathy.

11. Which chemotherapy agents are associated with pulmonary toxicity?

Although several chemotherapeutic drugs are associated with pulmonary toxicity, bleomycin is the most common causative agent, apparently because of formation of reactive oxygen metabolites and the subsequent inflammatory response in the lung. The initial reaction produces interstitial pneumonitis, which may progress to pulmonary fibrosis and death from hypoxia. The reported incidence of bleomycin pulmonary toxicity varies widely (0–50%) but averages 3–5% in most series. It increases dramatically after a total cumulative dose of 400 units (400 mg) is reached but can occur at any point during therapy or even several months after the last dose of bleomycin. Other factors that may increase the risk for this side effect include the concurrent or subsequent use of high oxygen concentrations, prior or subsequent mediastinal irradiation, age >70 years, and administration of single doses greater than 25 mg/m^2. The onset is insidious, consisting of cough, dyspnea, and occasional fever. Chest radiographic findings are nonspecific, and open lung biopsy may be required to differentiate bleomycin toxicity from other possible causes, such as infection and tumor infiltration. Once detected, bleomycin should be discontinued. Despite drug withdrawal, however, pulmonary symptoms may continue to worsen. Use of corticosteroids may be beneficial, especially if the toxicity is related to a hypersensitivity reaction. Other chemotherapy agents associated with pulmonary toxicity include busulfan, the nitrosoureas (carmustine [BCNU], lomustine [CCNU]), mitomycin C, methotrexate, and cyclophosphamide.

12. A 55-year-old white man with extensive small-cell lung cancer was admitted to the oncology service with a possible spinal cord compression. On physical examination, he reports numbness and tingling in his fingers and toes. What chemotherapy drugs can cause these effects?

Vincristine is the chemotherapy agent most commonly associated with neurotoxicity. This toxicity is most commonly manifested as a peripheral neuropathy, but the spectrum of vincristine neurotoxicity also includes autonomic neuropathy (constipation, abdominal pain, ileus, urinary retention) and cranial nerve palsies (jaw pain, ptosis, optic nerve neuropathy). Initially, the peripheral neuropathy consists of paresthesias in the fingers and toes, accompanied by a decrease and eventual loss of deep tendon reflexes (DTRs). The most severe cases involve impairment of motor function, including wrist drop, foot drop, gait abnormalities, and even quadriparesis. Vincristine neurotoxicity is reversible if it is detected early and if therapy is discontinued. Mild paresthesias are not an indication to stop vincristine therapy. If patients experience muscle weakness or difficulty with fine hand motions (buttoning their shirt, picking up small objects), however, vincristine therapy should be interrupted.

Another vinca alkaloid, vinblastine, is also associated with neurotoxicity, but not to the same degree as vincristine. Cisplatin also is associated with neurotoxicity, including ototoxicity, ocular toxicity, and peripheral neuropathy. The peripheral neuropathy caused by cisplatin is a cumulative, dose-related effect (total dose 300–600 mg/m^2) characterized mainly by sensory loss in a stocking-and-glove distribution. DTRs are usually decreased, but motor neuropathy is not common. The syndrome is usually reversible, but some patients have long-term sequelae. High-dose cytarabine (Ara-C) (>500 mg/m^2 dose) is also associated with severe and potentially fatal neurotoxicity. This toxicity, however, is usually characterized by cerebellar and central nervous system alterations rather than peripheral neuropathy. Other neurotoxic antineoplastic agents include paclitaxel (Taxol), hexamethylmelamine (altretamine, Hexalen), and procarbazine (Matulane).

13. Which chemotherapy agents are associated with hypersensitivity reactions?

Like other drugs, almost every chemotherapy agent has been reported to cause at least a few cases of allergic reactions. The chemotherapy drugs most commonly associated with hypersensitivity reactions are bleomycin, L-asparaginase and paclitaxel (Taxol). Although hyperpyrexia (with fevers up to 42°C) occurs in up to 30% of patients after the first few bleomycin treatments, true hypersensitivity reactions are rare. Nonetheless, the standard of practice at many institutions requires intradermal administration of a 1-unit (1-mg) test dose before the first dose of bleomycin. Patients receiving bleomycin should be premedicated with acetaminophen (Tylenol) to prevent fever.

L-asparaginase is associated with the highest incidence of hypersensitivity reactions. The overall incidence is as high as 40% for patients receiving single-agent therapy and 20% for patients receiving combination regimens, which often included corticosteroids. The reactions can occur at any time during treatment but are most likely during the second week of therapy. Test doses are associated with both false-negative and false-positive results and do not predict which patients will be affected. Some clinicians, however, still recommend that a 2-unit test dose be administered before the first dose of L-asparaginase and repeated any time there has been more than a 7-day lapse between doses. Commercially available L-asparaginase is derived from *E. coli*. For patients who experience allergic reactions, an *Erwinia*-derived product is available from the National Cancer Institute.

In the early development of paclitaxel, hypersensitivity reactions occurred in 84% of patients. Paclitaxel is formulated in a castor oil-based (cremophor-El) vehicle, which is believed to be the cause of the reactions. When patients are premedicated with dexamethasone, diphenhydramine (Benadryl), and an H2-antagonist (e.g., cimetidine [Tagamet]), the incidence of reactions is significantly decreased but not completely eliminated.

14. In a patient who has just experienced an extravasation of doxorubicin (Adriamycin), what should be done to prevent or minimize tissue damage?
Vesicants are drugs that can produce tissue necrosis on leakage outside of the vein (extravasation). Commonly used antineoplastics with vesicant potential include the anthracyclines (doxorubicin and daunorubicin), mitomycin C, nitrogen mustard (mechlorethamine), vincristine, and vinblastine. Once extravasation has occurred, several local maneuvers can decrease the extent of tissue damage. For most chemotherapy drugs, the most important intervention is application of ice to the affected area. The exception to this general rule is the application of heat to vinca alkaloid extravasations. Initially, the needle should be left in place, and an attempt should be made to aspirate drug from the site. If nothing can be aspirated, the needle should be removed. If fluid is aspirated, the needle can be left in place for instillation of specific antidotes, if applicable. Otherwise, the specific antidote can be injected locally to the affected area. Use of specific antidotes is controversial and is recommended for only a few chemotherapy agents. Examples include hyaluronidase (Wydase), which facilitates drug dispersion for vinca alkaloids, and sodium thiosulfate, which inactivates nitrogen mustard. Topical application of dimethylsulfoxide (DMSO) may be beneficial in anthracycline and mitomycin C extravasations. Despite appropriate measures, some patients still develop severe tissue damage and possibly functional loss. The key to management is prevention of extravasation through skilled and careful nursing techniques. Use of central venous catheters should be considered in patients with poor peripheral venous access.

USE OF ADJUNCTIVE PROTECTIVE AGENTS

15. Why is mesna given with ifosfamide?
Mesna (2-mercaptoethanesulfonate sodium [Na]) is used to prevent ifosfamide-induced hemorrhagic cystitis. Hemorrhagic cystitis is the dose-limiting side effect of ifosfamide and occurs to a lesser extent with cyclophosphamide. Both drugs undergo extensive hepatic metabolism. The inactive metabolite acrolein is believed to cause hemorrhagic cystitis by binding to and irritating the epithelial lining of the genitourinary tract. Although toxicity is usually limited to the bladder, the entire genitourinary system is at risk. The clinical spectrum of hemorrhagic cystitis ranges from mild bleeding to life-threatening hemorrhage. Long-term consequences include bladder fibrosis and malignancy. When used in standard doses, cyclophosphamide-induced urotoxicity can be easily prevented with oral hydration (2-3 liters/day) and frequent urination to decrease bladder contact time. High-dose cyclophosphamide regimens, as used in bone marrow transplantation, are associated with a higher risk of bladder toxicity. Preventive regimens include vigorous intravenous hydration, continuous bladder irrigation, mesna, or some combination of these interventions. The

incidence of hemorrhagic cystitis is higher with ifosfamide because more acrolein is formed. Mesna is a sulfhydryl compound that inactivates acrolein. Mesna and hydration should always be given with ifosfamide to prevent hemorrhagic cystitis. Because the plasma half-life of mesna is shorter than that of ifosfamide, the mesna is usually continued for 8–24 hours after the ifosfamide is administered. Once hemorrhagic cystitis occurs after either cyclophosphamide or ifosfamide, treatment consists of discontinuing the drug and providing intravenous hydration. Mild cases (microscopic hematuria) usually respond to this intervention alone. Severe cases are often refractory to treatment. Several agents (alum, silver nitrate, formaldehyde) have been used in bladder irrigation to treat severe or refractory hemorrhagic cystitis. Most recently the prostaglandins (dinoprost and dinoprostone) have been used with some success. Surgical intervention, including arterial ligation or cystectomy, is indicated for severe, refractory patients.

16. When is leucovorin rescue necessary with methotrexate therapy?
Methotrexate (MTX) is a folic acid antagonist that exerts its antineoplastic action by reversibly binding to the enzyme dihydrofolate reductase. This action depletes cells of reduced folate, which is necessary for numerous biochemical reactions, including formation of precursors required for DNA synthesis. Administration of leucovorin (folinic acid) after MTX supplies normal cells with reduced folate and rescues them from methotrexate toxicity. To avoid rescuing cancer cells, it is necessary to wait for 24–42 hours after administration of methotrexate before initiating leucovorin. If leucovorin rescue is delayed more than 42 hours, the rescue may not be complete, and toxicity occurs. Leucovorin rescue is usually not necessary for methotrexate doses <100 mg/m². For methotrexate doses of ≥100 mg/m², leucovorin rescue is given in divided doses for 24–72 hours or until serum concentrations of methotrexate fall below 0.01–0.05 μM. Leucovorin rescue prevents MTX-induced myelosuppression and mucositis. At high doses (>1 gm/m²), MTX is also nephrotoxic because of crystallization of MTX in renal tubules. Leucovorin does not protect against this side effect. Aggressive hydration and alkalinization of the urine are key to prevention of nephrotoxicity from high-dose MTX.

17. Why is leucovorin used with 5-fluorouracil therapy?
Leucovorin is commonly used with 5-fluorouracil (5-FU), especially in the treatment of gastrointestinal malignancies, such as colorectal cancer. The purpose of leucovorin in this setting, however, is not as a rescue agent. The active metabolite of 5-FU (5-FdUMP) exerts its cytotoxic effect by binding reversibly to thymidylate synthetase (TS). This action leads to depletion of thymidine, a necessary ingredient for DNA synthesis. Reduced folate is a necessary cofactor for the binding of 5-FdUMP to TS. Leucovorin is given with 5-FU to maximize enzyme binding and to enhance the anticancer activity of 5-FU. Although efficacy is increased, toxicity in the form of mucositis, diarrhea, and myelosuppression is also increased. As a result, dosages of 5-FU are lower when used with leucovorin than when 5-FU is given alone.

LATE COMPLICATIONS

18. How common are secondary malignancies from chemotherapy agents?
Advances in cancer treatment and chemotherapy have rendered several malignancies curable. As a result, both the number of long-term survivors of cancer and recognition of late complications of chemotherapy, including secondary malignancies and gonadal dysfunction, are increasing. The risk of cancers secondary to chemotherapy is difficult to evaluate, because much of the available data come from retrospective case reports. Although many types of solid tumors have been reported, acute nonlymphocytic leukemia (ANLL) accounts for over 50% of secondary malignancies. ANLL has been reported after successful treatment of Hodgkin's disease, non-Hodgkin's lymphoma, acute leukemias, multiple myeloma, breast cancer and ovarian cancer. Long-term survivors of Hodgkin's

disease who received radiation therapy and chemotherapy that included nitrogen mustard are the most recognized population; the risk of ANLL is 17.6% compared with 2.6% for the general population. The risk of ANLL is highest in the first few years after chemotherapy, with a mean time to diagnosis of 5 years (range 2–10 years). Chemotherapy-induced ANLL is usually refractory to standard treatment regimens. The antineoplastic agents most commonly associated with secondary cancer are the alkylating agents (melphalan, chlorambucil, nitrogen mustard, cyclophosphamide) and the nitrosoureas (carmustine [BCNU], lomustine [CCNU]). For curable tumors, the relatively small increased risk for secondary cancer is far outweighed by the benefits of increased survival in large numbers of patients. In less responsive tumors, the risk may not prove acceptable. Secondary malignancies are a particular concern in the setting of adjuvant chemotherapy.

19. Do all chemotherapy agents cause infertility?
Although gonadal dysfunction has been a known toxicity of antineoplastic agents for decades, it has received little consideration because it is not a life-threatening toxicity and most patients did not survive long enough to worry about reproductive potential. As with secondary malignancies, the alkylating agents are most often associated with gonadal dysfunction. The risk for infertility is related to sex of the patient, age at exposure, type of chemotherapy regimen, total dose administered, and duration of exposure. In postpubertal males, the primary toxicity appears to be at the lining of the seminiferous tubules, leading to reduced sperm counts, testicular atrophy, and infertility. The effects of sperm numbers and function are often reversible, but recovery may take 2–3 years after chemotherapy.

The type of chemotherapy regimen is an important determinant of infertility risk. For example, 100% of male patients receiving MOPP chemotherapy (*m*echlorethamine [*M*ustargen], vincristine [*O*ncovin], *p*rocarbazine, and *p*rednisone) for Hodgkin's disease experience azoospermia, and only 10% recover spermatogenesis. On the other hand, ABVD (doxorubicin [*A*driamycin], *b*leomycin, *v*inblastin, and *d*acarbazine [DTIC]) produces reversible azoospermia in only 35% of male patients treated for Hodgkin's disease. In women, germ-cell toxicity is more difficult to assess because of the inaccessibility of the ovary to biopsy and inability to measure the actual number of germ cells. Chemotherapy appears to induce gonadal dysfunction in women by causing ovarian fibrosis and follicle destruction. The clinical result is amenorrhea, with decreased levels of estradiol leading to menopausal symptoms such as hot flashes and vaginal dryness. Younger women seem to be more resistant to ovarian toxicity and are more likely to recover ovarian function after chemotherapy than older women. Patients with potentially curable cancers should be counseled regarding the risk of chemotherapy-induced infertility and the use of sperm or oocyte cryopreservation.

BIBLIOGRAPHY

1. Balmer CM, Valley AW: Basic principles of cancer treatment and cancer chemotherapy. In DiPiro JT, Talbert RL, Hayes PE, et al (eds): Pharmacotherapy: A Pathophysiologic Approach, 2nd ed. Norwalk, CT, Appleton & Lange, 1992, pp 1879–1929.
2. Blackwell S, Crawford J, et al: Colony-stimulating factors: Clinical applications. Pharmacotherapy 12(2 Pt 2):20S–31S, 1992.
3. Chabner BA, Collins JM (eds): Cancer Chemotherapy: Principles and Practice. Philadelphia, J.B. Lippincott, 1990.
4. Durivage HJ, Burnham NL: Prevention and management of toxicities associated with antineoplastic drugs. J Pharm Pract 4:27–48, 1991.
5. Gralla R, Weiss RB, Vogelzang NJ, et al: Adverse effects of treatment. In DeVita VT, Hellman S, Rosenberg SA (eds): Cancer: Principles and Practice of Oncology, 4th ed. Philadelphia, J.B. Lippincott, 1993, pp 2338–2416.
6. Loprinzi CL, Michalak JC, Schaid DJ, et al: Phase III evaluation of four doses of megestrol acetate as therapy for patients with cancer anorexia and/or cachexia. J Clin Oncol 11:762–767, 1993.
7. Mahood DJ, Dose AM, Loprinzi CL, et al: Inhibition of fluorouracil-induced stomatitis by oral cryotherapy

8. Perry MC (ed): Toxicity of chemotherapy. Semin Oncol 19:453–604, 1993.
9. Ries F, Klastersky J: Nephrotoxicity induced by cancer chemotherapy with special emphasis on cisplatin toxicity. Am J Kidney Dis 8:368–379, 1986.
10. Speyer JL, Green MD, Zeleniuch-Jacquotte A, et al: ICRF-187 permits longer treatment with doxorubicin in women with breast cancer. J Clin Oncol 10:117–127, 1992.

43. CANCER PAIN MANAGEMENT

Amy W. Valley, Pharm.D., BCPS, and Laura L. Boehnke, Pharm.D.

I found that when I didn't have Pain, I could forget I had Cancer.

Terminally ill cancer patient

1. Is cancer pain still a common problem?
Despite an improved understanding of the pathophysiology and the management of pain, approximately 60–90% of patients with advanced stages of cancer still suffer from moderate to severe pain. Barriers to adequate pain management have been identified and include poor pain assessment, reluctance of patients to report pain and to take prescribed pain medications, poor narcotic availability, and the health care professional's lack of basic skills in cancer pain management. If the basic principles of cancer pain management are employed, it is estimated that over 90% of cancer pain could be controlled.

2. What information is needed to assess pain in the cancer patient?
Of the barriers to adequate pain management listed in question 1, poor pain assessment is one of the most common. The following steps can be used to perform an appropriate pain assessment:

1. **Believe the patient's complaints of pain.** Patients with chronic cancer pain do not necessarily exhibit the usual signs associated with acute pain, such as tachycardia, perspiration, and anxiety. They are more likely to appear depressed.

2. **Perform a careful history and physical examination.** Evaluate each site of pain for intensity, quality, variation, and response to prior therapy. Some questions that may be asked to elicit this information include: Where is your pain? What is the pain like? It is a dull ache or a sharp stabbing or shooting pain? What makes the pain better/worse? When is the pain at its worst? Does the pain keep you awake at night or keep you from performing normal daily activities? The patient's current analgesic regimen should also be recorded.

3. **Use pain assessment tools to evaluate pain intensity.** The Visual Analog Scale (VAS) consists of a 10-cm line on which the patient makes a mark that corresponds to the level of pain being experienced.

No pain   Worst pain imaginable

The Visual Analog Scale

Patients who are unable to use the VAS may be asked to rate their pain on a scale of 0 to 10. This numerical rating scale uses the same descriptive parameters as the VAS.

4. **Individualize the therapeutic approach.** Continue to reassess pain and side effects frequently as the therapeutic regimen is individualized.

3. How is chronic pain different from acute pain?
Acute pain and chronic pain are two distinct syndromes. Acute pain is usually related to a specific event, has a well-defined onset, and is reversible. Acute pain requires temporary,

short-term treatment with agents that provide a rapid onset of action. Untreated chronic pain is usually irreversible and gets worse over time. Such pain requires long-term analgesic management with the principal goal of **pain prevention**. When analgesics are given routinely to prevent pain, a rapid onset of action is not necessary. Recognition of the differences between acute and chronic pain forms the foundation for the basic principles of cancer pain management. Although patients with cancer may experience acute pain, the basic management techniques are based on the prevalence of chronic pain in this patient population.

4. What are the basic principles of pain management in chronic cancer pain?

1. **Assess pain and treat the underlying cause if possible.** Approximately 70% of pain in cancer patients is due directly to the cancer. Therefore, treating the underlying cause may involve surgery, radiation, or chemotherapy.

2. **Match the choice of analgesic to the degree of pain.** See question 5.

3. **Titrate the analgesic regimen to patient response.** Give an adequate trial of the analgesic and maximize dosage before switching to another drug.

4. **Administer analgesic medications on a regular basis** (around-the-clock) to prevent pain rather than on an as-required (prn) basis. The prn schedule requires the patient to experience pain repeatedly before receiving medication, and it requires larger amounts of analgesics to control pain than an around-the-clock schedule. Prn dosing is indicated for the management of breakthrough pain during dosage titration.

5. **Use oral medications whenever possible.** Oral administration provides the same degree of analgesia as parenteral administration, facilitates patient independence and home care, and is much less expensive. Drugs with longer durations of action are preferred.

6. **Anticipate and treat side effects.** See questions 15 and 16.

7. **Consider adjuvant medications and nondrug measures to maximize efficacy.** See question 19.

8. **Be aware of tolerance.** Tolerance is usually manifested as a decrease in the duration of analgesic effect rather than a decrease in the overall degree of analgesia. Tolerance can often be managed by simpling increasing the narcotic dosage.

5. Do all patients with cancer need narcotics to control their pain?
Although narcotics are one choice for the management of cancer pain, other appropriate options exist. The choice of analgesic should match the degree of pain experienced by the patient. The World Health Organization (WHO) has developed a systematic approach, or "pain ladder," to assist in this process. For mild pain (the first step of the ladder), nonsteroidal anti-inflammatory drugs (NSAIDs) or acetaminophen (Tylenol) are effective choices. For moderate pain (the second ladder step), products that combine a weak opioid with a non-narcotic are indicated. The final step of the ladder for severe pain, or pain unresponsive to the previous measures, is the opiate, or narcotic, analgesics. Adjuvant analgesics should be added as needed for specific pain syndromes. (See question 19.)

6. What is the role of NSAIDs in cancer pain?
NSAIDs are very effective agents for cancer pain and act via inhibition of prostaglandin synthesis. This mechanism imparts a ceiling effect, or a maximum dosage above which there is no additional analgesia. These drugs are used as single agents to control mild pain and also are commonly used in combination with narcotics to treat moderate to severe pain. NSAIDs are particularly effective for the management of cancer pain due to bony metastases. Side effects of NSAIDs include gastrointestinal irritation and bleeding, antiplatelet effects, and renal toxicity. These agents must be used cautiously in patients with other risk factors for these complications, such as the elderly. Unlike aspirin, which irreversibly acetylates platelets, NSAIDs have antiplatelet effects that are reversible upon discontinuation of the drug. Nonacetylated salicylates, such as salsalate, have significantly fewer antiplatelet effects.

7. When should Tylox or Tylenol 3 be used to treat cancer pain?
The usefulness of combination agents such as Tylox or Tylenol 3 in patients with moderate cancer pain is well established. Most products combine a "weak" opioid, such as codeine, hydrocodone, or oxycodone, with a non-narcotic, such as aspirin or acetaminophen (Tylenol). Combination products do have a ceiling effect imparted by the non-narcotic component. Because there are no long-acting forms of combination products available, dosing is usually at 4- to 6-hour intervals.

8. Why do so many patients with cancer receive morphine instead of other narcotics?
Many opioid analgesics are available for the treatment of pain. When given in equipotent doses, all of these agents can provide effective analgesia. Morphine is considered the "gold standard" for cancer pain treatment for several reasons. It has a reasonable duration of analgesic activity (4–6 hours), and long-acting forms with a duration of 8–12 hours are available. In addition, morphine is formulated in a wide variety of dosage forms (see question 18), is the most readily available narcotic, and is one of the least expensive. Analgesics with agonist/antagonist properties, such as pentazocine (Talwin), are not commonly used to treat cancer pain because they may precipitate withdrawal in opioid-dependent patients and because they cause undesirable side effects.

Narcotic Analgesic Comparison

DRUG	ONSET* (min)	DURATION† (h)	PLASMA t ½ (h)	EQUIANALGESIC DOSES IM (mg)	EQUIANALGESIC DOSES ORAL (mg)
Codeine (various)	15–30	4–6	3	120	200
Fentanyl (Sublimaze, Duragesic)	7–8	1–2	1.5–6	0.1	N/A
Hydromorphone (Dilaudid)	15–30	4–5	2–3	1.5–2	7.5
Levorphanol (Levo-Dromoran)	30–90	6–8	12–16	2	4
Meperidine (Demerol)	10–45	2–4	3–4	75	300
Methadone (Dolophine)	30–60	6–8	15–30	10	20
Morphine (various)	15–30	4–6‡	2–3.5	10	30§
Oxycodone (Roxicodone)	15–30	4–6	ND	NA	30

* Onset of activity is delayed with oral administration.
† After IV administration. Duration of action may be longer with oral administration.
‡ Sustained-release products are available (MS Contin, Roxanol SR) that extend the duration of action to 8–12 hours.
§ With repeated dosing, the IV:po ratio is 1:3. Single-dose studies have shown ratio of 1:6.

9. What is the correct dosage of morphine for cancer pain?
Unlike the non-narcotic agents, the opiates do not possess an analgesic ceiling. Dosages can be progressively increased resulting in additional analgesic effects. The optimal dosage of morphine, or any other opiate, is the dosage that controls pain with minimal side effects. There is considerable variation in dosage requirements between patients. Opioid-naive patients are usually started at a low dosage, for example, 10 mg morphine orally every 4 hours or 30 mg long-acting morphine orally every 12 hours or an equivalent dosage of another narcotic. One study of long-acting morphine reported that 67% of patients with advanced cancer required a dosage of more than 120 mg per day for pain relief.

10. A 50-year-old woman with metastatic breast cancer is receiving hydromorphone (Dilaudid) 4 mg orally every 4 hours for her pain, but her primary oncologist wants to switch her to long-acting morphine for dosing convenience. What is an equivalent dose of morphine?
This patient is currently receiving a total of 24-mg per day of oral hydromorphone. According to the above table, it takes five times as much oral hydromorphone to achieve the same effects as parenteral hydromorphone. So the patient is receiving the equivalent of 4.8 mg per day of intravenous hydromorphone (24 mg PO ÷ 5 = 4.8 mg IV). According to

the table, 1.5 mg of parenteral hydromorphone is equivalent to 10 mg of parenteral morphine. Using simple proportions, 4.8 mg of parenteral hydromorphone is approximately equal to 32 mg of parenteral morphine. It takes three times as much oral morphine to get the same effect as parenteral morphine. So the patient is receiving approximately 96 mg per day of morphine (32 mg IV × 3 = 96 mg PO). Because the long-acting morphine tablets come in 30-mg tablets, a reasonable regimen would be 30 mg orally every 8 hours of long-acting morpine. A prn dose should also be provided to cover breakthrough pain during the dosage titration. A reasonable prn regimen is to calculate how much morphine the patient receives in a 2-hour period and to administer this amount every 2 hours prn. The number of prn doses used should be recorded and used to make future dosage titrations.

11. A 70-year-old man with pancreatic cancer who has been receiving morphine as an intravenous infusion by PCA pump (patient-controlled analgesia) is now ready to go home. What is an equivalent dosage of oral morphine?
PCA pumps allow the patient to activate a hand-held device that delivers a predetermined dosage of medication. To prevent overdosing, the dosage can be repeated only at certain time intervals, defined as the lockout interval. Additionally, these pumps permit delivery of a constant infusion of medication. They have the advantage of prompt delivery of prn doses and increased nursing convenience. To determine the dosage of morphine this patient needs, the total daily morphine dosage (constant infusion plus prn doses used) must be calculated and converted to an equivalent dosage of morphine using the above table as illustrated in question 10.

12. What are the advantages and disadvantages of methadone in cancer pain?
Methadone has a long duration of action and is one of the least expensive narcotic available. Its use is limited by poor availability in many pharmacies and by the complex pharmacokinetic profile of the drug. The plasma half-life of methadone (15–30 hours) is much longer than the duration of analgesia (6–8 hours). It takes four half-lives (4–5 days) for methadone plasma concentrations to reach steady-state levels. Therefore, when methadone is initiated, or when dosage changes are made, a period of 4–5 days must elapse before maximum pain control is seen and efficacy can be fully evaluated. In the meantime, the patient should be covered with prn doses of an immediate-acting narcotic with a shorter half-life, such as morphine. More rapid titration leads to accumulation of methadone, which can result in respiratory depression.

13. Why isn't meperidine (Demerol) a drug of choice for chronic pain control?
Meperidine has a very short half-life and duration of analgesia (2–3 hours), which makes long-term use inconvenient for the patient. The oral bioavailability of meperidine also is poor (see above table). In addition, meperidine's major metabolite, normeperidine, can produce central nervous system excitation and is eliminated renally. Tremors, agitation, and seizures have been reported in patients with renal insufficiency who received meperidine.

14. When is a fentanyl patch (Duragesic) an appropriate choice for pain control?
Fentanyl patches are an excellent option for patients who are not able to swallow or for patients who are noncompliant. Each fentanyl patch provides sustained drug release for 72 hours. The onset of action is delayed (12–24 hours until maximal effect), and patients should be covered with prn doses of an immediate-acting narcotic, such as morphine, during treatment initiation. After a patch is removed, fentanyl continues to be released from subcutaneous tissue for an additional 24 hours. Fentanyl patches are more expensive than long-acting morphine, which is another reason morphine is still considered first-line therapy for most patients.

15. How common is respiratory depression in patients with cancer?
Respiratory depression is rarely observed in patients who are tolerant to narcotics or in opioid-naive patients with unrelieved pain. Sedation almost always occurs before respiratory

depression becomes apparent. Tolerance develops to both respiratory depression and sedation. When respiratory depression does occur, it should be treated with a slow injection of naloxone (0.4 mg diluted in 10 ml normal saline) in order to avoid severe rebound pain. If the patient was receiving a long-acting opioid (methadone, long-acting morphine, or fentanyl patches), a prolonged naloxone infusion may be necessary.

16. What other side effects are associated with narcotic analgesics?
Sedation is a common side effect seen during treatment initiation or after dosage increases. However, tolerance develops to this side effect within a few days to a week. In patients who do not develop tolerance but have adequate pain control, a dosage decrease should be attempted. If a dosage decrease cannot be made, addition of a stimulant, such as methylphenidate (Ritalin) or dextroamphetamine should be considered.

Constipation is one of the most problematic side effects associated with narcotics. Tolerance does **not** develop to this side effect. All patients on chronic narcotic analgesics also should receive a regular bowel regimen that includes a stool softener and a stimulant laxative. The bowel regimen should be titrated to produce a bowel movement every 1–2 days. Lactulose and sorbitol are useful alternatives for refractory patients.

Nausea and vomiting occur in approximately 30% of patients during initiation of narcotic therapy or after dosing increases. Tolerance to this adverse effect develops in 5–10 days. Mild antiemetics such as oral prochlorperazine (Compazine) or scopolamine patches are effective for narcotic-induced nausea.

Other less common side effects of the narcotics include urinary retention, bladder spasm, pruritus, orthostatic hypotension, and dry mouth.

17. What are the differences between dependence and addiction?
Dependence is the physical, biologic need for a drug in order to prevent withdrawal symptoms on sudden discontinuation. Addiction is the psychological craving for a drug. When there is a physical impairment requiring chronic pain control (e.g., cancer), addiction is rarely seen. However, cancer patients do become physically dependent on narcotics. The distinction between physical dependence and addiction is an important one, because some patients will refuse narcotics because of fear of addiction, and some health care professionals wrongly avoid using opioids for the same reason.

18. What analgesic options are available for patients who cannot swallow?
The **sublingual and transdermal routes** are the simplest and least invasive methods of delivery in patients who are unable to swallow oral medications. Morphine is the narcotic usually employed for sublingual administration. The only narcotic available in the transdermal form is fentanyl (see question 14). Morphine and hydromorphone also are available as **rectal suppositories**.

Continuous intravenous infusions are also an alternative in patients who are unable to swallow. In patients without intravenous access, **subcutaneous infusions** may be employed. The intramuscular route is rarely necessary, because so many other less painful administration options exist. In general, parenteral administration is more expensive than the less invasive routes of administration listed previously (oral, sublingual, transdermal). In addition to the cost of the drug, the cost of infusion pumps, nursing care, and associated supplies must be considered.

Epidural and intrathecal administration is another option for patients who are not candidates for or who have failed systemic narcotic regimens. The advantages of spinal administration include long duration of action (6–24 hours) and lower incidence of systemic side effects such as sedation and respiratory depression. Disadvantages include the risk for infection and the need for expensive support services and equipment. Patient selection is the key to making best use of this invasive and costly analgesic option. Because 90% of patients can achieve pain control using basic principles (see question 4) and less invasive routes of administration, spinal administration has a limited role in cancer pain management.

19. Which adjuvant analgesics are most useful for managing neuropathic pain and other specific pain syndromes?
Neuropathic pain is characterized by an intense stabbing or shooting quality. The source of this type of pain is direct damage to nerves, nerve roots, or plexuses from tumor invasion or compression. Antidepressants (e.g., amitriptyline, nortriptyline) and anticonvulsants (carbamazepine) are the most effective adjuvant analgesics for control of nerve pain. They may be used alone for mild neuropathic pain or in combination with narcotics and anti-inflammatory agents for moderate to severe pain. The necessary doses are often much lower than those required for the treatment of depression or seizures. Corticosteroids may also be helpful for refractory pain.

Bone pain is common in patients with cancer that has either originated or metastasized to the bone. The usefulness of the NSAIDs is described in question 6. NSAIDs are effective alone in mild bone pain and have synergistic effects with the opioids in moderate to severe bone pain. Addition of NSAIDs to narcotic regimens may actually permit the use of lower narcotic doses and aid in minimizing narcotic side effects.

In addition to their activity in neuropathic pain, corticosteroids also are effective in the treatment of pain due to intracranial pressure and lymphedema.

BIBLIOGRAPHY

1. Cancer Pain Management Panel: Cancer Pain Management. Clinical Practice Guideline. Rockville, MD, Agency for Health Care Policy and Research, Public Health Service, U.S. Department of Health and Human Services (in press).
2. Foley KM: The treatment of cancer pain. N Engl J Med 313:84–95, 1985.
3. Levy MH: Pain management in advanced cancer. Semin Oncol 12:394–410, 1985.
4. Payne R, Max M, Sunshine A, et al: Principles of Analgesic Use in the Treatment of Acute and Chronic Cancer Pain, 2nd ed. American Pain Society, 1989.
5. World Health Organization: Cancer Pain and Palliative Care. Geneva, Switzerland, WHO, 1990.

44. INFECTIOUS COMPLICATIONS OF CHEMOTHERAPY

Patrick Moran, M.D.

1. What is the single most important risk factor in the development of infection in the cancer patient?
Neutropenia, identified as less than 500 polymorphonuclear neutrophils (PMNs) or band forms per cubic centimeter (cc), is the single most important identifiable risk factor for the development of fever and infection in the cancer patient. The risk of developing infection also is related to the duration of neutropenia (i.e., patients receiving more intensive chemotherapy who have prolonged neutropenia for more than a week).

2. Describe the classic signs and symptoms of infection in the neutropenic patient.
This is a significant problem. The absence of granulocytes may mask the classic signs of inflammation, making the diagnosis of infection difficult. A careful history must be taken and physical examination must be done in a scrupulous manner initially and repeated at regular intervals looking for possible sites of infection. Eye grounds should be examined for the cottony white lesions associated with invasive candidiasis, and the perianal area should be observed for any signs of tenderness or inflammation. Catheter exit sites, as well as the catheter tunnel, should be palpated for any sign of tenderness or inflammation.

3. What is the minimum evaluation for a patient who develops a fever while neutropenic?
In addition to the above-mentioned physical examination, a chest radiograph should be performed and cultures of blood, sputum (if productive), and urine should be obtained. If the patient has an indwelling catheter, cultures should be drawn through each port of the indwelling catheter, as well as peripherally, to try to determine if an infection is catheter related.

4. Is there a best initial coverage for a febrile neutropenic patient?
The primary consideration in choosing an empirical regimen for a febrile neutropenic patient is efficacy. Secondary considerations include the risk of emergence of resistance during therapy, the cost versus benefit ratio, and the patient's allergies. It is important to take into account the types of organisms that are commonly isolated at the center in which the patient is being treated. Possible regimens include two or three drug combinations containing an aminoglycoside (gentamicin, tobramycin, amikacin) and a cephalosporin or extended-spectrum penicillin. Monotherapy with a third-generation cephalosporin (e.g., ceftazidine or cefoperazone) or imipenem can be considered.

If *Enterobacter* species are commonly isolated, monotherapy with a cephalosporin should be avoided in view of the ease of induction of beta-lactamase in these organisms.

5. True or false? Once the patient has been examined, cultures have been drawn, and broad-spectrum antibiotics have been prescribed, that patient is on autopilot until the granulocyte counts recover.
False. If neutropenia continues, additions or modifications of antibiotic therapy are often required. Initial organisms may not be sensitive to the prescribed antibiotics or resistant organisms may emerge. Infection with nonbacterial pathogens, including viruses or invasive fungi, may occur. An appropriate treatment may be required for these organisms.

6. When should a fungal infection be considered in a neutropenic patient?
If a patient remains persistently febrile after 7 days of broad-spectrum coverage despite persistent attempts to identify a causative bacterial organism, antifungal therapy should be considered. In addition, if a patient has become afebrile on broad-spectrum antibiotic coverage but the fever recurs, fungal infection should be considered. Amphotericin B is the gold standard for treatment. Fluconazole is effective for thrush or esophagitis, but its value for systemic mycosis remains to be determined. Fluconazole is not effective against *Aspergillus, Mucor,* or *Candida krusei.*

7. If a neutropenic patient becomes afebrile, should antibiotics be discontinued?
No. As a general rule, antibiotics should not be discontinued until the granulocyte count rises above 500. If a patient is afebrile but remains neutropenic, stopping the antibiotics prior to recovery of the neutrophil counts is associated with a high degree of relapse of infection, fever, and hypotension.

8. What are the most common causative organisms of a catheter-related infection? Who is at risk?
Coagulase-negative staphylococci are the most common cause of a catheter-associated bacteremia; however, other organisms, as well as *Candida,* can be the cause of catheter-related infections. Patients who have indwelling catheters with normal neutrophil counts and those who are neutropenic are both at risk of catheter-related infection.

9. Do external catheters have a greater infection rate than subcutaneous catheters?
Although earlier studies show that the risk of infection may be somewhat lower in patients with a subcutaneously implanted catheter versus an exteriorized catheter, a prospective study showed no difference in the incidence of complications between the two types of devices.[4]

10. True or false? Suspected catheter-related infections require removal of the catheter.
If the infection is related to the catheter exit site, local wound care and oral antibiotics are often successful without catheter removal. Purulent infections of the catheter tunnel or pocket require caheter removal. Catheter-related sepsis, unless secondary to *Staphylococcus aureus* or *Candida*, can usually be managed with intravenous antibiotics.

11. What patient should receive *Pneumocystis* prophylaxis?
The risk of *Pneumocystis* infection is highest in patients receiving high-dose steroids for a prolonged period of time, as well as patients undergoing bone marrow transplantation and those who are HIV positive and undergoing cancer chemotherapy. Trimethoprim-sulfamethoxazole remains the best drug; a thrice weekly schedule is satisfactory.[7]

12. What is the role of prophylactic antibiotics?
Although an interesting idea investigated during the 1960s and 1970s, the use of antibiotics to prevent the emergence of bacterial infections has largely fallen into disuse because of lack of efficacy and the emergence of resistant organisms.

13. Discuss the indications for granulocyte transfusions.
The era of granulocyte transfusions has essentially passed. It has proved impractical to collect enough functional neutrophils to benefit neutropenic patients and the risk of complications is quite high. Such complications include pulmonary toxicity and the risk of transmission of infection.

14. How have colony-stimulating factors changed the management of cancer patients with infections?
Granulocyte and granulocyte-macrophage colony-stimulating factors (CSFs) stimulate bone marrow progenitor cells and increase the numbers of circulating granulocytes and macrophages. These factors shorten the duration and severity of neutropenia in patients receiving chemotherapy for a variety of solid and hematologic tumors. When CSFs are used, they have been associated with fewer infections. CSFs are well-tolerated; however, they are quite expensive. Using CSFs in patients who are at significant risk of infection through their prolonged neutropenia is probably beneficial.

BIBLIOGRAPHY

1. Benezra D, Kiehn TE, Gold JWM, et al: Prospective study of infections in indwelling central venous catheters using quantitative blood cultures. Am J Med 85:495, 1988.
2. DeVita VT, Hellman S, Rosenberg SA (eds): Cancer: Principles and Practices of Oncology. Philadelphia, J.B. Lippincott, 1993.
3. Hughes WT, Armstrong O, Bodey OP, et al: Guidelines for the use of antimicrobial agents in neutropenic patients with unexplained fever. J Infect Dis 161:381–396, 1990.
4. Kappers-Klunne MC, et al: Complications from long-term indwelling central venous catheters in hematologic patients with special reference to infection. Cancer 64:1747–1752, 1989.
5. Leischke GJ, Burgess AW: Granulocyte colony-stimulating factor and granulocyte-macrophage colony-stimulating factor. N Engl J Med 327:99–106, 1992.
6. Laszlo J (ed): Physicians' Guide to Cancer Care Complications. New York, Marcel Dekker, 1986.
7. Masur H: Prevention and treatment of Pneumocystis pneumonia. N Engl J Med 327:1853–1860, 1992.
8. O'Donnell JF, Coughlin CT, Lemarbre PJ: Oncology for the House Officer. Baltimore, Williams & Wilkins, 1992.
9. Pizzo PA: Management of fever in patients with cancer and treatment induced neutropenia. N Engl J Med 328:1323–1332, 1993.
10. Pizzo PA, Robichaud KJ, Gill FA, Witebsky FG: Empiric antibiotic and antifungal therapy for cancer patients with prolonged fever and granulocytopenia. Am J Med 72:101, 1982.

45. GASTROINTESTINAL COMPLICATIONS OF CHEMOTHERAPY

Patrick Moran, M.D.

1. What other causes of nausea and vomiting should be considered in a cancer patient in addition to chemotherapy?

Other common causes include narcotics and other medications, metabolic disturbances, especially hypercalcemia, bowel obstructions, and liver or brain metastasis.

2. Describe the pathophysiology of vomiting in the cancer patient.

This is a complex problem. It is believed to be related to stimuli to the vomiting center, which is located in the medulla. Closely allied to this is the chemoreceptor trigger zone that is sensitive to noxious substances (e.g., chemotherapy). Neurotransmitters, such as dopamine and serotonins, mediate the transmission of stimuli between the chemoreceptor trigger zone and the vomiting center.

3. Name two additional emetic problems in addition to acute chemotherapy-induced emesis.

The first problem is the development of delayed emesis, which occurs 24 hours or more after chemotherapy. This is most common with moderate to high doses of cisplatin or doxorubicin. Management consists of awareness of this problem and continuing patients on regular doses of antiemetics up to 4–5 days after chemotherapy administration.

The second problem is that of anticipatory emesis, which occurs when nausea and vomiting are experienced prior to the actual chemotherapy administration. This is a difficult problem. The best prevention is to treat nausea aggressively at the onset of therapy; however, it may respond to anxiolytics and behavior modification approaches.

4. How should antiemetic therapy be selected in the cancer patient?

Primary consideration is the emetogenic potential of the chemotherapy agents to be used. A regimen containing high-dose cisplatin will cause nausea in virtually 100% of patients treated, whereas 5-fluorouracil (5-FU) regimens commonly used in colon cancer have little emetagenic potential. The greater the potential for vomiting, the more aggressive the antiemetic regimen should be.

Emetogenic Potential of Common Chemotherapeutic Agents

HIGH	MODERATE	LOW
Cisplatin	Mitomycin C	Vinca alkaloids
Mechlorethamine	Doxorubicin (low dose)	5-Fluorouracil
Streptozotocin	Cytarabine	Etoposide
Dacarbazine	Procarbazine	Bleomycin
Cyclophosphamide	Methotrexate (high dose)	Melphalan
Daunorubicin	Lomustine	Methotrexate (low dose)
Doxorubicin	Methyl (CCNU)	L-Asparaginase
(moderate–high dose)	Carboplatin	Chlorambucil
	Mitoxantrone	
	Ifosfamide	

5. Which classes of drugs are active as antiemetics?

Phenothiazines act as dopamine antagonists, inhibiting the vomiting center. They are useful in outpatient regimens, causing mild to moderate nausea. Metoclopramide in low doses also acts primarily as a dopamine antagonist. Metoclopramide in high doses also acts as a serotonin antagonist, but its use is hindered by side effects.

A new class of medications, the serotonin antagonists, block serotonin receptors peripherally in the gastrointestinal tract as well as centrally in the medulla. These are well tolerated and have proved to be extremely effective in the treatment of chemotherapy-related emesis.

Other drugs used in combination with the above medications include benzodiazepines and corticosteroids.

For a more thorough discussion of this subject, refer to chapter 42.

6. What is stomatitis?

Stomatitis is a painful irritation of the oral mucosa produced by the effect of chemotherapeutic drugs on the rapidly dividing cells of the oral epithelium. Drugs commonly associated with this include methotrexate, 5-FU, doxorubicin, and bleomycin.

7. What can be done to prevent stomatitis?

It is sometimes unavoidable; however, the onset of severe oral lesions may indicate a need for prompt dosage reduction or discontinuance of therapy. Stomatitis related to methotrexate may be ameliorated by the use of oral leucovorin 24 hours after the administration of methotrexate (leucovorin rescue). Cooling of the mucosa with ice chips may reduce the exposure to mucositis-inducing drugs and may be helpful in prevention. A good oral hygiene regimen is important, although mouthwashes containing alcohol or hydrogen peroxide should be avoided.

8. Once mucositis has occurred, how should it be treated?

Mucositis can be extremely painful, and adequate analgesia, including opiate narcotics, is often needed. Yeast or herpes infections can contribute. An appropriate therapy should be instituted if these are suspected. Topical solutions such as KBX (Kaopectate [combination of kaolin and pectin], Benadryl [diphenhydramine], viscous Xylocaine [lidocaine] in a 1:1:1 formulation) may provide temporary relief of pain.

9. What is a "vincristine belly"?

It is constipation caused by autonomic neuropathy brought on by vincristine. It is especially prominent in elderly patients and can cause severe obstipation and possibly bowel obstruction. The condition can be managed prophylactically with a combination of laxatives and stool softener.

10. A neutropenic patient presents with fever and right lower quadrant abdominal pain with positive peritoneal signs. What are the diagnostic possibilities?

Certainly appendicitis is a consideration. Another entity is typhlitis, which is a potentially necrotizing infection of the cecum. It is best managed with the addition of anaerobic coverage to the broad-spectrum antibiotics and close monitoring for possible surgical intervention.

11. Name the three forms of hepatocellular injury possibly related to chemotherapy.

1. Chemical hepatitis
2. Veno-occlusive disease, which results from blockage of venous outflow in the small centrilobular hepatic vessels
3. Chronic fibrosis

12. True or false? Diarrhea is not a particularly severe complication of infusional 5-FU therapy.

False. In a patient receiving 5-FU therapy, the complaint of diarrhea must be taken seriously and evaluated carefully. Diarrhea in this situation may become watery or bloody and potentially life-threatening with a risk of dehydration and sepsis. The development of diarrhea should call for careful evaluation, possible temporary cessation of 5-FU therapy, and reinstitution of therapy at a lower dose when appropriate.

BIBLIOGRAPHY

1. Bleyer WA: New vistas for leucovorin in cancer chemotherapy. Cancer 63:995–1007, 1989.
2. DeVita VT, Hellman S, Rosenberg SA (eds): Cancer: Principles and Practices of Oncology. Philadelphia, J.B. Lippincott, 1993.
3. Einhorn LH, Nagy C, Werner K: Ondansentron: A new antiemetic for patients receiving cisplatin chemotherapy. J Clin Oncol 8:731–735, 1990.
4. Keidan RD, Fanning J, Gatenby RA, Weese JL: Recurrent typhlitis, a disease resulting from aggressive chemotherapy. Dis Colon Rectum 32:206–209, 1989.
5. Laszlo J (ed): Physicians' Guide to Cancer Care Complications. New York, Marcel Dekker, 1986.
6. Meyer BR, Lewin M, Drayer DE, et al: Optimizing metoclopramide control of cisplatin-induced emesis. Ann Intern Med 100:393–395, 1984.
7. O'Donnell JF, Coughlin CT, Lemarbre PJ: Oncology for the House Officer. Baltimore, Williams & Wilkins, 1992.
8. Rollins BJ: Hepatic veno-occlusive disease. Am J Med 81:297, 1986.
9. Starnes HF: Abdominal pain in neutropenic cancer patients. Cancer 57:616–621, 1986.

46. HEMATOLOGIC COMPLICATIONS OF CHEMOTHERAPY

Lori Jensen, M.D., and Marie E. Wood, M.D.

1. What are the general categories of hematologic complications from chemotherapy?
The most common hematologic complication of chemotherapy is myelosuppression resulting in neutropenia, thrombocytopenia, and less commonly anemia. For the majority of anticancer agents, myelosuppression is the most important dose-limiting toxicity. Other less common complications (specific to certain chemotherapeutic agents) include development of the hemolytic uremic syndrome, alterations in coagulation, and alterations in red blood cell morphology. A long-term hematologic complication with certain chemotherapeutic agents is the development of a secondary hematologic malignancy.

2. Why is the bone marrow generally more sensitive than other organs to the effects of chemotherapy?
Chemotherapeutic agents exert their major antitumor effect by affecting enzymes or substrates important in the tumor cell life cycle, the end result being impaired DNA synthesis. These agents are not tumor specific, and any cell that is actively dividing will be affected. The uncontrolled proliferation of tumor cells makes them more susceptible to the effects of chemotherapy than normal tissues, but tissues with high proliferative capacities also are affected; that is, the bone marrow, hair follicles, and gastrointestinal epithelium.

3. Why are there differences in the degree of depression of the three cell lines (i.e., neutropenia versus thrombocytopenia versus anemia) after the administration of chemotherapy?
The kinetics of the cell line (neutrophils, granulocytes, megakaryocytes) affected by a drug will determine the severity of the depression of that cell line. Few chemotherapeutic agents selectively depress the multipotent stem cell; most agents affect the cell lines after some degree of differentiation. Of the three cell lines, neutrophils have the shortest half-life

(6–8 hours). As a result, the granulocytic cell line is depressed earlier and to a greater degree than the other two cell lines. The half-life of platelets is 5–7 days; therefore, the mega-karyocytic cell line is usually less severely affected than the granulocytic cell line. Anemia from depression of red blood cell maturation is also seen; however, it is not generally clinically significant given the 120-day life of a red blood cell.

4. What factors affect the degree of cytopenia that develops after chemotherapy administration?
The degree of cytopenia that develops is determined both by the pharmacokinetics of the agent being administered as well as the degree of bone marrow reserve. Alterations in pharmacokinetics that increase drug delivery can cause more marked cytopenias. Examples of altered pharmacokinetics include variability in drug absorption, protein binding, and drug-drug interactions. Liver or renal disease can alter drug metabolism and/or excretion. Some drugs, such as methotrexate, accumulate in third-space fluids, resulting in prolonged release of the drug and causing severe cytopenias.

The degree of bone marrow reserve also is an important determinant in the development of postchemotherapy cytopenias. Several factors affect bone marrow reserve. Younger patients have more cellular bone marrow and, as a result, will have less severe cytopenias than older patients. Extensive tumor infiltration of the bone marrow, previous chemotherapy, or radiation therapy may result in more significant cytopenias. Nutritional status also is important. Patients who have a negative nitrogen balance or nutritional deficits of vitamin B12 or folate will be more sensitive to the myelosuppressive effects of the chemotherapy and less able to regenerate the bone marrow after chemotherapy.

5. What is the usual timing of the chemotherapy-induced myelosuppression?
As a general rule, cell cycle–specific agents produce a fairly rapid granulocytopenia followed by thrombocytopenia (7–14 days) with a relatively rapid recovery (14–21 days). Agents that are non–cycle-specific, that is, they exert their effect in cells that are in the resting phase (G_0), have a longer delay in onset, as well as a more prolonged granulocytopenia (recovery may take up to 4–6 weeks). Examples of these agents include certain alkylating agents (specifically the nitrosoureas carmustine and lomustine) as well as mitomycin C. These agents primarily affect the multipotent stem cell.

6. Discuss the role that colony-stimulating factors (CSFs) play in the treatment of neutro-penic fever.
Their role in the treatment of neutropenic fever has yet to be defined. Most studies to date have not been designed to answer the question of what role these agents play in the treatment of neutropenic fever but rather what role they play in the prevention of neutropenic fever. A randomized trial comparing granulocyte CSFs (G-CSF) versus placebo as an adjunct to the treatment of neutropenic fever has recently been completed, the results of which have not yet been published. Preliminary studies with relatively small sample sizes suggest that granulocyte-macrophage CSF (GM-CSF), when administered during a neutropenic fever, can shorten the duration of neutropenia. What impact this may have on length of hospital stay and patient morbidity or mortality is yet unknown.

7. What is thought to be the optimal timing for the administration of CSFs?
The optimal timing for the administration of the CSFs is still under investigation. Few studies have attempted to use G-CSF or GM-CSF simultaneously with chemotherapy because of the concern that increased toxicity would result from stimulating normal cell proliferation before metabolic clearance of the chemotherapeutic agents. In general, most studies start the cytokines within 24–48 hours after completion of chemotherapy, continue daily treatment until after the resolution of the neutropenia, and discontinue G-CSF or GM-CSF when the patient has a total white blood cell count of 5,000–10,000.

8. Do all patients with neutropenic fever need to be hospitalized?

Yes. The requirement for hospitalization of the neutropenic febrile patient has never been studied in a randomized prospective fashion, and it is considered standard care to admit these patients for observation and administration of intravenous broad-spectrum antibiotics.

9. What is thought to be the cause of the anemia of malignancy? How do chemotherapeutic agents cause anemia?

Patients with malignant tumors commonly have a mild to moderate normochromic-normocytic anemia that is multifactorial in etiology. Serum iron and total iron-binding capacity is generally low with an elevated ferritin, which indicates a block in the transfer of iron from stores to the erythroid precursor cells. Other potential causes for anemia include blood loss, marrow infiltration by tumor, or on occasion hemolysis. In addition, some patients with malignancies have demonstrated a blunted erythropoietin response. Erythropoietin levels may be elevated above the normal range but are inappropriately low for the given degree of anemia. How much this apparent blunted erythropoietin response contributes to the anemia is not known.

Chemotherapy contributes to the development of anemia by its direct toxic effect on erythroid precursors. It also has a direct toxic effect on the bone marrow microenvironment, which is important for hematopoiesis. Some agents have direct toxic effects on renal tubules that can adversely affect erythropoietin production.

10. Why do some patients receiving chemotherapy develop macrocytosis? Does this suggest a deficiency of folate or vitamin B12?

In vitamin B12 or folate deficient states, DNA synthesis is impaired, resulting in a nuclear maturation arrest relative to cytoplasmic maturation. This abnormality results in neutrophils with hypersegmented nuclei and macrocytic red blood cells. Cell cycle–specific chemotherapeutic agents that alter DNA synthesis also will impair nuclear maturation relative to cytoplasmic maturation. Examples of such agents are the folic acid antagonists (methotrexate, trimetrexate), antipyrimidines, antipurines, and some of the alkylating agents. Hydroxyurea impairs DNA synthesis by inhibiting conversion of ribonucleotides to their corresponding deoxy forms. An increase in the mean corpuscular volume (MCV) is expected with these agents, but vitamin B12 and folate levels are normal unless there is an independent nutritional or metabolic abnormality.

11. Define the hemolytic uremic syndrome (HUS) and describe its association with chemotherapeutic agents.

HUS consists of microangiopathic hemolytic anemia, thrombocytopenia, and renal failure. The syndrome can occur spontaneously, more commonly in children than in adults, but it also can be associated with the use of chemotherapeutic agents. Ninety percent of the chemotherapy-related cases have been associated with the use of mitomycin C. HUS is thought to be related to circulating immune complexes. With rare exceptions, coagulation studies are normal. The incidence of mitomycin C–associated HUS is about 4–15%, with the majority of cases occurring when total doses exceed 60 mg. Mortality exceeds 50%. Some evidence suggests that immunoperfusion of the patient's blood over a staphylococcal protein A (SPA) column may be beneficial. Other treatment modalities such as steroid use, dialysis, and plasmapheresis have not been shown to be helpful.

12. Which chemotherapeutic agents can alter coagulation and by what mechanism?

Mithramycin can cause an acquired platelet abnormality. Typically, the platelet count is normal, but the bleeding time is prolonged and clotting studies are normal. Platelet adenosine dinucleotide phosphate (ADP) levels are decreased, resulting in abnormal platelet aggregation studies. Clinically, these patients develop mucosal bleeding or oozing from wounds.

L-asparaginase globally impairs protein synthesis. Seventy percent of patients will have prolongation of the prothrombin time, partial thromboplastin time, or the thrombin time as a manifestation of decreased fibrinogen production. These clotting abnormalities do not appear to result in clinically significant bleeding.

Mitomycin C can cause the HUS (see question 11). Coagulation studies are usually normal; however, severe thrombocytopenia can result in a prolongation of the bleeding time.

13. What is the most common secondary malignancy that develops after treatment with chemotherapy? Which agents are thought to be important in the development of such malignancies?

The most common secondary malignancy associated with previous chemotherapy use is acute nonlymphocytic leukemia (ANLL). The diseases in which secondary malignancies have been observed are those which are treated with alkylating agents or nitrosoureas and for which there is prolonged survival. The most common examples include curable pediatric malignancies as well as Hodgkin's disease. Less common examples include ovarian cancer, multiple myeloma, breast cancer, non-Hodgkin's lymphoma, and gastrointestinal malignancies. Factors that alter the risk of development of a secondary malignancy are thought to include the chemotherapeutic agent used, the total amount of drug administered, the schedule of the administration, host immunity, and use of radiation therapy. The risk of leukemia appears to be highest within the first few years of completing treatment but can occur up to 10 years after treatment. The most common subtypes of ANLL seen in this population are acute myelomonocytic leukemia and erythroleukemia. A myelodysplastic period frequently precedes the acute leukemia. Chromosomal abnormalities are common; the most frequently encountered are deletions of chromosomes 5 and 7.

CONTROVERSIES

14. Should platelet transfusions be given when the platelet count drops below 20,000/μl?
For:
That is the way we have always done it!
Against:
There have been studies looking at the threshold for platelet transfusions. Most of these chose an arbitrary platelet count for transfusion or were done in the early days when aspirin was generally used. Although clearly the lower the platelet count is the greater the risk for bleeding, no studies have been able to identify a threshold platelet count. In fact, using a platelet count of 20,000/μl as a threshold for transfusion does nothing to prolong the patient's life. Some would argue that it takes away life with the attendant risks of any transfusion. The patients also are more likely to become refractory to platelet transfusions because of alloimmunization from multiple platelet donors. This can be a devastating consequence if the patient requires subsequent platelet transfusion due to bleeding. It seems logical to accept the algorithm proposed by Gmür et al.[7]:

    1. Routine platelet transfusion if the level is <5,000/μl
    2. Transfusion for platelet counts of 5,000–10,000/μl if fever or minor hemorrhage is present
    3. Transfusion for platelet counts of 10,000–20,000/μl if the patient is on heparin, is going to have surgery, or has additional coagulation abnormalities.

15. Should erythropoietin (EPO) be used for patients with chemothreapy?
For:
Avoiding red blood cell transfusions (with risk, cost, and discomfort to the patient) is a good thing.

EPO has been shown to be effective in patients with renal failure and myelodysplastic syndrome. Therefore, it is likely to be effective in patients with anemia due to chemotherapy.

Against:

There are no randomized studies clearly showing that EPO significantly increases the hemoglobin or decreases the transfusion requirement. It is expensive! Furthermore, patients need to learn to administer the drug via subcutaneous injection.

BIBLIOGRAPHY

1. Ahr DJ, Scialla SJ, Kimball DB Jr: Acquired platelet dysfunction following mithramycin therapy. Cancer 41:448–454, 1978.
2. Baer MR, Bloomfield CD: Controversies in transfusion medicine, prophylactic platelet transfusion therapy: Pro. Transfusion 32:377–380, 1992.
3. Beutler E. Platelet transfusions: The 20,000/μl trigger. Blood 81:1411–1413, 1993.
4. Chabner BA, Collins JM (eds): Cancer Chemotherapy: Principles and Practice. Philadelphia, J.B. Lippincott, 1990.
5. DeVita VT, Hellman S, Rosenberg SA (eds): Cancer: Principles and Practice of Oncology. Philadelphia, J.B. Lippincott, 1989.
6. Fleischman RA: Southwestern Internal Medicine Conference: Clinical use of hematopoietic growth factors. Am J Med Sci 305:248–273, 1993.
7. Gmür J, Burger J, Schanz U, et al: Safety of stringent prophylactic platelet transfusion policy for patients with acute leukemia. Lancet 338:1223, 1991.
8. Haskell CH (ed): Cancer Treatment. Philadelphia, W.B. Saunders, 1985.
9. Hoagland HC: Hematologic complications of cancer chemotherapy. In Perry MC (ed): The Chemotherapy Source Book. Baltimore, Williams & Wilkins, 1992, pp 498–507.
10. Miller LL: The Therapeutic Utility of G- and GM-CSF in Counteracting the Bone Marrow Suppression of Chemo- and Radiotherapy. ASCO Educational Book, 1993, pp 34–43.
11. Patten E: Controversies in transfusion medicine, prophylactic platelet transfusion resisted after 25 years: Con. Transfusion 32:381–385, 1992.
12. Platanias LC, et al: Treatment of chemotherapy-induced anemia with recombinant human erythropoietin in cancer patients. J Clin Oncol 9:2021–2026, 1991.
13. Platelet transfusion therapy. JAMA 257:1777, 1987.
14. Rothschild N, Erickson B, Sisk R, et al: Cancer-associated hemolytic uremic syndrome: Analysis of 85 cases from a National Registry. J Clin Oncol 7:781–789, 1989.
15. Sikora K, Halnan KE: Treatment of Cancer. London, Chapman and Hall, 1900.

47. COLONY-STIMULATING FACTORS

Malcolm Purdy, M.D.

1. What are colony-stimulating factors (CSFs)?

Blood is a self-renewing organ. Hematopoietic cells are unable to proliferate spontaneously and require the presence of factors obtained from the serum or the surrounding microenvironment of the cells to initiate and sustain proliferation. The first regulator to be discovered was erythropoietin. Subsequently numerous other factors have been identified. Granulocyte colony-stimulating factor (G-CSF) and granulocyte macrophage colony-stimulating factor (GM-CSF) were isolated from normal human serum and, in recombinant form and at pharmacologic doses, have reached clinical use. A number of other factors that stimulate the proliferation of all or specific hematopoietic cell lines are in testing for clinical use but presently are not approved for general release.

2. Why is the term "colony-stimulating factor" used?

The development of in vitro semisolid cultures of bone marrow progenitor cells allowed the evaluation of an individual cell's progeny, which forms clusters called colonies. The action of G-CSF on colony growth results in maturation of granulocytes. In the presence of GM-CSF, granulocytes and macrophages develop. In vitro cultures, however, do not always predict the scope of biologic effects when CSF is used in vivo. For example, at high doses (higher than clinically advisable) G-CSF may slightly increase lymphocytes, whereas GM-CSF may increase eosinophils. Complex interaction with other factors and the stromal environment of the bone marrow were not predictable from the semisolid cultures.

3. How do CSFs function?

CSFs act as ligands for specific receptors on the hematopoietic cell membrane. Cells that grow in response to G-CSF and GM-CSF have a receptor for each growth factor. The recombinant forms used clinically function much like natural G-CSF or GM-CSF but are given at supraphysiologic doses. Proliferation of progenitor cells, maturation of specific cells, and cell functions are enhanced by CSFs. G-CSF stimulates the phagocytic function of neutrophils, whereas GM-CSF also enhances the function of monocytes, macrophages, and eosinophils.

4. What happens clinically when G-CSF is given?

G-CSF given to normal people is associated with a transient leukopenia (within 1 hour of injection) followed by a sustained increase in neutrophils. These effects are due to (1) bone marrow release of mature neutrophils and (2) accelerated maturation of neutrophils in the bone marrow. The time for maturation of neutrophils decreases from 4 days to 1 day. Often the released neutrophils are less mature. The neutrophils continue to increase production until the second week of administration.

The effect of G-CSF is dose-related. Routinely used doses, 5 or 10 $\mu g/kg/day$, have little effect on other cell lines. Higher doses are associated with a 25% decrease in platelets.

5. What happens clinically when GM-CSF is given?

Transient leukopenia also occurs with each dose of GM-CSF, possibly accompanied by pulmonary sequestration of neutrophils. Unlike G-CSF, GM-CSF does not accelerate the rate of maturation of neutrophils from the bone marrow; instead, the half-life of a circulating neutrophil is prolonged from 8 to 48 hours. Proliferation of neutrophils and eosinophils is enhanced, and neutrophilia is seen in the blood.

6. Are there side effects to administering G-CSF or GM-CSF?

When G-CSF is administered after chemotherapy, the primary side effect is bone ache or pain in about 20% of people. Minor elevation of lactate dehydrogenase (LDH) and alkaline phosphatase has been reported. On rare occasions, vasculitis has been associated with administration. A few patients who receive G-CSF therapy for more than 1 year have reported splenomegaly, hair-thinning, thrombocytopenia, and persistent bone pain. The bone ache seems to precede recovery of peripheral neutrophil counts.

In certain individuals, first-dose effects of GM-CSF—even with doses of less than 1 $\mu g/kg$—may include flushing with hypotension, tachycardia, arterial oxygen desaturation, shortness of breath, and nausea. Readministration can result in the same syndrome, which is associated more commonly with intravenous administration but also occurs with subcutaneous administration. With doses above 20 $\mu g/kg$, thrombosis, fluid retention, and pleural effusions occur. GM-CSF should not be used in patients with idiopathic thrombocytopenia because it may lead to enhanced reactivation of the condition. Reactivation of other autoimmune processes also has been reported. Atrial fibrillation has been associated with administration after high-dose chemotherapy.

7. Describe clinical applications for GM-CSF or G-CSF in an oncology practice.
G-CSF and GM-CSF are used primarily to decrease anticipated morbidity from the severe neutropenia that accompanies myelosuppressive chemotherapy. They are given prophylactically 1 to 2 days after chemotherapy is completed. Therapy is continued through the period of neutropenia. In most instances, the neutrophil count decreases despite use of the CSF. Administration should be stopped when the absolute neutrophil count rises above 5,000–10,000 cells/μl. G-CSF is approved in the United States for this indication.

GM-CSF and G-CSF have been used to increase significantly the number of peripheral blood progenitors (or stem cells) used for autologous bone marrow transplants. GM-CSF is used after cylcophosphamide chemotherapy to obtain these stem cells; it is approved in the United States for this indication.

8. What is the natural history of chemotherapy-induced neutropenia without the use of growth factors?
The classic study of the significance of neutropenia, performed by Bodey and published in 1966, made two still important observations:

1. There is a definite relationship between the absolute granulocyte count and the incidence of infection. The risk increases significantly with an absolute neutrophil count below 1000 cells/μl. As the count drops to 500 and certainly to 100 cells/μl, the incidence of infection continues to increase.

2. The incidence of infection increases proportionally with duration of neutropenia. Two weeks of neutropenia at least doubles the incidence of infection.

9. How effective are GM-CSF and G-CSF in limiting chemotherapy-induced neutropenia?
This question has been addressed in clinical trials. The overall duration of chemotherapy-induced neutropenia can be shortened with G-CSF, resulting in fewer days in the hospital as well as fewer days on antibiotics. When GM-CSF is used in the setting of bone marrow transplant, days on antibiotics and days in the hospital again can be reduced. Neither agent improves survival rates.

10. Can G-CSF or GM-CSF shorten the duration of neutropenia once neutropenia has begun? Will either agent help patients with febrile neutropenia to recover faster?
No. At this time, no convincing evidence warrants the use of CSFs once neutropenia begins.

11. How can G-CSF and GM-CSF be used to mobilize stem cells?
The availability of GM-CSF and G-SCF has made practical the recovery of the earliest hematopoietic progenitor cells (stem cells) from peripheral blood. The stem cells can then be used in autologous bone marrow transplantation. Leukapheresis with centrifugation allows collection of the buffy coat fraction that contains the stem cells. The cells are cryopreserved and can be infused into the patient after high-dose chemotherapy or radiation therapy. Because the fraction contains the earliest precursor cells in greater numbers, hematopoiesis can be restored more rapidly. Stem cells are released in 100 times the usually small number of circulating stem cells, resulting in a dramatic reduction of neutropenic days.

12. What is the role of CSFs in nonmalignant disease?
Currently one of the most common uses of G-CSF and GM-CSF is support of individuals with acquired immunodeficiency syndrome (AIDS). Alone or in conjunction with erythropoietin, the CSFs increase neutrophil counts substantially and thus allow continued use of other bone marrow-suppressing agents. The CSF must be used continuously to remain effective.

Other indications include aplastic anemia; chronic, cyclic, and congenital neutropenia; and myelodysplasia.

CONTROVERSIES

13. Are CSFs worth the expense and risk?

The cost of CSFs is substantial. To date, no evidence suggests that using growth factors with standard chemotherapy decreases either mortality from neutropenia or the number of infectious episodes.

In the setting of autologous transplant, the ability of CSFs to increase the stem cell progenitors has reduced significantly the period of neutropenia. Studies to date allow no comment about reduction in mortality or morbidity due to CSFs.

14. Is there risk of tumor growth with CSFs?

The receptors for G-CSF and GM-CSF are present on the membrane surface of several tumors, including small cell lung cancer and acute myelogenous leukemia. Concern has been raised that use of growth factors may accelerate tumor growth, but no clinical evidence supports this theory.

15. Does proliferation of mature cells by CSFs deplete the hematopoietic stem cell? Are patients at risk for future bone marrow failure after use of CSFs?

The hematopoietic stem cell has been difficult to isolate. The kinetics of self-renewal of these cells has not been defined. Because CSFs seem primarily to drive terminal differentiation and proliferation, concern has been raised that the stem-cell population may be depleted with their use. During the 1–3 years that people with congenital neutropenia were treated with G-CSF, there were no indications of any depletion of the renewing ability of the bone marrow. Studies in mice suggest that administration in the setting of chemotherapy may deplete the stem cells.

16. Can G-CSF and GM-CSF be used to accelerate the recovery of aplastic bone marrow after therapy in acute leukemia?

Because CSF receptors have been found on myeloid leukemic cells, concern has been raised that their use after chemotherapy may drive the growth of any remaining leukemia cells. Published reports, however, suggest that this is not the case. There appears to be some earlier recovery of neutrophils with use of CSFs, but no randomized trial has confirmed their effectiveness in this setting.

17. What is on the horizon for hematopoietic growth factor therapy?

Combination therapy with erythropoietin and interleukin 3 (an earlier-acting, multipotent hematopoietic stimulating factor) is under review. A new factor that acts by a different mechanism, stem cell factor (also called c kit ligand or mast cell factor), is also under investigation for combination therapy with CSFs to combat chemotherapy-induced thrombocytopenia, which can be as great a problem as neutropenia. CSFs do not treat thrombocytopenia.

BIBLIOGRAPHY

1. Bell AJ, Jamblin TJ, Oscier DG: Peripheral blood stem cell autografting. Hematol Oncol 5:45, 1987.
2. Bodey GP, Buckly M, Sathe YS, Freireich EJ: Quantitative relationships between circulating leukocytes and infection in patients with acute leukemia. Ann Intern Med 64:328–340, 1966.
3. Crawford J, Ozer H, Stoller R: Reduction by granulocyte-stimulating factor of fever and neutropenia induced by chemotherapy in patients with small-cell lung cancer. N Engl J Med 325:164–170, 1992.
4. Dale DC, Bonilla MA, Davis MW, et al: A randomized controlled phase III trial of recombinant human granulocyte colony-stimulating factor (Filgrastim) for treatment of severe chronic neutropenia. Blood 81:2496–2502, 1993.
5. Groopman JE, Mitsuyasu RT, De Leo MJ, et al: Effect of recombinant human granulocyte-macrophage colony-stimulating factor on myelopoiesis in the acquired immunodeficiency syndrome. N Engl J Med 317:593, 1987.

6. Lieschke FJ, Bergess AW: Granulocyte colony-stimulating factor and granulocyte macrophage colony-stimulating factor. N Engl J Med 327:28–35, 1992.
7. Metcalf D, Morstyn G: Colony stimulating factors: General biology. In DeVita VT Jr, Hellman S, Rosenberg SA (eds): Biologic Therapy of Cancer. Philadelphia, J.B. Lippincott, 1991.
8. Nemunaitis J, Rabinowe SN, Singer JW: Recombinant granulocyte-macrophage stimulating factor after autologous bone marrow transplant for lymphoid cancer. N Engl J Med 324:1773–1778, 1991.
9. Souza LM, Boone TC, Gabrilove J, et al: Recombinant human granulocyte colony stimulating factor: Effects on normal and leukemic myeloid cells. Science 232:61, 1986.
10. Zsebo KM, Cohen AM, Murdock DC, et al: Recombinant granulocyte colony stimulating factor: Molecular and biological characterization. Immunobiology 172:175, 1986.

48. MONOCLONAL ANTIBODY THERAPY OF CANCER

Douglas K. Rovira, M.D.

1. What is a monoclonal antibody?
This term is applied to a purified antibody generated against a specific antigen or epitope.

2. How are monoclonal antibodies made?
Mice are immunized with purified antigen preparations, tumor extracts, or whole cells. Immunoglobulin-producing B lymphocytes from the spleens of the mice are then fused with an immortalized cell line to form hybridomas. Hybridomas can be grown in culture indefinitely and screened for production of the antibody of interest. The hybridoma clones that produce the antibody of interest can be purified and grown in culture in large quantities; the antibodies can be purified for clinical use.

3. What prize was awarded to Georges F. Köhler and Cesar Milstein for the development of the technique for producing monoclonal antibodies?
The Nobel Prize in Medicine and Physiology was awarded to Köhler and Milstein in 1984. Few discoveries have had such an immediate and profound influence on biologic research.

4. Why was this discovery so important?
Monoclonal antibodies have greatly advanced the ability to diagnose cancer correctly and specifically. This technology can also be used to mark the response of certain cancers to therapy. Most recently monoclonal antibodies have been used to treat cancer.

5. Within the field of oncology, what are some of the cellular targets for production of monoclonal antibodies?
Oncofetal antigens, usually lost during embryogenesis, are present on some cancers, such as alphafetoprotein (AFP) in testicular cancer and carcinoembryonic antigen in colon cancer. **Differentiation antigens** are tissue-specific and are variably expressed as mature cells; examples include the common acute lymphocytic leukemia antigen (CALLA) present on immature lymphocytes; the T-cell receptor present on mature T lymphocytes; and the human milk-fat globule antigen present on breast ductal epithelial cells. Cancer cells may express abnormal amounts or mutated **protein products of oncogenes,** such as the *HER-2/neu* oncogene in breaast cancer or the *ras* oncogene in colon cancer.

6. How are monoclonal antibodies used to diagnose cancer?

When monoclonal antibodies are conjugated to peroxidases, a color reaction can identify whether the antigen is present on the surface of the tumor cells. A panel of monoclonal antibodies can be used to identify the immunophenotype of the tumor. This technology has been applied to typing lymphomas and leukemias; it also may be helpful in typing carcinomas of unknown origin.

7. How have monoclonal antibodies been helpful in staging and monitoring various cancers?

Certain antigens expressed on the surface of tumor cells may be shed into the bloodstream, such as AFP or the β chain of human chorionic gonadotropin (β-HCG) in testicular cancer and CEA in colon cancer, to name a few. Identification of elevated levels of tumor antigens in the bloodstream may be a clue to diagnosis. A decrease over time while an individual undergoes treatment may suggest a response to therapy.

Monoclonal antibodies also can be useful in staging cancer, but this technology is in an earlier stage of development. If the monoclonal antibody is tagged to a radionuclide and injected into the patient, an image can be produced, similar to a bone scan, that identifies metastatic disease.

8. What are the toxicities of monoclonal antibodies?

Because monoclonal antibodies are foreign particles, they produce a reaction similar to other foreign particles. Some patients develop fevers, chills, and hypersensitivity reactions that on rare occasions result in anaphylaxis. Organ damage can result from nonspecific binding of the monoclonal antibodies to nontumor tissue.

When the monoclonal antibody is bound to a toxin or radionuclide, then toxicities specific to those agents can be expected.

9. Have monoclonal antibodies been used to treat cancer? If so, how?

Yes. Many monoclonal antibodies that bind to antigens expressed on the surface of tumor cells have been identified. As a method of treatment, these antibodies have been used alone as well as conjugated to toxins or radionuclides. With a few exceptions, the overall results have been disappointing.

10. Why has monoclonal antibody therapy yielded such disappointing results?

Barriers to effective monoclonal antibody therapy are many:

1. Cross-reactivity of the monoclonal antibody with normal antigens
2. Expression of the tumor antigen on normal cells
3. Binding kinetics of the antibody to the cell surface
4. Weak affector mechanisms such as antibody-dependent cell-mediated cytotoxicity or complement-mediated cytotoxicity
5. Large tumor burden
6. Circulating tumor antigen, which prevents monoclonal antibody binding to the cell surface
7. Modification of the tumor antigen by the tumor cell so that the cell no longer binds the monoclonal antibody
8. Production of human antimouse antibodies (HAMA) by the patient, which inactivate the monoclonal antibody before it reaches the tumor cell.

11. Are there ways to limit the formation of HAMA?

Patients may be treated with immunosuppressive agents to halt the production of HAMAs. This approach may lead to infectious complications and therefore do more harm than good. Alternatively, using recombinant DNA technology, some investigators have spliced the hypervariable region (the part that recognizes antigen) of a mouse monoclonal antibody to the rest of a human IgG molecule. The humanization of the antibody overcomes the HAMA barrier and allows multiple dosing. In addition, because the affector mechanisms are regulated by the constant region of the molecule, a humanized antibody may be more effective.

12. What are immunotoxins? How have they been used therapeutically?
Immunotoxins are monoclonal antibodies conjugated to toxins. Lethal compounds such as ricin A, diphtheria toxin, and *Pseudomonas* exotoxin are altered and bound to monoclonal antibodies. Various investigators have been able to achieve cell killing with very small amounts of these compounds. The toxicity profile is increased, as expected, mainly because of nonspecific binding. Early results in heavily treated patients with refractory cancer have been promising.

13. Can radionuclide conjugated monoclonal antibodies be used therapeutically?
Yes. Radionuclides that are beta emittors cause lethal DNA damage. The clinically used radionuclides are capable of inducing this damage over a relatively large area. For example, iodine-131 has a path length of 8 mm and yttrium-90 a path length of 5.3 cm. These and other radionuclides have been conjugated to monoclonal antibodies and administered to patients as a therapeutic agent. The results have been promising, especially in the treatment of lymphomas, and larger trials are being designed.

14. What is it about lymphomas that makes them a good potential target for monoclonal antibody therapy?
Lymphoma represents a clonal expansion of cells, all of which express the same immunoglobulin on their surface. This homogeneous cell-surface antigen makes an attractive target for monoclonal antibody production.

15. Can the lymphoma cells change the surface immunoglobulin they produce?
Unfortunately, yes. Thus the cells will no longer bind the specific monoclonal antibody.

16. Is there a future for monoclonal antibody therapy?
Yes. Despite early discouraging results, investigations continue in the following areas:
    1. Treatment of minimal residual disease. Because monoclonal antibody therapy is difficult to use in treating bulky disease, it may be more effectively used as adjuvant therapy or with small residual disease after other modalities.
    2. Purging for bone marrow transplantation. One of the limitations of autologous bone marrow transplanation has been the infusion of bone marrow contaminated with cancer cells. Purging the bone marrow with monoclonal antibodies may resolve this problem.
    3. Combination with conventional chemotherapy, radiation therapy, or other biologic response modifiers.

17. What other creative strategy can be used to cure human cancer with antibodies?
B-cell lymphomas express immunoglobulin on their surface. Because they are clonal, the immunoglobulin molecules are identical on every cell. In addition, antibodies can be formed to the variable regions (idiotypes). Thus, if the antibody expressed on the patient's lymphoma is purified and administered to the patient with the appropriate adjuvant, it may serve as a vaccine. A recent study has shown that 7 of 9 patients treated with this technique have developed sustained, specific immune responses to their tumors.

BIBLIOGRAPHY

1. Dienhart D, Schmelzer R, Lear J, et al: Imaging of non-small lung cancers with a monoclonal antibody, KC-4G3, which recognized a human milk globule antigen. Cancer Res 50:7068, 1990.

2. Frankel A: Immunotoxin therapy of cancer. Oncology 7:69, 1993.
3. Goldenberg DM: Monoclonal antibodies in cancer detection and therapy. Am J Med 94:297, 1993.
4. Grossbard ML, Press OW, Appelbaum FR, et al: Monoclonal antibody-based therapies of leukemia and lymphoma. Blood 80:863–878, 1992.
5. Kaminski M, Zasadny K, Francis I, et al: Radioimmunotherapy of B-cell lymphoma with [Iodine-131] anti-B1 (anti-CD20) antibody. N Engl J Med 329, 459, 1993.
6. Köhler G, Milstein C: Continuous culture of fused cell secreting antibodies of pre-defined specificity. Nature 256:495, 1975.
7. Kwak LW, Campbell M, Czerwinski D, et al: Induction of immune responses in patients with B-cell lymphoma against the surface-immunoglobulin idiotype expressed by their tumors. N Engl J Med 327:1209, 1992.
8. Milstein C: Monoclonal antibodies. Sci Am 243:66, 1980.
9. Press O, Eary J, Appelbaum F, et al: Radiolabeled-antibody therapy of B-cell lymphoma with autologous bone marrow support. N Engl J Med 329:1219, 1993.
10. Reichmann L, Clark M, Walkmann H, et al: Reshaping human antibodies for therapy. Nature 332:323, 1988.
11. Schlom J: Antibodies in cancer therapy: Basic principles of monoclonal antibodies. In DeVita V, Hellman S, Rosenberg S (eds): Biologic Therapy of Cancer. Philadelphia, J.B. Lippincott, 1991, pp 464–481.

49. BONE MARROW TRANSPLANTATION

Scott I. Bearman, M.D.

1. What are indications for bone marrow transplantation?
Historically, indications for bone marrow transplantation have included hematologic malignancies, such as acute myelogenous leukemia (AML), chronic myelogenous leukemia (CML), acute lymphocytic leukemia (ALL), and Hodgkin's and non-Hodgkin's lymphoma. Other indications include aplastic anemia, congenital immune deficiencies, such as Wiskott-Aldrich syndrome and severe combined immunodeficiency syndrome (SCIDS), and inborn errors of metabolism, such as Gaucher's disease. The fastest growing area of bone marrow transplantation involves the use of high-dose chemotherapy with autologous marrow or stem cell support for solid tumors, including advanced or high-risk breast cancer, neuroblastoma, and advanced ovarian cancer.

2. What are the different types of bone marrow transplantation?
There are three major types of bone marrow transplantation:
1. **Autologous marrow transplantation:** the patient provides his or her own marrow.
2. **Syngeneic marrow transplantation:** marrow is provided by an identical twin.
3. **Allogeneic marrow:** marrow is provided by another individual, usually a human leukocyte antigen identical (HLA-identical) sibling.

3. Technically, how is marrow obtained for transplantation?
First, bone marrow is "harvested" from the patient or the bone marrow donor. Usually under general anesthesia, 1–2 liters (L) of marrow is aspirated from the posterior iliac crests by multiple aspirations. The marrow is filtered to remove bone particles and large globules of fat and then placed in transfusion bags.

4. What happens to marrow after it is "harvested"?
Autologous marrow is cryopreserved for later use. Allogeneic and syngeneic marrow are infused into the recipient immediately after harvest, without freezing. The marrow is infused through a central venous catheter.

5. How is the patient treated?

Patients who undergo bone marrow transplantation are treated with high-dose chemotherapy with or without total body irradiation. These high doses are administered with the intention of completely eradicating the tumor. Unfortunately, high-dose chemotherapy or chemoradiotherapy will destroy the patient's own bone marrow. Therefore, marrow must be given to the patient or he or she will have no functioning marrow, with the fatal risks of infection and bleeding.

6. With autologous marrow transplantation, how can you be sure you do not reinfuse tumor cells?

The simple answer is that you cannot be completely sure. Marrow from patients with hematologic abnormalities are almost always harvested when the patient is in remission. In addition, many strategies exist that attempt to deplete the marrow of tumor cells. These include treating the marrow with chemotherapy, treating the marrow with a monoclonal antibody directed against an antigen specific for the tumor, or selecting primitive marrow stem cells using adsorption techniques. All of these methods have advantages and disadvantages. Although there have been several studies that suggest that the relapse rate after autologous marrow transplantation for AML and non-Hodgkin's lymphoma is reduced when marrow is purged, many studies have shown no benefit from purging autologous marrow.

7. Is bone marrow transplantation dangerous?

Yes. Because high doses of chemotherapy or chemoradiotherapy are used to "condition" the patient, there will be a period of marrow aplasia lasting 1–3 weeks. During this time, the patient will be at risk for infection and hemorrhage. In addition, high-dose chemotherapy or chemoradiotherapy may be toxic to normal tissues, including the bladder, heart, liver, lungs, kidneys, and central nervous system. Depending on the patient's overall condition, the chemotherapy or chemoradiotherapy regimen used and the compatibility in tissue typing between donor and recipient, anywhere from 5–25% of patients will have a fatal complication of the transplant.

8. What is graft-versus-host disease (GVHD)?

GVHD is a clinical syndrome characterized by skin rash, enteritis, and elevated liver function tests (predominantly transaminases) that follows an allogeneic marrow transplant. In GVHD, the immunocompetent new marrow recognizes the recipient as foreign tissue causing an immune-mediated (T-cell) reaction in the skin, gut, and liver. GVHD occurs in approximately 40% of patients who receive HLA-identical sibling transplants and may occur in greater than 80% of patients who receive marrow from a family member who is not HLA-identical or marrow from an unrelated marrow donor. GVHD that begins within 80 days after the marrow reinfusion is usually referred to as acute GVHD. GVHD that begins more than 100 days after marrow reinfusion is called chronic GVHD. Chronic GVHD occurs most commonly in patients who had acute GVHD. The clinical manifestations of chronic GVHD, like acute GVHD, include rash, enteritis, and hepatitis. However, the skin involvement may resemble scleroderma. In addition, patients with chronic GVHD may have oral and ocular sicca (dry mouth and eyes). Patients with chronic GVHD are more likely to develop infection with encapsulated microorganisms than patients without GVHD.

9. Can GVHD be prevented or treated?

All patients who undergo allogeneic marrow transplantation receive prophylactic treatment for GVHD. These regimens use single or multiple immunosuppressive agents, such as cyclosporine A, methotrexate, corticosteroids, or antithymocyte globulin. Another strategy to prevent GVHD is to deplete the donor marrow of T lymphocytes, which mediate the GVHD response. Unfortunately, many studies of T-cell depletion showed that it was more likely to result in rejection of the transplanted marrow. GVHD can be mild, requiring no therapy, or it can be severe, requiring profound immunosuppressive therapy. Approximately 50% of patients respond to initial therapy for GVHD. Those who do not respond are treated on secondary regimens, on which approximately 40% respond.

10. What are the results of bone marrow transplantation for AML?
When discussing the results of marrow transplantation for AML, one must first consider the results with conventional chemotherapy. Approximately 60–80% of patients with AML enter complete remission with induction chemotherapy. Unfortunately, only 20–30% of patients with AML are cured with conventional-dose chemotherapy. When marrow transplantation was first performed for AML, it was done for refractory disease. Despite the apparent hopelessness of this situation, marrow transplantation cured about 10% of patients. When marrow transplantation was applied to patients with very sensitive disease, in whom the burden of leukemia was low (i.e., first complete remission), the results were much superior, with long-term disease-free survival of 45–55%. First complete remission has generally become the accepted time to perform marrow transplantation for AML, particularly when an HLA-identical sibling exists to provide the marrow. In the United States, marrow transplantation for AML was usually delayed until first untreated relapse or second complete remission when an HLA-identical sibling did not exist. In this situation, the sources of marrow would include the patient's own marrow (autologous transplant), marrow from family members not perfectly matched with the patient, or marrow from an unrelated donor having the same HLA typing as the patient. Patients who receive transplants in untreated first relapse or second complete remission have a disease-free survival of about 25%. The potential advantage of waiting until first relapse or second remission is that patients who are already cured with conventional chemotherapy are not subjected to the risks of marrow transplantation. In addition, the overall cure rate may be similar, because 20–30% of patients with AML are cured with conventional-dose chemotherapy. These results must be contrasted with data, largely from Europe, showing that autologous marrow transplantation in first complete remission may be just as good as allogeneic marrow transplantation in first remission. There are too few data regarding unrelated donor transplants to speculate whether they are superior to autologous transplants.

11. How successful is marrow transplantation for CML?
Marrow transplantation is the only therapy that can cure CML. Although interferon may induce clinical and cytogenetic remissions, there are no data to suggest that the overall results of interferon are equivalent or superior to marrow transplantation. Virtually all results in CML have been obtained with allogeneic or syngeneic marrow. Autologous marrow transplantation studies in CML are in their infancy. We recommend that any patient with CML have tissue typing studies on themselves and their family members as soon after diagnosis as possible. Data from the Fred Hutchinson Cancer Research Center in Seattle have suggested that the results of marrow transplantation for chronic phase CML depend, in part, on the duration from diagnosis to transplant, with the best results in patients whose transplant is performed within 1 year of diagnosis. Overall, disease-free survival for chronic-phase CML after marrow transplant is 55–75%. For patients who are transplanted in accelerated-phase CML or blast crisis, the results are about 20% and 10%, respectively. Failure of marrow transplantation for chronic-phase CML is usually due to treatment-related toxicities, whereas failure for patients with accelerated- or blast-phase CML is due to relapse.

12. What is the "graft versus leukemia" effect?
The graft versus leukemia effect refers to the observation that the relapse rates after marrow transplantation for leukemia are lower in patients who received allogeneic marrow, in whom GVHD is common, compared with patients who received syngeneic marrow, where GVHD does not occur, because the donor and recipient are genetically identical. In fact, if

only patients who receive allogeneic marrow are considered, those who do not develop GVHD have a higher incidence of relapse than patients who develop GVHD. This effect may be present in lymphoma as well. Because of these observations, some groups are attempting to induce GVHD in recipients of autologous marrow, because they do not develop GVHD and, consequently, do not enjoy a graft versus leukemia effect.

13. Should high-dose chemotherapy with autologous marrow support be considered for patients with advanced or high-risk breast cancer?
Simply put, yes. Stage IV, or metastatic, breast cancer is incurable with conventional-dose chemotherapy. The prognosis for patients with primary breast cancer, that is, cancer limited to the breast with or without involved axillary lymph nodes, is inversely proportional to the number of lymph nodes involved at the time of diagnosis. Patients who are "node negative" enjoy a reasonably good prognosis, with a 5-year survival and disease-free survival >75%. Patients who have four or more involved lymph nodes usually do poorly, with 5-year disease-free survivals of <50%. For those who have 10 or more involved nodes, the prognosis is even worse, with only 20–30% of patients being alive and disease free at 5 years. The use of high-dose chemotherapy for such patients has been very encouraging. A number of studies have reported the disease-free survival at 3 years for metastatic breast cancer to be between 20% and 25% for patients with sensitive disease treated with high-dose chemotherapy and autologous marrow and/or peripheral blood progenitor cell support. It appears from the earliest of these studies that almost all relapses occur within the first 2 years after transplant. Patients who are free of disease at 2 years may enjoy a durable remission.

The results for patients with high-risk primary breast cancer, that is, 10 or more involved nodes, is even more striking. In a study from Duke University and the Cancer and Leukemia Group B, the disease-free survival for patients with high-risk primary breast cancer treated with high-dose chemotherapy and autologous marrow support is 72%. Although this study is not very mature, with only half of the patients being 3 years from transplant, the data are extremely encouraging. There have been no relapses in this study after 28 months, with the longest survivor being more than 5 years from transplant.

14. What are some future directions of bone marrow transplantation?
Gene therapy, specifically the introduction of new or altered genes, will require a cell population capable of self-replication as well as differentiation. The hematopoietic stem cell fits this description and will likely be the vehicle for this therapeutic approach. Newer and more effective methods of cell separation will permit the selection of marrow cell populations that preceded clonogenic tumor stem cells. For example, AML may involve a "committed" progenitor only of the myeloid lineage. It is theoretically possible to select a more primitive "uncommitted" progenitor cell that is not leukemic. Finally, it is becoming possible to expand stem cells in the laboratory. Thus, marrow transplants in the future may only require a small amount of marrow to be harvested. By becoming more sophisticated about the growth of progenitor cells in the laboratory, it may be possible to do marrow transplantation where the entire period of absolute neutropenia is eliminated. Furthermore, they may provide a way to administer autologous white blood cell transfusions to patients undergoing conventional dose chemotherapy.

BIBLIOGRAPHY

1. Bearman SI, Appelbaum FR, Buckner CD, et al: Regimen-related toxicity in patients undergoing bone marrow transplantation. J Clin Oncol 6:1562–1568, 1988.
2. Blaese RM: Development of gene therapy for immunodeficiency: Adenosine deaminase deficiency. Pediatr Res 22(Suppl 1):S49–S55, 1993.
3. Buckner CD, Clift RA, Appelbaum FR, et al: Effects of treatment regimens on post marrow transplant relapse. Semin Hematol 28(Suppl 4):32–34, 1991.

4. Clift RA, Buckner CD, Appelbaum FR, et al: Allogeneic marrow transplantation in patients with acute myeloid leukemia in first remission. A randomized trial of two irradiation regimens. Blood 76:1867–1871, 1990.
5. Goldman JM, Gale RP, Horowitz MM, et al: Bone marrow transplantation for chronic myelogenous leukemia in chronic phase. Increased risk for relapse associated with T-cell depletion. Ann Intern Med 108:806–814, 1988.
6. Gribben JG, Freedman AS, Neuberg D, et al: Immunologic purging of marrow assessed by PCR before autologous bone marrow transplantation for B-cell lymphoma. N Engl J Med 325:1525–1534, 1991.
7. Peters WP: High-dose chemotherapy and autologous bone marrow support for breast cancer. In DeVita VT Jr, Hellman S, Rosenberg SA (eds): Important Advances in Oncology. Philadelphia, J.B. Lippincott, 1991, pp 135–150.
8. Shpall EJ, Stemmer SM, Johnston CF, et al: Purging of autologous bone marrow for transplantation: The protection and selection of the hematopoietic progenitor cell. J Hematother 1:45–54, 1992.
9. Sullivan KM, Storb R, Buckner CD, et al: Graft-versus-host disease as adoptive immunotherapy in patients with advanced hematologic neoplasms. N Engl J Med 320:828–834, 1989.
10. Sullivan KM, Agura E, Anasetti C, et al: Chronic graft-versus-host disease and other late complications of bone marrow transplantation. Semin Hematol 28:250–259, 1991.
11. Thomas ED: Bone marrow transplantation: Past experiences and future prospects. Semin Oncol 19(Suppl 7):3–6, 1992.
12. Thomas ED, Clift RA, Fefer A, et al: Marrow transplantation for the treatment of chronic myelogenous leukemia. Ann Intern Med 104:155–163, 1986.

50. PRINCIPLES OF RADIATION THERAPY

Deborah A. Waitz, M.D.

1. What is the difference between x-rays and gamma rays?
X-rays and gamma rays have identical properties and nature but are produced in different ways. X-rays are produced extranuclearly—for example, when electrons are accelerated to high energies in a linear accelerator and directed onto a target of high atomic number, such as tungsten. Gamma rays are produced intranuclearly when, as a result of interactions of particles within the nucleus, a particle gains sufficient energy to escape.

2. What are some of the particles employed in radiation therapy?
Electrons, negatively charged particles, are most frequently employed in the clinical setting. They are produced in a linear accelerator and exit the machine without striking a target. The electron beam is used to treat superficial tumors, whereas x-rays or gamma rays are used to treat deep-seated tumors. Less commonly encountered, because of their use in limited and specifically indicated settings, are positively charged protons, alpha-particles (helium nuclei), heavy-charged ions (carbon, neon, argon, silicon), pi-mesons, and neutrons.

3. Which portion of the cell cycle is the most sensitive and which the most resistant to ionizing radiation?
Actively growing mammalian cells have a cycle consisting of four stages: mitosis, gap (G) 1, DNA synthesis, and gap (G) 2. The cell cycle is most sensitive to radiation during mitosis and G2, which immediately precede it. The greatest resistance to radiation is found in the late phase of DNA synthesis.

4. How are x-rays produced in a linear accelerator?
X-rays are produced when electrons injected into an accelerator tube gain energy by interacting with the electromagnetic field of microwaves and strike a target. The results of

the interaction of the accelerated electron with the nuclei of the target atoms are a photon and a deflected electron with lesser energy. The photons (x-rays) pass through a flattening filter and are shaped by collimators before exiting the treatment head of the machine and striking the patient.

5. How is the dosage of ionizing radiations in tissue expressed?

Absorbed dose—i.e., the mean energy imparted by ionizing radiations per unit of mass of the absorbing material—is a measure of the biologically and clinically important effects of the applied radiation. Dose is expressed in units of grays (Gy); 1 Gy equals 1 joule of energy per kilogram of mass. The gray is divided into units of one hundred centigrays (cGy); 1 cGy is equal to the rad, a previous measure of dose.

6. How do photons (x-rays and gamma rays) interact with biologic material, ultimately resulting in cellular damage?

Photons are indirectly ionizing; that is, they themselves produce no biologic or chemical damage within the cell. For photon energies characteristic of linear accelerators, the radiations are thought to interact with atoms or molecules such as water to produce highly reactive, short-lived free radicals, which then diffuse to critical structures, such as DNA and possibly cell membranes, and disrupt cellular chemical bonds.

7. What are the two types of radiation techniques most commonly used?

The two common techniques are teletherapy and brachytherapy. Teletherapy (tele = distant) refers to treatment administered from a distance, as with a machine. Brachytherapy (brachy = short) refers to treatment by radiation sources placed close to or in the treated volume. Implanted sources may be left in place (permanent implants employing gold-198 or iodine-125) or removed (temporary implants employing cesium-137, iridium-192, or cobalt-60).

8. What steps are involved in planning for radiation treatments?

1. The volume is delineated precisely by means of physical examination and diagnostic imaging as well as other techniques. Careful consideration must be given to the tolerance of normal tissues through which the radiation beam may transit.

2. The various potential techniques and field arrangements are evaluated by the radiation oncologist, medical physicist, and dosimetrist, often with computer plans.

3. A simulation is performed, with diagnostic-quality radiographs of the area to be treated on a unit with the same geometry as the treatment machine. The area to be treated is filmed with the number, size, and orientation of fields previously planned.

4. Patient immobilization devices and beam-modifying devices are constructed.

9. How are radiation treatments specified?

The radiation oncologist writes a prescription for a course of radiation in the therapy chart. This prescription constitutes direction and authorization to the radiation technologist who administers the treatments. Contained in the prescription are the identifying name of the area to be treated, the dose per fraction of radiation, number of doses per day (in the case of hyperfractionated regimens) or per week, the beam energy, field arrangement, and total dose. Directions for patient monitoring, such as requests for blood tests and weight checks, are often included with the prescription.

10. How are blocks employed in radiation treatment?

Blocks are structures interposed between the radiation beam and the patient. Their purpose is to shape the treatment field to permit inclusion of the desired volumes while excluding as much uninvolved tissue as possible. The commonly used method begins with localizing radiographs of the treatment area obtained during the planning session. The radiation oncologist then indicates on the films the structures to be excluded. The films become a template for styrofoam sheets on which the regions to be blocked are cut out and the deficits filled with Cerrobend, an alloy of bismuth, lead, tin, and cadmium, with a low melting point. Once the Cerrobend has cooled, it is broken out of the styrofoam sheets, fastened onto a lucite tray, labeled with the patient's name and orientation instructions, then stored in the treatment room for use with that patient.

11. What techniques are used to modify the radiation beam for a more uniform distribution of the administered dose?

Beam-modifying devices (which serve a different function from the blocks described above) serve to shape the field, exclude normal tissue, and result in greater uniformity or adequacy of dose in the treated region. Such devices consist of bolus, wedge filters, and compensating filters. Bolus refers to tissue-equivalent material that is placed directly on the patient in the treated area. The result is to increase the dose to the skin and other superficial structures beneath the bolus, as required, to ensure adequate treatment. This technique also may be used to even out irregular surface contours so that the beam traverses a uniform plane. Materials used for bolus include slabs of synthetic plastic polymers, blocks of paraffin wax, and wet gauze. Wedge filters bend the radiation beam relative to the incident angle to achieve a smoother dose distribution at a specified depth. The most commonly employed wedges are 15°, 30°, 45°, and 60°, although custom wedges for other angles can be devised. Wedges often are considered when the beam is incident on a sharply sloping surface such as the superior thorax. The wedge is oriented in the beam so that the thickest portion (heel) overlies the most attenuated tissue in the treated area. Compensating filters of aluminum, brass, wax, or lucite are placed in the radiation beam, rather than directly on the patient, to compensate for irregular tissue contours.

12. What is a portal film?

To ensure that radiation treatments are administered as planned at simulation, radiographs are obtained on the treatment machine to verify accuracy of field size and location as well as patient positioning. These radiographs, called portal or check films, are usually obtained for every field weekly and repeated whenever adjustments in blocks or field parameters are requested. Portal films differ in appearance from conventional diagnostic-quality radiographs, because they are obtained with energies in the megavoltage range that the linear accelerator produces for treatment rather than in the kilovoltage range (as in the normal chest radiograph). At such high energies, soft tissue and bone have equivalent absorption and appear similar.

13. What is fractionation? Why are radiation treatments fractionated?

Fractionation refers to the division of a total radiation dose into multiple smaller increments. This practice is based on radiobiologic experiments performed earlier in the century, which demonstrated that a given level of desired radiation effect (for example, sterilization of experimental animals by scrotal irradiation) could be obtained with lesser toxicity by dividing the dose into daily fractions. In clinical terms, fractionated radiotherapy allows a greater level of tumor control for an acceptable degree of normal tissue toxicity than single large doses.

14. What constitutes conventional fractionation?

Conventional radiotherapy with curative intent generally refers to daily treatment with 5 fractional doses per week of about 200 cGy each. The required total dose is a function of the mass (occult, microscopic, or macroscopic) and histology of the tumor and for the most part has been determined empirically.

15. What are possible alternatives to conventional fractionation?

Alternatives currently under evaluation include hyperfractionation and acelerated fractionation. Hyperfractionation entails dividing a standard or somewhat larger total dose into smaller-than-usual individual fractions administered twice daily; the total treatment time in weeks remains about the same. The goal of this approach is twofold: (1) to minimize the toxicity of late-responding normal tissues, which are more sensitive to individual fraction size, and (2) to maximize total dose for a greater probability of tumor eradication. Accelerated fractionation refers to an identical or somewhat smaller total dose administered in a shorter time interval to address potential repopulation of the tumor during treatment. This approach may entail two or more daily treatments of smaller-than-conventional fractions.

16. What is hyperthermia?
Hyperthermia is the clinical application of heat above 42.5° Celsius to tumors, which kills cells either independently or through enhancement of the cytotoxic effects of chemo- or radiotherapy. The specific advantages of hyperthermia are twofold: (1) it is effective against cell populations that may be present in an hypoxic, low-pH, and nutritionally lacking environment, and (2) it acts preferentially in the S phase of the proliferative cycle, which is resistant to radiotherapy. Postulated targets of hyperthermia are the cell membrane and intracellular structures, including the nucleus and components of the cytoplasm. Power deposition in tissue is accomplished by radiofrequency, microwave, and ultrasound applicators. Use of this modality is hampered by difficulties in the uniform heating of large or deep-seated tumors and by accurate measurement of heat distribution.

17. Give examples of acute-reacting and late-reacting normal tissues.
The kinetics of differentiation and proliferation are important determinants of acute and late toxicity; a given tissue may demonstrate components of both. Acute-reacting tissues, which may manifest toxicity during or several weeks after a course of treatment, include skin (desquamation), bowel mucosa, platelets, and leukocytes. Late-reacting tissues, which may give evidence of radiation injury months to years after treatment, include skin (fibrosis), spinal cord, bone, bone marrow, or viscera such as lung, liver, kidney, breast, and gonads.

18. What is meant by radiosensitivity and radiocurability? Are they correlated?
Radiosensitivity, or its converse, radioresistance, expresses the degree and speed with which a tumor responds during treatment. Radiocurability reflects the likelihood of tumor eradication, given the restraints imposed by factors such as normal tissue tolerance. The two concepts are not predictably correlated: a tumor may be extremely radiosensitive and radioincurable (e.g., leukemia and myeloma) or relatively radioresistant and radiocurable (e.g., squamous cell carcinomas of the head, neck, and cervix). An example of a neoplasm that is both radiosensitive and radiocurable is Hodgkin's lymphoma. Renal cell carcinomas and malignant melanomas are essentially radioresistant and radioincurable.

19. How does a palliative course of radiation therapy differ from a course with curative intent?
The goal of palliative therapy is relief of symptoms that impair function or comfort or pose a reasonable risk of doing so in a foreseeable interval. Palliative regimens are distinguished by larger daily fractions (>200 cGy, often 250–400 cGy), shorter duration of treatment time (a few weeks), and lower total doses (2,000–4,000 cGy). Larger doses per fraction increase the risk of toxicity to late-reacting tissues, but this risk is balanced by the decreased time demands on patients with limited life expectancies.

BIBLIOGRAPHY

1. Beahrs OH, Henson DE, Hutter RV, Kennedy BJ (eds): Manual for Staging of Cancer, 4th ed. Philadelphia, J.B. Lippincott, 1992.
2. DeVita VT, Hellman S, Rosenberg SA (eds): Cancer: Principles and Practice of Oncology, 4th ed. Philadelphia, J.B. Lippincott, 1993.

3. Hall AJ: Radiobiology for the Radiologist, 3rd ed. Philadelphia, J.B. Lippincott, 1988.
4. Johns HE, Cunningham JR: The Physics of Radiology, 4th ed. Springfield, IL, Charles C Thomas, 1983.
5. Levitt SH, Khan FM, Potish RA (eds): Technological Basis of Radiation Therapy, 2nd ed. Philadelphia, Lea & Febiger, 1992.
6. Million RR, Cassisi NJ (eds): Management of Head and Neck Cancer, 2nd ed. Philadelphia, J.B. Lippincott, 1994.
7. Moss WT, Cox JD (eds): Radiation Oncology, 6th ed. St. Louis, C.V. Mosby, 1989.
8. Niederhuber JE (ed): Current Therapy in Oncology. St. Louis, C.V. Mosby, 1993.
9. Perez CA, Brady LW (eds): Principles and Practice of Radiation Oncology, 2nd ed. Philadelphia, J.B. Lippincott, 1992.

51. RADIATION ONCOLOGY: THERAPEUTICS

Deborah A. Waitz, M.D.

1. What is the role of radiation therapy in the management of early-stage invasive breast cancer?
An alternative to mastectomy in many women with stage T1 (<2 cm) or T2 (>2 and <5 cm) tumors is conservation surgery, usually by means of wide local excision of the primary lesion and axillary dissection, followed by radiation to the breast with or without treatment of the regional lymphatics. Survival rates have been shown to be equivalent to those for mastectomy in randomized trials conducted by the National Surgical Adjuvant Breast Project, the National Cancer Institutes of both the U.S. and Italy, EORTC, Guy's Hospital (England), the Danish Breast Cancer group, and the Gustave-Roussy Institute (France) in the 1970s and 1980s. Five-year local control rates for T1 and T2 lesions are generally greater than 85%; 5-year survival rates are equivalent when axillary lymph nodes are negative but drop to about 70% when nodes are involved.

2. What factors are involved in the selection of patients for conservation management of breast cancer?
The patient must be motivated to conserve her breast and willing to undertake a course of treatment that is more prolonged than mastectomy alone. The efficacy of conservation management is appropriate for lesions up to 5 cm in size, but factors such as breast size and body habitus are important. Complete excision of a lesion in a small breast may result in suboptimal cosmesis because of significant soft-tissue deficit; in the obese or pendulous-breasted patient it may have a similar result because of subsequent fibrosis and retraction. Factors associated with increased risk of local recurrence but not constituting an absolute contraindication to treatment include age less then 35 years, high histologic or nuclear grade, vascular or lymphatic invasion, and extensive intraductal component (>25%) within the tumor. Conservation management is not appropriate in the presence of multicentricity, diffuse microcalcifications (as noted on mammogram), pregnancy, a history of collagen vascular disease (which may be exacerbated during treatment), or prior radiation to the affected site.

3. How is radiation administered to the breast after conservation surgery? What are the expected acute and potential long-term toxicities?
Radiation is administered with paired medial and lateral tangential photon portals; separate fields are added for treatment of the regional lymphatics as indicated. Typical doses to the whole breast are in the range of 4,500–5,000 cGy (45–50 Gy) over 5–6 weeks,

followed by a boost employing electrons to the operative bed of 1,000–2,000 cGy (10–20 Gy) in 1–2 weeks, depending on whether the surgical margins are clear or microscopically involved. Acute, reversible toxicities from radiation include skin reactions, ranging from erythema to dry or moist desquamation or rarely ulceration, and fatigue. Long-term toxicities, though rare, include nonreversible edema of the breast or arm, breast or muscle fibrosis, pneumonitis, rib fracture, brachial plexopathy, and secondary malignancies.

4. Is postoperative radiation therapy ever indicated for patients who undergo mastectomy for early-stage disease?

Adjuvant radiation to the chest wall and regional lymphatics is frequently recommended for patients known to have factors that predict significant risk of local recurrence after mastectomy alone. These factors include a primary lesion >5 cm, skin or muscle involvement, close or positive surgical margins, >4 involved axillary lymph nodes, or extranodal extension of tumor into the axillary soft tissues.

5. What is the role of radiation therapy in locally advanced breast cancer without distant metastases?

Patients with stage T3 (>5 cm), T4 (involvement of the chest wall, edema, ulceration, satellite nodules, inflammatory carcinoma), N2 (metastasis to fixed ipsilateral axillary nodes), or N3 (metastasis to ipsilateral internal mammary lymph nodes) disease may be managed with a combination of chemotherapy, surgery, and radiation. This protocol usually entails several cycles of multiagent chemotherapy, after which the patient is assessed for resectability. If mastectomy is possible, it is followed by radiation to the chest wall and regional lymphatics to decrease the risk of local recurrence. Should surgery not be possible after chemotherapy, radiation to the intact breast may be given in an attempt to render the patient operable.

6. What acute toxicities may be observed while patients are undergoing abdominal or pelvic radiation therapy?

Patients receiving abdominal or pelvic radiation may experience nausea, vomiting, or anorexia if significant portions of the stomach or small intestine are treated. Change in bowel habits with increased stools, diarrhea, bloating, cramping, proctitis, or tenesmus may occur with treatment of the colon and rectum. Urinary symptoms such as urgency, frequency, and dysuria can be seen with treatment of the bladder and urethra. Skin irritation may be expected if the scrotal, penile, or anal regions are included in the field. Fatigue is common, and the blood count should be followed closely for acute decrements in white cells and platelets from the effect of radiation on nucleated elements in the bone marrow.

7. What are some of the clinical settings in which radiation is administered with palliative intent?

The indications for palliative radiation are locally advanced disease when tumor size or extent precludes a reasonable rate of cure; functional status inadequate to withstand full-course, definitive treatment; or presence of metastatic lesions. Common clinical settings include (1) invasion of the bladder with bleeding or obstruction from recurrent or advanced carcinomas of the bowel, bladder, prostate, or cervix; (2) obstruction of the esophagus intrinsically or extrinsically by lesions originating in the esophagus, lung or elsewhere; (3) pain or neurologic impairment from lesions involving the central or peripheral nervous system; (4) pain or loss of osseous integrity from lesions in bone; (5) airway obstruction, hemoptysis and pain from lung tumors; and (6) swelling, compression, and pain from lymph node metastases.

8. In which clinical situations is radiation therapy indicated urgently or emergently?

Compression of the spinal cord or peripheral or cranial nerves is frequently seen late in the course of metastatic disease; it also may be noted with localized tumors or at presentation.

Predictors of treatment outcome include the severity of neurologic deficit, time-course of symptom progression, and histology of the tumor. A relatively favorable constellation of factors includes mild deficits of gradual onset in a patient with a radioresponsive tumor, whereas a profound, rapidly progressing deficit in a patient with a radioresistant tumor constitutes an unfavorable situation.

Compression of the airway with obstruction, hemoptysis, stridor, and dyspnea may occur with tumors involving the lung and mediastinum. Obstruction of the superior vena cava, most commonly seen with lymphomas and primary lung tumors, may present with edema, venous engorgement, and respiratory distress.

9. Is the use of radiation ever appropriate in the management of benign disease?
Radiation therapy may be an option in a number of benign diseases when previous attempts at medical or surgical management have proved unsuccessful or in the rare instance when a nonneoplastic entity threatens to compromise life or function. Most patients treated in this setting are adults; children are considered only in exceptionally compelling circumstances. Sites of benign disease most often involve the eye, bone, skin, blood vessels, and soft tissues. Orbital entities are Grave's exophthalmos and pterygium. Osseous lesions may include recurrent heterotopic bone formation after hip arthroplasty, unresectable bone cysts, and ameloblastomas. Radiation may be administered after scar resection in patients known to form keloids; for hemangiomas of the eye, brain, skin, liver, and vertebral column; for treatment of Peyronie's disease; and for prevention of gynecomastia in men receiving estrogen therapy for prostate cancer. Historical applications of radiation have included treatment of bursitis, tendinitis, and parotitis.

10. How is radiation therapy used in the management of tumors of the head and neck?
Small localized tumors are generally suitable for treatment by means of surgery or radiation alone, with the other modality reserved for disease persistence or significant risk of local recurrence. Locally advanced tumors usually have been approached with a combination of surgery and pre- or postoperative radiation. A growing body of clinical evidence suggests equivalent control rates and possible organ conservation with use of hyperfractionated radiotherapy or a combination of chemotherapy and radiotherapy.

11. What are the important pretreatment evaluations for patients who are to receive radiation therapy to the head and neck?
For dentulous patients a pretherapy dental evaluation is paramount, particularly if the proposed radiation portals encompass the salivary glands, jaw, or teeth. Restorative dental work or extractions should be completed as necessary and allowed to heal before the start of treatment. Edentulous patients may benefit by inspection and adjustment of dentures. A nutritional assessment also should be performed, because the patient may require placement of a tube into the stomach or small bowel before treatment if significant compromise is present. A thorough social history should note whether or not the patient uses tobacco or alcohol, and the physician should encourage strongly the cessation of their use, with emphasis placed on their role in carcinogenesis. If the proposed radiation portals encompass the orbits or ears, a baseline audiometric and ophthalmologic assessment is reasonable. Neuropsychometric evaluation is helpful in patients, particularly children, receiving treatment to the brain. Hormone assays are considered when deficits are known to exist before treatment or when the portals involve the pituitary, hypothalamus or thyroid glands.

12. What symptoms can patients expect while undergoing radiation to the head and neck?
When the parotid glands are treated, an acute, transient parotitis may occur. Saliva soon becomes scant and viscous because of decrements in the serous component of glandular secretion. This results in xerostomia, with increased risk of dental caries, and contributes, along with the effect of radiation on the taste buds, to dysgeusia. Radiation doses to the

major salivary glands in excess of 3,000 cGy are associated with permanent salivary dysfunction, although dysgeusia usually resolves within several months. Mucosal reaction can cause pain and dysphagia, placing the patient at risk for dehydration and poor nutritional intake. Skin reactions such as erythema and desquamation may accompany treatment to the cervical lymphatics; they are often pronounced when the beam strikes the patient tangentially or at a site where the contour is thinner, as in the upper neck, especially if beam-compensating devices are not used. Fatigue is common when treatment volumes are large. Inclusion of significant portions of the brain or brainstem may cause nausea, vomiting, and decreased sense of well-being. Alopecia is noted over treated regions of the face and scalp.

13. How is radiation used in the management of rectosigmoid adenocarcinomas?
Tumors confined to the mucosa or bowel wall have a low risk of local recurrence after surgery alone and are appropriately managed by low anterior resection or abdominoperineal resection. If the tumor invades perirectal tissues or adjacent viscera and/or if regional lymph node metastases are present, the risk of local recurrence is significantly increased. Postoperative radiation to the pelvis in the range of 4,500-5,000 cGy over 5-6 weeks has been shown to reduce the risk of recurrence from >20% to <10%. However, an advantage in survival has not been demonstrated. Pelvic radiation administered preoperatively also has been observed to decrease risk of local recurrence for tumors deemed to be primarily resectable; it has been used alone or in conjunction with chemotherapy in attempts to render unresectable or marginally resectable tumors operable.

14. Is there an organ-conserving alternative to abdominoperineal resection in patients with anal carcinoma?
A combination of chemotherapy and radiation is an alternative to abdominoperineal resection for most patients. The few contraindications include a previous history of pelvic irradiation, extensive destruction of the anal sphincter with fecal incontinence, or ano-vaginal fistulae. The usual chemotherapeutic agents are 5-fluorouracil and mitomycin C, and the radiation volume encompasses the primary lesion and the pelvic and inguinal lymph nodes. Most series report an 80% or greater rate of complete response; few patients require subsequent surgery for complications or relapse.

15. What are the major advantages of radiotherapy compared with prostatectomy in the treatment of localized carcinoma of the prostate?
Radiotherapy affords the opportunity to treat electively the regional lymphatics in the pelvis; the risk of their occult involvement increases with stage and grade. The overall risk of bowel and bladder complications, specifically incontinence and proctitis, is generally <5%. Rates of impotence are about 30-40%, whereas conventional prostatectomy renders virtually all patients impotent. For patients undergoing a nerve-sparing prostatectomy, the rate of potency retention is 85% in experienced hands, although the rate of positive surgical margins is slightly higher. Radiation therapy obviates the risks associated with surgery, including anesthetic complications, blood loss, and infection; the time required to complete radiation, however, is about 6½-7 weeks for external beam treatment. An alternate technique is a permanent interstitial implant of the prostate with iodine-125 or gold-198. Local control and survival at 5 and 10 years are equivalent with radiation or surgery.

16. What is the value of thoracic radiation in the management of small cell carcinoma of the lung?
Small cell lung cancer is a systemic disease for which chemotherapy is the mainstay of treatment. For patients receiving chemotherapy alone, up to 80% experience relapse in the chest. Thoracic radiation of 5,000 cGy over 5-5½ weeks reduces this rate to about 35-50%. In addition, several randomized studies have demonstrated improvement in mean and

long-term survival in patients receiving both treatments. Thoracic radiation can be given concomitantly with chemotherapy or after chemotherapy for patients who have sustained a complete or partial response.

17. When is radiation considered for patients who have undergone thoracotomy for early-stage, non-small cell lung cancer?

Postoperative radiation therapy is recommended for patients who have metastasis to the hilar or mediastinal lymph nodes or positive surgical margins. It may be recommended as well for patients who have not received a surgical staging of the mediastinum at the time of resection of the primary lesion. A randomized study demonstrated improved local control in patients with nodal involvement who received postoperative radiation to the mediastinum; survival, however, is not improved.

18. What is a superior sulcus tumor? What role does radiation therapy play in its management?

A superior sulcus tumor is a lesion that involves the apex of the lung. Pancoast's syndrome (brachial plexopathy, shoulder pain) and Horner's syndrome (ptosis, meiosis, and anhydrosis) may be present. If the tumor is considered potentially curable by resection, a course of preoperative radiation of 4,500 cGy over 5 weeks may be administered 4–5 weeks before surgery. Unresectable tumors and other locally advanced non-small cell lung cancers may receive definitive radiation with shrinking fields to 6,500 cGy over 6½–7 weeks. Several series have demonstrated that definitively radiated tumors of the superior sulcus may afford a long-term survival of >20%, which is superior to the rate usually seen with locally advanced lung lesions in other locations.

19. What is the overall survival rate in patients with high-grade astrocytomas? What can be gained by radiation therapy?

Survival in patients with high-grade astrocytomas is among the most dismal in oncology: <10% are alive in 5 years. Randomized studies have demonstrated a significant increase in survival (7–10 months) in patients who receive radiation therapy of 5,000 cGy after surgery. Prognostic factors include age, Karnofsky status, histology, extent of surgical resection, and symptom duration. A relatively favorable constellation of factors includes age younger than 60 years, good performance status, >6-month history of symptoms, successful surgical debulking, and a lesion of lower grade than a glioblastoma multiforme. A poor situation involves an elderly patient with a glioblastoma multiforme who presents with a short history of symptoms and a limited performance status and has received only a biopsy. The standard approach uses external beam radiotherapy to treat focal fields (i.e., the tumor and several centimeters of margin instead of the whole brain) with doses up to 6,000 cGy.

20. Are radiation strategies other than external beam fractions of 180–200 cGy/day to a total dose of 6,000 cGy under investigation for treatment of primary or recurrent high-grade astrocytomas?

Treatment modalities to supplant or supplement conventional radiation therapy include altered fractionation schedules, interstitial implants, and radiosurgery. Both hyperfractionation and accelerated fractionation (see previous chapter for definitions) have been used in phase II studies with acceptable toxicity and equivalent or a slight trend toward better results compared with conventional therapy. Temporary removable implants using iodine-125 have been placed into stereotactically localized lesions as part of a planned tumor boost or into lesions recurring after conventional radiation. Localization with a stereotactic frame and computed tomography or magnetic resonance imaging permit treatment of small intracranial volumes in a single large fraction with great precision. Linear accelerators with either rotational beams or the gamma-knife (a stationary array of multiple intersecting beams from sources of cobalt-60) are commonly used to deliver this treatment.

21. What is a mantle field?
The mantle field is a radiation portal designed to permit inclusive treatment of all major supradiaphragmatic lymph node regions at risk for involvement in Hodgkin's disease. The field encompasses the superior cervical lymphatics and extends inferiorly to the supra- and infraclavicular, axillary, and mediastinal lymph nodes. Two beams are used, one passing from anterior to posterior and the other from posterior to anterior.

22. What is an inverted-Y field?
The inverted-Y field is the infradiaphragmatic counterpart to the mantle field described above. It is designed to permit irradiation of the lymphatics of the paraaortic, pelvic, inguinal, and femoral lymph node regions in a single field. When the extent of disease does not require or the patient's hematologic tolerance does not permit treatment of the entire inverted-Y field, it may be divided into two separate regions, paraaortic and pelvic.

23. When is radiation therapy considered in the treatment of nonmelanoma carcinomas of the skin?
Radiation therapy is part of the therapeutic armamentarium for squamous and basal cell carcinomas of the skin, along with surgical resection, Moh's chemosurgery, cryotherapy, and electrodesiccation and curettage. Indications for primary radiation therapy include lesions whose removal is expected to result in functional or cosmetic deficit (such as lesions of the lip, nose, eye, or eyelid), locally advanced lesions, tumors involving regional lymph nodes, lesions recurring after surgery, or lesions in patients who are medically inoperable or decline resection.

24. What is Karnofsky Performance Status?
The Karnofsky Performance Status (KPS) is one of several commonly encountered indices of functional ability. It is frequently used to provide a standardized assessment of patients considered for inclusion in protocols or to characterize patients at diagnosis, during treatment, or at follow-up. Initial KPS score has prognostic value in patients with tumors of the lung and brain. The Karnofsky scale runs in increments of 10 from 0 (death) to 100 (no impairment) and can be divided into three broad ranges:
    100–80: normal activity without need of special assistance and no or minimal symptoms of disease
    50–70: unable to work but able to live at home and capable of self-care, although varying degrees of assistance may be required
    10–40: incapable of self-care, requiring acute or chronic care in a hospital or institutional setting, with marked or rapidly progressing disease processes.

25. How is radiation used in the conservation approach to sarcomas of soft tissues and bone?
A combination of surgery (wide resection) and radiation with or without chemotherapy is often an alternative to amputation or radical resection with sarcomas of the bone and soft tissues. Important principles in the selection of conservation surgery include the ability to resect the primary lesion, biopsy site, and any potentially contaminated tissues. The operative site is radiated after wound healing is complete. A shrinking field technique is used, with a total dose of 6,000–7,000 cGy over 6½–7½ weeks, depending on whether the surgical margins are negative or involved.
    When the tumor is not primarily resectable, preoperative chemotherapy, radiotherapy (of about 5,000 cGy), or both may be used in an attempt to render the lesion operable. If wide local excision is performed without radiation, local recurrence rates of 50% are not unusual. The risk of local recurrence with conservation surgery and pre- or postoperative radiation is usually <15%.

26. When is whole-body or hemibody radiation used?

Whole-body radiation therapy is sometimes an element in the conditioning regimens of patients undergoing bone marrow transplants. Radiation may serve several functions in this setting, including eradication of tumor cells and destruction of host cellular elements, such as stem cells and lymphocytes, to lessen the risk of rejection when the transplant is allogeneic rather than autologous or syngeneic. It also has been used to induce remissions in low-grade malignant lymphomas of advanced stage or chronic lymphocytic leukemia. Hemibody radiation may be considered for the palliation of symptoms, primarily pain, in patients with lesions at multiple sites, as in malignant lymphoma, multiple myeloma, and prostate carcinoma.

BIBLIOGRAPHY

1. Beahrs OH, Henson DE, Hutter RV, Kennedy BJ (eds): Manual for Staging of Cancer, 4th ed. Philadelphia, J.B. Lippincott, 1992.
2. DeVita VT, Hellman S, Rosenberg SA (eds): Cancer: Principles and Practice of Oncology, 4th ed. Philadelphia, J.B. Lippincott, 1993.
3. Hall AJ: Radiobiology for the Radiologist, 3rd ed. Philadelphia, J.B. Lippincott, 1988.
4. Johns HE, Cunningham JR: The Physics of Radiology, 4th ed. Springfield, IL, Charles C Thomas, 1983.
5. Levitt SH, Khan FM, Potish RA (eds): Technological Basis of Radiation Therapy, 2nd ed. Philadelphia, Lea & Febiger, 1992.
6. Million RR, Cassisi NJ (eds): Management of Head and Neck Cancer, 2nd ed. Philadelphia, J.B. Lippincott, 1994.
7. Moss WT, Cox JD (eds): Radiation Oncology, 6th ed. St. Louis, C.V. Mosby, 1989.
8. Niederhuber JE (ed): Current Therapy in Oncology. St. Louis, C.V. Mosby, 1993.
9. Perez CA, Brady LW (eds): Principles and Practice of Radiation Oncology, 2nd ed. Philadelphia, J.B. Lippincott, 1992.

52. HYPERCALCEMIA OF MALIGNANCY

Fred D. Hofeldt, M.D.

1. What are the signs and symptoms of hypercalcemia?

They are frequently nonspecific but include irritability, weakness, fatigue, anorexia, nausea, vomiting, constipation, photophobia, and polyuria. The polyuria is caused by a hypercalcemia-induced nephrogenic diabetes insipidus. Severe hypercalcemia may be associated with central nervous system and cardiac depression with progressive stupor, coma, and shock. Hypercalcemia causes a shortening of the QT interval, a prolonged PR interval, and T wave changes on electrocardiography. The hypercalcemic patient may manifest nephrolithiasis or nephrocalcinosis. Many patients undergoing preventive care evaluations may be incidentally discovered to have a high serum calcium on routine chemistry panel.

2. In a sick patient with a low albumin level, what is the correction for the serum calcium?

As a rule, approximately 45% of the measured serum calcium is protein bound and 55% is diffusible. The protein-bound fraction is greatest for albumin compared with globulin. For a serum calcium of 10 mg/dl, approximately 0.8 mg/dl will be protein bound to globulin and 3.7 mg/dl protein bound to albumin. For a low albumin state, the correction is that 1 gm of albumin will bind 0.8 mg of calcium.

For example: If the measured serum calcium is 7.6 mg/dl and albumin is 2.4 gm/dl, what is the corrected calcium? (Assume a normal serum albumin is 4.0 gm/dl.)

$$
\begin{array}{rl}
4.0 & \text{Normal level} \\
-\ \underline{2.4} & \text{Patient value} \\
1.6 & \text{Difference} \\
\times\ \underline{0.8} & \text{Amount calcium bound per gram of albumin} \\
1.28 & \text{Add this to measured calcium to adjust for low albumin state} \\
+\ \underline{7.6} & \\
8.88 & \text{mg/dl equals corrected calcium value}
\end{array}
$$

Hence, the calcium is adjusted into the normal range and is appropriately low for the level of hypoalbuminemia.

3. How is hypercalcemia evaluated when the serum albumin or total protein is elevated?

$$
\text{Corrected serum calcium} = (\text{measured serum calcium}) \div \left(\frac{0.6 + \text{total serum protein}}{19.4} \right)
$$

4. What conditions cause hypercalcemia?
The following causes of hypercalcemia need to be considered in any patient in whom there is a bonafide elevation of serum calcium as documented on at least three repeat determinations:

Primary hyperparathyroidism
   Sporadic (90–95% of all cases of hyperparathyroidism)
   Familial syndromes (multiple endocrine neoplasia [MEN] types I and II)
      MEN I (tumors of pituitary, pancreas, and parathyroid)
      MEN IIa (medullary thyroid carcinoma, hyperparathyroidism, pheochromocytoma)
      MEN IIb (medullary thyroid carcinoma, pheochromocytoma, mucosal neuromas, marfanoid habitus, and parathyroid hyperplasia)
Neoplastic diseases
   Local osteolysis (breast and lung carcinoma metastatic to bone and myeloma)
   Humoral hypercalcemia of malignancy
Endocrine disorders
   Hyperthyroidism
   Adrenal insufficiency
   Benign familial hypocalciuric hypercalcemia

Medications
   Thiazide diuretics
   Vitamin D and rarely vitamin A
      intoxication
   Milk-alkali syndrome
   Lithium
Granulomatous diseases
   Sarcoidosis
   Berylliosis, tuberculosis, coccidio-
      idomycosis, histoplasmosis

Miscellaneous
   Immobilization (associated with
      high bone turnover rates such as
      in children or in patients with
      Paget's disease)
   Recovery phase of acute renal failure
      (rare)
   Idiopathic hypercalcemia of infancy
      (rare)
   Dehydration (due to hemoconcentration)

5. Which two medical conditions account for most cases of hypercalcemia?
Of the many causes of hypercalcemia listed above, the most common are malignancy (45%) and hyperparathyroidism (45%). The large differential diagnosis includes the other 10% of the causes of hypercalcemia. Hence, from a practical approach, the evaluation of hypercalcemic disorders can be broken into two categories, such as parathyroid hormone-mediated versus non–parathyroid hormone–mediated hypercalcemia.

6. What are the renal actions of parathyroid hormone (PTH)?
PTH has many actions on the renal proximal tubule. It causes increased renal loss of phosphate with phosphate wasting and hypophosphatemia. There is an increased tubular

reabsorption of calcium. However, because the filtered load of calcium is high and the normal tubule reabsorption capacity of calcium is approximately 95% ± 2%, patients with hyperparathyroidism experience only mild hypercalciuria; whereas in malignancy where PTH is suppressed, there is renal calcium wasting, and urinary calciums of 400–600 mg per 24 hours may be seen.

Excessive PTH causes a type II renal tubular acidosis, which manifests as a hyperchloremic metabolic acidosis. PTH also stimulates renal gluconeogenesis and causes aminoaciduria. PTH acts as a trophic factor for renal 1α-hydroxylase regulation with generation of 1,25-dihydroxyvitamin D from its precursor 25-hydroxyvitamin D.

7. How can understanding these actions of PTH assist in distinguishing between hypercalcemia of malignancy and hyperparathyroidism?
Hypophosphatemia is seen in only 40–60% of patients with hyperparathyroidism, and its presentation varies considerably depending on dietary phosphate intake. A chloride >104 mmol/L suggests hyperparathyroidism, as does a serum bicarbonate in the mildly acidotic range. A chloride/phosphate ratio of >33 suggests hyperparathyroidism. An elevated PTH level is diagnostic. Today's generation of immunoradiometric (IRMA) and immunochemiluminometric PTH assays are highly specific for the patient with primary hyperparathyroidism and in most cases enable differentiation between patients with non–PTH-mediated hypercalcemia, particularly those with malignancies. The table below summarizes these differences.

Hypercalcemia

PTH MEDIATED	NON–PTH MEDIATED
Laboratory Values	
Low phospahte (<2.4 mg/dl)	↓, N, or ↑
High chloride (>104 mEq/dl)	Generally <100 mEq/dl
Mild metabolic acidosis	Metabolic alkalosis
High Cl/PO₄ (>33)	<33
High PTH	Low
Specific Diseases	
Hyperparathyroidism*	1. Neoplasia with/without humoral hypercalcemia of malignancy
	2. Other non-PTH causes (see previous table)

*Remember BFHH (benign familial hypocalciuric hypercalcemia).

8. Does a 24-hour urine calcium measurement help in evaluating a hypercalcemic patient?
Yes. Before establishing the diagnosis of hyperparathyroidism, it is important that benign familial hypocalciuric hypercalcemia be eliminated from consideration. This familial autosomal dominant condition frequently affects family members with nonspecific symptoms, which may suggest a clinically significant disorder. However, when they are evaluated, they have a calcium/creatinine excretion of <0.01. These patients may have enlarged parathyroid glands due to increases in the amount of fat within the parathyroid glands. Parathyroidectomy does not cure the hypercalcemia. The calcium/creatinine ratio (Ca/Cr) is calculated as follows:

$$\text{Calcium/creatinine} = \frac{\text{Calcium urine} \times \text{Cr plasma}}{\text{Creatinine urine} \times \text{Ca plasma}*}$$

*equals total calcium, not ionized fraction

A value >0.01 is seen in other hypercalcemic disorders; a value <0.01 is seen in benign familial hypocalciuric hypercalcemia.

9. Which malignancies are associated with hypercalcemia?

Hypercalcemia may occur in association with various malignancies, especially adenocarcinoma of breast, kidney, and pancreas, and squamous cell cancer of lung. It also is seen with hematologic malignancies such as multiple myeloma, lymphoma, and adult T-cell acute leukemia. Other less commonly associated malignancies include islet cell carcinoma, pheochromocytoma, and squamous cell cancer of the esophagus, stomach, penis, parotid, and urothelium.

10. What percentage of cancer patients have hypercalcemia?

Hypercalcemia occurs in 10–20% of patients with cancer. It may be seen more frequently with certain tumors such as in 20–40% of patients with multiple myeloma, 40–50% of patients with type C virus-induced T-cell lymphoma, and 8–15% of patients with bronchogenic carcinoma, where it may be seen in up to 23% of patients with the epidermoid tumor type. This hypercalcemia is associated with poor life expectancy.

11. Discuss the mechanism for hypercalcemia in malignancy.

The malignant tumor may be primarily invasive in bone, which locally activates bone reabsorption, or the tumor may be in a distal site, and resorption is stimulated by humoral substances that active the osteoclast directly or indirectly. Immobilization may contribute to the hypercalcemia.

12. What are the mediators of humoral hypercalcemia of malignancy?

Tumors may produce cytokines (osteoclastic-activating factor) to include interleukin-1, tumor necrosis factor, lymphotoxin, and colony-stimulating factor or other humoral substances such as prostaglandins of the E series, 1,25-dihydroxyvitamin D, transforming growth factors, and the more recently described PTH-like or PTH-related peptide. 1,25-dihydroxyvitamin D has been implicated in the hypercalcemia of melanoma and Hodgkin's and non-Hodgkin's lymphoma.

13. Define PTH-related peptide.

PTH-related peptide (PTHrP) was recently extracted and identified by complementary DNA probes to be produced by certain malignancies. These peptides are a larger molecular species than PTH but retain homology to the PTH molecule, which allows it to imitate some of the actions of the parathyroid hormone, particularly activation of bone resorption, phosphate renal wasting, and generation of renal cyclic adenosine monophosphate. However, most often the Cl/PO_4 is <33 in these malignancies.

14. What could be a mechanism of hypercalcemia in a patient with squamous cell carcinoma of the lung?

PTHrP has been identified and elevated serum values have been seen in hypercalcemic patients with squamous cell carcinoma of the lung. Similar PTHrP findings have been observed in patients with small-cell and anaplastic lung carcinoma, melanoma, and renal and breast carcinoma.

15. Is there a level of hypercalcemia that is considered critical?

Patients may manifest their symptoms quite variably to any elevated serum calcium level. However, a serum calcium in excess of 14 mg/dl should be considered a critical value and that patient treated under intensive monitoring. In this setting, symptomatic hypercalcemia may include the symptoms of profound weakness, impaired mental function, nausea, and vomiting and central nervous system depression leading to stupor, lethargy, or coma.

16. What are the immediate therapeutic options to treat severe hypercalcemia?

Urgent Therapy of Hypercalcemia

Saline
Generally safe with 200–300 ml/h but may need over 10 L/d with careful monitoring. Use NS:D5W alternate 4:1 ratio with 20 mEq KCl/bottle (can follow urinary K^+, Na^+, and volume in order to document losses). May need 15 mg magnesium/hr.

Saline plus furosemide
With aggressive management, 80–100 mg furosemide intravenously every 1–2 hours and replace urinary electrolytes.[16] Less urgent management, 40 mg furosemide every 4–6 hr.[16] Before using furosemide, be sure patient is adequately hydrated.

Calcitonin
4–8 IU/kg subcutaneously every 6–12 hours.

Calcitonin plus glucocorticoids
4–8 IU units/kg every 6–12 hours. Prednisone, 40–60 mg/d.

Intravenous diphosphonates
IV etidronate (Didronel) at dose of 7.5 mg/kg, with 3 L of saline given over 24 hours and repeat daily for 3 days. Intravenous APD (Aredia), 60–90 mg as single 24-hour infusion with adequate saline hydration. Allow a minimum of 7 days to elapse before retreatment.

Gallium nitrate
(Avoid use if creatinine >2.5 mg/dl) Give 100–200 mg/m^2 of body surface in 1,000 ml NS over 24 hours daily for 5 days

Intravenous phosphate
Given as 1,000 mg elemental phosphate (0.16 mM/kg) over 8–12 hours during each 24-hour period. *Caution:* can cause hypotension. Avoid use if serum phosphate elevated.

Dialysis

Intravenous EDTA
Avoid use because of formation of insoluble calcium compounds that damage kidney

17. What are the therapeutic options for management of chronic hypercalcemia of malignancy?

Chronic Therapy for Hypercalcemia*

Mobilization

Oral phosphates
1,000–2,000 mg of elemental phosphate (start K-Phos, 3 tablets, three times daily). Avoid use if elevated serum phosphate.

Mithramycin (may also be used in semiacute situations)
25 μg/kg in 50 ml D5W given as infusion over 3 hours.

Glucocorticoids
Prednisone, 50–60 mg/day.

Diphosphonates
Oral etidronate (Didronel) 5–20 mg/kg/day.

*Adjunct therapy in addition to treatment of primary cause.

BIBLIOGRAPHY

1. Attie MF: Treatment of hypercalcemia. Endocrinol Metab Clin North Am 18:807–828, 1989.
2. Bilezician JP: Management of acute hypercalcemia. N Engl J Med 326:1196–1203, 1992.
3. Blind E, Schmidt-Gayk H, Scharla S, et al: Two-site assay of intact parathyroid hormone in the investigation of primary hyperparathyroidism and other disorders of calcium metabolism compared with a midregion assay. J Clin Endocrinol Metab 67:353, 1988.
4. Burtis WJ, Brady BS, Onloff JJ, et al: Immunochemical characterization of circulating parathyroid hormone-related protein in patients with humoral hypercalcemia of cancer. N Engl J Med 322:1106–1112, 1990.
5. Danks JA, Ebeling PR, Hayman J, et al: Parathyroid hormone-related protein: Immunohistochemical localization in cancers and in normal skin. J Bone Miner Res 4:273, 1989.
6. Henderson JE, Shustik C, Kremer R, et al: Circulating concentrations of parathyroid hormone-like peptide in malignancy and in hyperparathyroidism. J Bone Miner Res 5:105, 1990.

7. Insogna KL, Broadus AE: Hypercalcemia of malignancy. Ann Rev Med 38:241–256, 1987.
8. Lufkin EG, Kao PC, Heath H: Parathyroid hormone radioimmunoassays in the differential diagnosis of hypercalcemia due to primary hyperparathyroidism or malignancy. Ann Intern Med 160:559, 1987.
9. Malette LE: The parathyroid polyhormones. Endocrine Rev 12:110–118, 1991.
10. Marchant DJ: Estrogen-replacement therapy after breast cancer: Risks versus benefits. Cancer 71:2169–2176, 1993.
11. Mundy GR: Hypercalcemia of malignancy revisited. J Clin Invest 82:1–6, 1988.
12. Mundy GR: The hypercalcemia of malignancy. Kidney Int 31:142, 1987.
13. Ralston SH, Gallacher SJ, Patel U, et al: Cancer-associated hypercalcemia: Morbidity and mortality. Ann Intern Med 112:499, 1990.
14. Warrell RP: Etiology and current management of cancer-related hypercalcemia. Oncology 6:37–43, 1992.
15. Wright CDP, Mansell RE, Gazet JC, et al: Effect of long-term tamoxifen treatment on bone turnover in women with breast cancer. Br Med J 306:429–430, 1993.
16. Suki WN, Yium JJ, Von Minden MD, et al: Acute treatment of hypercalcemia with furosemide. N Engl J Med 283:836–840, 1970.

53. PARANEOPLASTIC NEUROLOGIC SYNDROMES

James Kelly, M.D.

1. What is the definition of paraneoplastic?

Paraneoplastic disturbances are remote effects of the neoplasm not related to direct invasion or compression from the tumor or to metastatic spread. Although paraneoplastic neurologic syndromes are the focus of this chapter, paraneoplasia may include hormonal, biochemical, or hematologic disturbances associated with malignancy.

2. What is the incidence of paraneoplastic syndrome?

In some reports, syndromes related to remote effects of neoplasm occur in as many as 10% of patients with tumors, but in other reports the incidence is 5–7%.

3. What is the most common type of cancer associated with paraneoplastic syndrome?

Lung cancer accounts for the majority of cases, although gastrointestinal, breast, gynecologic, and prostate cancers are widely recognized as capable of producing remote neurologic effects.

4. What are the typical neurologic features of paraneoplastic syndromes?

Virtually any level of the central and peripheral nervous systems can be affected, but cerebellar and neuropsychiatric features predominate. Common clinical presentations are agitation and confusion with memory dysfunction, ataxia, nystagmus or dysarthria, peripheral sensory loss, generalized weakness, and visual dysfunction. Neurologic paraneoplastic syndromes are frequently the most debilitating aspect of a cancer patient's disease process.

Clinical Presentations of Paraneoplastic Neurologic Syndromes

Limbic encephalitis	Polyradiculoneuropathy (chronic inflammatory
Brainstem encephalitis	demyelinating polyneuropathy or acute
Cerebellar ataxia	inflammatory demyelinating polyneuritis)
Myelitis	Myasthenia gravis
Peripheral neuropathy	Necrotizing myopathy

5. What is the work-up for paraneoplastic syndrome?
Work-up includes a detailed history of what typically is a subacute onset of progressive dysfunction of the nervous system. Detailed examination of the affected central or peripheral nervous system offers information about the level of involvement. Neuroimaging, especially magnetic resonance imaging (MRI) scan, has been useful in detecting evidence of inflammatory changes in the central nervous system. Analysis of spinal fluid by lumbar puncture is frequently useful and in most cases demonstrates a mononuclear pleocytosis. Electroencephalographic (EEG) abnormalities have been detected in many cases of encephalopathy due to paraneoplastic effects. A negative work-up, however, does not entirely rule out paraneoplastic syndrome, and frequently autopsy results are the only confirmation of the diagnosis. Serologic markers for cerebellar degeneration (anti-Purkinje cell or anti-Yo) and encephalopathy (anti-Hu or anti-Ri) are now commercially available in the form of tests for the presence of auto-antibodies in either blood or spinal fluid.

6. Does this syndrome ever precede other signs of cancer?
Yes. It is not uncommon for features of paraneoplastic syndrome to precede other symptoms of neoplasm by weeks or months. If paraneoplastic syndrome is suspected, a thorough work-up for any evidence of underlying cancer is warranted.

7. Can this problem be treated?
Most authors suggest that early detection and treatment of underlying cancer is the single best way to halt or even to reverse certain aspects of paraneoplastic syndrome. There have been reports of successful treatment with plasma exchange or immunosuppressive therapy. Unfortunately, in many cases, it is not possible to reverse the effects of paraneoplastic syndrome. All too often, the neurologic effects can be treated only symptomatically, despite association with relatively treatment-responsive tumors.

8. Is neuroimaging useful?
MRI scan is particularly useful in demonstrating abnormalities in the temporal lobes associated with limbic encephalitis, even if computed tomography (CT) scan with contrast has been normal.

9. Describe the difference between neurologic symptoms of paraneoplastic syndrome and neurologic side effects of chemotherapy or radiation treatments.
This may be the most difficult clinical issue in any patient who already has been treated for cancer and exhibits cranial nerve damage, cerebellar ataxia, myelopathy, peripheral neuropathy, or even myopathy. Chemotherapy or radiation treatment is the more likely etiology if the agent or modality is known to cause the symptom in question.

10. What other neurologic disorders must be considered in the differential diagnosis?
Other neurologic conditions associated with cancer include multiple cerebral infarctions, disseminated intravascular coagulation, nonbacterial thrombotic endocarditis that produces emboli, hemorrhage related to coagulopathy, and thrombocytopenia. On rare occasions, B-cell lymphoma produces encephalopathic changes through disseminated intravascular lymphomatosis.

11. Are there autonomic or endocrine features of paraneoplastic neurologic syndrome?
Yes. Various hypothalamic dysfunctions have been reported; the most common are orthostatic hypotension and syndrome of inappropriate secretion of antidiuretic hormone (SIADH).

12. What are the pathologic findings in paraneoplastic neurologic syndrome?
 Neuronal loss
 Perivascular mononuclear infiltrates
 Demyelination and focal atrophy of the area of the nervous system involved

CONTROVERSIES

13. Can paraneoplastic syndrome exist without associated malignancy?
For:
Virtually every type of neurologic paraneoplastic syndrome has been described in patients in whom no malignancy was detected on autopsy. Further studies may prove associations between other etiologic agents and so-called paraneoplastic findings, much as the true cause of progressive multifocal leukoencephalopathy (PML) was determined to be Jakob-Creutzfeldt (JC) virus rather than malignancy, as earlier thought.
Against:
The fact that no malignancy is detected at autopsy may reflect incomplete or flawed pathologic evaluation in these rare cases.

BIBLIOGRAPHY

1. Brown RH: Paraneoplastic neurologic syndromes. In Wilson JD, Braunwald E, Isselbacher KL, et al (eds): Harrison's General Principles of Internal Medicine, 12th ed. New York, McGraw-Hill, 1991, pp 1641-1645.
2. Kalkman PH, Allen S, Birchall IWJ: Magnetic resonance imaging of limbic encephalitis. Can Assoc Radiol J 44:121-124, 1993.
3. Newman NJ, Bell IR, McKee AC: Paraneoplastic limbic encephalitis: Neuropsychiatric presentation. Soc Biol Psychiatry 27:529-542, 1990.
4. Peterson K, Rosenblum MK, Kotanides H, Posner JB: Paraneoplastic cerebellar degeneration. I. A clinical analysis of 55 anti-Yo antibody-positive patients. Neurology 42:1931-1937, 1992.
5. Veilleux M, Bernier JP, Lamarche JB: Paraneoplastic encephalomyelitis subacute dysautonomia due to an occult atypical carcinoid tumor of the lung. Can J Neurol Sci 17:324-328, 1990.

---

54. ENDOCRINE PARANEOPLASTIC SYNDROMES

William J. Georgitis, M.D., COL, MC

---

1. What are endocrine paraneoplastic syndromes?
A syndrome is an aggregate of signs and symptoms associated with any morbid process or disease. Endocrine paraneoplastic syndromes or "ectopic" hormone syndromes present with hormone-related manifestations, either remote or systemic, of a neoplasm not directly attributable to the physical effects of the primary tumor or its metastases.

2. Why is it important to recognize endocrine paraneoplastic syndromes?
Recognition may help direct the search for primary tumors or aid in the early detection of recurrence. Tumor products may serve as disease markers and even permit detection of otherwise occult neoplasms. Differentiating a paraneoplastic syndrome from disseminated cancer may permit curative or palliative treatments. For example, ketoconazole, aminoglutethimide, or metyrapone can relieve devastating symptoms due to ectopic adrenocorticotropic hormone (ACTH) even when the cancer is incurable.

3. What mechanisms cause endocrine paraneoplastic syndromes?
Paraneoplastic syndromes result from circulating biologically active substances—almost all of which are polypeptides. Tumor-associated peptides can be detected frequently in many types of malignancy, but clinical manifestations from those tumor products are relatively uncommon. Not all immunoassayable peptides are biologically active. There are two major

pathogenic paradigms—random genetic "derepression" and the "endocrine-cell" theory. The derepression model implicates transformations in neoplastic cells releasing structural genes from normal inhibition. Enhanced production of enzymes, intact hormones, or hormonally active polypeptides results in clinically evident paraneoplastic syndromes. With the endocrine-cell theory, proliferation in tumors of endocrine cells normally present in the tissue of origin explains the excess hormone production. An example is amine precursor uptake and decarboxylation (APUD) cells, which are cells of neuroectodermal origin with distinct structural and cytochemical features capable of elaborating a wide array of substances.

4. Does a paraneoplastic syndrome indicate malignancy?
Not always. Oncogenic osteomalacia, a rare syndrome with bone pain, muscle weakness, and radiologic features of osteomalacia, has been cured by removal of benign mesenchymal tumors. However, oncogenic osteomalacia has been associated with prostate cancer and squamous cell lung cancer.

5. Does resolution of paraneoplastic phenomena after tumor removal indicate cure?
Sometimes not. Paraneoplastic symptoms and signs may resolve when the concentrations of substances causing the paraneoplastic findings fall below a threshold level. With regrowth of the tumor, hormone levels may again rise above the clinical detection threshold, indicating that a cure was not achieved.

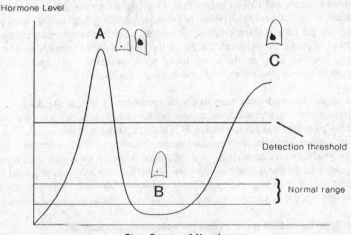

Time Course of Neoplasm

An endocrine paraneoplastic syndrome is recognized when a tumor produces enough biologically active hormone to cause clinical signs and symptoms (A). Resolution of the syndrome may occur when therapy for the malignancy succeeds in reducing hormone levels below the detection threshold (B). The paraneoplastic syndrome may reappear when hormone levels again rise with tumor recurrence (C).

6. Are there effective treatments to palliate paraneoplastic syndromes?
Yes. Because the symptoms and signs result from excesses of biologically active substances, treatments directed at decreasing production, removal, or blocking the actions of these humoral factors can benefit the patient. Effective treatment modalities can include surgery, radiation therapy, medications, and plasmapheresis.

7. Which endocrine paraneoplastic syndrome was first reported?
In 1928, W.H. Brown reported Cushing's syndrome with small-cell lung carcinomas as, "A case of pluriglandular syndrome: diabetes of bearded women." In addition to the proopiomelanocortin-derived ACTH molecule, small-cell carcinoma also can produce a variety of hormonally active peptides. For example, small-cell lung cancer can cause

hyponatremia due to inappropriate antidiuretic hormone secretion or gynecomastia from chorionic gonadotropin. About half of ectopic ACTH cases result from small-cell lung cancers. Other tumors presenting with Cushing's syndrome include pheochromocytoma, thymoma, medullary thyroid carcinoma, and carcinoid tumors.

8. Can ectopically produced parathyroid hormone (PTH) cause hypercalcemia?
Rarely. An elevated level of PTH is diagnostic of primary hyperparathyroidism, a common outpatient diagnosis in middle-aged, asymptomatic hypercalcemic patients. A low PTH level is consistent with humoral hypercalcemia of malignancy. There are a few convincing case reports of hypercalcemia due to PTH production by malignancies.

Hypercalcemia in patients with cancer without bony metastases now appears to be due to humoral substances with parathyroidlike actions. These substances, designated as PTH-like, share sequence homology with PTH. Biologic effects, including hypercalcemia, hypophosphatemia, and phosphaturia, result from activation of PTH receptors. A variety of tumor types, including renal, bladder, adenocarcinomas, lymphomas, and squamous cell lung and head and neck cancers, can impersonate hyperparathyroidism by producing PTH-like peptides.

9. Which tumors are associated with erythrocytosis?
Erythrocytosis is seen in approximately 50% of renal carcinomas, 20% of cerebellar hemangioblastomas, and 15% of benign renal cysts and adenomas. It has also been reported in association with a variety of other neoplasms, including hepatomas, uterine fibroids, virilizing ovarian tumors, lung cancers, thymomas, pheochromocytomas, paragangliomas, and parotid fibrous histiocytomas. Excess erythropoietin is often the cause. The kidney, in the adult, and the liver, in the fetus, make erythropoietin, thus explaining the major association of erthrocytosis with renal and hepatic neoplasms.

10. Can signs of an endocrine paraneoplastic syndrome be seen in the skin?
Hyperpigmentation can result from excess production of peptides with the melanocyte-stimulating hormone sequence, including ACTH and lipotropin. Hirsutism in women, usually severe with masculinization due to male-range testosterone levels, can result from excess androgen production of adrenal or ovarian tumor origin. Excess glucagon from islet cell glucagonomas in the distal pancreas has been associated with a curious polymorphous, often evanescent rash termed necrolytic migratory erythema. Glossitis, dystrophic nails, anemia, diabetes, and weight loss are additional features of this often slowly developing syndrome.

11. Can hyperthyroidism result from a paraneoplastic mechanism?
Yes. Human chorionic gonadotropin (hCG) has sufficient sequence homology in its beta-chain with thyroid-stimulating hormone (TSH) to cause excess thyroid hormone production by stimulating the thyrotropin receptor—a form of cross-activation or "specificity spillover at the hormone receptor."[1] Sensitive assays for TSH performed in women without thyroid disease have shown that hCG secreted by the placenta stimulates thyroid hormone production during pregnancy. hCG levels must be very high to cause overt thyrotoxicosis. Thyroxine levels correlate with the very high hCG levels from trophoblastic tumors, including choriocarcinoma and hydatidiform moles in women. Rare cases of hyperthyroidism in men with testicular trophoblastic tumors or choriocarcinoma have been reported.

12. Does acromegaly often result from growth hormone–releasing hormone (GHRH)?
Very rarely. Nonpituitary tumors can produce acromegaly and pituitary somatotroph hyperplasia by elaborating GHRH. As a rule, acromegaly is caused by growth hormone from large pituitary adenomas. Tumors reported to produce GHRH include carcinoids, pancreatic islet cell neoplasms, and gastric, breast, and ovarian carcinomas. In fact, the 44–amino acid sequence of GHRH was characterized from extracts of tumors from patients with GHRH-dependent acromegalic syndrome. A study screening for excess serum GHRH

levels in 177 asymptomatic patients failed to detect a single case, implying that ectopic GHRH production must be a rare cause of acromegaly.

13. Have other hypothalamic peptides been produced by tumors?
Yes. Corticotropin-releasing hormone (CRH), in association with ectopic ACTH, and somatostatin have been found in nonpituitary tumors. Thyroid-releasing hormone (TRH) and luteinizing hormone–releasing hormone (LHRH) have not yet been reported.

14. What is the most common ectopic hormone produced?
Adrenocorticotropic hormone (ACTH).

15. Is ectopic ACTH easily recognized?
Sometimes yes. A patient presenting with a pulmonary mass, hyperpigmentation, hypo-kalemia, weight loss, and muscle weakness should readily have the diagnosis of ectopic ACTH-induced Cushing's syndrome confirmed with appropriately elevated ACTH and cortisol levels. Primary adrenal insufficiency due to adrenal metastases should have low serum cortisol levels. Metastatic involvement by lung and breast cancer is common at autopsy, but failure of cortisol secretion requires destruction of 90% or more of the gland and has rarely been reported.

Sometimes no. Consult an endocrinologist! Ectopic ACTH can be notoriously difficult to distinguish from ACTH-producing pituitary adenomas causing Cushing's syndrome (Cushing's disease). Plasma ACTH levels can be normal or only mildly elevated in both. In cases of ectopic ACTH from carcinoid tumors and bronchial adenomas, cortisol may suppress with high-dose dexamethasone, the expected response for pituitary-dependent Cushing's syndrome. Simultaneous sampling for plasma ACTH from peripheral and petrosal veins draining the pituitary separates ectopic from eutopic ACTH but requires skillful specialists to perform the procedure and is not appropriate for every case.

16. What hormones and resulting signs and symptoms can be associated with pancreatic islet cell tumor?
There are five islet cell tumor types and etiologic hormones.

Islet Cell Tumor Syndromes

TUMOR	HORMONE	EPONYM	MANIFESTATIONS
Insulinoma	Insulin		Hypoglycemia
Gastrinoma	Gastrin	Zollinger-Ellison syndrome	Hyperacidity, peptic ulcers
VIPoma	Vasoactive intestinal polypeptide (VIP)	Werner-Morrison syndrome	Diarrhea
Glucagonoma	Glucagon		Rash, diarrhea, anemia, glucose intolerance
Somatostatinoma	Somatostatin		Abdominal pain, diarrhea, weight loss, hyperemia, gallbladder disease

BIBLIOGRAPHY

1. Fradkin JE, Eastman RC, Lesniak MA, et al: Specificity spillover at the hormone receptor—Exploring its role in human disease. N Engl J Med 320:640, 1989.
2. Odell W, Wolfsen A, Yoshimoto Y, et al: Ectopic peptide synthesis: A universal concomitant of neoplasia. Trans Assoc Am Physicians 90:204, 1977.
3. Patel AM, Peters SG: Paraneoplastic syndromes associated with lung cancer. Mayo Clin Proc 6:278, 1993.
4. Wallach PM, Flannery MT, Stewart JM: Paraneoplastic syndromes for the primary care physician. Prim Care 19:727, 1992.

55. SPINAL CORD COMPRESSION

Alice Luknic, M.D., and Catherine E. Klein, M.D.

1. Why do I need to know about spinal cord compression in patients with cancer? Isn't this something for the oncology specialist to deal with?

Spinal cord compression is one of the true emergencies encountered in patients with cancer. To prevent permanent paralysis and incontinence, it must be immediately recognized, evaluated, and treated by the clinic or emergency room physician to whom the patient presents. To refer these patients to their primary oncologist will delay the diagnosis and frequently result in permanent loss of function. In addition, 10–40% of patients who present with an acute spinal cord compression were not previously known to have cancer, and this is the initial manifestation.

2. How is spinal cord compression recognized?

As more than 90% of patients who develop spinal cord compression from cancer have back pain, the combination of back pain and a known diagnosis of cancer should immediately bring this diagnosis to mind. Once the diagnosis is considered, further history, physical examination, and radiologic evaluation can help to establish or rule out the diagnosis.

3. Which tumors are the most likely to cause spinal cord compression?

Prostate cancer, breast cancer, and lung cancer together account for more than 50% of cases. Other common tumors associated with spinal cord compression include lymphomas, melanomas, renal cell cancers, sarcomas, and multiple myeloma. In children, sarcomas, neuroblastomas, and lymphomas are the tumors most likely to cause this condition.

4. Give the most common symptoms of spinal cord compression.

Back pain, often increased by movement or with a Valsalva maneuver, coughing, or recumbency is found in about 95% of affected patients and is usually the first symptom. Pain is commonly at the site of the involved vertebral body, but may be radicular in nature, localizing the lesion to within one or two vertebral levels. Weakness, sensory loss, and changes in bowel or bladder function usually follow the onset of pain but may progress very rapidly to complete paralysis.

5. How should patients with signs and symptoms of spinal cord compression be evaluated?

They need emergent evaluation. History and physical and careful neurologic examinations are important in localizing the level of a cord lesion. Plain spine radiographs are abnormal in at least two-thirds of patients with spinal cord compression, and these radiographs are 85% accurate in predicting the presence or absence of epidural metastases. Unfortunately, normal films do not exclude the diagnosis.

Bone scans are more sensitive than plain films in detecting spine metastases and can increase the yield of the plain radiographs. In patients with acute symptoms and progressive signs, scans are not employed, as their specificity is not high enough.

The standard procedure for diagnosis and localization has been the myelogram, which introduces a contrast medium into the subarachnoid space. This is usually supplemented with a computed tomographic (CT) scan. If a complete block is demonstrated, additional puncture needs to be done rostrally (usually cervical) to determine adequately the upper extent of the lesion. Recently magnetic resonance imaging (MRI) has been used increasingly to replace the more invasive CT myelogram and to better delineate paravertebral masses.

6. Is there a role for steroids in spinal cord compression?

Yes. Steroids reduce surrounding edema and may dramatically improve symptoms until imaging and therapy are initiated. Dexamethasone is usually employed, initially in doses of 10–100 mg IV, followed by 4–24 mg every 6 hours either intravenously or orally. Whether higher doses are really better is unknown, and generally they are reserved for patients with severe or rapidly deteriorating symptoms. Steroids should be tapered fairly quickly once therapy begins, as the long-term side effects are significant, and steroid-induced proximal myopathy may be particularly troublesome in these patients who may already have some weakness.

7. What are the treatment options for patients with spinal cord compression?

The goal of therapy in these patients is to maintain ambulation and to prevent loss of bowel or bladder function, so emergent decompression of the cord is imperative. Radiation to the region of involvement has generally been the mainstay of therapy. Although surgery with decompressive laminectomy (removal of the spinous process and laminae above and below the site of compression) may sound more immediately beneficial, many studies have now shown that surgery is no better in most instances than is radiation, and the morbidity of surgery is sizable. Surgery is usually reserved for patients who fail to respond to, or relapse after, radiotherapy.

Chemotherapy is used only occasionally in patients with very drug-sensitive tumors. Most experience with this approach has been in children with Ewing's sarcoma or neuroblastoma.

Most patients with spinal cord compression have tumors that are not curable, but treatment of the underlying tumor is appropriate if possible. Patients with prostate cancer can greatly benefit from orchiectomy, for example.

8. Can the outcome following treatment for spinal cord compression be predicted?

The most valuable prognostic factor predicting the outcome of patients who present with spinal cord compression is their neurologic status at the time they present. Almost all patients who are ambulatory at presentation remain ambulatory, but only 25% of patients who are nonambulatory regain the ability to walk. Fewer than 10% of paraplegic patients will walk again after therapy.

9. Diagram the anatomy of an epidural metastasis.

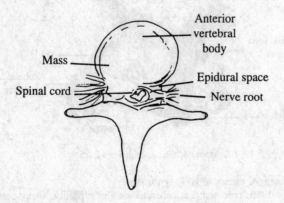

BIBLIOGRAPHY

1. Boogerd W, van der Sande JJ: Diagnosis and treatment of spinal cord compression in malignant disease. Cancer Treat Rev 19:129, 1993.
2. Byrne TN: Spinal cord compression from epidural metastases. N Engl J Med 327:614, 1992.
3. Grant R, Papadopoulos SM, Greenberg HS: Metastatic epidural spinal cord compression. Neurol Clin 9:825, 1991.
4. Grossman SA, Lossignol D: Diagnosis and treatment of epidural metastases. Oncology 4:47, 1990.
5. Murray PK: Functional outcome and survival in spinal cord injury secondary to neoplasia. Cancer 55:197, 1985.
6. Sorensen PS, Borgesen SE, Rohde K, et al: Metastatic epidural spinal cord compression: Results of treatment and survival. Cancer 65:1502, 1990.
7. Weissman DE: Glucocorticoid treatment for brain metastases and epidural spinal cord compression: A review. J Clin Oncol 6:543, 1988.

56. SUPERIOR VENA CAVA SYNDROME

Alice Luknic, M.D., and Catherine E. Klein, M.D.

1. Briefly describe the pathophysiology of a superior vena cava (SVC) syndrome.
A superior vena cava syndrome results when flow of blood in the superior vena cava is obstructed either from thrombosis within the vessel or from compression of the vein externally. Often a combination of the two processes occurs. The superior vena cava drains the head, neck, arms, and upper thorax. It runs through the middle mediastinum in a narrow space surrounded by lymph nodes, the trachea, the aorta, the right mainstem bronchus, the pulmonary artery, and the sternum. Abnormal enlargement of any of these structures can compress the vein and result in SVC syndrome.

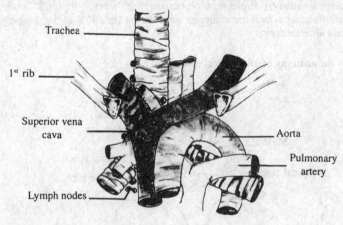

Trachea

1st rib

Superior vena cava

Aorta

Pulmonary artery

Lymph nodes

Anatomy of the superior vena cava

2. Name some "benign" causes of SVC syndrome.
Old series from the 1950s reported that tuberculosis and syphilitic aneurysms of the aorta were common "benign" causes of this syndrome. Today, benign causes account for around 20% of SVC syndrome, and many are due to central venous catheters or pacemakers and related thrombosis. Mediastinal fibrosis from infection, sarcoidosis, benign tumors, and inflammatory diseases account for most of the remaining benign cases.

3. What are the most common causes of SVC syndrome?

Today, 75% to 85% of cases of SVC syndrome have a malignant etiology, with lung cancer accounting for up to 80%. Small-cell lung cancer is the most frequent cell type. Most of the remaining cases are due to lymphoma or other mediastinal malignancies, either primary or metastatic.

4. Why is SVC syndrome called an "oncologic emergency"?

SVC syndrome has long been considered a life-threatening medical emergency justifying often empirical therapy in the absence of a defined etiology. This approach, however, has been challenged. Although obstruction of the vena cava can lead to severe edema of the upper body, including the head, with headaches, visual disturbances, and dizziness, only very rarely do these symptoms progress to laryngeal edema, seizures, coma, or death. In the absence of these true emergencies, time should be taken to establish the diagnosis. Diagnostic procedures, including bronchoscopy or mediastinoscopy, are not only safe but are important in designing appropriate therapy.

5. How do patients present with SVC syndrome?

Patients on presentation usually complain of an insidious onset of dyspnea, facial puffiness, a sense of fullness in the head, and often a cough. Slowly evolving obstruction allows collaterals to form and diminishes the severity of symptoms.

6. What are the usual physical findings in the patient with SVC syndrome?

Two-thirds of patients with SVC syndrome have engorgement of the neck veins and of the veins over the chest wall. These represent important collateral circulation as do the internal mammary veins, lateral thoracic veins, azygous vein, paraspinous veins, and the esophageal veins. Half of patients will have facial edema and one-fourth will have plethora and peripheral cyanosis.

7. What is the usual radiographic appearance of a patient with SVC syndrome?

Remarkably, about 15% of patients with SVC syndrome will have a normal chest radiograph. Superior mediastinal widening is seen in 66% and 25% have a pleural effusion. Right hilar mass is seen in 10–20% of patients. Computed tomographic (CT) scanning can further delineate the involved mediastinal structures and often give additional information about the presence and extent of any thrombosis.

8. How are patients with SVC syndrome managed?

Following a diagnosis of malignancy, patients are offered therapy depending on the histologic type of cancer. Patients with small-cell lung cancer, lymphoma, or germ cell tumors are generally treated with chemotherapy, as these are drug-sensitive tumors. Patients with non–small-cell lung cancer usually receive radiation therapy. Surgery is rarely considered unless the process is due to a retrosternal thyroid goiter or an aneurysm. Anticoagulation is used in addition when there is evidence of thrombosis.

BIBLIOGRAPHY

1. Abner A: Approach to the patient who presents with superior vena cava obstruction. Chest 103:3945, 1993.
2. Adelstein DJ, Hines JD, Carter SG, Sacco D: Thromboembolic events in patients with malignant superior vena cava syndrome and the role of anticoagulation. Cancer 62:2258, 1988.
3. Armstrong BA, Perez CA, Simpson JR, Hederman MA: Role of irradiation in the management of superior vena cava syndrome. Int J Radiat Oncol Biol Phys 13:531, 1987.
4. Bell DR, Woods RL, Levi JA: Superior vena cava obstruction: A 10-year experience. Med J Austr 145:566, 1986.
5. Yahalom J: Superior vena cava syndrome. In DeVita VT, Hellman S, Rosenberg SA (eds): Cancer: Principles and Practice of Oncology, 4th ed. Philadelphia, J.B. Lippincott, 1989, p 2111.
6. Yellin A, Rosen A, Reichert N, Lieberman Y: Superior vena cava syndrome: The myth—the facts. Am Rev Respir Dis 141:1114, 1990.

57. NEUTROPENIC FEVER

Miho Toi, M.D., and Madeleine Kane, M.D., Ph.D.

1. What is neutropenia?

Neutropenia is defined as an absolute decrease in the number of circulating, terminally differentiated neutrophils. The lower limit of normal in the white population is about $1,800/\mu l$, and $1,400/\mu l$ in the black population. Clinical problems are generally not seen above $1,000/\mu l$. Clinically significant neutropenia occurs with an absolute neutrophil count (ANC) below $1,000/\mu l$. Serious bacterial infections are very likely with a neutrophil count below $500/\mu l$.

2. What are the treatment-related causes of neutropenia?

Idiosyncratic neutropenia caused by certain medications is abrupt in onset and can be very severe. Fatal cases of agranulocytosis have been reported. Common offending agents are:

Sulfonamides (trimethoprim-sulfamethoxazole)	Aspirin
Penicillins	Acetaminophen
Antithyroid drugs	Gold
Anticonvulsants (phenytoin, carbamazepine)	Levamisole
Antipsychotics (clozapine)	Penicillamine
Procainamide	Barbiturates
Phenothiazines	Benzodiazepines

Withdrawal of the causative agents will usually restore granulocyte counts within 7–14 days.

Neutropenia also can be the predictable result of cancer chemotherapy. Cancer chemotherapy, such as leukemic induction therapy, causes severe neutropenia. A leukemic patient may already be neutropenic because of the leukemia prior to the treatment. Therapy-related neutropenia tends to be prolonged and may occur almost immediately. In other types of chemotherapy, neutropenia occurs 7–14 days (also known as the "nadir") after chemotherapeutic agents such as anthracyclines, cyclophosphamide, VP16, vinblastine, and nitrogen mustard are given. With nitrosoureas, mitomycin C, and melphalan, neutropenic nadirs may occur at 4–6 weeks.

3. What are the disease-related causes of neutropenia?

There are both benign and malignant causes of neutropenia. Benign causes are:

Infections. Acute infections, such as gram-negative and viral infections, can cause transient neutropenia. Persistent agranulocytosis may accompany chronic infections, such as mycobacterial infection.

Autoimmune disorders. Neutropenia is caused by an immune destruction of neutrophils, and sometimes myeloid progenitors. Patients present with usually mild neutropenia and require no therapy. Examples include polymyositis, systemic lupus erythematosus, and Felty's syndrome (rheumatoid arthritis, neutropenia, splenomegaly).

Splenomegaly. Increased sequestration of neutrophils in an enlarged spleen causes neutropenia. Examples include chronic liver disease causing congestive splenomegaly, Gaucher's disease, myeloid metaplasia, and idiopathic splenomegaly.

Chronic idiopathic neutropenia. This condition is more common in women. Patients present with absolute neutrophil counts below $1,000–2,000/\mu l$. Bone marrow biopsies often reveal many early myeloid precursors, but reduced numbers of late metamyelocytes and mature granulocytes. The clinical course can be either (1) asymptomatic even when the white blood cell count approaches zero or (2) symptomatic with pyoderma *(Staphylococcus* *aureus, Escherichia coli),* and otitis media (pneumococci or *Pseudomonas aeruginosa*) in children.

Chronic cyclic neutropenia. Neutrophil counts oscillate periodically with the nadir occurring at about 3-week intervals. At the nadir, the neutrophil count falls below 100 cells/ μl. Patients are often symptomatic with fever, buccal, labial, or lingual ulcers, cervical adenopathy, carbuncles, cellulitis, infected cuts with lymphangitis, chronic gingivitis, and abscesses of the axillae or groin. Life-threatening complications are rare. Patients are successfully treated with granulocyte colony-stimulating factor.

Nutritional deficiencies. Folic acid, vitamin B12, or copper deficiency can cause suppressed or ineffective granulopoiesis. Starvation may cause neutropenia. Correcting the nutritional deficiency will resolve neutropenia.

Malignant causes are lymphoma, acute lymphocytic leukemia, multiple myeloma, hairy cell leukemia, T-cell leukemia, and myelodysplastic syndrome. Granulopoiesis is suppressed secondary to abnormal immune function or marrow infiltration by malignant cells. Neutropenia may also occur secondary to bone marrow infiltration by solid tumors such as lung cancer, prostate cancer, and breast cancer.

4. How do you determine the etiology of neutropenia?
History and physical examination need to include the oral cavity and the perianal area, looking for ulcerations. Careful review of current medication history must be obtained. Bone marrow biopsies can often aid in finding the cause of neutropenia. Complete blood counts, including platelet count, should be ordered. Possible laboratory studies are antineutrophil antibody assay, antinuclear antibody assay, immunoglobulins (IgG, IgA, IgM), and antiviral antibody studies. Nutritional deficiency states can be assessed by obtaining folate, vitamin B12, and iron levels. For more information see chapters 9 and 10.

5. Discuss the complications of neutropenia.
Severe neutropenia can cause life-threatening infections (ANC <500/μl). The clinical presentation of neutropenic patients can be misleading because of an impaired inflammatory response. Neutropenic patients tend to form less pus, lack pneumonic consolidation on either physical examination or chest radiograph, and are less likely to present with exudate, swelling, heat, and regional adenopathy (indicative of local inflammatory response). Neutropenic patients with potential infection require careful and frequent evaluation. The primary sites of infections are the gastrointestinal tract and sites of invasive procedures (e.g., bone marrow aspiration, vascular access device placement).

6. What is a neutropenic fever?
A neutropenic fever is defined as neutropenia with <1,000 granulocytes/μl with a new oral temperature of 38°C two times or of 38.5°C once in 12 hours.

7. How should a patient with neutropenia and fever be evaluated?
Detailed history and physical examination are essential. The most commonly affected sites need to be judiciously evaluated (i.e., periodontium, pharynx, lower esophagus, lung, perineum, skin lesions, bone marrow aspiration sites, vascular catheter exit sites, and fingernails). Multiple bacteriologic and fungal cultures must be obtained prior to the initiation of antibiotics. These cultures are (1) blood culture (two peripheral sites when a patient does not have an indwelling catheter or one peripheral site and each lumen of indwelling catheter) must be obtained, ideally prior to the initiation of antibiotics; (2) urinalysis and culture (urinalysis may be normal due to the absence of granulocytes); (3) sputum culture; (4) throat swab; and (5) culture of anterior nares and rectum. Cultures of anterior nares may isolate methicillin-resistant *Staphylococcus aureus* or *Aspergillus* species. Rectal cultures may isolate *Pseudomonas aeruginosa*, multiple drug-resistant gram-negative bacilli, *Candida* species, or *Salmonella* species. Other accessible sites of potential infection should be aspirated or biopsied. Appropriate material obtained should be sent for Gram

stain, culture, and histologic examination. Diarrheal stool should be tested for *Clostridium difficile* toxin, and bacterial, viral, or protozoal agents.

Complete blood counts, serum transaminases, sodium, potassium, creatinine, and urea nitrogen levels must be obtained prior to antibiotic initiation. A chest radiograph also is needed. Facial sinus radiographs must be obtained if the patient complains of facial pain or swelling. Cranial computed tomography (CT) and lumbar puncture should be done when the patient presents with neurologic signs and symptoms. Cerebrospinal fluid must be cultured and Gram stained, because meningeal inflammation and pleocytosis may be absent in neutropenic patients with meningitis.

8. What are the causative organisms of a neutropenic fever?
In patients with neutropenic fever, organisms are documented in only 40% of cases and bacteremia 50% of the time. Eighty percent of isolates are *Pseudomonas, Staphylococcus, Escherichia coli,* or *Klebsiella. Candida* is isolated in 5%, and anaerobes and viruses are relatively uncommon. Initial infection is usually caused by endogenous flora (85%). Subsequently, patients who received courses of broad-spectrum antibiotics may acquire antibiotic-resistant bacteria, filamentous fungi, and/or yeast.

Principal causative organisms are:
Gram-negative bacteria *(E. coli, Klebsiella pneumoniae,* and *P. aeruginosa)*
Gram-positive bacteria (coagulase-positive staphylococci, e.g., *S. epidermidis* or *S. aureus)*
Group D streptococci (e.g., *S. faecalis*) and α-hemolytic streptococci (e.g., *S. mutans* or *S. viridans)*
Anaerobic bacteria (e.g., *Bacteroides fragilis, Clostridium* spp)
Mycobacteria

9. How should a patient with a neutropenic fever be treated?
After appropriate cultures are done, empirical broad-spectrum antibiotic therapy needs to be started *immediately*—this means within 1–2 hours of determining that the patient has a neutropenic fever. The choices of antibiotics are:

1. **Aminoglycoside** (e.g., gentamicin, tobramycin, and amikacin) **with antipseudomonal beta-lactam** (eg., ticarcillin, azlocillin, mezlocillin, piperacillin) **or a third-generation antipseudomonal cephalosporin** (e.g., cefoperazone, ceftazidime). Aminoglycoside serum levels need close observation and dosage adjustments are required to ensure efficacy and to avoid drug toxicity (i.e., renal toxicity, ototoxicity).

2. **Two beta-lactam drugs** (e.g., third-generation cephalosporin and antipseudomonal penicillin) can be used safely. The disadvantages are high cost and questionable reliability in treating staphylococcal infections.

3. **Vancomycin, aminoglycoside, and antipseudomonal beta-lactam** should be used in patients with indwelling central venous catheters. Addition of vancomycin will add better gram-positive coverage, particularly for methicillin-resistant *S. aureus.*

4. **Monotherapy** (third-generation cephalosporin or a carbapenam) can be used effectively in neutropenic patients with mild or moderate renal dysfunction as an initial treatment. Monotherapy should be used only in neutropenic patients with limited periods of neutropenia, because of higher failure rate and emergence of resistance.

Antibiotics can be adjusted when a causative organism is isolated, but broad-spectrum coverage should be continued. If other signs and symptoms of inflammation emerge during the initial course of antibiotics (e.g., abdominal pain, pulmonary infiltrate, drainage of catheter sites), antibiotics may be changed or other antibiotics can be added. Changes of antibiotics are required when side effects occur.

For patients with central venous catheters, indications for removal are tunnel infection, septic emboli, and nonpatent catheter. Central venous catheter removal should be considered with infection due to *Bacillus* spp. or *Corynebacterium* of the JK group and fungemia due to *Candida* spp., because they respond poorly to antibiotics.

When patients become afebrile within 3 days of treatment, appropriate antibiotics should be continued (1) until cultures become negative, (2) until all sites of infection have resolved, (3) until all signs and symptoms of infection have resolved, and (4) for a minimum of 7 days.

Antiviral therapy should be added when skin or mucous membrane lesions caused by herpes simplex or varicella-zoster virus present. Afebrile neutropenic patients should be treated with acyclovir when they have a positive viral culture.

10. What do you do if the fever persists despite broad-spectrum antibiotic coverage and the patient is still neutropenic?

Reassessment is needed when fever persists in neutropenic patients for more than 3 days. Hidden sites of infection (i.e., sinus, perianal area, and oral cavity) need to be reevaluated. Blood and appropriate cultures need to be repeated. Causative organisms and their antibiotic sensitivities should be evaluated. Possible inadequate serum or tissue antibiotic level should be considered. Emergence of a second bacterial infection should be assessed by repeating all cultures. Addition of an antifungal agent (e.g., amphotericin B) after 3–4 days needs to be considered, especially when the patient continues to appear toxic.

If neutropenia is prolonged, consider stopping and observing the patient closely when (1) there is no fever for at least 7 days and antibiotics have been administered for 14 days; (2) all signs of infection are resolved; or (3) no mucositis is present and skin is intact.

11. What is to be done if the fever persists despite broad-spectrum antibiotic coverage and neutropenia is resolved (2 days of granulocyte count >500/μl)?

Febrile patients need to be reassessed in essentially the same manner as the neutropenic febrile patients. Repeat blood and other appropriate cultures should be done. Causative organisms, their antibiotic sensitivities, and serum drug levels need to be checked. Drug fever is one of the possible causes of fever. Discontinuation of antibiotics for 24 hours can be considered, and it is necessary to reculture if patients continue to be febrile.

12. What are granulocyte colony-stimulating factor (G-CSF) and granulocyte-macrophage colony-stimulating factor (GM-CSF)?

Both G-CSF and GM-CSF are lineage-specific hematopoietic growth factors. The details of these growth factors are discussed in Chapter 47.

G-CSF is an 18-kilodalton (kd) protein, encoded by a gene on the long arm of chromosome 17, which stimulates proliferation of granulocyte progenitor cells and activates neutrophil function. It is produced by monocytes, macrophages, endothelial cells, and fibroblasts. G-CSF production is induced by interleukin-1, tumor necrosis factor alpha (TNF-α), and/or endotoxin.

GM-CSF is a glycoprotein of 14 to 35 kd encoded by a gene located on the long arm of chromosome 5. GM-CSF stimulates clonal growth of multipotential colony-forming units, erythroid burst-forming units, megakaryocyte colony-forming cells, granulocyte-macrophage progenitor cells, and eosinophil colony-forming cells. GM-CSF is produced by mast cells, T lymphocytes, endothelial cells, fibroblasts, and thymic epithelial cells. Its production is induced by interleukin-1, TNF-α, and phorbol esters.

13. What is the role of G-CSF and GM-CSF in the treatment of neutropenia with or without fever?

G-CSF and GM-CSF have been used in patients with cyclic neutropenia and drug-induced neutropenia. Neutropenia induced in patients with cancer has also been treated by G-CSF and GM-CSF. They are used when a patient has documented neutropenic fever with a previous cycle of chemotherapy and dose reduction is not desired. When a patient presents with neutropenic fever, it is too late to use these growth factors. Growth factors are not usually used in leukemia.

BIBLIOGRAPHY

1. Hoffman R, Benz EJ Jr, Shattil SJ, et al (eds): Hematology: Basic Principles and Practice. New York, Churchill Livingstone, 1991.
2. Hughes WT, Armstrong D, Bodey GP, et al: Guidelines for the use of antimicrobial agents in neutropenic patients with unexplained fever. J Infect Dis 161(3):381–386, 1990.
3. Joshi JH, Schimpff SC, Tenney JH, et al: Can antibacterial therapy be discontinued in persistently febrile granulocytopenic cancer patients? Am J Med 76:450–457, 1984.
4. Karp JE, Dick JD, Angelopulos C, et al: Empiric use of vancomycin during prolonged treatment-induced granulocytopenia. Am J Med 81:237–242, 1986.
5. Rubin M, Hathorn JW, Marshal D, et al: Gram-positive infections and the use of vancomycin in 550 episodes of fever neutropenia. Ann Intern Med 108:30–35, 1988.
6. Sugar AL: Empiric treatment of fungal infection in the neutropenic host. Arch Intern Med 150:2258–2264, 1990.
7. Wade JC: Antibiotic therapy for the febrile granulocytopenic cancer patient: Combination therapy vs. monotherapy. Rev Infect Dis 11(Suppl 7):S1572–S1581, 1989.

58. LEUKOSTASIS

Miho Toi, M.D., and Madeleine Kane, M.D., Ph.D.

1. Define leukostasis.

Leukostasis is an accumulation of large myeloblasts in the microvessels which often results in organ dysfunction. Pulmonary and cerebral circulation are most often affected, frequently with serious consequences. Renal and penile circulation can also be affected. Cardiac chamber involvement has been reported.

2. Who gets leukostasis?

Those who present with a blast count >50,000/μl are at significantly increased risk for pulmonary leukostasis. Patients with acute myelogenous leukemia (AML) and elevated peripheral blood blast counts are at increased risk for cerebral hemorrhage from leukostasis. Fatal cerebral hemorrhage is found more frequently in AML than acute lymphocytic leukemia (ALL) for all age groups. Despite advancements in treatment and supportive care, leukostasis continues to cause early death and fatal complications prior to or in the first days of treatment. The development of leukostasis in patients with acute leukemia is still a poor prognostic sign.

3. What causes leukostasis?

Excessive numbers of immature leukocytes (leukemic blasts) seriously affect circulation by obstructing microcirculation or by forming white blood cell thrombi in small vessels. The inelasticity of the large leukemic blasts leads to plugging of the microcirculation. This can take place in the lung, brain, and other less critical organs. The leukemic blasts may compete for oxygen in the microcirculation and result in local tissue hypoxia and organ dysfunction. As leukostasis becomes advanced, endothelial injury occurs, vessel walls are damaged, and tumor cells invade the surrounding tissue. In the pulmonary circulation, leukocyte thrombi and plugging of pulmonary microvascular channels lead to vascular rupture and infiltration of the lung parenchyma. In the brain, tumor nodules can form in the perivascular white matter when circulating blasts are >300,000/μl. Vessels exhibiting stasis of leukemic blasts and local intravascular growth of leukemic cells also are seen. Under such conditions, the risk for cerebral hemorrhage increases substantially.

4. What would one expect to find on a lung biopsy performed on a patient with AML and white blood cell count of 100,000 and 50% blasts?

Vascular engorgement and accumulation of large aggregates of leukemic cells would be found. The involved vessels would have leukemic cells occupying most or all of the lumen. Fibrin strands would be inconspicuous or absent. Degenerating leukemic blasts in the pulmonary parenchyma may be seen. In some cases, leukemic infiltration of pulmonary parenchyma and hemorrhage also may be seen.

5. Will the patient with chronic lymphocytic leukemia (CLL) develop leukostasis?

A typical patient with CLL presents with a leukocytosis consisting of small mature lymphocytes. Large immature blast cells are usually responsible for leukostasis. There are few cases of leukemic thrombi or aggregates observed in autopsy series of patients with CLL with leukocyte counts over $300,000/\mu l$, but these findings were not clinically significant.

6. Can leukostasis be prevented?

It is difficult to prevent leukostasis, but the risk of developing leukostasis can be decreased with appropriate treatments to reduce the number of leukemic cells. When leukemic patients present with a blast count $>50,000/\mu l$ and without signs or symptoms of leukostasis, they should be adequately hydrated, urine should be alkalized, and allopurinol should be administered. When adequate diagnostic work-up is completed, leukemic patients should be treated as soon as possible. The details of treatment (i.e., chemotherapy, leukapheresis) are listed below.

7. How can one determine whether a patient with acute leukemia who is short of breath has pneumonia, immunocompromised infection, or pulmonary leukostasis?

When a patient presents with shortness of breath, neutropenia, and blast counts $>50,000/\mu l$, this individual needs to be treated for both immunocompromised pulmonary infection as well as pulmonary leukostasis. The diagnosis of pulmonary leukostasis is a diagnosis of exclusion in this situation. Infectious causes need to be excluded by vigorous diagnostic methods: blood cultures for bacteria and fungi, and other appropriate cultures. Detailed history and physical examination are required. However, signs and symptoms of pulmonary leukostasis can also be suggestive of pneumonia in an immunocompromised individual. A leukemic individual with neutropenia or pulmonary leukostasis, or both, can present with shortness of breath, progressive dyspnea, tachypnea with diffuse bilateral rales, hypoxia, and diffuse interstitial infiltrate on chest radiograph. Fever, hypercapnia, hypoxia, and progressive respiratory acidosis may also be present in both cases.

8. How is leukostasis diagnosed?

Patients with pulmonary leukostasis often present with a sudden onset of shortness of breath, progressive dyspnea, tachypnea with diffuse bilateral rales, hypoxia, and diffuse interstitial infiltration on chest radiograph. Fever is often present. Poor prognostic signs are hypercapnia, hypoxia, and progressive respiratory acidosis. Patients with intracerebral leukostasis present with stupor, delirium, dizziness, tinnitus, ataxia, visual blurring, papilledema, and retinal venous distention. Priapism and renal insufficiency have been reported.

9. What can be done for the patient before the oncologist makes the diagnosis and begins definitive treatment?

When a patient with AML presents with blast counts $>50,000/\mu l$, it should be considered an emergency, and immediate therapy should be instituted. During the history and physical examination, specific questions for leukostasis need to be addressed. Intensive monitoring, cautious but vigorous hydration, urine alkalinization, and allopurinol administration need to be started. Cytologic evaluation of cerebrospinal fluid may reveal central nervous system involvement. Immediate blood transfusion should **not** be administered until the blast count is decreased to <100,000/μl. Specific treatments may include chemotherapy, leukapheresis, and cranial irradiation.

10. How is leukostasis treated?

Leukostasis is relatively difficult to treat. Chemotherapy should be instituted immediately; however, its effect on the white blood count is relatively slow in comparison with leukapheresis. In AML and CML with a significantly elevated peripheral blood blast count, hydroxyurea (3 gm/m² of body surface area daily orally for 2 days) may be used. Anthracyclines and cytosine arabinoside have been used successfully to reduce the blood counts in AML. Vincristine, L-asparaginase, and prednisone have been used in ALL with high peripheral blood blast counts.

Leukapheresis can decrease the white blood cell count by 20–60% in a few hours. The risk of uric acid nephropathy can be reduced by immediate initiation of leukapheresis, without waiting for the allopurinol to take effect. This reduces the tumor burden and minimizes the complications of hyperuricemia, hypocalcemia, and hyperphosphatemia. However, effects of leukapheresis are temporary and other therapies (such as chemotherapy) should be administered as well. Leukapheresis has been used as a single agent to control leukemia in pregnancy until chemotherapy can be used more safely. In most cases, leukapheresis is a benign procedure, but fatal disseminated intravascular coagulation by fragmented leukemic cells has been reported. Leukapheresis can be used to reduce the white cell count when a patient is anemic and needs to be transfused to avoid the increase in blood viscosity due to correction of anemia.

When a peripheral blood blast count is in the 50,000–300,000/μl range, the principal risk is symptomatic leukostasis, whereas at levels higher than this intracranial hemorrhage is the major complication seen. Leukapheresis is indicated when symptoms of leukostasis are present. There are some who support emergency leukapheresis when blast counts are between 50,000 and 100,000/μl. This should be evaluated in each case with consideration of the rate of increase of the blast count and the morphologic type of leukemia.

If the blast count is >300,000/μl, it is likely that there are tumor nodules in the brain parenchyma. This increases the risk of sudden intracranial hemorrhage. Although the reduction of blast counts through leukapheresis has not been proved to reduce the risk of cerebral hemorrhage, it is reasonable to try. Leukapheresis alone is not adequate therapy, as it will not affect the tumor nodules in the brain. Cranial radiation (600 rads in a single fraction) has been shown to be effective in destroying intracerebral foci of leukemic cells and thus preventing intracerebral leukostasis and intracerebral hemorrhage. When symptoms of leukostasis are absent, the patient can be immediately treated with chemotherapy.

11. If the patient is severely anemic and has evidence of leukostasis, which should be treated first and why?

Leukostasis needs to be treated first. Immediate blood transfusion should **not** be administered until the peripheral blood blast count decreases to <100,000/μl. Extreme leukocytosis itself may result in increased blood viscosity. Increased viscosity may cause impaired blood flow and in the accumulation of cells in the small vessels, particularly in the central nervous system (CNS), the lungs, and the kidneys, which further contributes to tissue damage. If the patient also is anemic, the whole blood viscosity may be lower than expected. Correction of anemia by transfusion prior to the leukocyte count reduction may precipitate neurologic or respiratory deterioration (owing to leukostasis).

12. Which patients with AML are at the greatest risk and why?

Leukostasis is more commonly seen in AML than in ALL. High-risk subtypes of AML include monocytic subtypes (French-American-British [FAB] classification M4 and M5) and microgranular variant of acute promyelocytic leukemia (FAB M3). The increased risk of leukostasis in monocytic subtypes is probably associated with the extreme leukocytosis seen, as well as the tendency of the blast cells to infiltrate tissues. In promyelocytic leukemia, leukostasis is probably associated with very high percentages of blast cells.

Clinically significant cases of leukostasis are found most commonly in CML. Very rarely, leukostasis in prolymphocytic leukemia and hairy cell leukemia is reported when these conditions present with extremely high leukemic cell counts. It appears that patients with marked leukocytosis associated with a lymphoproliferative neoplasm are at risk for leukostasis.

BIBLIOGRAPHY

1. Creutzig U, Ritter J, Budde M, et al: Early death due to a hemorrhage and leukostasis in childhood acute myelogenous leukemia. Cancer 60:3071–3079, 1987.
2. Freireich EJ, Thomas LB, Frei E, et al: A distinctive type of intracerebral hemorrhage associated with "blastic crisis" in patients with leukemia. Cancer 13:146–154, 1960.
3. Lester TJ, Johnson JW, Cuttner J: Pulmonary leukostasis as the single worst prognostic factor in patients with acute myelocytic leukemia and hyperleukocytosis. Am J Med 79:43–48, 1985.
4. Lichtman MA, Rowe JM: Hyperleukocytic leukemias: Rheological, clinical, and therapeutic considerations. Blood 60:279–283, 1982.
5. McKee LC, Collins RD: Intravascular leukocyte thrombi and aggregates as a cause of morbidity and mortality in leukemia. Medicine 53:463–478, 1974.
6. Megaludis AM, Winkelstein A, Zeigler ZR, Miller TR: Leukostasis: A phenomenon of prolymphocytic leukemia. Am J Hematol 32:146–147, 1989.
7. Ng MH, Tsang SS, Ng HK, et al: An usual case of hairy cell leukemia: Death due to leukostasis and intracerebral hemorrhage. Hum Pathol 22:1298–1302, 1991.
8. Preston FE, Sokol RJ, Lilleyman JS, et al: Cellular hyperviscosity as a cause of neurological symptoms in leukaemia. Br Med J 1:476–478, 1978.
9. Price TH: Plateletpheresis and leukapheresis. In Rossi EC, Simons TL, Moss GS (eds): Principles of Transfusion Medicine. Baltimore, Williams & Wilkins, 1991.
10. Van Rybroek JJ, Olson JD, Burns CP: White cell fragmentation after therapeutic leukapheresis from acute leukemia. Transfusion 27:353–355, 1987.
11. Wiernik PH, Serpick AA: Factors effecting remission and survival in adult acute nonlymphocytic leukemia (ANLL). Medicine 49:505–513, 1970.

59. ANXIETY AND DEPRESSION IN CANCER PATIENTS

Nathan A. Munn, M.D., and Ann D. Futterman, Ph.D.

1. What are the psychological stages dying patients go through?
The classic stages of dying are denial, anger, bargaining, depression, and acceptance (DABDA). Patients vary widely on the progression through these stages, and there may be a spectrum of other emotions that patients feel; for example, anxiety. Remember that the stages are only a guideline; they can occur in a variety of orderings, reorderings, and arrangements, and some people never experience some of the stages.

2. How does a 5-year-old patient view death compared with an older child?
Children younger than age 5 view death as a "great sleep," like Snow White or Sleeping Beauty. They are curious but not usually sad or frightened of it, because death is not understood as final or irreversible. From ages 5 to 9, death may be seen as final (e.g., the person won't return), but there is no biologic understanding. Death is often personified as a shadowy figure, like a ghost or devil, where a supernatural force takes the person away. Although adolescents have the cognitive capacity to understand death, they view themselves

as invulnerable: for example, "I will live forever." As a result, death is accompanied by feelings of shock, outrage, and injustice.

3. How does a physician determine if a patient is competent to make medical decisions, including refusal of care?

Competency is task specific, for example, refusing chemotherapy or surgery, and should not be confused with general mental status. To determine competency, a physician must review the following:

    Ability to understand pertinent information about treatment

    Ability to communicate options concerning treatment (e.g., risks and benefits of treatment versus no treatment)

    Presence of any psychiatric symptoms that could inhibit rational thinking (e.g., paranoia, suicidal ideation, or delirium)

4. How common are psychiatric illnesses in patients with cancer?

Approximately one-half of all cancer patients have or develop a psychiatric illness. In order of frequency, these include:

    Adjustment disorders

    Major affective disorders

    Organic mental disorders

    Personality disorders

    Anxiety disorders

Each of these disorders is treatable using psychotherapeutic and/or psychopharmacologic interventions.

5. What complicates the differential diagnosis of depression in patients wiht cancer?

Depressed mood can be caused by psychiatric illness (e.g., adjustment disorder, major depression, dysthymia), thyroid and other endocrine dysfunction, brain lesions (CNS tumor, stroke, encephalopathy), and medication side effects. It is difficult to diagnose major depression because the physical symptoms of depression—decreased energy, anorexia, sleep disturbance, and weight loss—also are characteristic of cancer per se. Thus, it is necessary to examine psychological symptoms—depressed mood, anhedonia, hopelessness, suicidal ideation—when diagnosing depression in patients with cancer or other medical illnesses.

6. Are antidepressants effective in depressed patients dying of cancer who are understandably depressed?

Yes! Even though a major depression may seem "understandable" given a grave situation, antidepressants are still effective in relieving depressive symptoms and improving quality of life.

7. Do patients with cancer have an increased risk of committing suicide?

Patients with cancer have a moderately increased risk of suicide: it is more common in the first year after diagnosis. Risk factors are:

    Uncontrolled pain

    Advancing illness

    Any psychiatric illness (e.g., major depression, adjustment disorder, delirium)

    Preexisting psychiatric history

    History of previous suicide attempts or family history of suicide.

8. What is a delirium and what are possible etiologies?

Delirium is characterized by a reduced ability to maintain attention, disorganized thinking, fluctuating level of consciousness, disorientation and disturbances in perceptions, and alterations in the sleep-wake cycle and memory. There are numerous differential diagnoses for delirium; a helpful mnemonic is I WATCH DEATH.

Causes of Delirium (I Watch Death)

I	=	Infection	Encephalitis, meningitis, syphilis
W	=	Withdrawal	Alcohol, barbiturates, sedatives-hypnotics
A	=	Acute metabolic	Acidosis, alkalosis, electrolyte disturbance, hepatic failure, renal failure
T	=	Trauma	Heat stroke, postoperative state, severe burns
C	=	CNS pathology	Abscesses, hemorrhage, normal pressure hydrocephalus, seizures, stroke, tumors, vasculitis
H	=	Hypoxia	Anemia, carbon monoxide poisoning, hypotension, pulmonary/cardiac failure
D	=	Deficiencies	Vitamin B12, hypovitaminosis, niacin, thiamine
E	=	Endocrinopathies	Hyper(hypo)adrenalcorticism, hyper(hypo)glycemia
A	=	Acute vascular	Hypertensive encephalopathy, shock
T	=	Toxins/drugs	Medications, pesticides, solvents
H	=	Heavy metals	Lead, manganese, mercury

From Wise MG: Delirium. In Hales RE, Yudofsky SC (eds): Textbook of Neuropsychiatry. Washington, DC, American Psychiatric Press, 1987.

9. When is anxiety considered abnormal in patients with cancer?
If anxiety is so great that it disturbs the patient's functioning or ability to understand or cooperate, it would be helpful to either prescribe anxiolytics or have the patient learn a behavioral technique, such as relaxation and imagery.

10. What are some anxiety disorders that may complicate cancer treatment?
First, the physical symptoms of panic disorder may complicate care in that they can be interpreted, for example, as a myocardial infarction, pulmonary emboli, or neurologic disorders, and possibly lead to unnecessary procedures. Second, agoraphobia (fear of being in places or situations from which escape might be difficult, or help might be unavailable in the event of a panic attack) could lead to a patient's being handicapped in seeking treatment or being able to comply with treatment. Third, obsessive compulsive disorder may cause severe anxiety in patients with cancer, especially in germ-free environmental situations.

11. How does psychiatric status interact with cancer pain?
Patients with a psychiatric diagnosis are more likely to report pain. However, psychological factors are too often used to explain why there is pain when medical aspects have not been fully addressed.

12. What are some of the psychiatric treatment modalities for cancer pain?
Strategies include decreasing mood disturbance (with psychopharmacologic agents), providing psychosocial interventions (e.g., support, coping), and behavioral interventions (e.g., relaxation, hypnosis, cognitive therapy, communication, self-observation, documentations).

13. Does giving patients with cancer opiates frequently turn them into opiate addicts?
No. The chance of patients with cancer becoming dependent on opiates is very small.

14. Why do some patients with cancer feel nauseous or vomit before their chemotherapy?
Following the development of postchemotherapy nausea, many patients (as many as 65%) begin to experience anticipatory nausea and/or vomiting (ANV). This is thought to be an example of classic conditioning, a biologic adaptive phenomenon, where cues associated with chemotherapy (e.g., smells of the hospital, the appearance of the clinic, strong-tasting foods, the "thought" of chemotherapy) are conditioned to the unconditioned response of postchemotherapy nausea and vomiting.

15. Why do some patients lose their appetite for specific foods over the course of chemotherapy?
At least half of all cancer patients suffer from treatment-related food aversion. This can occur after a single pairing of food ingestion and malaise from foods (approximately 24 hours before or after chemotherapy). A novel-tasting food item ingested around the time of chemotherapy is more likely to elicit aversion than a habitual food item.

16. What is the difference between active and passive euthanasia?
Active euthanasia is when steps are taken to assist in a patient's death. Passive euthanasia is not implementing care that might prolong a patient's life (such as feeding tubes or intubation). Active euthanasia is illegal, whereas passive euthanasia is generally legal.

17. What is a normal grief reaction to the death of a loved one? How is a normal reaction distinguished from a pathologic one?
Normal grief is characterized by decreased appetite, sleep disturbance, depressed mood, and crying. Pathologic grief is usually of a longer duration. It is characterized by negative self-evaluations (hopeless, worthless, thoughts of suicide) and prolonged disruption of daily functioning.

18. How long after a death of a loved one with resulting pathologic grief should antidepressants be prescribed?
This is a difficult question, but most physicians would say 4 to 6 months.

CONTROVERSIES

19. Is there a link between major depression and the development and/or progression of cancer?
The literature on the relationship between depression and cancer has been contradictory, at best. One possibility is that major depression poses a greater risk for patients with cancer because it directly interferes with immune processes. Clinically, many patients believe that their emotional states actually caused their cancer and leads them to feel guilty. Frequently, these patients are relieved when informed of the inconclusive data on this topic.

20. Do psychosocial interventions prolong cancer remission rates?
This is another subject currently under investigation. Two important recent studies have found that structured psychiatric intervention groups for patients with postsurgical stages I and II malignant melanoma and breast cancer result in increased survival time.

BIBLIOGRAPHY

1. Appelbaum PS, Grisso T: Assessing patients' capacities to consent to treatment. N Engl J Med 319:1635–1638, 1988.
2. Breitbart W, Holland JC: Psychiatric complications of cancer. In Brain MC, Carbone PP (eds): Current Therapy in Hematology Oncology—3. Philadelphia, B.C. Decker, 1988, pp 268–274.
3. Hendin H, Klerman G: Physician-assisted suicide: The dangers of legalization. Am J Psychiatry 150:143–145, 1993.
4. Fawzy FI, Cousins N, Kemeny ME, et al: A structured psychiatric intervention for cancer patients. I. Changes over time in methods of coping and affective disturbance. Arch Gen Psychiatry 47:726–732, 1990.
5. Futterman AD, Munn NA: Affective states and cancer: New perspectives from psychoneuroimmunology. Cancer Invest (in press).
6. Kubler-Ross E: On Death and Dying. New York, Macmillan, 1969.
7. Wise MG: Delirium. In Hales RE, Yudofsky SC (eds): Textbook of Neuropsychiatry. Washington, DC, American Psychiatric Press, 1987, pp 89–103.

60. TERMINATION OF TREATMENT

Joyce S. Kobayashi, M.D.

1. Does a patient have the right to refuse potentially lifesaving medical treatment?

It is a well-established principle in the law of informed consent that an adult patient "of sound mind" (legally competent) may refuse any treatment at any time, even if family or medical practitioners disagree with that decision. Others may attempt to persuade the patient through discussion, but the fact that the decision may seem "irrational" does not negate the patient's ability to make that decision unless the patient is irrational or incompetent. Where there is doubt or clinical concern about the patient's competence, psychiatric consultation might be considered for an assessment of the patient's mental status, judgment, and suicidality.

Any significant treatment intervention requires a process of informed consent between the patient and physician, even if it is the standard treatment for a condition. A patient may at any time decide that the demands of a treatment—for whatever reason—outweigh the potential benefits, or that he or she wishes to allow "nature to take its course" and terminate all formal medical therapy.

The best guarantee for defining the sometimes elusive line between the limits of intervention and the final termination of treatment, for patient and physician alike, is an ongoing treatment relationship in which there is sufficient trust, communication, and respect that treatment can be tailored to the needs of the individual. The physician must find a balance between being encouraging to a patient about the potential benefits of even palliative therapy, and not being misleading to the patient who wishes to believe every intervention may lead to a cure.

2. What should a physician do if the termination of treatment seems premature?

When a patient wishes to terminate treatment at a time that seems premature relative to the general prognosis, a physician should consider whether depression, avoidance, denial, fear, anger, or some other emotional factor might be overwhelming the patient's judgment. Although clinical evaluation of suicidality must be considered in every wish to terminate care, any wish to terminate treatment should not be presumed to be suicidal. Giving support to the anxious patient whose refusal of treatment has more to do with fear than with the particulars of the treatment itself, for example, may be better clinical management than lengthy discussions of the risks and benefits of the treatment.

On the other hand, for a patient who continues to seek even highly questionable therapies in an advanced terminal condition, the most caring treatment may be in helping the patient work toward acceptance of the illness and an understanding of the prognosis.

Lack of trust, sociocultural miscommunications, personality conflicts, or other factors may complicate the doctor-patient relationship, and these should also be recognized as potentially affecting the process of treatment decision making for either the patient or physician.

Unless the patient is depressed to the point of impaired judgment, unrealistic to the point of being delusional, or in a confusional state, the patient's decisions must be respected. Any competent patient has the right to refuse any medical treatment for his or her own reasons.

3. Why are the physician's attitudes toward death important?

The oncologist or treating physician must understand his or her own attitudes toward disease, suffering, death, and dying to avoid interfering with the patient's values, attitudes, and decisions. Physicians often believe that their role is to intervene with disease processes.

Not doing anything or terminating treatment may be more difficult for physicians than for the patients who have to live through the treatment regimens, their often rigorous requirements, and their sometimes debilitating side effects. Conversely, a physician might think treatment should be terminated because the patient has a quality of life unacceptable to him or her, or because of guilt about the side effects or sequelae of his or her recommended treatment protocol.

In other cases, a patient may consider a standard alternative therapy more acceptable even though the physician recommends another as more effective. The physician must accept that his or her criteria of efficacy may not be equivalent to the patient's standard of acceptability.

4. How can the physician balance paternalism with patient autonomy?
Physician paternalism might be defined as a stance of benevolence and caring for the patient in which the physician wishes to make treatment decisions in the patient's best interests. Society has requested that, in most cases, a physician should take a paternalistic position in overriding the suicidal patient's wishes.

Paternalism, however, must be balanced with respect for patient autonomy—the capacity of the adult patient to make decisions for himself or herself. It is sometimes difficult for physicians to accept that autonomy must mean the ability to make or consider decisions other than those the physician might recommend.

5. What constitutes informed consent?
There are three elements to the informed consent process. It must be voluntary, informed, and competent.

While questions may be raised about whether prisoners are able to give voluntary consent to research protocols, for example, this element particularly highlights the requirement that the patient must be free from coercion in making any treatment decision.

Most physicians realize they are negligent if they do not fully inform their patients of treatments and their potential side effects, but they often forget that fully informed patients must know about alternative therapies, even if they are less effective.

The competent patient must understand the nature of the illness, the nature of the treatment or procedure proposed, and the consequences of consenting to or refusing the treatment. It is important to remember that there is a logical fallacy or circular reasoning in thinking that any patient who refuses treatment must be incompetent. This may be easier to recognize in theory, however, than in the immediate clinical situation when the physician may experience anger or feel "affronted" in having well-intentioned, well-reasoned recommendations "rejected."

Remembering that informed consent is a process of communication and decision making, rather than a single point of discussion noted by a signature on a form, facilitates flexibility in responding to individual patient needs, and leads to improved mutual trust and respect.

6. When may the physician make the decision to terminate care?
If there is a clear medical consensus that a patient is in a terminal phase, and further treatment would only serve to prolong the acute dying process, the treatment would in this sense be considered medically futile, and there is no ethical obligation to continue treatment. Although minor "improvements" in laboratory values, for example, might be possible, there would be no clinically meaningful target for reversibility, and the patient would inevitably and predictably die regardless of those changes. In this case, the physician may decide to terminate treatment because further interventions would be medically futile. Treatment might be continued for clinical concerns, such as allowing family members to gather in anticipation of the patient's death.

The physician must be very cautious, however, not to confuse medical futility with a sense of futility about the quality of life the individual is leading under the circumstances.

If there is any potential for some degree of medical improvement in a clinically significant process, then the decision becomes that of the patient or his or her decision maker, as he or she is the only one who can balance the potential benefits of treatment with the quality of his or her life.

7. What are advance directives for health care?

An advance directive for health care is a legal document or instrument that a patient may establish in anticipation of possible incapacitation (and while still competent to give informed consent). This document assures that medical decisions made when the patient is incapacitated are consistent with his or her wishes. Although legislation varies from state to state, and not all states allow these alternatives to medical decision making, there are three general types of advance directives: a living will, a durable power of attorney for health care, and a cardiopulmonary resuscitation (CPR) directive.

8. What is a living will?

A living will is a document that specifies what kind of care a person wishes to have under certain stated circumstances, generally in terminal states. A common element of living wills sets a limit on the time which the person writing the living will wishes to be on mechanical life support systems, for example. This might relieve any agent or proxy decision maker from the responsibility of making a decision to terminate care that would result in the patient's death. A living will also protects the patient's wishes not to be left on mechanical support beyond whatever limit he or she feels would maintain his or her dignity.

9. What is a durable power of attorney for health care?

A durable power of attorney for health care is a legal instrument that empowers a specific person or agent to be a substitute medical decision maker for a patient who has become incapacitated. Rather than specifying the conditions under which a patient prefers a particular decision, the patient, while still competent, designates an individual who will make whatever decisions are necessary in the event of incapacitation. It is presumed that the individual designated will have a sense of what decisions the patient would have made for himself or herself under those circumstances. Although the durable power of attorney allows much more flexibility than the living will because of the difficulty inherent in attempting to specify treatment decisions in a wide range of circumstances, many use the living will as well in order to address issues of termination of care, including nutrition and hydration.

10. What is a CPR directive?

A few states currently allow an individual to register an advance directive specifying the wish for no CPR in the event of cardiopulmonary arrest. This is often reassuring to elderly patients, for example, who wish to be allowed to die if their hearts stop beating or they stop breathing for any reason. This differs from other directives in requiring an order from a physician, and it is best utilized in the context of an ongoing doctor-patient relationship. It also can clarify whether or not paramedics should be called, or if an attempt should be made to transfer the patient to a hospital, in the event of a cardiopulmonary arrest.

11. If the patient has not established an advance directive and is incompetent to give informed consent, who should make decisions for the patient?

Some states specify or accept a hierarchy of proxy decision makers in the event of incapacitation, such as the spouse, the adult children, the parents, the siblings, or the next nearest relative of the patient. The person "highest" in this ordering, or a person agreed on by all those involved, would be the decision maker. If the medical team is uncomfortable with this designation because of questions as to the competence or genuineness of the relationship, for example, a petition to the courts for formal guardianship might be considered. Some courts have the capacity to designate a guardian even under emergent circumstances. For significant, nonemergent medical treatment for the incompetent patient, a physician should identify a specific substitute decision maker and document this in the medical record.

12. Does decision making regarding termination of medical treatment always include or exclude withdrawal of nutrition and hydration?

States may or may not allow the withdrawal of nutrition and hydration by health care personnel in cases such as a persistent vegetative state, which is not considered medically futile. The decision of the United States Supreme Court in the case of Nancy Cruzan to allow her legal guardians (parents) to withdraw nutrition and hydration and allow her to die affirmed the right of individual states to legislate the parameters of decision making in the termination of medical treatment.

13. What is the role of hospital ethics committees in cases of refusals or termination of medical treatment?

Individual hospital ethics committees vary significantly in their scope and function, but they are often used in providing a broad-based forum for the discussion of difficult cases, such as conflicts of opinion between the family and health care team. Providing an avenue for impartial review and improved communication can often make involvement of the legal system unnecessary. In some hospitals, ethics committees have a role in educating staff about the use of advance directives and in standardizing a policy and institutional history about such issues.

14. What is the ethical difference between withholding and withdrawing treatment?

Although opinions on any question of this complexity vary, many ethicists now argue that withholding and withdrawing major treatment interventions are ethically equivalent. Withdrawing ventilatory support provides a useful illustration of this dilemma, because "turning off" the respirator "feels" so fundamentally different from never having initiated it.

One argument favoring this approach is the model of a "clinical trial" of ventilatory support. If there is a question as to how well a patient might do with ventilation, a trial period of treatment will add critical clinical information to the ultimate usefulness of the ventilator for that particular patient. This would not be possible if treatment could be initiated only under the condition that it would never subsequently be terminated. If it becomes clear that the patient will not be able to survive without remaining on the ventilator, the withdrawal of treatment at that point (equivalent to the decision not to use ventilatory support) is now based on more knowledge than would have been available if the treatment had never been initiated.

15. Who should make the decision to terminate care?

The most important clinical issue regarding the question of "terminating care" is that the patient, family, and medical staff all understand that the termination of care refers to a limitation of specific forms of medical treatment, and **not** the withdrawal of all treatment, particularly the withdrawal of caring by the staff.

A basic and mutual understanding of "comfort care" measures must accompany any discussion of termination of major medical treatment. Addressing specific concerns about pain control and about the fact that the patient will not be abandoned by the staff must be done with great care. Physicians and nursing staff must be equally committed to maintaining the comfort of the patient and not feel as if the decision to terminate care at any point means "giving up" care of the patient.

The decision to terminate care may be made, under different circumstances, by the patient, the patient's advance directive, a legally designated substitute decision maker such as a proxy, the person designated as the power of attorney for health care, a legal guardian, or at times by the physician.

BIBLIOGRAPHY

1. Bedell S, Delbanco TL: Choices about cardiopulmonary resuscitation in the hospital: When do physicians talk with patients? N Engl J Med 310:1089–1093, 1984.
2. Callahan D: Setting Limits. New York, Simon & Schuster, 1987.
3. Council on Ethical and Judicial Affairs: Guidelines for the Appropriate Use of Do-Not-Resuscitate Orders. JAMA 265:1868–1871, 1991.
4. Danis M, Southerland LI, Garrett JM, et al: A prospective study of advance directives for life-sustaining care. N Engl J Med 324:882–887, 1991.
5. Davidson KW, Hackler C, Caradine DR, et al: Physicians' attitudes on advance directives. JAMA 262:2415–2419, 1989.
6. The Hastings Center: Guidelines on the Termination of Life-Sustaining Treatment and the Care of the Dying: A Report by the Hastings Center, New York, 1987.
7. Lantos JD, Singer PA, Walker RM, et al: The illusion of futility in clinical practice. Am J Med 87:81–84, 1989.
8. Marsh FH: Informed consent and the elderly patient. Clin Geriatr Med 2(3):501–510, 1986.
9. Medicine and Biomedical and Behavioral Research: Deciding to Forego Life-Sustaining Treatment: A Report on the Ethical, Medical and Legal Issues in Treatment Decisions. Washington, DC, Government Printing Office, 1983.
10. Schuster DP: Everything that should be done—Not everything that can be done. Am Rev Respir Dis 145:508–509, 1992.
11. Youngner SJ: Who defines futility? JAMA 260:2094–2096, 1988.

61. HOSPICE CARE

Georgia Lee Caven, R.N., B.S., O.C.N.

1. How did hospices originate?

Hospices were first established by Catholic nuns in Ireland in the 19th century. They arose in the United States approximately 17 years ago. Since then nearly 1830 hospices have been established across the country.

2. What is a hospice?

Originally, the term "hospice" referred to a haven or safe place for wayfarers and travelers. It assured them of food, warmth, lodging, and other basic comforts. In other words, these safe stations were a refuge. Later, hospices were designed to be an extension of hospital care for the terminally ill. Now, many thousands of people are given support during their terminal illness so that they may die in a safe, nonjudgmental environment and in a dignified manner.

3. Who qualifies for hospice?

Any child, adolescent, or adult who is diagnosed with a terminal illness and whose life expectancy is estimated in days, weeks, or months may qualify for hospice care.

4. What makes the hospice model unparalleled?

Their unique philosophy of health care delivery brings a new and distinctive precedent to medical care. Care is directed toward the patient *and* the family as the unit of care in the home or in a care facility. It is provided by an interdisciplinary team of professionals and trained volunteers with 24-hour on-call provision. The focus is on control of symptoms and pain—not cure. The large staff of volunteers is an integral part of the hospice concept.

Hospice care replaces the sense of helplessness that propagates the "high tech, low touch" approach to terminal illness with a philosophy that recognizes dying as a normal process of living. It defies the concept that terminal illness is an intrusion into life and focuses on maintaining the quality and dignity of the remaining life . . . neither hastening nor postponing death.

5. How does a patient or family access hospice care?
The patient or family must personally contact the hospice. There must be a life expectancy of less than 6 months. A physician referral is mandatory. The emphasis must change from curative to palliative interventions. There must be a 24-hour care coordinator in the home. There must be a signed statement from the patient or family agreeing to care directed toward the terminal illness, as well as a signed DNR (do not resuscitate) order.

6. What benefits are included in a hospice plan?
Hospice benefits cover the medical equipment, supplies, medications, laboratory tests, and costs related to medical treatment of the terminal illness, as well as bereavement support for the family. Although discouraged and rarely needed, the benefits also cover a hospital admission related to the terminal illness.

7. Do diagnosis-related groups (DRGs) interfere with requirements for hospitalization that may be necessitated during hospice care?
Patients who are receiving their care through a hospice and via funding by Medicare Hospice Benefits are not required to meet normal criteria of DRGs. They may be admitted to the hospital for symptom and pain control should that become necessary.

8. Do insurance companies reimburse for hospice care?
Medicaid, Medicare, some health maintenance organizations, and many private insurance plans will subsidize hospice costs for the terminally ill.

9. When is it an appropriate time for referral to hospice?
Referral is appropriate when no further treatment is available or desired and care is redirected toward palliation. When the patient becomes weak enough to require medical overseeing in the home, it is reasonable to initiate hospice. It also is a sensible referral if the family is having difficulty adjusting to and coping with the terminal illness of their loved one.

10. When is inpatient hospice appropriate?
Inpatient hospice may be required when a patient is unable to manage self-care and activities of daily living (ADL). When there is no care provider at home, and when pain is out of control and may require continuous infusion of analgesics, as well as professional monitoring, one should consider an inpatient hospice setting. As always, this should be discussed with the patient and/or family.

11. Does the family benefit from hospice?
Most hospice centers provide bereavement support to all immediate family members for 1–3 years after the patient's death. In the first year after death, there is a heightened predilection to illness, as demonstrated by a 40% increase in the mortality rates of widows. Other sequelae include increased alcoholism and reactive depression, which can be allayed by continued follow-up by hospice staff.

12. Give the interventions that may be appropriate under most hospice programs.
Tube feedings, antibiotics, and chemotherapy or radiation therapy for palliation only may all be acceptable interventions in a hospice setting.

13. What treatments are generally inappropriate under the hospice concept?
Dialysis, ventilators, hyperalimentation, and extensive antibiotic or antiviral therapy are unacceptable treatment plans.

14. What is the *most* important clinical factor in estimating survival time?
Karnofsky's performance scale (KPS) is the most reliable clinical factor in estimating survival time. Most patients in the very terminal stages of their disease hover at the lower end of the KPS. However, survival time decreases with age, with an extremely high or low heart rate, with immobility, and with nutritional depletion.

15. Is spirituality a necessary component when caring for hospice patients?
Medical personnel have historically avoided the spiritual aspects of care by focusing on physical, social, psychologic, and financial elements of care. Yet, it is the medical profession's obligation to be cognizant of the spiritual roots of their clients. In doing so, the staff may facilitate the patient's ability to access this source of peace and assuredness.

> The things we are going through either make us sweeter, better, nobler men and women or they make us more captious and fault finding, more insistent upon our own way. The things that happen either make us fiends, or they master our character. It depends entirely upon the relationship we are in to God.[1]

16. What do terminal patients want from the medical staff?
Patients want to be seen as living, not actively dying. They *want* the emphasis to be on living, encouraging openers in communicating feelings (especially about death and dying). They think physicians are caring who spend time talking with them and do not rush them, explain the treatment and situation in detail, and treat them with dignity and respect. Studies suggest that patients don't fear death as much as they fear pain, isolation, mutilation, and physical deterioration. Medical staff can work closely with hospice personnel to minimize these fears.

17. Who are members of a hospice staff?
Physicians, registered nurses, registered dietitians, social workers, pastoral care, psychiatrists, nutritionists, rehabilitation specialists, bereavement counselors, and volunteers all collaborate to make the hospice interdisciplinary team operate successfully.

18. What is the average stay in hospice?
The average stay is 30 to 45 days.

19. Discuss when to initiate social services for a patient in need of hospice care.
Depending on the area of the country one resides, the policy of hospice may not accept patients without a third-party pay source.
Social workers should be consulted as soon after a cancer diagnosis as possible in order to gain Medicaid or Medicare eligibility. This can defray problems and delays at the end-stage disease when patients can't be transferred as a result of a lack of pay source.

20. Explain a living will and a durable power of attorney.
As of December 1991, the federal law has ordered that all health care agencies that are reimbursed by Medicare ask patients if they have either a living will or durable power of attorney for health care issues. A living will is a legal document that may indicate a patient's wish to die a natural death without extraneous interventions by medical staff. The living will is easily revoked by speaking with one's physician but is infrequently rescinded.

BIBLIOGRAPHY

1. Chambers O: My Utmost for His Highest. Grand Rapids, MI, Discovery House, 1963, p 143.
2. Conrad N: Spiritual support for the dying. Nurs Clin North Am 20:415–420, 1985.
3. Fitzgibbon C: Learning to let go. Nursing 46(40):21–23, 1991.
4. Franks L, Cassady: When a patient dies. RN 29: 1984.
5. Hill F: Caring for the terminally ill. Nursing 4(34):9–22, 1991.
6. Kubler-Ross E: What is it like to be dying? Am J Nurs 54–62, 1971.

7. Millison MB, Dudley JR: The importance of spirituality in hospice work: A study of hospice professionals. Hospice J 6(3):63, 1990.
8. Scheideberg D: How can you be so sure my baby's dead? RN 30: 1984.
9. Schonwetter RS, Teasdale TA, et al: Estimation of survival time in terminal cancer patients: An impedance to hospice admission? Hospice J 6(4):65–79, 1990.
10. Tyner R: Elements of empathic care for dying patients and their families. Nurs Clin North Am 20:393–401, 1985.
11. Ufema J: Grieving families, Let your heart do the talking. Nursing 81:80–83, 1981.
* Some data obtained from marketing pamphlets for Hospice of Metro Denver by approval of Shirley Jennett, RN, MSN, Administrator of Hospice of Metro Denver.

V. Solid Tumors

62. HEAD AND NECK TUMORS

Steven B. Aragon, D.D.S., M.D., and Arlen Meyers, M.D., M.B.A.

SINONASAL TUMORS

1. What is the most common malignancy of the sinonasal tract?
Squamous cell carcinoma accounts for more than 70% of the malignant lesions of the sinonasal tract. The most common site involved is the maxillary sinus, which is involved in about 70% of cases, followed by the nasal cavity in 20% and the ethmoid cavity in about 10%. Primary carcinomas of the frontal or sphenoid sinuses are rare.

2. List the most common signs and symptoms of patients with sinonasal tumors.
Unilateral nasal obstruction (48%)   Nasal discharge (37%)
Facial or palatal swelling (41%)   Epistaxis (35%)
Facial pain (41%)

3. Do environmental factors play a role in sinonasal tract malignancies?
Yes. Nickel-refining processes have been implicated in squamous cell and anaplastic carcinomas, with a 250 times greater incidence than the general population and with a latent period of 18–36 years. Furniture workers exposed to hardwood dust have an increased incidence of adenocarcinoma of the ethmoid sinus.

4. What are the most common metastatic tumors to the sinonasal tract?
The most common primary sources are kidney, breast, and lung, from which carcinomas metastasize to the maxillary, ethmoid, frontal, and sphenoid sinus in descending order.

5. Discuss the treatment options for sinonasal carcinomas.
Surgery is the mainstay treatment and is often combined with radiation therapy for positive margins and perineural and perivascular invasion. Radiation alone may be used for unresectable lesions, lymphoreticular tumors, or poor surgical candidates. Chemotherapy currently is used mostly in palliation.

ORAL CAVITY

6. The oral cavity comprises which structures?
The oral cavity is the region from the vermilion border of the lips to the junction of the hard and soft palates superiorly and the circumvallate papillae inferiorly. Included are the lips, buccal mucosa, alveolar ridges, retromolar trigone, anterior two thirds of the tongue (oral tongue), floor of the mouth, and the hard palate.

7. What is the most common oral cancer? What risk factors are associated with oral cancer?
Squamous cell carcinoma represents over 95% of the oral malignancies. Others include minor salivary gland tumors, sarcomas, lymphomas, and melanomas. According to 1987

National Cancer Institute statistics, oral cancer comprises 4% of cancers in men and 2% in women. Smoking and alcohol ingestion are strongly linked to oral cancer and their concomitant use appears to have a synergistic effect. Excessive use of both tobacco and alcohol results in a 15-fold increased risk of oral cancer compared with those who abstain from both of these substances. Patients cured of their original cancer who continue to smoke have about 40% chance of developing a second head and neck primary. About 95% of the patients are over the age of 40, with an average age of 60 years.

8. Which areas of the oral cavity are most often associated with malignancy?
Excluding the lip, over 75% of the cases involving the oral cavity involve only 10% of the oral cavity—the anterior floor of the mouth along the gingivobuccal sulcus and lateral border of the tongue to the retromolar trigone and the anterior tonsillar pillar. This may be due to the flow and pooling of carcinogens in these areas.

9. What treatment modalities are available for oral cancer?
In general, radiation therapy and surgical therapy offer equal cure rates for small (T1) lesions. Radiation therapy can often result in superior speech and swallowing; however, this must be balanced with diminution of taste and xerostomia and its duration of treatment (usually 6 weeks of treatment). Furthermore, radiation therapy alone for floor of mouth cancers has been associated with complications involving the mandible in over 40% of cases. Surgical therapy is more definitive and rapid with equal cure rates and preserves function, and it is therefore generally the most common treatment. Combined therapy (surgical and radiation) provides better cure rates for larger and more advanced (stages III and IV) cancers than either modality alone.

OROPHARYNGEAL CANCER

10. The oropharynx comprises which structures?
The base of tongue (posterior to the circumvallate papillae), soft palate, uvula, the tonsillar pillars, tonsillar fossa, tonsils, and posterior pharyngeal wall. Waldeyer's ring is lymphatic tissue that lines the nasopharynx and oropharynx and is made up of the pharyngeal (adenoid), palatine, and lingual tonsils.

11. What are the most common malignancies of the oropharynx? Where are they located?
Again, squamous cell carcinoma is the most common malignancy in the oropharynx, and the tonsil and tonsillar fossa are the most common locations. Waldeyer's ring is a common site for head and neck lymphomas and accounts for about 16% of oropharyngeal malignancies. The remaining malignancies are the same as for oral carcinoma (see question 2).

12. Give the prognosis for base of tongue carcinoma.
The prognosis is often poor because of late diagnosis and regional metastasis to the cervical lymph nodes, which is about 70% owing to the delay in diagnosis. Bilateral cervical metastasis is not unusual and occurs in about 30% of these patients. Symptoms often include dysphagia, odynophagia, referred otalgia, "hot potato voice," and trismus. Approximately 50% of patients requiring a total glossectomy for treatment will require a laryngectomy to prevent aspiration.

13. Are there differences between cancers occurring on the anterior tongue and those on the posterior tongue?
The majority of cancers on the anterior tongue (oral tongue) occur on the middle portion of the lateral border. Seventy-five percent of these lesions are T2 or smaller, whereas <5% of tongue base tumors are T1 lesions. About 40% of oral tongue cancers present with cervical metastasis, whereas up to 70% of base of tongue lesions will do so. Lymphatic

drainage of oral tongue cancers are usually unilateral unless near the midline, whereas base of tongue cancers exhibit bilateral lymphatic spread.

14. Explain the basic work-up for head and neck tumors.
A complete history and physical examination (thorough head and neck examination) is completed first. Diagnosis is confirmed by histologic examination of the lesion in question. Cervical lymphadenopathy can be evaluated with fine-needle aspiration. A chest radiograph is performed to rule out pulmonary metastasis. Bronchoscopy, direct laryngoscopy, and esophagoscopy (triple endoscopy) are done for staging purposes and to rule out synchronous malignancies that may occur in 10% of these patients. Other imaging studies which may prove useful include magnetic resonance imaging (MRI), computed tomography (CT) of the head and neck, panoramic evaluation of the mandible, angiography, and dental radiographs.

15. What is the main cause of treatment failure and death in patients who present with early-stage head and neck cancers?
Second primaries are the chief cause of failure in these patients. Daily treatment with isotretinoin is effective in preventing second primary tumors in patients previously treated for squamous cell carcinoma. Isotretinoin does not, however, prevent recurrences of the original tumor in local, regional, or distant sites.

NASOPHARYNX

16. Give the anatomic boundaries of the nasopharynx.
The nasopharynx extends from the base of skull to the soft palate. The nasopharynx includes the eustachian tube, the torus tubarius (the cartilaginous crescent-shaped posterior lip of the eustachian tube), and the fossa of Rosenmüller (lateral nasopharyngeal recess), which is the most common site of nasopharyngeal carcinoma.

17. Which malignancies are found in the nasopharynx?
Malignancies of the nasopharynx can be divided into three main groups under light microscopy:
   Squamous cell carcinomas (keratinizing, nonkeratinizing, and undifferentiated) (71%)
   Lymphomas (18%)
   Miscellaneous cancers consisting of adenocarcinomas, plasma cell myelomas, adenoid cystic carcinomas, melanomas, and fibrosarcomas (11%)

18. Describe the World Health Organization (WHO) classification system of nasopharyngeal carcinomas.
The WHO divides the squamous cell carcinomas into three entities:
   Squamous cell carcinomas (WHO type 1) (25%)
   Nonkeratinizing carcinomas (WHO type 2) (12%)
   Undifferentiated carcinomas (WHO type 3) (63%)

19. What are the clinical signs and symptoms of nasopharyngeal carcinoma?
Unilateral neck mass (60%) and aural fullness (41%) are the most common signs and symptoms. Other findings include hearing loss (37%), epistaxis (30%), nasal obstruction (29%), head pain (16%), and ear pain (14%). Adults with unilateral serous otitis media c a cranial nerve VI palsy should have a careful examination of the nasopharynx.

20. Describe tests that are helpful in the work-up of nasopharyngeal carcinoma (NPC).
A CT scan displays skull base invasion, which occurs in about 25% of cases. Immunologic and biochemical investigations have confirmed that the Epstein-Barr virus (EBV) is associated with nasopharyngeal carcinoma. Indirect immunofluorescence for immunoglobulins and antibodies to viral capsid antigen (VCA) and to the diffuse component of the early

antigen (EA) are most sensitive for diagnosis of nasopharyngeal carcinoma (the VCA [IgG] is the more specific test of the two). The antibody-dependent cellular toxicity (ADCC) is predictive of prognosis. The polymerase chain reaction (PCR) can be used to test for the presence of EBV genomes in metastatic squamous cell carcinoma of the neck obtained by fine-needle aspirate.

21. How is nasopharyngeal carcinoma treated?
The initial treatment of choice is external-beam supravoltage radiation with a dose between 6500 and 7000 cGy.

LIP CANCER

22. How common is lip cancer?
Lip cancer is the most common malignant tumor of the oral cavity, accounting for 25–30% of the cases. About 90% of lip carcinomas are squamous cell and about 90% of these occur on the lower lip.

23. What is keratoacanthoma?
Keratoacanthoma is a benign, self-limiting epithelial lesion that can mimic squamous cell carcinoma. It appears as an ulcerated, circumscribed lesion with elevated or rolled margins, a keratinized central region, and an indurated base. It has a rapid initial growth phase and may be present for weeks or even months. Incisional biopsy is important for lesions that are present for several weeks to rule out squamous cell carcinoma.

24. Are other tumors associated with the lips?
Basal cell carcinoma is the second most common malignancy of the lips. It is actually more common in the upper lip than squamous cell carcinoma. These are very slow-growing tumors and rarely metastasize.

Minor salivary gland tumors are more commonly (85% of the cases) associated with the upper lip. The most common minor salivary gland neoplasm is a pleomorphic adenoma, which is a benign neoplasm. Only 17% of minor salivary gland tumors are malignant, including melanoma, microcystic adenexal carcinoma, Merkel's cell carcinoma, malignant fibrous histiocytoma, and malignant granular cell tumors.

25. What negative prognostic factors are important with respect to lip cancers?
Large primary tumor (>3 cm)	Poorly differentiated histology
Cervical node metastasis	Mandibular invasion
Recurrent tumors	Commissure lesions
Perineural invasion	

Primary lip cancers <2 cm have a 5-year survival rate of about 90%, whereas larger tumors such as those involving the mandible have a 5-year survival rate of <50%. The larger the primary tumor, the more likely a recurrence (e.g., a recurrence rate of 40% for lesions >3 cm). Cervical nodal metastases decreases survival to between 25% and 50%. Well-differentiated squamous cell lesions have a higher survival rate (86–95%) than poorly differentiated lesions (38–62%). Recurrence reduces the 5-year survival to <50%. Perineural invasion also is associated with a poor outcome.

HYPOPHARYNGEAL CANCER

26. The hypopharynx comprises which structures?
The hypopharynx extends from the hyoid bone superiorly to the inferior border of the cricoid cartilage inferiorly. It is subdivided into three regions: the piriform sinus (fossa), the postcricoid region, and the posterior hypopharyngeal wall.

27. What areas of the hypopharynx are most commonly involved?
Pyriform sinus (70%)
Postcricoid area (15%)
Posterior pharyngeal wall (<15%)

28. Does hypopharyngeal cancer have unique pathologic characteristics?
As in the other areas of the aerodigestive tract, epidermoid carcinoma accounts for 95% of the lesions. Most of the remaining 5% are adenocarcinomas. Submucosal spread is common and is more prevalent as the tumor approaches the cervical esophagus. Satellite tumors, or "skip areas," also are more common in this region. Cervical lymph node metastasis is common, occurring in 75% of piriform sinus lesions, 40% of postcricoid lesions, and 60% of posterior hypopharyngeal wall lesions.

29. How is hypopharyngeal cancer managed?
Radiation therapy alone may be used for small lesions (T1 and T2), with surgery being reserved for salvage should the primary radiotherapy fail. Combined surgery and radiotherapy are used for larger lesions. Treatment of the cervical lymphatics by radiation therapy or neck dissection is often required because of the high incidence of grossly involved or occult metastatic lymph nodes.

LARYNGEAL CARCINOMA

30. What is the most common benign neoplasm of the larynx?
Squamous papillomas are the most common benign laryngeal neoplasm, accounting for about 80% of benign laryngeal tumors. They are generally divided into juvenile- and adult-onset papillomas. Juvenile papillomas may have a viral etiology and commonly occur in infancy or childhood and present as hoarseness or stridor. Juvenile papillomatosis may be very aggressive, requiring multiple surgical procedures for control and protection of the airway.
Adult-onset papillomas are commonly solitary and less aggressive than their juvenile counterpart. In many cases, a single surgical procedure may produce a cure.

31. Discuss the signs and symptoms associated with laryngeal neoplasms.
Hoarseness is the cardinal sign of laryngeal cancer. Dyspnea and stridor occur later when associated with airway obstruction. Pain may be confined to the throat or it may be referred to the ipsilateral ear. Dysphagia (difficulty swallowing) and odynophagia (painful swallowing) are present with extralaryngeal involvement. Chronic cough and hemoptosis also are frequently present.

32. What are the important functions of the larynx?
Airway protection   Phonation
Respiration   Sphincteric action (Valsalva maneuver and lifting)

33. What is the most common laryngeal cancer? Where is it located?
Carcinoma of the glottic region (true vocal cords) is the most common type of laryngeal carcinoma (50–75% of the cases). Because it interferes with phonation, it is often diagnosed earlier than cancers in other areas of the aerodigestive tract.

34. Are there causes of vocal cord paralysis other than glottic cancer?
Vocal cord paralysis is a sign of a disease and not a diagnosis. It may be due to a lesion anywhere from the cerebral cortex throughout the pathway of the vagus nerve to the muscles of the larynx. Surgical trauma is the most common cause of unilateral and bilateral vocal cord paralysis, most often occurring following thyroidectomy. Other surgical procedures associated with vocal cord paralysis include lung resection, carotid artery and cervical spine operations, mediastinoscopy, laryngectomy, radical neck dissection, and

cardiac surgery. Other causes include malignancy (lung, esophageal, thyroid), trauma, inflammation (pulmonary tuberculosis, jugular thrombophlebitis, thyroiditis, meningitis, influenza), neurologic disorders (cerebrovascular disease, Parkinson's disease, multiple sclerosis, poliomyelitis, amytrophic lateral sclerosis, and epilepsy), and idiopathic causes.

SALIVARY GLAND NEOPLASMS

35. Which salivary glands are responsible for most of the neoplasms?
About 80% of all salivary gland neoplasms arise in the parotid gland, 10–15% in the submandibular gland, and remaining in the sublingual gland and minor salivary glands. The smaller the gland of origin, the more likely the tumor may be malignant. Approximately 80% of parotid tumors are benign, whereas 50% of the submandibular and less than 40% of the sublingual and minor salivary glands are benign.

36. In children, what is the most common salivary gland tumor?
Hemangioma is the most common benign tumor and pleomorphic adenoma is the most common type of benign epithelial tum r in children. Other benign tumors include lymphangioma, lymphoepithelial tumor, and Warthin's tumor. Most of the malignant tumors arise in the parotid gland (85%), and approximately 50% of these are mucoepidermoid carcinoma.

37. In adults, what is the most common parotid gland tumor?
Pleomorphic adenoma is the most common tumor of the parotid gland in adults. In fact, this benign neoplasm is the most common tumor for each of the salivary glands and makes up about 65% of all salivary gland tumors. The second most common benign tumor of the parotid is Warthin's tumor (papillary cystadenoma lymphomatosum), which accounts for 6–10% of all parotid neoplasms. Other benign entities include oncocytoma, monomorphic adenoma, and benign lymphoepithelial lesion.

38. What is the most common malignancy of the parotid gland?
Mucoepidermoid carcinoma. It accounts for 6–9% of all major salivary gland neoplasms, and 50–60% of these are located in the parotid. Other malignancies include malignant mixed tumor, acinic cell carcinoma, adenocarcinoma, squamous cell carcinoma, undifferentiated carcinoma, and lymphoma.

39. What is the most common malignancy of the submandibular gland and minor salivary glands?
Adenoid cystic carcinoma. Perineural invasion is a typical feature of this neoplasm, which may make eradication of this tumor difficult. Adenocarcinoma most frequently occurs in the minor salivary glands followed by the parotid gland. The remainder of the malignant tumors includes the same entities as the parotid gland.

40. How accurate is fine-needle aspiration in the diagnosis of head and neck and salivary gland neoplasms?
Although the results are dependent on the skill, expertise, and experience of the cytopathologist, fine-needle aspiration for squamous cell carcinoma of the head and neck has been reported to be >90% accurate. The diagnostic accuracy for salivary gland neoplasms is somewhat less, between 60% and 80%. Use of fine-needle aspiration has not been associated with tumor seeding on the needle tract.

41. What is the treatment of choice for salivary gland neoplasms?
Surgical excision. Most parotid lesions are present in the region of the tail and are superficial to the facial nerve and therefore amenable to a superficial parotidectomy with identification and preservation of the facial nerve. Occasionally, the deep lobe may be involved, requiring a total parotidectomy. Submandibular gland lesions are usually limited

to the gland, and gland excision is the treatment of choice. Malignant tumors of the submandibular gland may extend beyond the gland to important structures such as the marginal branch of the facial nerve, hypoglossal nerve, lingual nerve, mandible, tongue, and floor of the mouth.

BIBLIOGRAPHY

1. Baden E: Prevention of cancer of the oral cavity and pharynx. CA 37:49–62, 1987.
2. Bailey JB: Head and Neck Surgery—Otolaryngology. Philadelphia, J.B. Lippincott, 1993.
3. Baker SR, Krause CJ: Carcinoma of the lip. Laryngoscope 90:19–21, 1980.
4. Feinmesser R, Miyazaki I, et al: Diagnosis of nasopharyngeal carcinoma by DNA amplification of tissue obtained by fine needle aspiration. N Engl J Med 326:17–21, 1992.
5. Larson DL, Lindberg RD, Lane E, Goepfert H: Major complications of radiotherapy in cancer of the oral cavity and oropharynx. Am J Surg 146:531–536, 1983.
6. Lee KJ: Essential Otolaryngology, 5th ed. New York, Medical Examination, 1991.
7. Lippman SM, Hong WK: Second malignant tumors in head and neck squamous cell carcinoma: The overshadowing threat for patients with early-stage disease. Int J Radiat Oncol Biol Phys 17:691–694, 1989.
8. Neel HB, Taylor WF, Pearsen G: Prognostic determinants and a new view of staging for patients with nasopharyngeal carcinoma. Ann Otol Rhinol Laryngol 94:529–537, 1985..
9. Paparella MM, Shumrick DA (eds): Otolaryngology, 3rd ed. Philadelphia, W.B. Saunders, 1991.
10. Regezi, Sciubba: Oral Pathology: Clinical-Pathological Correlations. Philadelphia, W.B. Saunders, 1989.
11. Waun KH, et al: Prevention of second primary tumors with isotretinoin in squamous-cell carcinoma of the head and neck. N Engl J Med 323:795–801, 1990.

63. BREAST CANCER

Scot M. Sedlacek, M.D.

1. What does lobular carcinoma in situ (LCIS) represent?

Despite the fact that carcinoma is a part of its name, it is now believed that LCIS does not represent malignancy but rather a marker for a woman who is at increased risk for the development of breast cancer. Some pathologists are attempting to change the name to **lobular neoplasia,** which also includes atypical lobular hyperplasia. In women with the diagnosis of lobular neoplasia, both breasts are at risk, and most of the cancers that occur are actually infiltrating ductal carcinoma and not infiltrating lobular carcinoma.

2. Now knowing the significance of LCIS on a breast biopsy, what recommendations should be made concerning therapy?

Because LCIS is only a marker for the high risk of developing breast cancer, the woman should be placed on a close follow-up program consisting of monthly breast self-examination, yearly mammography, and every 6 months a physician-conducted physical examination. If there are other significant risk factors along with the diagnosis of LCIS, such as a first-degree relative with breast cancer, and the woman is unwilling to accept this markedly increased risk, the other option for treatment is bilateral prophylactic total mastectomies. This surgical procedure is thought to reduce the risk of breast cancer to as close to 0% as possible.

3. How does ductal carcinoma in situ (DCIS) typically present and what is the appropriate treatment?

DCIS typically presents as abnormal calcifications seen on a mammogram. Prior to 1985, the standard of care was mastectomy with or without an axillary dissection. This modality carried close to a 99% cure rate. The incidence of positive lymph node metastases in pure DCIS is 0–2%, thus making it difficult routinely to recommend this procedure for all women. The National Surgical Adjuvant Breast Project (NSABP) protocol B-17 was published in 1993 and demonstrated that women with DCIS that can be excised with negative surgical margins have a 5.1% risk per year of local breast recurrence with lumpectomy alone but only a 2.1% risk per year with lumpectomy followed by breast irradiation. Thus, breast conservation with radiation therapy offers a woman a high likelihood of retaining her breast and minimal risk of ultimately dying from breast cancer. Either breast conservation with irradiation or total mastectomy is an appropriate option for women with DCIS.

4. Is there currently any role for hormone receptors and/or DNA analysis in DCIS?
No. The most important issue for the pathologist in evaluating a case of suspected DCIS is whether there are any areas of invasive cancer. Therefore, all of the tissue is processed for histologic examination and none preserved fresh for estrogen/progesterone receptor and/or DNA analysis. This information was of no value when the standard treatment for DCIS was total mastectomy, with nearly 99% of women cured of this disease process. Now that breast conservation is being employed more frequently for this disorder, these prognostic factors may play a role in determining the risk of local recurrence and possibly which cases are likely to recur as the more worrisome infiltrating ductal carcinoma.

5. What surgical procedure is more aggressive and therefore offers a woman her best chance to be alive and free of cancer in 10 years: modified radical mastectomy (MRM) or lumpectomy with radiation therapy (RT)?
For the woman with a cancer in her breast that is small enough (4 to 5 cm maximum diameter) to be excised with negative surgical margins and who is left with sufficient residual breast tissue for an acceptable cosmetic result, postoperative RT to the breast offers her the *same* long-term prognosis for survival as the woman who has her entire breast removed. These therapies obviously are quite different, with certain advantages and disadvantages that a woman and her physician should discuss. The advantages and disadvantages of the two options are outlined below.

	Advantages	Disadvantages

Mastectomy	No need for RT
	No need for ipsilateral
	  mammograms
		No breast
		May need breast
		  reconstruction

Lumpectomy/RT	Have a breast
	No need for breast
	  reconstruction
		Need RT for 5–6 weeks
		Risk of local recurrence
		Still needs mammograms
		  of irradiated breast

6. Is inflammatory breast cancer (redness and swelling of the overlying skin) a surgical emergency that warrants excision prior to further rapid growth by this most aggressive malignancy?
On the contrary, attempts at complete surgical excision are fraught with complications and poor outcomes due to the cancer rapidly spreading through the skin and lymphatics. Initially, some form of biopsy should be performed to diagnose the process, including determinations of hormone receptors. This should be followed by neoadjuvant or induction chemotherapy in an attempt to cytoreduce the tumor. A multimodality approach such as chemotherapy → surgery → chemotherapy → RT → hormonal therapy has improved outcome in a disease that in the past carried a 0–2% 5-year survival rate to one with a 50–65% 5-year survival rate.

7. What are the indications for RT in women treated with MRM?
  1. Large T3 (>5 cm) primary tumors
  2. Any T4 (skin or chest wall involvement) primary tumors
  3. Inflammatory breast cancer (T4d)
  4. ≥4 lymph nodes involved with cancer
  5. Spread of the cancer outside of the lymph node capsule into the surrounding perinodal fat
  6. Positive surgical margin
Any of these six clinicopathologic findings place a woman at significant (>20%) risk for local/regional recurrence on the chest wall postmastectomy such that RT should seriously be entertained.

8. In women treated with MRM but without postoperative RT who then develop a local recurrence on the chest wall, what therapeutic and diagnostic options should be considered?
  1. Attempts should be made to excise the entire recurrence with negative surgical margins to provide the best chance for local control.
  2. A metastatic work-up should be performed (bone scan, chest radiograph, and computed tomography [CT] scan of the abdomen) since one third to one half of women will have demonstrable metastatic deposits at the time of their local recurrence.
  3. RT should be administered not only to the site of recurrence but to the entire chest wall and draining lymph node chains, because they also are at risk of multifocal recurrence.
  4. "Adjuvant" chemotherapy or hormonal therapy? Approximately 20% of patients at risk following an isolated local recurrence will develop metastatic disease each year. Therefore, by 10 years, 93% of women have developed metastases and will ultimately die of their cancer. Owing to these ominous figures signifying that a local recurrence portends dissemination, attempts at preventive treatments with chemotherapy and/or hormonal therapy have been made but the effect remains largely unstudied.

9. Which patients should be considered for postoperative adjuvant chemotherapy and/or hormonal therapy?
This is a difficult question to answer. What is being done in clinical practice does *not* always reflect the results of clinical trial outcomes. The facts are:
  1. The initial studies from 10–20 years ago demonstrated the benefit of adjuvant chemotherapy in preventing and/or delaying the recurrence of breast cancer in premenopausal, lymph node (LN)–positive women. There also was a demonstrable improvement in overall survival.
  2. Tamoxifen (an antiestrogen hormonal agent) was proved to improve disease-free survival (DFS) and overall survival (OS) in trials first reported in 1985.
  3. More recent studies now are expanding the applicability of postoperative chemotherapy to pre- and postmenopausal and LN+ and LN– women. Likewise, adjuvant tamoxifen has shown benefit in pre- and postmenopausal and LN+ and LN– women.
  4. The combination of chemotherapy and tamoxifen is currently being studied to determine whether they have an additive, synergistic, or antagonistic interaction. Early results suggest an additive benefit of combination adjuvant therapy.

10. Although adjuvant tamoxifen has been shown to improve DFS and OS, what other benefits are obtained from this hormonal agent?
  • Decreases chest wall recurrences by 50%
  • Decreases breast recurrences in lumpectomy/RT–treated patients by 50%
  • Decreases new contralateral breast cancers by 50%
  • Prevents calcium loss from the bone
  • Improves lipid profile (decreases total cholesterol by lowering low-density lipoprotein [LDL] levels)
  • Induces vaginal secretions in one-third of postmenopausal women
  • Possibly decreases the incidence of ovarian cancer by 50%

11. What are the potential downsides to adjuvant tamoxifen?
- Exacerbation of preexisting hot flashes
- Menstrual irregularity in premenopausal women
- Vaginal discharge related to a resumption of vaginal secretions
- Increased incidence of endometrial cancer; approximately a 1/1500 chance per year
- Increased incidence of phlebitis or thromboembolic disease; approximately a 1/800 chance per year
- Cost of $75 to $80 per month
- Depression in 1% to 10% of patients
- Retinal effects, which are rare and usually reversible
- Increased estrogen levels in young premenopausal women leading to PMS-like symptoms

12. How should the patient with metastatic disease be approached in relationship to her treatment?

Because the current treatment of metastatic breast cancer is not curative, the goal of the physician caring for these women is **palliation!** The average woman with spread of her breast cancer will live 18–24 months. This figure has not changed during the last 50 years of advances in cancer therapy.

The first goal in these patients is to find the patient who will respond to hormonal manipulations. Hormone treatments have much fewer toxic side effects than chemotherapy. Even a woman whose cancer was hormone receptor negative has a 10% chance of objective disease regression and a 20–30% chance of disease stabilization with hormone therapy. Hormone therapy includes tamoxifen, megesterol acetate, aminoglutethimide/hydrocortisone, diethylstilbestrol (DES) and/or halotestin. As long as the patient does not have immediately life-threatening disease such as significant liver involvement and/or lymphangitic spread in the lung, an attempt at hormonal therapy should be considered.

Radiation to a few sites of bony metastases can quickly palliate the woman with significant pain. Care must be taken to limit the total area of RT. With extensive RT, the bone marrow becomes permanently damaged, which may prohibit the use of other systemic modalities such as chemotherapy. Chemotherapy also may be used to treat all sites of spread, including bones.

CONTROVERSIES

13. Every woman with invasive breast cancer should be offered adjuvant tamoxifen.

For:

When you review the list of potential benefits already demonstrated in women with invasive breast cancer, which include many effects totally unrelated to her cancer, an argument can be made that tamoxifen can positively affect a woman's life and therefore should be offered to all women with breast cancer. Although tamoxifen has largely been offered only for estrogen receptor (ER)–positive breast cancers in the United States, two large studies in the United Kingdom (NATO and Scottish Trials) have shown the same benefit in DFS and OS in ER– tumors. One researcher has even stated that ER– women receive even more benefit than ER+ women because of their higher risk of recurrence. If a woman experiences untoward side effects from the medication, then she can decide whether these adverse reactions are not worth the potential benefits and discontinue the drug.

Against:

The absolute reduction of risk of metastatic disease in women who already have a high likelihood of being "cured" of their breast cancer does not warrant the cost of this therapy. In a group of LN– women with breast cancer, tamoxifen could decrease the risk of recurrence from 24% to 18%. This 25% reduction in recurrences translates into a benefit for 6/100 women at a monetary cost of nearly $900/year/patient. The potential life-threatening effects of tamoxifen such as pulmonary embolus and endometrial carcinoma, along with the cost of the diagnostic work-ups for women with complaints in their lower legs and those with postmenopausal bleeding, are not insignificant. Psychologically, women who take tamoxifen also are constantly being reminded of their diagnosis of breast cancer. The use of tamoxifen also leads to the use of even more medications to control side effects such as clonidine/vitamin E/bellargal-S for hot flashes, mild anxiety medications for PMS symptoms, and mood elevators for tamoxifen-associated depression.

14. High-dose chemotherapy with autologous bone marrow transplant, or more appropriately described as stem-cell rescue, should be available to all qualifying women.
For:
Because the prognosis of metastatic breast cancer is an average survival of 18–24 months with 98% of patients having died by 10 years and with all of these women requiring some form of therapy for the rest of their lives, high-dose chemotherapy with stem-cell rescue offers a 15–20% chance for long-term DFS without the need for further therapy. These women who have been followed for up to 10 years post-transplant in a sustained remission are very likely *cured* of their breast cancer, which is a term never before used in the treatment of metastatic disease. The issue of cost is greatly exaggerated, because it already costs $30,000 to $100,000/year to treat a woman with metastatic breast cancer. The cost of loss of productivity must also be figured into the equation, because the women who qualify for high-dose chemotherapy with stem-cell rescue are younger with many more years of potential productivity.
Against:
How can this country in times of runaway health care costs and astronomical budget deficits be spending approximately $150,000 per patient to treat a disease with only a 15–20% chance of long-term DFS. This therapy also carries a significant upfront mortality of between 5% and 15%, depending on the particular institution, thus potentially shortening the life of a woman who would normally have lived 18–24 months. For those women who actually survive the treatment, some of them are left with significant long-term side effects. Until a large, multi-institutional, randomized study has been conducted comparing conventional therapy with high-dose chemotherapy and stem-cell rescue, this treatment modality must still be considered experimental.

BIBLIOGRAPHY

1. Baum M, Brinkley DM, Dossett JA, et al: Controlled trial of tamoxifen as single adjuvant agent in management of early breast cancer. Analysis at six years by Nolvadex Adjuvant Trial Organisation. Lancet 1:836, 1985.
2. Early Breast Cancer Trialist's Collaborative Group: Systemic treatment of early breast cancer by hormonal, cytotoxic, or immune therapy. Lancet 1:1, 71, 1992.
3. Fisher B, Costantino J, Redmond C, et al: A randomized clinical trial evaluating tamoxifen in the treatment of patients with node-negative breast cancer who have estrogen-positive tumors. N Engl J Med 320:479, 1989.
4. Fisher B, Costantino J, Redmond C, et al: Lumpectomy compared with lumpectomy and radiation therapy for the treatment of intraductal breast cancer. N Engl J Med 328:1581, 1993.
5. Fisher B, Redmond C, Poisson R, et al: Eight-year results of a randomized clinical trial comparing total mastectomy and lumpectomy with or without irradiation in the treatment of breast cancer. N Engl J Med 320:822, 1989.
6. Harris JR, Lippman ME, Veronesi U, Willett W: Breast cancer. N Engl J Med 327:319, 390, 473, 1992.
7. Love RR, Mazess RB, Barden HS, et al: Effects of tamoxifen on bone mineral density in postmenopausal women with breast cancer. N Engl J Med 326:852, 1992.
8. Love RR, Newcomb PA, Wiebe DL, et al: Lipid and lipoprotein effects of tamoxifen therapy in postmenopausal women with node negative breast cancer. J Natl Cancer Inst 82:1327, 1990.
9. Mansour EG, Gray R, Shatila AH, et al: Efficacy of adjuvant chemotherapy in high-risk node-negative breast cancer. An Intergroup Study. N Engl J Med 320:485, 1989.
10. Sedlacek S: The effect of tamoxifen on serum lipids in premenopausal women with breast cancer. Breast Cancer Res Treat 23:168, 1992.

64. LUNG CANCER

Karen Kelly, M.D.

1. What is the incidence of lung cancer and lung cancer deaths in both men and women in the United States?
In the United States, lung cancer is the leading cause of cancer deaths. It is estimated that 170,000 Americans are diagnosed with lung cancer each year and greater than 85% of these patients will die from their disease. Recently, lung cancer surpassed breast cancer as the leading cause of cancer deaths among women. This observation correlates with the increase in the number of women who smoke. In contrast, the number of men who smoke is decreasing. Even if a cigarette smoker quits smoking today, his or her risk of developing lung cancer declines but at 15 years the risk is still 1.5 (with 1.0 the risk for a nonsmoker).

2. Besides smokers, who else gets lung cancer?
Persons exposed to asbestos (such as shipyard workers and insulators) and radon (from underground mining or previous radiation therapy) are at greater risk for lung cancer. Other substances that have been associated with lung cancer include arsenic, nickel-cadmium, chromium, and chloromethyl ether. Underlying lung disease with scarring or chronic obstructive pulmonary disease (COPD) predisposes patients to lung cancer. Passive smoking exposure accounts for 3–5% of all cases of lung cancer. Remember, these risks are dramatically increased in smokers versus nonsmokers.

3. Patients with lung cancer often present with nonspecific pulmonary complaints such as cough, dyspnea, chest pain, hemoptysis, and/or weight loss. What test would raise your suspicion for lung cancer?
A mass on a chest radiograph. Although 85% of patients have symptoms from their disease, 15% of patients will be asymptomatic and an incidental mass will be discovered on a routine chest radiograph. Once a mass has been identified, the patient is presumed to have lung cancer until proved otherwise.

4. What other symptoms could a patient with lung cancer present with?
A variety of paraneoplastic syndromes are associated with lung cancer. Paraneoplastic syndromes are defined as signs and symptoms related to a peptide hormone secreted by the tumor. The most common are hypercalcemia associated with squamous cell lung cancer and hyponatremia associated with small-cell lung cancer. Treatment of the underlying tumor usually reverses the clinical manifestations of the paraneoplastic syndrome. In addition, return of the paraneoplastic syndrome can be the first sign of recurrence. Evidence of a paraneoplastic syndrome is not synonymous with metastatic disease. Documentation of metastatic lesions is crucial to avoid subjecting a patient to a palliative therapy when curative intervention is available and vice versa.

5. Does it matter what histologic type of lung cancer a patient has?
Yes. The management of the patient is based on whether the patient has small cell lung cancer (SCLC) versus non–small cell lung cancer (NSCLC). Chemotherapy is the cornerstone of treatment for all patients with small cell histology, whereas surgery, radiation, and/or chemotherapy may be recommended for patients with NSCLC. SCLC accounts for 20% to 25% of all lung cancers; therefore, NSCLC occurs in the majority of patients. NSCLC can be subdivided into squamous cell carcinoma (30%), adenocarcinoma (30%), large cell undifferentiated (15%), and bronchoalveolar (1% to 3%).

6. How does lung cancer spread?

The route of spread for NSCLC is to the peribronchial and hilar lymph nodes and then to mediastinal lymph nodes. Distant sites of metastases include the opposite lung, liver, bone, brain, and adrenal glands. More than half the patients will present with extrathoracic spread. Two thirds of the patients with SCLC will present with extensive-stage disease. Common sites of involvement include the liver, lung, bone, bone marrow, and brain.

7. What tests can be used to identify areas of spread of lung cancer?

All patients require a complete history and physical examination, a routine complete blood cell count, and blood chemistries. For patients with NSCLC, a staging work-up includes computed tomographic (CT) scan of the chest and abdomen, bone scan, and a brain scan. If there is no evidence of metastatic disease and the patient is considered *medically and surgically operable,* then mediastinoscopy should be performed to stage the chest accurately. For patients diagnosed with SCLC, the following additional tests are required: CT scan of the chest and abdomen, bone scan, brain scan, and bilateral bone marrow biopsies.

8. What are the stages of lung cancer?

The current staging schema for NSCLC uses the TNM classification that is designed to determine the extent of disease, which can then be used to determine treatment and assess prognosis. T describes the primary tumor, N identifies lymph node involvement, and M represents metastatic disease. The stages for NSCLC are:

Stage I (T1N0M0, T2N0M0): A tumor <3 cm (T1) or >3 cm with or without extension to the visceral pleura (T2) and at least 2 cm from the carina, which is not accompanied by lymph node or metastatic spread

Stage II (T1N1M0, T2N1M0): A tumor of any size as described in stage I but with extension into intrabronchial lymph nodes (N1)

Stage IIIa (T3N0M0, T1-2N2M0): A tumor of any size that extends into the parietal pleura, chest wall, or mediastinal pleura (T3) and/or hilar or ipsilateral mediastinal lymph node involvement (N2)

Stage IIIb (T4 with any N or any T with N3): A tumor of any size that invades mediastinal structures (heart, great vessels, esophagus, vertebrae) (T4) and/or involves contralateral hilar, mediastinal, or supraclavicular lymph nodes (N3)

Stage IV (any T or N with a M): A tumor with evidence of distant metastasis. SCLC is staged as either limited or extensive disease.

Limited stage: Disease confined to one hemithorax, mediastinal, hilar, or supraclavicular areas that could be encompassed within a single radiation therapy port

Extensive stage: Any disease spread outside the previously stated areas

9. What are the accepted treatment modalities for lung cancer?

For stages I and II NSCLC, surgical resection of the lobe of the lung containing the tumor is the standard of care. Patients with stage IIIa disease represent a very heterogeneous population. Patients with T3N0 tumors do very well with surgical resection alone, but patients with mediastinal lymph node involvement (T1-3N2) do not. Trials are under way to determine if combined modality with chemotherapy plus radiation therapy with or without surgery is advantageous. For patients not eligible for trials, the use of chemotherapy with radiation or surgery is a rational approach. Patients with stage IIIb disease are currently treated with radiation therapy alone; however, efforts to improve survival with radiation and chemotherapy look promising. Patients with metastatic disease are offered chemotherapy or the best supportive care.

Concurrent administration of radiation therapy and chemotherapy is the treatment of choice for patients with limited-stage SCLC. Unlike patients with NSCLC, patients with extensive-stage SCLC should all receive chemotherapy, because the majority of patients will respond. Chemotherapy has clearly been shown to improve survival from 1 month without treatment to 9 to 12 months with drug therapy.

10. Does staging of lung cancer affect survival?

Yes. The following survival curve clearly demonstrates the effect of stage on 5-year survival in patients with NSCLC.

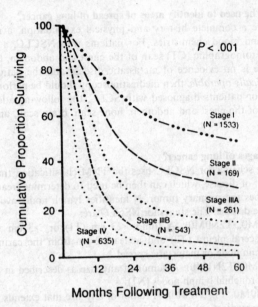

Survival of NSCLC patients by clinical stage. (From Mountain CF: A new international staging system for lung cancer. Chest 89(Suppl):225S–233S, 1986, with permission.)

This holds true for patients with SCLC as well:
Limited SCLC: 5% to 10% (5 years) 15 months (median)
Extensive SCLC: 0% to 1% (5 years) 9 months (median)

11. Are there any tests that can detect lung cancer at an early, curative stage?

No. The 1960s screening trials using chest radiography and sputum cytology in a high-risk population of male smokers did not show any survival benefit and cannot be recommended. To date, no trial has evaluated chest radiography alone, and a nationwide study is currently under way. Attempts to reevaluate sputum with more sensitive staining techniques also is ongoing and shows promising results.

CONTROVERSIES

12. Should patients with stage IV NSCLC receive chemotherapy?

For:
Patients with this diagnosis want therapy.
Patients who respond to chemotherapy live longer than patients who do not respond.
Patients who respond to therapy have a better quality of life.
Response can be predicted. Patients with good performance status, weight loss <5%, female sex, and minimal tumor burden are more likely to respond to chemotherapy.

Six trials of best supportive care versus combination chemotherapy have demonstrated a prolongation in survival in favor of the chemotherapy arm; however, this was not statistically significant in all of the trials.

The randomized trials of best supportive care versus combination chemotherapy are flawed by their small patient accruals that do not allow for a small increase in survival to be detected.

Against:

Although some trials have shown a survival advantage, it is only in terms of weeks (7–17).

The response rate with the most active regimen (a platinum-containing regimen) is 20–30% with rare complete responders (<5%).

The drug regimens are toxic.

BIBLIOGRAPHY

1. Bunn PA: Lung Cancer: Current Understanding of the Biology, Diagnosis, Staging, and Treatment. 1992.
2. Gazdar AF, Linnoila RI: The pathology of lung cancer—Changing concepts and newer diagnostic techniques. Semin Oncol 15:215–225, 1988.
3. Hinson JA, Perry MC: Small cell lung cancer. CA Cancer J Clin 43:216–225, 1993.
4. Ihde DC: Chemotherapy of lung cancer. N Engl J Med 327:1434–1441, 1992.
5. Martini N: Operable lung cancer. CA Cancer J Clin 43:201–214, 1993.
6. Mountain CF: A new international staging system for lung cancer. Chest 89(Suppl):225S–233S, 1986.
7. Mountain CF: Therapy of stage I and stage II non-small cell lung cancer. Semin Oncol 10:71–80, 1983.
8. Tockman MS, Gupta OK, Myer JD, et al: Sensitive and specific monoclonal antibody recognition of human lung cancer antigen on preserved sputum cells: A new approach to early lung cancer detection. J Clin Oncol 6:2685–2693, 1988.
9. Van Raemdonck DE, Schneider A, Ginsberg RJ: Surgical treatment for higher stage non-small cell lung cancer. Ann Thorac Surg 54:999–1013, 1992.

65. ESOPHAGEAL CANCER

Justin D. Cohen, M.D.

1. What is the most common cell type in esophageal cancer?

From 90–95% of primary esophageal cancers are squamous cell carcinomas. The remainder are almost all adenocarcinomas with rare leiomyosarcomas or melanomas. Benign leiomyomas are uncommon, and metastases to the esophagus from other organs are surprisingly rare.

2. Does the incidence of esophageal cancer vary much geographically?

Esophageal cancer actually has the greatest geographic variation of any major type of malignancy. The annual incidence varies dramatically from 0.7:100,000 to 436:100,000. A monstrous "esophageal cancer belt" cuts a broad swath from east to west across the entire continent of Asia. This and many other areas of high incidence are associated with dietary carcinogen and promoter exposures.

3. What causes esophageal cancer in the United States?

Smoking, usually with the important promoter effect of alcohol, causes most esophageal cancer in the United States. These risk factors and esophageal cancer are more frequent in lower socioeconomic groups.

4. Which other groups are at increased risk?
Roughly 7% of patients with achalasia and 5% of patients with lye stricture will develop esophageal squamous cell carcinoma at some point. Individuals with a metaplastic columnar lined lower esophagus (Barrett's esophagus), **particularly those with high-grade dysplasia,** are at increased risk for adenocarcinoma of the gastroesophageal junction.

5. How do most esophageal cancer patients present?
The majority present because of dysphagia or odynophagia. Interestingly, symptoms usually develop only after the luminal circumference has decreased to 30–50% of normal.

6. What are the best radiographic measures of resectability of esophageal cancer?
Tumor bulk, extent of invasion, resectability, and curability all correlate strongly with the length of tumor defect seen on barium or air contrast esophagram or computed tomographic (CT) scan. Some 40% of tumors <5 cm in length are localized, 25% are locally advanced, and 35% have distant metastases. Only 5–10% are localized when tumor length is >5 cm. CT scans add important detail regarding erosion into adjacent structures and the possibility of lymph node and hepatic metastases.

7. If surgery is considered for esophageal cancer, what other preoperative evaluations are useful?
Many patients are heavy smokers with related pulmonary and cardiac disease. Congestive heart failure, significant symptoms of cardiac ischemia, or advanced pulmonary disease usually exclude surgical resection. Formal pulmonary function testing, an electrocardiogram, nutritional assessment (e.g., serum albumin), and careful history are important. The possibility of alcoholic liver disease, related coagulopathy, or portal hypertension should be considered. Liver function enzymes are occasionally useful.

8. Are synchronous or metachronous second malignancies a significant problem in esophageal cancer?
Patients with esophageal squamous cell carcinomas have a 5–12% incidence of simultaneous or metachronous malignancies. These primarily include lung cancers and squamous cell carcinomas of the head and neck. Three fourths of synchronous malignancies are symptomatic.

9. Can esophageal cancer be surgically controlled?
In some studies, as many as 30% of patients with localized disease will have 5-year disease-free survival. Even with positive regional lymph node metastases (including celiac nodes), as many as 10–15% of patients who survive esophagectomy may live 5 years without recurrent disease. More extensive disease is almost invariably incurable and therapy should focus on maintaining swallowing. For most patients, optimal chance of long-term tumor control and optimal palliation are both served by aggressively acting to control the primary tumor in the esophagus.

10. Is esophageal cancer ever considered cured?
Most oncologists consider 5-year disease free survival a cure in this disease. However, *some* studies have suggested that as many as 78% of patients free of cancer 5 years postoperatively may ultimately die of recurrent esophageal cancer.

11. Does nutrition affect the surgical outcome of esophageal cancer?
In formal studies, patients have had fewer postoperative complications if given 5 days of preoperative nutritional support. Enteric feeding has been shown to work as well as parenteral feeding and is the route of choice.

12. How large should surgical margins be in esophageal cancer?
Esophageal cancer can spread surprisingly far beyond grossly visible tumor following the extensive lymphatic network of the esophagus. Nests of cancer cells can be 8 cm beyond

visible tumor—right in the middle of what appears to be normal esophagus. Tumors that appear localized to the cervical esophagus often have metastases to celiac lymph nodes! For these reasons, esophageal cancers are generally treated with subtotal or total esophagectomy if technically practical. "Segmental resections" have up to 45% incidence of local anastomotic recurrence.

13. What are advantages and disadvantages of surgery for esophageal cancer?
Depending on surgical skill and patient selection, surgery alone offers 5-year disease free survival of 2–20% (combining localized and more extensive disease patients) but with mortality of 4–30%. Thus, excluding marginal surgical candidates is a critical concern. Complications related to surgery include stricture, adhesions, perforation, fistula, or hemorrhage. Surgery is difficult for high thoracic and cervical esophageal cancers, an area where radiation therapy is still practical.

14. What are advantages and disadvantages of radiation therapy in esophageal cancer?
Radiotherapy will restore swallowing in 60–80% of patients, may cure 2–10%, and rarely causes mortality. However, like surgery, radiotherapy can produce stricture, adhesions, perforation, fistulas or hemorrhage. Radiation also tends to produce a shorter duration of palliation and can take 6–8 weeks to complete, a serious limitation when median survival with radiation alone is only 24 weeks.

15. Are there contraindications to radiation therapy for esophageal cancer?
Individuals with airway fistula, mediastinitis, or hemorrhage have very short survival and often do even worse if irradiated. These patients are candidates only for minimal palliative interventions such as gastrostomy tubes.

16. Which drugs are effective against esophageal cancer?
Esophageal cancers, both squamous and adenocarcinomas, have complete and partial responses in 20–40% of patients treated with single-agent cisplatin, mitomycin C, 5-fluorouracil, or bleomycin. Other drugs have produced 10–20% response rates.

17. How long do chemotherapy responses last in patients with esophageal cancer?
Those who respond to single agents generally do so for 2–3 months. Combinations of drugs (e.g., cisplatin + bleomycin, cisplatin + 5-fluorouracil) produce median response durations of 6–8 months. Occasional patients respond for more than 12 months.

18. What is the best way to treat new esophageal cancers?
Recently, radiotherapy combined with chemotherapy, for example, cisplatin plus 5-fluorouracil, has produced results easily comparable to surgery alone and with very infrequent mortality. Increasingly, it appears that combining radiation, chemotherapy, and surgery may offer optimal chances for palliation and cure.

BIBLIOGRAPHY

1. Aggestrup S, Holm JC, Sorensen HR: Does achalasia predispose to cancer of the esophagus? Chest 102:1013–1016, 1992.
2. Elias D, Mankarios H, Lasser P, et al: Epidermoid cancers of the operated esophagus: High incidence of associated neoplasia. Presse Med 21:652–656, 1992.
3. Herskovic A, Martz K, al Serraf M, et al: Combined chemotherapy and radiotherapy compared with radiotherapy alone in patients with cancer of the esophagus. N Engl J Med 326:1593–1598, 1992.
4. Mamontov AS, Kiseleva ES, Kucharenko VM, Zimina HS: Combined therapy of thoracic esophageal cancer. Semin Surg Oncol 8:21–26, 1992.
5. Pera M, Trastek VF, Carpenter HA, Allen MS, et al: Barrett's esophagus with high grade dysplasia: An indication for esophagectomy? Ann Thorac Surg 54:199–204, 1992.

6. Toh Y, Kuwano H, Tanaka S, et al: Detection of human papillomavirus DNA in esophageal carcinoma in Japan by polymerase chain reaction. Cancer 70:2234–2238, 1992.
7. Tytgat GN, Hameeteman W: The neoplastic potential of columnar lined (Barrett's) esophagus. World J Surg 16:308–312, 1992.

66. GASTRIC CANCER

Justin D. Cohen, M.D.

1. How is the incidence of gastric cancer changing in the United States?
The incidence of gastric cancer has declined strikingly in the past three decades, perhaps owing to changes in diet and food preservation methods.

2. What dietary, medical, and social factors are associated with gastric cancer?
Gastric cancer is associated with consumption of smoked or salted foods and aflatoxin. There may be a small (twofold) increase in risk with cigarette smoking. Immigrants from Japan (and probably other high-risk areas such as Chile) and their children, asbestos workers, and lower socioeconomic groups also are at increased risk. Gastric cancer is as much as 20-fold more common in patients with pernicious anemia. Finally, gastric resection for peptic ulcers is associated with an increased incidence of gastric cancer one to three decades later. It no longer appears that blood group A or atrophic gastritis per se is associated with gastric cancer. However, bacterial growth in atrophic gastritis with production of carcinogenic N-nitroso products may be an important factor in many gastric cancers. There is strong evidence that *Helicobacter pylori* colonization may be an important causative factor.

3. What cell types of gastric cancer are common?
Roughly 95% of gastric cancers are adenocarcinomas. Squamous cell carcinomas, carcinoid tumors, lymphomas, and leiomyosarcomas comprise the remainder.

4. What is the typical appearance of a gastric cancer?
A stereotypical gastric carcinoma exceeds 2 cm in diameter and has borders raised above the surrounding mucosa. However, gastric cancers can appear quite benign both radiograph-ically and endoscopically, can be polypoid (about 10%), or can present in a "scirrhous" pattern with a thickened, rigid gastric wall (linitis plastica) because of diffuse infiltration by anaplastic cells.

5. Does tumor appearance relate to prognosis of gastric cancer?
Polypoid lesions tend to be better differentiated and have an above-average prognosis. Linitis plastica is clinically very aggressive and is almost invariably fatal.

6. Is there a premalignant lesion in gastric cancer?
Studies in Japan suggest that intestinal metaplasia of the stomach is a premalignant lesion that tends to correlate with well-differentiated and sometimes polypoid tumors. Anaplastic or scirrhous carcinomas are associated less with metaplasia.

7. Are gastric polyps or ulcers precursors to cancer?
Most gastric polyps do not contain or lead to cancer. Cancer occurs in roughly 40% of villous polyps but rarely or never in hyperplastic, adenomatous, or hamartomatous polyps. Gastric ulcers do not predispose to gastric cancer. However, ulceration can develop next to cancer. Presumably for this reason, cancer is identified in up to 3% of *resected* gastric ulcers.

8. Where in the stomach does gastric cancer arise?
Most tumors occur in the lower third of the stomach. The cardia has the lowest incidence.

9. Can gastric cancers be multicentric?
A second gastric tumor is *grossly* apparent in over 2% of patients. Careful histologic examination reveals multicentric disease in about 20% of gastric resection specimens.

10. How often is gastric cancer localized?
Cancer is limited to the stomach in about 8% to 11% of patients with a typical population that is not screened for gastric cancer. In one series, overall 5-year disease-free survival was 7% but was 30% in patients with localized disease.

11. Can screening improve prognosis of gastric cancer?
Tumors have clearly been less extensive and survival has been higher in endoscopically screened Japanese. However, gastric cancer causes 40% of all cancer deaths in Japan. In the United States, screening has merit only for individuals at especially increased risk; for example, in individuals with pernicious anemia and in immigrants from Japan or Chile.

12. What is the role of surgery in gastric cancer?
Increasingly, it appears that total gastrectomy may offer a better chance of cure than does subtotal gastric resection—including for localized tumors. The much less morbid subtotal gastrectomy is usually preferable when the objective is only palliation. Thus, gross metastatic disease must be carefully excluded before pursuing a "curative" resection. Unfortunately, local and regional recurrence are the norm even after surgery with curative intent.

13. Is adjuvant chemotherapy or radiation useful in gastric cancer?
At present, there is no proven role for adjuvant chemotherapy. Adjuvant radiation has also produced interesting but not definitive results. Ironically, gastric cancer is relatively sensitive to radiation and to a number of drugs and drug combinations; for example, cisplatin, 5-fluorouracil, doxorubicin, mitomycin C, and nitrosoureas. Combinations of these drugs have produced complete and partial responses in up to 50% of patients with metastatic disease. Because most "completely" resected gastric cancers recur locally, there is a strong rationale for these patients participating in studies of adjuvant chemotherapy with or without radiation.

BIBLIOGRAPHY

1. Bartram CI: Imaging of the stomach and duodenum. Curr Opin Radiol 4:26–31, 1992.
2. Bonenkamp HJ, Sasako M, Kampschoer GH, van de Velde CJ: The surgical treatment of gastric cancer with special reference to systematic lymph node dissection. Cancer Treat Res 55:339–356, 1991.
3. Caygill CP, Hill MJ: Malignancy following surgery for benign peptic disease: A review. Ital J Gastroenterol 24:218–224, 1992.
4. Elder JB, Knight T: Surgical suppression of gastric acid secretion. Lessons from long-term followup studies. Scand J Gastroenterol 188(Suppl):26–32, 1991.
5. Leichman L, Berry BT: Cisplatin therapy for adenocarcinoma of the stomach. Semin Oncol 18(Suppl 3):25–33, 1991.
6. Lise M, Nitti D, Marchet A, Fornesiero A: Adjuvant treatment for gastric cancer. Anticancer Drugs 2:433–445, 1991.
7. Macdonald JS: Gastric cancer: Chemotherapy of advanced disease. Hematol Oncol 10:37–42, 1992.
8. Rohde H: Staging of gastric cancer: Clinical, surgical, and pathological. Cancer Treat Res 55:91–106, 1991.
9. Smith JW, Brennan MF: Surgical treatment of gastric cancer: Proximal, mid, and distal stomach. Surg Clin North Am 72:381–399, 1992.
10. Tepper JE: Combined radiotherapy and chemotherapy in the treatment of gastrointestinal malignancies. Semin Oncol 19:96–101, 1992.
11. Weese JL, Nussbaum ML: Gastric cancer—Surgical approach. Hematol Oncol 10:31–35, 1992.

12. Wils JA: Perspectives in chemotherapy of advanced gastric cancer. Anticancer Drugs 2:133–137, 1991.
13. Young GP, Demediuk BH: The genetics, epidemiology and early detection of gastrointestinal cancers. Curr Opin Oncol 4:728–735, 1992.

67. COLORECTAL CARCINOMA

Allen L. Cohn, M.D.

1. What is the incidence of colorectal carcinoma in the United States?

Each year, approximately 155,000 new cases of colorectal carcinoma are diagnosed in the United States. This represents 15% of all cancers. Cancer of the large intestine affects approximately 1 in every 20 people in the United States.

2. What are some of the inherited syndromes associated with colorectal carcinoma?

Familial adenomatous polyposis syndrome is an autosomal dominant trait with approximately 90% penetrance and affects approximately 1 person in 7000. Virtually 100% of patients affected by this syndrome will develop a colorectal cancer if no intervention takes place. Gardner's syndrome is an autosomal dominant trait that occurs at approximately one-half the frequency of familial adenomatous polyposis. Patients afflicted with this syndrome have many adenomas in the small and large intestines. Oldfield's syndrome is similar to Gardner's syndrome except patients also have multiple sebaceous cysts in addition to polyposis and adenocarcinoma of the colon. Turcot's syndrome is less common and is inherited as an autosomal recessive trait. Patients with this syndrome develop malignant tumors of the colon and central nervous system.

3. Are any familial cancer syndromes associated with colorectal cancer?

Yes. There are two hereditary non–polyposis colorectal cancer syndromes. The first is inherited as an autosomal dominant trait with 90% penetrance. Patients present with multiple colon cancers at an early age. The second syndrome also is inherited as an autosomal dominant trait. Patients develop early onset of adenocarcinomas of the colon, ovary, pancreas, breast, bile duct, and ureters. First-degree relatives of patients afflicted with this syndrome have a sevenfold increase in cancer risk.

4. Is inflammatory bowel disease associated with an increased risk of colorectal carcinoma?

Yes. Patients with ulcerative colitis have about a 30-fold increase in the risk of colorectal cancer if no intervention takes place. Patients with Crohn's disease may have some increased risk of colorectal carcinoma but not to the degree associated with ulcerative colitis.

5. What preoperative evaluation should be done prior to surgery for suspected or confirmed colorectal carcinoma?

All patients should have a complete blood count, liver function tests, carcinoembryonic antigen (CEA) level, chest radiograph, and colonoscopy to rule out any synchronous primary tumors as well as polyps. In addition, a CT scan of the abdomen and pelvis should be done to rule out any metastatic disease.

6. What is the Astler-Collier modification of the Duke's staging system for colorectal carcinoma?

Stage A is tumor penetration that is confined to the mucosa of the intestine. Duke's stage B1 is a tumor that penetrates into the muscularis layer. Duke's stage B2 is tumor penetration through the muscularis into the serosa or perirectal fat. Duke's stages C1 and C2 represent Duke's stages B1 and B2, respectively, with lymph node involvement. Duke's stage D represents metastatic disease.

7. What is the TNM staging system for colon carcinoma?
The TNM staging system looks at the size of the primary tumor (T), regional lymph node involvement (N), and metastatic disease (M). T1 represents invasion into the submucosa, T2 is invasion into the muscularis propria, T3 is invasion into the serosa or perirectal fat, and T4 is invasion into the free peritoneal cavity or into a contiguous organ. N0 would represent no metastatic disease to regional lymph nodes, and N1 represents one to three positive lymph nodes. N2 would be four or more positive lymph nodes. M0 represents no metastatic disease present, and M1 is the stage when distant metastasis are present. Stage I cancer comprises T1–T2 and N0 tumors, corresponding to Duke's stage A. Stage II corresponds to Duke's B cancers, (T3–T4 and N0). Stage III is made up of any T stage and node-positive tumors (N1–N3) corresponding to Duke's stage C. Metastatic tumors are stage IV.

8. How are the patterns of metastatic spread different for rectal and colon carcinomas?
Colon cancer typically will metastasize to regional nodes and the liver owing to the fact that the venous drainage is through the portal system. Distal rectal cancers are more likely to have isolated lung metastasis, because the venous drainage of the distal rectum is through the inferior and medial hemorrhoidal veins and not the portal system.

9. What is the primary treatment for tumors of the colon and rectum?
Surgery is the primary treatment for most cases. Hemicolectomy is the surgery of choice for colon carcinomas. Low anterior resection or abdominal perineal resection is the surgery of choice for rectal carcinomas depending on the proximity of the tumor to the anal sphincter. For small rectal tumors near the sphincter, there are sphincter-sparing approaches such as a transanal resection, posterior proctectomy, or a coloanal pull through.

10. Are there any adjuvant treatments for colon cancer after surgical resection?
Recent studies have shown a survival benefit for patients with Duke's stage C colon cancer treated with adjuvant 5-fluorouracil and levamisole. There has been a trend toward improved survival for Duke's stage B, but this is not statistically significant.

11. Are there any adjuvant treatments for rectal cancer?
Studies using the combination of postoperative radiation therapy combined with chemo-therapy with 5-fluorouracil have shown improved survival rates as well as decreased local relapse rates for Duke's stages B2 and C rectal cancers.

12. Does surgery play any role in the treatment of isolated liver metastasis?
Patients with solitary liver metastasis or several metastases confined to one lobe of the liver are candidates for hepatic resection with intent to cure. There is about a 20% 5-year survival in patients who are resected for cure.

13. Is chemotherapy effective for metastatic disease?
The combination of 5-fluorouracil and leucovorin is the standard chemotherapy for metastatic disease. There are many different treatment regimens available, yielding response rates between 25% and 35%, with little overall effect on survival.

BIBLIOGRAPHY

1. American Joint Committee on Cancer: Manual for Staging of Cancer, 3rd ed. Philadelphia, J.B. Lippincott, 1982.
2. DeVita VT, Hellman S, Rosenberg SA (eds): Cancer: Principles and Practice of Oncology, 4th ed. Philadelphia, J.B. Lippincott, 1993.

3. Erbe RW: Inherited gastrointestinal polyposis syndromes. N Engl J Med 294:1101–1104, 1976.
4. Huges KS, et al: Resection of the liver for colorectal carcinoma metastases: A multi-institutional study of patterns of recurrence. Surgery 100:778, 1986.
5. Lynch HT, Smyrk T, Watson P, et al: Hereditary colorectal cancer. Semin Oncol 18:337–366, 1991.
6. Moertel CG, Fleming TR, Macdonald JS, et al: Levamisole and fluorouracil for adjuvant therapy of resected colon carcinoma. N Engl J Med 322:352–356, 1990.
7. O'Connell M, Wieand H, Krook J, et al: Lack of value of methyl-CCNU (MeCCNU) as a component of effective rectal cancer surgical adjuvant therapy: Interim analysis of Intergroup Protocol 86-47-51. Proc Am Soc Clin Oncol 10:134, 1991 (abstr).
8. Olson RM, Perencevich NP, Malcom AW, et al: Patterns of recurrence following curative resection of adenocarcinoma of the colon and rectum. Cancer 45:2969–2974, 1980.
9. Poon MA, O'Connell MJ, Wieand HS, et al: Biochemical modulation of fluorouracil with leucovorin: Confirmatory evidence of improved therapeutic efficacy in advanced colorectal cancer. J Clin Oncol 9:1967–1972, 1991.
10. Roh MS: Hepatic resection for colorectal liver metastases. Hematol Oncol Clin North Am 3:171–184, 1989.

68. TUMORS OF THE LIVER AND BILIARY TREE

Louis A. Morris, M.D., and Stephen E. Steinberg, M.D.

LIVER

1. What is the most common type of liver malignancy?

Metastatic tumor involvement to the liver accounts for the majority of hepatic malignancies. The liver is a common site of metatastic spread in many common cancers, including those originating in the lung, breast, and gastrointestinal tract.

2. In what areas of the world is hepatoma (hepatocellular carcinoma) common and why?

Although relatively rare in the United States, hepatoma is one of the most common fatal malignancies in the world, causing more than a million deaths each year. It is most common in sub-Saharan Africa and the Far East, where hepatitis B is endemic. Epidemiologic studies have shown a 30-fold increased risk of hepatoma in HBsAg-positive patients.

Not all types of chronic hepatitis B infections are associated with the same risk of developing hepatocellular carcinoma. The highest risk of developing chronic hepatitis B and cirrhosis appears to be in those infections acquired vertically; that is, from mother to newborn infant. In contrast, in parenterally acquired hepatitis B, >90% of patients will clear the virus and not develop chronic hepatitis B.

3. Name other risk factors for the development of a hepatoma. Is cirrhosis of the liver a prerequisite?

Cirrhosis of the liver regardless of etiology is a major risk factor for hepatoma. This would include cirrhosis as a result of alcoholic liver disease, hemochromatosis, autoimmune chronic active hepatitis, alpha$_1$-antitrypsin deficiency, hepatitis C infection, and other rarer genetic conditions such as hereditary tyrosinemia and glycogen storage diseases. Other agents implicated in the pathogenesis of hepatocellular carcinoma include aflatoxin B$_1$ (especially in southern China and Africa) and exogenous steroids, including long-term use of oral contraceptives and high doses of anabolic steroids.

4. How do patients with hepatocellular carcinoma present?
Typically, the usual presenting symptoms are right upper quadrant pain, fatigue, abdominal swelling, and elevated bilirubin. Unusual presentations include massive bleeding into the peritoneum (hemoperitoneum), as these tumors can be quite vascular; and variceal hemorrhage secondary to portal hypertension resulting from invasion by tumor into the portal vein. The tumor also can invade the inferior vena cava and cause acute Budd-Chiari syndrome. Any acute change in an otherwise stable patient with cirrhosis should bring to mind the possibility of a superimposed hepatoma.

5. Which paraneoplastic syndromes are associated with hepatocellular carcinoma?
Rarely, patients have paraneoplastic syndromes associated with this tumor, including erythrocytosis, hyperthyroidism, hypercalcemia, hypertrophic pulmonary osteoarthropathy, and rarely hypoglycemia (usually a late sign).

6. What tumor markers are useful in the evaluation of hepatocellular carcinoma?
Alpha-fetoprotein (AFP) is an embryonic protein that can be markedly elevated in primary hepatocellular carcinoma approximately 70% of the time. Serum AFP levels appear to correlate with tumor size, as those patients with levels >500 ng/dl had larger tumors than those with levels <300 ng/dl. The use of this tumor marker has been mostly in screening high-risk populations and diagnosing tumor recurrence after resection. Although high levels correlate with hepatocellular carcinoma (and germ cell tumors), it needs to be remembered that lower elevations can occur with benign liver disease (e.g., exacerbation of hepatitis) and other gastrointestinal malignancies. In addition, false-negative values can be obtained with small tumors.

7. Name the most sensitive imaging modality for diagnosing small liver tumors.
Ultrasound and computed tomography (CT) are probably equivalent in diagnosing small tumors, imaging tumors as small as 2 cm. Ultrasound has proved useful in screening protocols in high-risk populations such as Alaskan Eskimos and Asian hepatitis B carriers.

8. Describe the recommended screening protocol developed for the early detection of hepatocellular carcinoma. Are there groups that are considered at increased risk and therefore should be screened on a regular basis?
The National Institutes of Health has issued a screening program for the detection of early tumors based on the tumor doubling time and the use of AFP and ultrasound as complementary tools. Screening is only recommended for those deemed to be at high or moderate risk for the development of hepatocellular carcinoma. Those at high risk are those with replicative hepatitis B virus infections (e antigen or hepatitis B DNA positive), for example, chronic active hepatitis or vertically acquired carrier state; and cirrhosis, particularly in nonwhite males. Hepatoma is a relatively slow-growing adenocarcinoma compared with others such as breast and colon cancer. This is important in that the disease can be present for years if not decades before it becomes clinically evident. In studies of serial ultrasound measurements in patients with primary hepatocellular carcinoma, the mean doubling time ranged from 1 month to 14 months with a median of 4 months. It is therefore recommended that these patients have serum AFP levels checked every 3–4 months and abdominal ultrasound every 4–6 months. Those at moderate risk (nonreplicative adult-acquired hepatitis B infection, e.g., surface antigen positive) are recommended to undergo yearly ultrasound and have AFP levels checked every 3–4 months.

9. What is the mortality for patients undergoing surgical resection of hepatocellular carcinoma? What are the factors that limit resectability of the primary tumor?
The only treatment that offers a chance for cure is surgical resection, which reinforces the importance of screening to detect small resectable tumors. Small tumors in patients without underlying liver disease have a 5-year survival as high as 85% in some series. Because these tumors occur against a background of chronic liver disease, the functional capacity of the

remaining liver is a major factor limiting the resectability of the tumor. Other factors that limit resectability include presence of metastasis (e.g., lung, porta hepatis, adrenal, inferior vena cava, and portal vein), size and location of the tumor (e.g., multicentric tumors), and presence of malignant lymph nodes. In most series, the rate of resectability is approximately 25%, and the 5-year survival rate of patients whose tumors are resected also is 25%. The overall 5-year survival rate is 10%.

10. Is there a role for orthotopic liver transplantation in the treatment of hepatoma?
In selected patients, liver transplantation appears to be useful, although tumor recurrence is common. Patients with tumors found incidentally during orthotopic liver transplantation for other reasons have a lower rate of recurrence because their tumors are usually small and have not metastasized.

BILIARY TREE

11. What is a Klatskin tumor?
In 1965, Klatskin described 13 patients with primary bile duct cancers (cholangiocarcinoma) occurring at the hepatic duct bifurcation. Cholangiocarcinoma at this location became known as a Klatskin tumor.

12. How does the location of a cholangiocarcinoma affect its prognosis?
Disseminated disease is found in 5–10% of patients at presentation. About 50–60% of cholangiocarcinomas occur in the common hepatic duct at the bifurcation (Klatskin tumors), or the intrahepatic ducts. Owing to unresectability, there are few if any disease-free survivors in these patients. Mid and distal common bile duct each account for 15–20% of cholangiocarcinomas. Five-year disease-free survivals following radical pancreaticoduodenectomy (Whipple procedure) may range from 25–40%.

13. Name the risk factors for the development of cholangiocarcinoma.
Strong associations for the development of cholangiocarcinoma have been found and include sclerosing cholangitis, cystic abnormalities of the bile duct, a radiocontrast agent called thorium dioxide and the liver fluke *Clonorchis sinensis*. Ulcerative colitis (even in the absence of sclerosing cholangitis) and gallstones may also represent risk factors. Most cholangiocarcinomas occur in older age groups without obvious risk factors. These may be more indolent, allowing 1- to 2-year survivals even in the absence of curative treatment. In contrast, tumors occurring in younger age groups with risk factors appear to be more aggressive.

14. How does the medical or surgical treatment of ulcerative colitis affect the natural history of primary sclerosing cholangitis and/or the development of cholangiocarcinoma?
The incidence of cholangiocarcinoma in patients with primary sclerosing cholangitis and chronic ulcerative colitis is severalfold higher than that of the general population and these patients present two decades earlier than the usual patients (40–45 years of age). They have usually had a long duration of colitis involving the entire bowel. The medical and surgical treatment of colitis does not appear to change the course of primary sclerosing cholangitis or the overall risk of developing biliary duct cancer.

15. How often is cholangitis the presenting sign of cholangiocarcinoma?
Rarely. The obstructing lesion serves to isolate undrained areas of the biliary tree from bacterial contamination. The most common presenting symptom is jaundice. In addition, pruritus and mild abdominal discomfort are frequently seen. Weight loss may occur as a result of steatorrhea secondary to absent bile salts (due to biliary obstruction) and/or the systemic effects of the tumor. Physical examination is usually only significant for jaundice and excoriations, although ascites and abdominal tenderness will occasionally be seen. Courvoisier's gallbladder may be present with distal lesions.

16. How often does CT scan or abdominal ultrasound show the primary tumor?
The CT or ultrasound findings that are suggestive of cholangiocarcinoma include a dilated intrahepatic biliary tree, a normal, dilated, or collapsed gallbladder (depending on the site of involvement), and a normal pancreas. Usually, it will spread along tissue planes as opposed to forming a mass lesion. As a result, the tumor itself is only seen in 20% of patients by ultrasound and 40% by CT scan, and these in later stages.

17. How can benign bile duct lesions be distinguished from malignant ones preoperatively?
It is often difficult to establish a preoperative diagnosis of cholangiocarcinoma by percutaneous needle aspiration biopsy or endoscopically obtained biopsies or brushings. The yield is approximately 50% with these modalities. Fortunately, the clinical presentation will almost always provide a clear distinction between benign and malignant strictures. It is therefore not always necessary (or possible) to establish a tissue diagnosis prior to surgery or palliative intervention. An important exception are those patients with primary sclerosing cholangitis in whom disease-related strictures may be indistinguishable from cholangiocarcinoma.

18. What is the role of liver transplantation in the treatment of cholangiocarcinoma?
The results of liver transplantation for cholangiocarcinoma have been disappointing with a <10% 2-year survival without tumor recurrence. At present, there is no role for orthotopic liver transplantation for this disease.

GALLBLADDER

19. What is the most important risk factor for the development of carcinoma of the gallbladder?
Gallbladder cancer accounts for two thirds of all cancers arising in the extrahepatic biliary tree. The majority of patients have gallstones present at diagnosis, suggesting a pathogenic mechanism. In addition, it appears that the risk of cancer is increased in those patients with large (>2.5 cm) stones. It needs to be remembered, however, that the vast majority of patients with gallstones will not develop gallbladder cancer, and except for the patient with a very large stone, cholecystectomy is not recommended for the prevention of gallbladder cancer.

20. What is a "porcelain" gallbladder?
Diffuse calcification in the wall of the gallbladder can make it radioopaque and this has been called a "porcelain" gallbladder. This risk of associated malignancy in this uncommon lesion has been reported from 3% to 20%. It is often considered an indication for cholecystectomy.

AMPULLARY CANCER

21. Which patients are at higher risk for ampullary tumors (tumors of the major papilla of Vater)?
Patients at risk for the development of duodenal villous adenomas and ampullary adenocarcinomas are those with familial adenomatosis polyposis syndromes, including Gardner's syndrome. Patients with carcinomas of the colon associated with hereditary cancer syndromes also are at increased risk.

22. Why should the diagnosis of ampullary cancer be considered in patients who present with progressive painless jaundice?
It is important to distinguish ampullary cancer from pancreatic carcinoma and cholangiocarcinoma because of prognosis. If confirmed with endoscopic retrograde cholangiopancreatography (ERCP), pancreatoduodenectomy affords a cure rate as high as 75% in some series.

BIBLIOGRAPHY

1. Blumgart LH, Benjamin IS: Liver resection for bile duct cancer. Surg Clin North Am 69:323–337, 1989.
2. Bosma A: Surgical pathology of cholangiocarcinoma of the liver hilus (Klatskin tumor). Semin Liver Dis 10:85–90, 1990.
3. Colombo M, De Franchis R, Ninno ED, et al: Hepatocellular carcinoma in Italian patients with cirrhosis. N Engl J Med 325:675–680, 1991.
4. Di Bisceglie AM, Rustgi VK, Hoofnagle JH, et al: Hepatocellular carcinoma. Ann Intern Med 108:390–401, 1988.
5. Ebara M, Ohto M, Shinagawa T, et al: Natural history of minute hepatocellular carcinoma smaller than three centimeters complicating cirrhosis: A study in 22 patients. Gastroenterology 90:289–298, 1986.
6. McMahon BJ, Lanier AP, Wainwright RB, Kilkenny SJ: Hepatocellular carcinoma in Alaska Eskimos: Epidemiology, clinical features, and early detection. In Popper H, Schaffner F (eds): Progress in Liver Diseases. Vol IX. New York, Harcourt Brace Jovanovich, 1990, pp 643–655.
7. McMahon BJ, London T: Workshop on screening for hepatocellular carcinoma. J Natl Cancer Inst 83:916–919, 1991.
8. Roslyn JJ: Cancer of the gallbladder and bile ducts. In Kaplowitz N (ed): Liver and Biliary Diseases. Baltimore, Williams & Wilkins, 1992, pp 658–672.
9. Sheu JC, Sung JL, Chen DS, et al: Early detection of hepatocellular carcinoma by real-time ultrasonography: A prospective study. Cancer 67:660–666, 1985.
10. Wanebo HJ, Falkson G, Order SE: Cancer of the hepatobiliary system. In DeVita VT, Hellman S, Rosenberg SA (eds): Cancer: Principles and Practice, 3rd ed. Philadelphia, J.B. Lippincott, 1989, pp 836–874.
11. Wands JR, Blum HE: Primary hepatocellular carcinoma. N Engl J Med 325:729–731, 1991.
12. Yeo CJ, Pitt HA, Cameron JL: Cholangiocarcinoma. Surg Clin North Am 70:1429–1447, 1990.

69. PANCREATIC CANCER

Louis A. Morris, M.D., and Stephen E. Steinberg, M.D.

1. List the known and suspected risk factors for pancreatic cancer. Is caffeine a risk?
The cause of pancreatic cancer remains unknown. The most clearly established risk factor for the development of pancreatic cancer is cigarette smoking with a relative risk of approximately 2. Another risk factor appears to be the high-fat Western diet with a protective effect afforded by a diet high in fruits and vegetables. Other less clearly established risk factors or associated conditions include diabetes mellitus and chronic pancreatitis, but cause and effect have not been elucidated. Caffeine has been extensively studied as a risk factor and no prospective studies have confirmed that a statistically significant risk exists.

2. The pancreas consists of endocrine and exocrine (ductal and acinar) cells. What is the cell type from which most pancreatic cancers originate?
Approximately 95% of pancreatic tumors occur within the exocrine portion of the pancreas. Ductal adenocarcinoma (i.e., arising from ductal epithelium) makes up approximately 80–90% of pancreatic neoplasms. Rarer tumors include those that originate from the islets of Langerhans (insulinoma, glucagonoma, VIPoma [vasoactive intestinal polypeptide secreting tumor], and nonsecreting islet cell tumors). The pancreas also can be the site of metastasis from other malignancies but these are of little to no clinical significance. In addition, cystic neoplasms may arise from the pancreas. These are usually large and filled with mucinous secretions and may be multilocular. Those lined with benign columnar epithelium are called cystadenomas, and those with malignant epithelium are called

cystadenocarcinomas. The significance of these latter tumors are that they are usually localized and cured with surgery approximately 50% of the time.

3. How does the typical patient with pancreatic carcinoma present? What determines the clinical presentation?

The most important determinant of the clinical presentation is the location of the tumor. Tumors of the head of the pancreas may be discovered relatively early, because even a small tumor may obstruct the common bile duct, whereas tumors of the body and tail more often are discovered because of their larger size and/or metastasis. Since cancers of the head of the pancreas can frequently obstruct the common bile duct, patients often present with progressive painless jaundice and pruritus. Tumors of the body and tail of the organ are not discovered until the enlarging mass causes pain or duodenal obstruction. This pain is often described as unremitting "gnawing" epigastric pain radiating to the back. Long-standing and/or more aggressive disease may present as metastatic disease: malignant ascites or carcinomatosis, liver metastasis, or even malignant pleural effusions. Weight loss occurs in nearly all patients and may be related to maldigestion (absent bile salts and pancreatic enzymes due to obstruction), intestinal obstruction, and systemic tumor effects that diminish appetite and alter metabolism. Less commonly, pancreatic cancer can present as new-onset diabetes mellitus or acute pancreatitis.

4. What is Courvoisier's sign?

Courvoisier's sign is an enlarged, palpable, nontender right upper quadrant mass (the distended gallbladder) resulting from biliary obstruction secondary to carcinoma of the head of the pancreas. This occurs in less than a third of patients at presentation.

5. What is Trousseau's sign?

Spontaneous and recurrent venous thrombosis, also referred to as migratory thrombophlebitis, is sometimes encountered in pancreatic carcinoma as well as other adenocarcinomas. It frequently occurs at unusual sites and may be difficult to suppress with anticoagulation. It appears to be part of the spectrum of disseminated intravascular coagulation and nonbacterial thrombotic endocarditis. Ironically, Trousseau diagnosed his own fatal disease as cancer of the pancreas when he developed migratory thrombophlebitis.

6. What is Sister Mary Joseph's sign? Who was she?

Patients with advanced gastrointestinal malignancies, particularly pancreatic and gastric, may have an enlarged periumbilical lymph node. Sister Mary Joseph, Dr. Mayo's surgical scrub nurse, noted that the finding of a periumbilical mass on prepping the abdomen prior to surgery portended a poor prognosis.

7. What is the classic description of stool color that is occasionally seen with pancreatic cancers or carcinoma of the ampulla of Vater?

Silver stools. Pale or acholic stools are caused by biliary obstruction, and when blood is added to an acholic stool, the stool takes on a silver color. The majority of patients with pancreatic carcinoma are guaiac positive.

8. Name the most sensitive test for detecting pancreatic carcinoma. What is the classic sign seen with this test?

Endoscopic retrograde cholangiopancreatography is reported to be very sensitive in the diagnosis of pancreatic cancer with a normal pancreatogram seen in only 2.8% (i.e., false negatives = 2.8%). The duct can be seen to be encased or obstructed by tumor or extravasation of contrast may be seen. When the malignancy is in the head of the pancreas, one can see dilation of both the common bile duct and pancreatic duct. This finding is referred to as the double-duct sign. It is not pathognomonic and on rare occasions may be seen with benign disease.

Computed tomographic (CT) scan and ultrasound (US) detect pancreatic tumors 2 cm or larger. They can detect dilation of the pancreatic duct and biliary tree and metastasis to the liver. US is less expensive and can help differentiate obstructive from nonobstructive jaundice, whereas CT can accurately delineate retroperitoneal anatomy.

9. Under what circumstances are tumor markers helpful in the *diagnosis* of pancreatic carcinoma?
The tumor-associated antigen CA-19-9 has been widely studied. Although intermediate values (<100 U/mL) lack specificity, the higher the CA-19-9 level, the greater its specificity in diagnosing pancreatic cancer, so that at serum concentrations >1000 U/mL, the positive predictive value approaches 100%. Although the overall sensitivity is 81%, the fact that small tumors frequently do not have elevated levels of CA-19-9 reduces it utility as a screening test.

10. Should all patients with pancreatic carcinoma have percutaneous aspiration biopsy performed?
Percutaneous aspiration biopsy can be performed with CT or US guidance. It is a very specific way of confirming the diagnosis or identifying rarer tumors (e.g., lymphoma, islet cell tumors). Sampling error may be significant, and a negative biopsy does not exclude the diagnosis, as the tumor (especially smaller ones) can be missed. A tissue diagnosis obtained by needle aspiration is appropriate for patients under consideration for surgical resection, chemotherapy, or radiation therapy. Patients may on occasion undergo palliative procedures to alleviate obstruction without a prior tissue diagnosis.

11. What percentage of patients who present with pancreatic carcinoma have a potentially resectable tumor?
At the time of diagnosis >85% of pancreatic tumors have extended beyond the organ and patients with such tumors are not candidates for curative surgery. Tumors >4 cm in size are rarely resectable. Because tumors that are located in the body and tail of the pancreas remain "silent" until later in the course, patients with these tumors tend to have a poorer prognosis. In large series, only 5–22% of patients have potentially resectable tumors, and of patients with resected tumors, the 5-year survival is only 10%. For all patients coming to surgery, therefore, the 5-year survival is about 1%.

12. Which procedures can be helpful in assessing the resectability or operability of the tumor?
The poor surgical results have led to attempts to identify a subset of patients with early disease who are more likely to benefit from an attempt at curative resection. To this end, some experts have advocated laparoscopy as a means of diagnosing extrapancreatic involvement that does not show up on CT and US examinations. In up to 40% of patients with no extrapancreatic involvement on CT, tumors are found to be unresectable on the basis of small metastasis seen at laparoscopy. Angiography also has been used to assess resectability, because involvement of major vessels is a contraindication to curative surgery.

13. Name the most common sites of metastasis.
Liver and peritoneum (carcinomatosis).

14. What is removed with the Whipple procedure?
The standard operation for pancreatic cancer is the Whipple operation, which involves the resection of the distal stomach, common bile duct, gallbladder, duodenum, the pancreas to the midbody en bloc and a truncal vagotomy. In some cases, the distal stomach and pylorus can be preserved and vagotomy is then unnecessary. Potential complications such as pancreatic and biliary fistulas, hemorrhage, and infection can occur, but in experienced hands the operative mortality should be about 5%.

15. What are the problems associated with pancreatic carcinoma that most often require palliation? How are these problems best managed?
Growth of the primary tumor may cause duodenal obstruction with intractable nausea and vomiting; this is best managed with surgical bypass. Obstruction of the bile duct, also from the enlarging mass, is best treated with endoscopically placed internal stents.

16. Is there a role for chemotherapy or radiation therapy in the treatment of pancreatic cancer?
Results of trials with radiation therapy and chemotherapy have been disappointing, and their role has mainly been confined to that of palliation. Clinical trials are ongoing.

BIBLIOGRAPHY

1. Brennan MF, Kinsell AT, Friedman M: Cancer of the pancreas. In DeVita VT, Hellman S, Rosenberg SA (eds): Cancer: Principles and Practice, 3rd ed. Philadelphia, J.B. Lippincott, 1989, pp 800–835.
2. Castillo CF, Warshaw AL: Diagnosis and preoperative evaluation of pancreatic cancer, with implications for management. Gastroenterol Clin North Am 19:915–933, 1990.
3. Gordis L: Consumption of methylxanthine-containing beverages and risk of pancreatic cancer. Cancer Lett 52:1–12, 1990.
4. Gudjonsson B: Cancer of the pancreas: 50 years of surgery. Cancer 60:2284–2303, 1987.
5. Merrick HW III, Dobelbower RR: Aggressive therapy for cancer of the pancreas: Does it help? Gastroenterol Clin North Am 19:935–962, 1990.
6. Shemesh E, Czerniak A, Nass S, Klein E: Role of endoscopic retrograde cholangiopancreatography in differentiating pancreatic cancer coexisting with chronic pancreatitis. Cancer 65:893–896, 1990.
7. Steinberg W: The clinical utility of the CA 19-9 tumor-associated antigen. Am J Gastroenterol 85:350–355, 1990.
8. Warshaw AL, Castillo CF: Pancreatic carcinoma. N Engl J Med 326:455–465, 1992.

70. OVARIAN CANCER

Helen Frederickson, M.D.

1. What is the incidence of ovarian cancer? Which women are at an increased risk for developing the disease?
The incidence of ovarian cancer increases with age. Lifetime incidence is 1 in 70 women (1.4%). The median age at diagnosis is 61 years. Reproductive factors related to the risk of developing ovarian cancer include an increased risk in nulliparous women and a protective effect of oral contraceptive users. Thus, the probability of developing ovarian cancer is related to the total number of ovulatory cycles.

Patients with breast cancer have a twofold increase in risk of developing ovarian cancer. A small percentage of ovarian cancer is familial, with patients in true familial ovarian cancer families having a 50% risk (autosomal dominant) of developing the disease.

Environmental factors play an unknown role in development of ovarian cancer. Ovarian cancer has its highest incidence in industrialized countries. This may be related to the high animal fat diets in these countries.

2. How does the typical patient with ovarian cancer present?
The majority of patients have vague abdominal complaints. Early satiety and abdominal bloating signal ascites and commonly omental spread of the disease. Usually a pelvic mass is present. Serum CA125 levels are elevated in 80% of patients with epithelial cancers. Seventy-five percent of patients present with stage III disease.

3. Is there a screening test for ovarian cancer?
No. Pelvic examination may detect an ovarian cancer before it becomes disseminated, but there are no data on the frequency with which ovarian cancer is detected in the asymptomatic woman by pelvic examination. Ultrasonography is not sufficiently specific to be useful as a screening procedure in asymptomatic women. The specificity of ultrasound diagnosis may be improved by transvaginal sonography and color-flow Doppler studies, but to date there are no data to imply a decrease in mortality in a screened population.

CA125 is not a good "screening" test, as the incidence of the disease in the general population is so low that the majority of positive tests are false positives.

Even in women with two first-degree relatives with ovarian cancer (i.e., true familial ovarian cancer syndrome with a risk of 50%), the ability of "screening tests" to detect earlier-stage ovarian cancer has not been established.

4. How is ovarian cancer staged?
Surgical staging in the absence of obvious stage III disease includes (1) peritoneal washings, (2) multiple peritoneal biopsies (in the upper abdomen); bilateral colic gutters and diaphragm assessment (may be by Pap smear); in the pelvis, bilateral pelvic sidewall, cul-de-sac, and bladder peritoneum; (3) pelvic and para-aortic node sampling; and (4) infracolic omentectomy.

Stages
I   Confined to the ovaries
IA   Confined to a single ovary
IB   Both ovaries involved
IC   No gross spread beyond the ovaries
        Malignant cells are present in cytologic washings or in ascites
        Tumor extends to the ovarian surface
        Tumor is ruptured at surgery
II   Tumor spread in the pelvis beyond the ovaries
IIA   Spread to the uterus or fallopian tube
IIB   Spread to the other pelvic structures
IIC   Malignant cells present in cytologic washings or in ascites
        Tumor is ruptured at surgery
III   Extrapelvic spread confined to abdominal cavity or inguinal nodes
IIIA   No gross spread beyond the pelvis, with microscopic implants to the
            upper abdomen
IIIB   Gross intra-abdominal extrapelvic implants <2 cm
IIIC   Gross intra-abdominal extrapelvic implants >2 cm
        Retroperitoneal spread to pelvic or aortic lymph nodes or the
            inguinal nodes
IV   Distant spread

5. Why is aggressive cytoreductive surgery pursued in the initial treatment of advanced-stage ovarian cancer?
Survival of patients with smaller residual disease is improved over patients with larger residual disease despite identical chemotherapeutic regimens postoperatively. This relates to the Goldie-Coldman hypothesis that predicts smaller tumor nodules are more likely to be chemosensitive than larger nodules owing to a higher percentage of spontaneous mutations to a resistant phenotype in larger nodules. Most gynecologic oncologists consider maximal nodule diameter of <2 cm as "optimal" debulking.

6. Which chemotherapy regimens are used postoperatively?
Presently, platinum-based chemotherapeutic regimens are the first-line chemotherapy for ovarian cancer. Studies comparing single-agent chemotherapy with combination therapy

have suggested that combination therapy prolongs survival and progression-free interval. Until recently, the standard chemotherapeutic regimen has been the combination of cisplatin plus cyclophosphamide (Cytoxan). The doses of cisplatin ranged from 50 mg/m^2 to 100 mg/m^2. The major dose-limiting toxicity of cisplatin is neurotoxicity. Carboplatin is an analogue of cisplatin and has less neurotoxicity, thus being more suitable for dose-intensity studies. The activity of the new drug paclitaxel (Taxol) in previously treated patients has led to studies using combinations of platinum and taxol as first-line therapy. These preliminary data suggest this combination may be slightly better than cisplatin and Cytoxan in suboptimally debulked patients. The optimal length of therapy has not been established. A prospective randomized trial compared 5 cycles with 10 cycles of platinum-based therapy and showed no statistical difference.

7. Is there a role for a second-look laparotomy?

Yes. When a patient is part of a research protocol for either first- or second-line therapy. In about half of patients with a complete clinical response (including a negative CA125), malignancy will be found at the time of the second look. In 25-30% of patients with a negative second-look laparotomy, tumor will recur. Surgical assessment of residual disease remains the only way to determine treatment effectiveness and thus the only way to determine the benefit of new treatment regimens. The survival benefit of second-look laparotomy has not been proven.

8. What is the prognosis of patients with ovarian cancer?

The 5-year survival for patients with stage III or IV disease is only 25-30%. The most common cause of death is related to ascites, bowel obstruction, and essentially a slow "starvation." Distant metastases, including bone, lung, liver, and brain, are unusual.

The 5-year survival of patients with stage I disease is 80%. Grade I stage I tumors have a 95% 5-year survival.

9. Is there any benefit to secondary debulking (at second-look laparotomy or in recurrence after first-line therapy)?

The benefit of secondary debulking has not been proven. Patients who progress on platinum therapy are unlikely to survive regardless of further therapy. Patients with bulky residual at second surgery also are unlikely to survive, but some studies suggest that if bulky disease can be converted to microscopic residual, patients may have a survival advantage with second-line treatments.

10. What second-line therapies are available?

Patients with minimal residual disease after second surgery are candidates for intraperitoneal chemotherapy. The most common agent used for intraperitoneal therapy is cisplatin. After intraperitoneal salvage, 50% to 75% of patients survive 2-4 years. More recently the new drug paclitaxel (Taxol) has become available for second-line therapy. Thirty percent of platinum-resistant patients respond to paclitaxel, with an average response duration of 7 months. Other second-line drugs include hexamethylmelamine, VP-16, and 5-fluorouracil. Whole abdominal radiation therapy has had significant response rates in patients with small-volume disease, but the rate of bowel obstruction after this therapy is about 20-30%.

11. What is the significance of an ovarian tumor of low malignant potential?

Tumors of low malignant potential (or borderline malignancies) are epithelial tumors of the ovary with an excellent prognosis but histologic features of cancer. Even if the tumor has spread to the abdomen, the 5-year survival is still 80%. Patients may, however, die of disease after as long as 20 years. These tumors do not benefit from adjuvant chemotherapy in early- or advanced-stage disease. The indolent clinical course of these tumors suggests a low growth fraction and thus accounts for their lack of responsiveness to chemotherapy.

BIBLIOGRAPHY

1. Bast RC, Klug TL, St John E, et al: A radioimmunoassay using a monoclonal antibody to monitor the course of epithelial ovarian cancer. N Engl J Med 309:883, 1983.
2. The Cancer and Steroid Hormone Study of the Centers for Disease Control and the National Institute of Child Health and Human Development: The reduction in risk of ovarian cancer associated with oral contraceptive use. N Engl J Med 316:650, 1987.
3. Goldie JH, Coldman AJ: A mathematic model for relating the drug sensitivity of tumors to their spontaneous mutation rate. Cancer Treat Rep 63:1727, 1979.
4. Granai CO: Ovarian cancer—unrealistic expectations. N Engl J Med 327:197, 1992.
5. Griffiths CT, Parker LM, Fuller AF: Role of cytoreductive surgical treatment in the management of advanced ovarian cancer. Cancer Treat Rep 63:235, 1979.
6. Potter ME, Partridge EE, Hatch KD, et al: Primary surgical therapy of ovarian cancer: How much and when? Gynecol Oncol 40:195, 1991.
7. Potter ME, Hatch KD, Soong SJ, et al: Second-look laparotomy and salvage therapy: A research modality only? Gynecol Oncol 44:3, 1992.

71. CARCINOMA OF THE UTERINE CERVIX AND ENDOMETRIUM

Helen Frederickson, M.D.

1. What are the presenting signs of cervical carcinoma?

The most frequent symptom is a bloody discharge presenting as postcoital bleeding, intermenstrual bleeding, or menorrhagia. Symptoms of more advanced disease include backache, leg pain, leg edema, or hematuria.

2. What are the risk factors for cervical carcinoma?

Established risk factors include first coitus at a young age, multiple sexual partners, and lower socioeconomic status. Human papillomavirus probably acts as a cofactor in cervical carcinogenesis.

3. How is the diagnosis of cervical cancer made?

All cervical lesions should be biopsied regardless of the Papanicolaou (Pap) smear. Pap smear and colposcopically directed biopsies are used in microscopic or occult lesions. Cervical biopsy consistent with microinvasion requires a cone biopsy to rule out frankly invasive carcinoma.

4. Which patients are candidates for primary surgical management? What is the appropriate response if paraaortic nodes are positive on frozen section?

Patients with stage I and stage IIA cervical carcinomas are candidates for primary surgical treatment. If paraaortic nodes are positive, usually the procedure is abandoned and the patient treated with primary radiation therapy.

5. How does a radical hysterectomy differ from a simple hysterectomy? Are the ovaries always removed at the time of radical hysterectomy?

In a radical hysterectomy, the uterine artery is ligated at its origin from the internal iliac artery; uterosacral ligaments are resected toward the sacrum; the cardinal ligaments are resected at the pelvic sidewall; and the upper one-third of the vagina is removed. Pelvic lymphadenectomy is routinely performed. Ovaries may be preserved with this procedure; this is the major advantage of surgery over radiation therapy in the young patient.

6. What is the alternative to surgical therapy for early-stage disease? Is there a difference in rates of cure?

Primary radiation therapy can be used to treat early-stage carcinoma of the cervix with the same survival rates as surgery.

7. What is the theory on which radiation therapy for cervical cancer is based?

The cervix is accessible to application of radiation techniques and is surrounded by normal tissue (cervix and vagina) that is highly radioresistant. The anatomy of the cervix allows delivery of intracavitary doses of 10,000 rads to the tumor. Because the dose of radiation decreases by the inverse square of the distance from the source, the bowel and bladder are protected by packing them away.

8. What is the most common location of recurrence after radical hysterectomy? After radiation therapy?

After radical hysterectomy, approximately one-third of recurrences are in the pelvic sidewall and approximately one-fourth in the central pelvis. Recurrence after radiation therapy is in the parametrial area 43% of the time.

9. What is the prognosis for a patient with persistent or recurrent cervical carcinoma?

The 1-year survival rate is 10–15%. This is compared to the overall survival by stage:

Stage I—80–85%
Stage III—25–35%
Stage II—60–65%
Stage IV—8–14%

10. Which patients are candidates for pelvic exenteration?

Pelvic exenteration for recurrent carcinoma of the cervix is indicated only when the pelvic recurrence is centrally located. The triad of unilateral leg edema, sciatic pain, and ureteral obstruction indicates unresectable disease.

11. Does chemotherapy have a role in treatment of recurrent cervical cancer?

Chemotherapy traditionally has had low response rates and short duration. The prognosis for patients with unresectable recurrent disease is so poor that new combinations of chemotherapeutic agents are under evaluation. Cisplatin has been shown to be the most effective single agent against squamous cell carcinoma. The use of chemotherapeutic agents (cisplatin, 5-fluorouracil, and hydroxyurea) as radiosensitizers to increase rates of survival and/or cure in patients with poor prognosis is under evaluation. The combination of bleomycin, ifosfamide, and cisplatin has shown initially encouraging results in recurrent disease. To date, the use of chemotherapy as neoadjuvant therapy has shown no significant improvement over standard therapies.

12. What is the incidence of endometrial carcinoma? How does the incidence compare with other gynecologic malignancies?

The incidence of endometrial carcinoma is about 72/100,000 women per year. It is the most common gynecologic malignancy.

13. Describe the evidence that estrogens play a role in carcinogenesis in endometrial adenocarcinoma.

Endometrial carcinoma is associated with disorders characterized by chronic production of endogenous estrogen in the absence of progesterone. The risk of developing endometrial carcinoma is increased 7 times in postmenopausal women who have a uterus and take estrogens without progesterone. Other studies show a relative risk of 3 for women who use unopposed estrogens contrasted with a relative risk of 15 for patients who are 30 or more pounds overweight.

14. What is the most common presenting symptom of endometrial carcinoma?

Abnormal uterine bleeding is the most common presenting symptom. Any postmenopausal bleeding is considered abnormal. Any increase in menstrual bleeding (i.e., more frequent or heavier menses) or intermenstrual spotting deserves an endometrial biopsy in the perimenopausal period.

15. How useful is the Pap smear in screening and diagnosing endometrial carcinoma?

The Pap smear is not useful as a screening test for endometrial carcinoma; only one-third of patients with endometrial carcinoma have an abnormal Pap smear. If endometrial cells are present on a Pap smear in a postmenopausal woman, she should have an endometrial biopsy.

16. How is the diagnosis of endometrial carcinoma made?

An endometrial biopsy is used to diagnose endometrial carcinoma. The biopsy may be done with any of the multiple devices for office biopsies or with dilatation and curettage (D&C). Staging is now surgical, and adjuvant therapy is determined by surgical pathology findings.

17. How does endometrial carcinoma spread?

Endometrial carcinoma arises from the glands of the endometrium; initial growth is slow. As the tumor grows, it eventually invades the underlying myometrium. Extrauterine spread occurs by lymphatics and blood. Lymphatic invasion results in metastasis to the parametrial, pelvic, aortic, or inguinal nodes. Hematogenous spread usually results in pulmonary metastasis but may involve bone and liver. Peritoneal implants may be caused by lymphatic spread or by transtubal or transmural penetration.

18. What is the incidence of pelvic node metastases in patients with disease limited to the uterus? What is the incidence of metastases to paraaortic nodes?

Overall, 9.3% of patients have positive pelvic nodes, but in patients with grade 1 tumors the incidence is <2%. Patients with grade 3 tumors have an incidence of positive pelvic nodes as high as 30%. Overall, paraaortic nodes are positive in 5.4% of patients, but almost never in patients with grade 1 tumors. The incidence of positive paraaortic nodes in patients with grade 3 tumors is as high as 15%, even in the presence of negative pelvic nodes.

19. How is endometrial carcinoma treated?

Endometrial carcinoma is treated with initial surgical staging, including peritoneal cytology, total abdominal hysterectomy, bilateral salpingo-oophorectomy, and pelvic and paraaortic node sampling. Many surgeons, however, sample nodes on the basis of grade and depth of myometrial invasion. The results of surgical staging determine use of adjuvant radiation, chemotherapy, and hormonal therapy.

20. What are the most common sites of recurrence in patients treated with radiation therapy? In patients treated with surgery alone?

The most common sites of recurrence in patients who receive adjuvant radiation therapy are the lung, abdomen, liver, and bone. The most common site of recurrence in patients treated with surgery alone is the vaginal apex. Pelvic wall and parametrium are also areas of recurrence when no radiation has been given.

21. What is the role of hormonal therapy in endometrial carcinoma?

Patients with advanced or recurrent endometrial carcinoma and positive progesterone or estrogen receptors may be treated with high doses of progestin therapy in addition to surgery and radiation. Responses may be slow and not apparent for 3 or more months. As long as the disease remains stable, therapy is continued. The mean duration of response for progestin therapy in patients with recurrent or metastatic endometrial carcinoma is about 10–12 months. The level of progesterone receptors varies with the degree of tumor differentiation

22. How effective are chemotherapeutic agents in advanced endometrial carcinoma?
The overall rate of response with current agents is about 20–30%. Unfortunately, the duration of response is short. Cisplatin and Adriamycin appear to be the most effective agents for endometrial adenocarcinoma.

23. What is uterine papillary serous adenocarcinoma? How does it commonly spread?
Papillary serous adenocarcinoma is a variant of endometrial carcinoma, characterized by histology that resembles ovarian serous carcinoma. Like ovarian carcinoma, this variant tends to spread intraperitoneally but has a higher incidence of nodal spread.

BIBLIOGRAPHY

1. Bokhman JV: Two pathogenic types of endometrial carcinoma. Gynecol Oncol 15:10, 1983.
2. Buxton EJ, Meanwell CA, Hilton C, et al: Combination bleomycin, ifosfamide and cisplatin chemotherapy in cervical cancer. J Natl Cancer Inst 81:359–361, 1989.
3. Chambers JT, MacLusky N, Eisenfield A, et al: Estrogen and progesterone receptor levels as prognosticators for survival in endometrial cancer. Gynecol Oncol 31:65, 1988.
4. Creasman WT, Morrow CP, Bundy BN, et al: Surgical pathology spread patterns of endometrial cancer: A Gynecologic Oncology Group study. Cancer 60:2035, 1987.
5. Delgado G, Bundy B, Zairo R, et al: A prospective surgical pathological study of Stage I squamous carcinoma of the cervix: A Gynecologic Oncology Group study. Gynecol Oncol 35:314, 1989.
6. International Federation of Gynecology and Obstetrics (FIGO): Corpus cancer staging. Int J Gynecol Obstet 28:190, 1989.
7. Jefferey JR, Krepart GV, Lotocki RJ: Papillary serous adenocarcinoma of the endometrium. Obstet Gynecol 67:670, 1986.
8. Keys H, Bundy B, Stehman FB, et al: Adjuvants to radiation therapy in the treatment of locally advanced carcinoma of the cervix: The Gynecologic Oncology Group (GOG) experience. In Salmon SE (ed): Adjuvant Therapy of Cancer, 6th ed. Philadelphia, W.B. Saunders, 1990, pp 544–555.
9. Marrow CP, Panel Report: Is pelvic irradiation beneficial in the postoperative management of stage IB squamous cell carcinoma of the cervix with pelvic lymph node metastasis treated by radical hysterectomy and pelvic lymphadenectomy? Gynecol Oncol 37:74, 1990.
10. Perez CA, Camel HM, Kuske RR, et al: Radiation therapy alone in the treatment of carcinoma of the uterine cervix: A 20-year experience. Gynecol Oncol 23:127–140, 1986.
11. Potter MD, Alvarez R, Shingleton HM, et al: Early invasive cervical cancer with pelvic lymph node involvement: To complete or not to complete radical hysterectomy? Gynecol Oncol 37:78, 1990.
12. Rubin GL, Peterson HB, Lee NC, et al: Estrogen replacement therapy and the risk of endometrial cancer: Remaining controversies. Am J Obstet Gynecol 162:148, 1990.
13. Weiss NS, Szekely DR, English DR, Schweid AI: Endometrial cancer in relation to patterns of menopausal estrogen use. JAMA 242:261, 1979.
14. Yazigi R, et al: Adenosquamous carcinoma of the cervix: Prognosis in Stage IB. Obstet Gynecol 75:1012, 1990.

72. TESTICULAR CANCER

David H. Garfield, M.D.

1. What is included in the differential diagnosis of a new, scrotal mass in a young man?

Epididymitis	Orchitis
Spermatocele	Infarction
Hydrocele	Trauma

Benign tumor of the testis, epididymis, or tunica albuginea

2. What is the most common solid tumor in men aged 28 to 32?
A germ cell tumor.

3. How many new cases of testicular cancer occur in the United States every year?
6000, or an incidence of 5/100,000.

4. What is most well-documented risk factor for testicular cancer?
Cryptorchidism. It is associated with 10% of all germ cell tumors with a 30-fold relative risk.

5. Can cryptorchidism be eliminated as a risk factor for testicular cancer?
Yes. If orchidopexy is performed before the age of 6.

6. What is the etiology of germ cell tumors?
Unknown.

7. What percentage of solid testicular masses are malignant?
95%.

8. What percentage of testicular tumors are of germinal origin?
97%.

9. Can the diagnosis of testicular cancer be made by blood tests?
No. Although, typically, alpha-fetoprotein and/or beta human chorionic gonadotropin levels are elevated in nonseminomatous germ cell tumors, an orchiectomy must be performed for diagnosis.

10. Can the diagnosis of testicular cancer be made by biopsy, as with other cancers, thereby preserving the testes?
No. A radical inguinal exploration with high ligation of the cord followed by orchiectomy is carried out. Vascular control should be achieved prior to manipulation of the tumor. Open biopsy is absolutely contraindicated, as is scrotal exploraton.

11. Explain why transscrotal biopsy of the testis is contraindicated.
Transscrotal biopsy is contraindicated for two reasons: (1) the biopsy technique may cause implantation of the tumor into the scrotum; that is, a surgically induced metastatic site; and (2) the biopsy procedure significantly alters the lymphatic drainage of the scrotum, affecting the recurrence rate and overall prognosis.

12. How are germ cell tumors classified?
Seminoma and nonseminoma are the major categories.

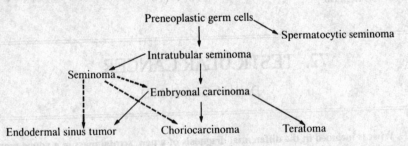

Proposed scheme of histogenesis of germ cell tumors. Solid lines represent generally accepted paths of differentiation; dashed lines are hypothetical. (From Brodsky GL: Pathology of germ cell tumors. Hematol Oncol Clin North Am 5:1098, 1991, with permission.)

13. Why is the distinction between seminoma and nonseminoma important?
Seminomas tend to be less aggressive, both locally and with regard to distant metastases. Seminomas are exquisitely radiosensitive; both classes are equally chemosensitive.

14. Which *pure* germ cell tumor is the most common?
Seminoma (27% in World Health Organization series).

15. What are the subtypes of nonseminomatous germ cell tumors (NSGCT)?

Embryonal carcinoma   Choriocarcinoma
Endodermal sinus tumor   Mixed germ celltumor
Teratoma

16. Which is the most common of all germ cell tumors?
Mixed germ cell tumor, composed of a mixture of elements in any combination, accounts for about 50% of all testicular tumors.

17. What is the most common NSGCT?
Over two-thirds of nonseminomas are mixed germ cell tumors.

18. What is the most common combination of NSGCT?
Embryonal carcinoma plus teratoma.

19. Which is the most aggressive type of germ cell tumor?
Pure choriocarcinoma.

20. How often is pure choriocarcinoma seen?
In <1% of all germ cell tumors.

21. Where else is choriocarcinoma seen?
It is most commonly seen as a small component of mixed tumors, in which its presence has little bearing on clinical behavior and outcome. Choriocarcinoma also can be seen in the placenta, in which case it is easily cured with single-agent chemotherapy.

22. Why is staging of testicular cancer important?
To determine prognosis and treatment.

23. Describe the stages.

Stage A: Disease limted to the testis
Stage B: Spread to retroperitoneal lymph nodes
Stage C: Supradiaphragmatic extension and pulmonary or other visceral organ involvement

Staging of Testis Tumors

WALTER REED GENERAL HOSPITAL		SKINNER	
IA	Confined to testis; no clinical or radiographic evidence of spread	A	Same as Walter Reed IA but includes no positive nodes on lymph node dissection
IB	Same as IA but at lymph node dissection; metastases to iliac or paraaortic nodes	B	Disease below diaphragm, normal chest roentgenogram and mediastinum
II	Disease below diaphragm/no spread to visceral organs; clinical or radiographic evidence of metastases to paraaortic, femoral, inguinal, and iliac lymph nodes	B_1	Fewer than 6 positive nodes that are well encapsulated and no extension to retroperitoneal fat
III	Disease above diaphragm or spread to body organs (clinical, roentgenogram)	B_2	6 or more positive lymph nodes that are well encapsulated and/or retroperitoneal fat extension
		B_3	Bulky abdominal mass (exceeding 5 cm)

From Richie JP: Surgical aspects in the treatment of patients with testicular cancer. Hematol Oncol Clin North Am 5:1130, 1991, with permission.

24. What percentage of patients with NSGCTs present with stage C tumors?
Stage C tumors account for 20%. Forty percent are stage A and 40% are stage B.

25. Toward what end should the staging work-up be directed?
The staging work-up will guide the treatment plan. Patients with stage A or early B disease are treated by retroperitoneal lymph node dissection (RPLND). In some cases, surveillance alone is adequate for stage A. The patient with advanced stage B or C disease will need a cisplatin-based combination chemotherapy regimen.

26. What studies should be performed in the staging work-up?
Chest radiography. If that is normal, computed tomography (CT) of the chest and abdomen and alpha-fetoprotein (AFP) and β-hCG testing should be performed.

27. When is a bipedal lymphangiogram useful?
In the work-up of seminoma. There is a 95% correlation with surgical findings. If the lymphangiogram is negative, surgery is not necessary and radiation or chemotherapy may be deferred. If the lymphangiogram is positive, abdominal radiation therapy is given.

28. What percentage of patients with recurrent NSGCTs have normal AFP and β-hCG?
10%.

29. What percentage of patients with NSGCTs with clinical stage A disease (normal CT scan and serum markers) will have retroperitoneal lymph node involvement?
30%.

30. For patients with clinical stage A NSGCT, RPLND will cure what percentage with positive nodes?
50–60%.

31. What percentage of patients with NSGCTs whose lymph nodes were negative by RPLND will develop recurrent disease?
10%.

32. What percentage of those whose nodal disease was resected will have recurrences?
40–50%.

33. If patients with stage A and resected B NSGCTs are followed closely every month for 12 months and every 2 months for the second 12 months, virtually all those who have recurrences will have minimal disease. What percentage of patients who have recurrences will be cured with cisplatin combination chemotherapy?
99%.

34. When do most recurrences occur following initial therapy for germ cell tumors?
In the first 24 months.

35. What percentage of patients with NSGCTs, clinical stage A, who undergo RPLND will have no disease found?
70%.

36. What is the main complication of bilateral RPLND?
Retrograde ejaculation and sterility (uniformly).

37. A sympathetic nerve-sparing RPLND procedure has now been developed. What percentage of patients can maintain normal ejaculation?
80%.

38. Patients with stage B are cured by RPLND how often?
50–60%.

39. If patients with stage B are treated by RPLND, is it better to give them two prophylactic (adjuvant) courses of cisplatin, VP-16, and bleomycin following surgery or closely follow them (as in question 33) and treat *if* there is recurrence?
It doesn't matter, because the outcome is the same—very good.

40. If a patient with an NSGCT has elevated tumor markers following orchiectomy and an abnormal CT scan with abnormal nodes <3 cm in diameter, how should he be treated?
RPLND with sympathetic nerves being spared.

41. What if RPLND cannot be done?
Three courses of cisplatin, VP-16, and bleomycin should be administered.

42. And if the lymph nodes are >3 cm?
Three courses of cisplatin, VP-16, and bleomycin should be administered.

43. What is the most effective, least toxic chemotherapy for patients with "minimal or moderate" extensive stage C disease?
Three courses (9 weeks) of cisplatin, VP-16, and bleomycin.

44. For patients with "advanced extensive" disease, what is the most effective, least toxic chemotherapy?
Four courses (12 weeks) of cisplatin, VP-16, and bleomycin.

Treatment Arms of Southeastern Cancer Study Group Trial Comparing PVB and PVP-16B

R	Cisplatin, 20 mg/m^2/d × 5 every 3 wk × 4
A	Vinblastine, 0.15 mg/kg days 1 and 2 every 3 wk × 4
N	Bleomycin, 30 U weekly × 12
D	
O	
M	
I	Cisplatin, 20 mg/m^2/d × 5 every 3 wk × 4
Z	VP-16, 100 mg/m^2 × 5 every 3 wk × 4
E	Bleomycin, 30 U weekly × 12

From Loehrer PJ Sr: Current Therapy in Hematology-Oncology, 4th ed. Philadelphia, B.C. Decker, 1992, p 302, with permission.

45. How many patients with stage C disease treated with cisplatin combination therapy will relapse?
25%.

46. When is surgery to be contemplated after chemotherapy?
When a residual retroperitoneal mass ≥3 cm is seen by CT scan. It could represent residual tumor, benign teratoma, or scar tissue.

47. Where else is surgery to be considered?
A residual lung mass, especially if the tumor markers have normalized. It, too, may represent a former teratocarcinoma now transformed into a benign teratoma. If not removed, it could degenerate back into a teratocarcinoma.

48. Of all patients with metastatic NSGCTs, 50–70% can obtain a complete remission with chemotherapy. Can surgery improve on this?
Yes. Another 10–15% can be made tumor free by surgical removal of residual tumor.

49. What percentage of patients in complete remission by any means will relapse?
10–20%.

50. Is there a risk with general anesthesia in patients who have received chemotherapy for germ cell tumors?
Postoperative respiratory failure is occasionally seen in patients who were treated with bleomycin. Postoperative care must, therefore, be more careful than usual.

51. Does bleomycin cause other toxicity long term?
Bleomycin together with vinblastine (Velban), and probably enhanced by cisplatin, may produce Raynaud's phenomenon.

52. Can the use of bleomycin be avoided?
Four courses of cisplatin and VP-16 are probably equivalent to three courses of the same two drugs with bleomycin in patients with a favorable prognosis.

53. Radiation therapy is the treatment of choice for seminomas up to what stage?
Patients with clinical stage A disease are given 2500 rad (2500 cGy) to the infradiaphragmatic nodes, although surveillance is advocated by some. The same radiation therapy is used for "nonbulky" stage B disease.

54. Is it necessary to radiate the mediastinum prophylactically?
No.

55. What is the treatment for a patient with "bulky" stage B seminoma?
Radiation therapy or chemotherapy with cisplatin, VP-16, and bleomycin.

56. What about stage C disease?
The same chemotherapy as for advanced extensive NSGCT.

Treatment Recommendations

CLINICAL SETTING	STANDARD THERAPY	INVESTIGATIVE THERAPY
Nonseminomatous Germ Cell Tumor (NSGCT)		
Stage A	Retroperitoneal lymphad-enopathy (modified or nerve-sparing)	Surveillance (including first year): CT scan of abdomen every 2 mo, chest radiograph and markers (AFP, βhCG, LDH) qmo × 1 yr. Second year: Abdominal CT scan q4mo with chest radiograph and serum markers every 2 mo
Stage B1 or B2 (S/P RPLND)	Observation with PVP-16B on relapse or two cycles of PVP-16B as adjuvant	None
Stage B3 or C Minimal or moderate	PVP-16B × 3 cycles or cisplatin plus etoposide × 4 cycles plus resection of residual disease	Ongoing trials to minimize toxicity
Advanced	PVP-16B × 4 cycles plus resection of residual disease	Clinical trials ongoing, such as VIP (etoposide, ifosfamide plus cisplatin) versus PVP-16B Early integration of high-dose chemotherapy with autologous bone marrow transplant

Table continued on following page.

Treatment Recommendations (Continued)

CLINICAL SETTING	STANDARD THERAPY	INVESTIGATIVE THERAPY
Seminoma		
Stage A	Infradiaphragmatic radiotherapy (2,500 cGy)	Surveillance (including first year): CT scan of abdomen every 2 mo, chest radiograph and markers (AFP, βhCG, LDH) qmo × 1 yr. Second year: Abdominal CT q4mo with chest radiograph and serum markers every 2 mo.
Stage B1 or B2	Infradiaphragmatic radiotherapy (2,500 cGy)	
Stage B3 (palpable or >10 cm)	Infradiaphragmatic radiotherapy or cisplatin-based combination chemotherapy	Management of residual mass is controversial (observe, resect, radiotherapy)
Stage C	PVP-16B × 4 cycles or other cisplatin-based combination therapy	Same as NSGCT clinical trials; based on tumor extent ("good risk" vs. "poor risk")

From Loehrer PJ Sr: Current Therapy in Hematology-Oncology, 4th ed. Philadelphia, B.C. Decker, 1992, p 305, with permission.

57. Where else may germ cell tumors arise?

Most frequently, in midline structures such as mediastinum and retroperitoneum.

58. What is the prognosis of extragonadal germ cell tumors in relation to their testicular counterparts?

Stage for stage, it is the same as with regard to chemosensitivity, although patients tend to present with more advanced disease.

59. What is in the differential diagnosis of extragonadal germ cell tumors?

They may be confused with adenocarcinomas, sarcomas, lymphomas, and melanomas. The germ cell tumors are much more curable and are treated with different chemotherapy. The diagnosis can be made by testing for βhCG and AFP.

60. What is the reproductive capacity of patients with germ cell tumors treated with chemotherapy?

Ninety-six percent of patients have azoospermia following four courses of cisplatin-based combination chemotherapy. However, eventually one-half of patients will have normal sperm counts and motility.

61. Have congenital anomalies been seen in the offspring of patients who have had germ cell tumors treated with chemotherapy?

No.

62. Will patients whose disease is resistant to first- and second-line chemotherapy invariably die of their disease?

No. Some patients may have their retroperitoneal and pulmonary metastases resected and never have recurrences. Alternatively, 15–30% of patients with resistant disease who receive two courses of high-dose carboplatin and VP-16 followed by autologous bone marrow transplantation may also be cured.

Acknowledgment. The author acknowledges with thanks the contribution of Kelly Mack, RN, MSN, OCN for her assistance in the review and preparation of this manuscript.

BIBLIOGRAPHY

1. Brodsky GL: Pathology of testicular germ cell tumors. Hematol Oncol Clin North Am 5(6):1095–1126, 1991.
2. Einhorn LH: Testicular cancer as a model for curable neoplasm: The Richard and Hinda Rosenthal Foundation Award Lecture. Cancer Res 41(3):275–280, 1981.
3. Holleb AL, Fink DJ, Murphy GP: American Cancer Society Textbook of Clinical Oncology. Atlanta, American Cancer Society, 1991.
4. Loehrer PJ: Testicular cancer. In Brain MC, Carbone PP (eds): Current Therapy in Hematology-Oncology, 4th ed. Philadelphia, B.C. Decker, 1992.
5. Loehrer PJ, Sledge GW, Einhorn L: Heterogeneity among germ cell tumors of the testis. Semin Oncol, 1985, pp 304–316.
6. Loehrer PJ, Williams SD, Einhorn LH: Testicular cancer: The quest continues. J Natl Cancer Inst 80(17):1373–1382, 1988.
7. Murphy BR, Breeden ES, Donahue JP, et al: Surgical salvage of chemorefractory germ cell tumors. J Clin Oncol 11:324–329, 1993.
8. Nichols CR, Andersen J, Lazarus HM, et al: High-dose carboplatin and etoposide with autologous bone marrow transplantation in refractory germ cell cancer: An Eastern Cooperative Oncology Group Protocol. J Clin Oncol 10:558–563, 1992.
9. Nichols CR, Williams SD, Loehrer PJ, et al: Randomized study of cisplatin dose intensity in poor-risk germ cell tumors: A Southeastern Cancer Study Group and Southwest Oncology Group Protocol. J Clin Oncol 9:1163–1172, 1991.
10. Oliver RTD, Ong JYH, Ostrowski MJ, et al: Surveillance, prophylactic radiotherapy or adjuvant carboplatin in the management of stage I seminoma. Abstract 22, 7th International Conference on the Adjuvant Therapy of Cancer, Tucson, AZ, 1993.
11. Richie JP: Surgical aspects in the treatment of patients with testicular cancer. Hematol Oncol Clin North Am 5(6):1127–1142, 1991.
12. Williams SD, Birch S, Einhorn LH, et al: Disseminated germ cell tumors: Chemotherapy with cisplatin plus bleomycin plus either vinblastine or etoposide. A trial of the Southeastern Cancer Study Group. N Engl J Med 316:435–440, 1987.
13. Williams SD, Stablein DM, Einhorn LH, et al: Immediate adjuvant chemotherapy versus observation with treatment at relapse in pathological stage II testicular cancer. N Engl J Med 317:433–438, 1987.

73. RENAL AND BLADDER CANCER

Frank J. Mayer, M.D., and L. Michael Glode, M.D.

RENAL CELL CARCINOMA

1. What is the approximate annual incidence and yearly death rate from renal cell carcinoma in North America?

Incidence: 25,000/yr (approximately)

Mortality: 10,000/yr (approximately)

2. What is the classic triad of symptoms with which patients with renal cell carcinoma present? Approximately what percentage of patients present with this triad?

Hematuria, flank pain, and palpable flank mass comprise the classic triad of renal cell carcinoma. Whereas in the past 30–40% of patients presented with one of the above symptoms or signs, now only 10% of patients present with all three. With the advent of more frequent abdominal imaging with computed tomography (CT) and ultrasound, detection of asymptomatic, small renal cell carcinomas has increased considerably. Thus, fewer patients are expected to present with any of the symptoms of the triad.

3. Which paraneoplastic syndromes commonly occur in association with renal cell carcinoma? Name the presumptive agents causing each syndrome.

Syndrome	Agent
Erythrocytosis	Erythropoietin
Hypercalcemia	PTH-like substance
Stouffer's syndrome (abnormal liver function tests without liver metastasis)	Unknown
Hypertension	Renin

4. What neovascular feature of renal cell carcinoma makes this tumor unique among neoplasms?

Although many tumors demonstrate angiogenesis, renal cell carcinoma often produces tumor thrombi that extend into the renal vein or vena cava. These thrombi may extend even into the right atrium. On rare occasions, the tumor thrombus outgrows its blood supply and undergoes autonecrosis.

5. Give the tumor, node, and metastasis (TNM) system for staging renal cell carcinoma.

T_1 Tumor confined by capsule, <2.5 cm
T_2 Tumor confined by capsule, >2.5 cm
T_{3a} Tumor confined by perirenal (Gerota's) fascia, may involve ipsilateral adrenal gland
T_{3b} Tumor confined by perirenal (Gerota's) fascia, with tumor thrombus in renal vein or vena cava
T_4 Tumor invades contiguous structures, (e.g., colon, liver, spleen)
N_+ Regional or distant lymphatic metastasis(es)
M_+ Distant metastases (liver, lung, bone, brain)

6. What are the most common sites of metastasis of renal cell cancer?

Liver, lung, bone, brain, and regional lymphatics.

7. What is the natural history of untreated metastatic renal cell cancer?

Most patients succumb within 1 year of diagnosis. On rare occasions, patients with biopsy-proved solitary metastases have demonstrated spontaneous regression and enjoy long-term survival, probably because of host immunosurveillance and tumor necrosis.

8. Is renal cell carcinoma sensitive to either chemotherapy or radiotherapy?

Renal cell carcinoma is neither chemosensitive nor radiosensitive. Most renal cell carcinomas can be shown to express the multiple drug-resistance gene, which codes for production of a glycoprotein that causes calcium-channel–mediated efflux of chemotherapeutic agents.

9. Is renal vein or vena cava tumor always a poor prognostic feature of renal cell carcinoma?

Patients treated with complete en-bloc resection of the kidney and its tumor thrombus enjoy a survival rate equal to that of patients who have the identical stage of renal primary tumor without tumor thrombus. Incomplete resection of the tumor thrombus is associated with shortened survival (6 months–1 year). These patients are at risk of sudden death due to pulmonary embolism. Adjunctive or palliative renal arterial embolization is often used, although the technique is controversial.

10. What is the generally recommended approach to the management of a patient with a clinically staged T_2 lesion of the kidney, normal contralateral kidney, solitary (biopsy-proved) pulmonary metastasis, and no other evidence of disease?

Because renal cell carcinoma is generally resistant to chemotherapy, most urologists attempt radical nephrectomy and segmental resection of the isolated pulmonary metastasis.

Long-term survival with this approach is possible, although many patients ultimately relapse with metastases elsewhere. The approaches outlined in question 11 are a reasonable option in a research setting.

11. Name the immunotherapeutic approaches that have shown promise in the management of metastatic renal cell carcinoma.

Interleukin and interferon alpha, used either separately or in concert, have shown modest efficacy in treating renal cell carcinoma. The technique of harvesting patient blood and superinducing the cell fraction with lymphokine-activated killer cells is no longer actively practiced.

Research with tumor-infiltrating lymphocyutc therapy continues to show moderate promise. The tumor or metastasis is excised, and the lymphocytes contained in the cancer are surperinduced with lymphokines and reinfused into the patient's blood stream. Durable response rates of about 33% have been obtained, although this therapy is highly toxic.

BLADDER CANCER

12. Identify the two major histologic subtypes of bladder cancer seen in North America. On a percentage basis, what is their respective contribution to the total annual number of primary bladder cancer cases?

Transitional cell carcinoma (TCC) comprises about 92% of the roughly 50,000 cases of bladder cancer diagnosed annually in the United States. Squamous cell carcinoma is the next most common variant of bladder cancer in the United States, accounting for 3–7% of all cases.

13. What are the purported etiologic factors associated with the development of TCC of the bladder?

Up to one-third of all cases of bladder cancer may be due to cigarette smoking. A dose-response relationship has been proposed, because the risk for bladder cancer increases with increased duration of smoking and increased number of cigarettes smoked (on average). Exsmokers have a lowered incidence of cancer compared with active smokers.

Occupational exposures may be responsible for up to one-third of newly diagnosed cases of bladder cancer. Rehn demonstrated in 1895 that aniline dyes were linked to bladder malignancies. In general, the aromatic amines, such as 2-naphthylamine, 4-aminobiphenyl, and 4, 4 diaminobiphenyl have been shown to act as carcinogens in the urothelium.

Several other studies have tried to link coffee and artificial sweetener (saccharin, cyclamates) to the development of bladder cancer. The pervasive use of these two substances in modern society makes it exceedingly difficult to implicate either in the formation of TCC of the bladder. Laboratory studies in rodents used excessively high doses of sweeteners to induce tumor formation. To achieve the same dose with human consumption would be quite difficult.

Up to 10% of patients treated with cylcophosphamide and followed for more than 10 years may develop bladder cancer. The metabolite, acrolein, is felt to be the agent responsible for tumor initiation. Pelvic irradiation also has been linked to the development of TCC of the bladder.

14. What is the mechanism of bladder carcinogenesis?

A significant proportion of products inhaled through the pulmonary system or ingested through the alimentary tract are filtered through the renal system, concentrated in the urine, and then stored in the urinary bladder for several hours. It is believed that ingested carcinogens, which bathe the bladder epithelium, initiate a change in the genome of the epithelial cells. Alterations on chromosome 9 may be associated with the development of bladder cancer. Promotion of oncogenes or inactivation of tumor suppressor genes may be the second step in the transformation to the cancerous state.

15. What are the presumed etiologic factors associated with the development of primary squamous cell carcinoma of the bladder in North America? How do they contrast with etiologic factors for the same disease in the Nile River valley?

Chronic irritation can induce squamous metaplasia of the bladder mucosa (epithelium). Although squamous metaplasia is not a premalignant condition, ongoing irritation of the mucosa by a bladder calculus or indwelling bladder catheter may promote malignant change. Up to 10% of paraplegics with long-term indwelling catheters develop bladder cancer, usually squamous cell carcinoma.

In the Nile River valley, endemic infestation by the fluke *(Schistosoma haematobium)* has been linked to the development of chronic cystitis in field workers and other infected individuals. The worm burrows through the sole of the bare foot of individuals wading in the Nile River. The chronic infection eventually leads to squamous cell carcinoma of the bladder. The bilharzial variant of squamous cell carcinoma is usually well-differentiated, occurs in younger individuals, and generally has a better prognosis than the nonbilharzial variant, which carries a very poor prognosis.

16. What is the embryologic progenitor of the urachus? What is the most common histologic type of cancer arising in this structure?

The allantois gives rise to the urachus, a thin fibrous cord connecting the umbilicus to the bladder dome. Urachal carcinomas are usually adenocarcinomas arising in an incompletely obliterated urachus. They are quite rare, presenting as a bloody or mucoid mass draining into the bladder or via the umbilicus. Even with radical extirpation, the prognosis is poor, because the tumor is usually disseminated at diagnosis.

17. Outline the TNM system for staging bladder cancer.

T_0	No tumor in specimen
T_{is}	Carcinoma in situ
T_a	Noninvasive (mucosal) papillary tumor
T_1	Invasion of lamina propria (submucosa) only
T_2	Superficial invasion of muscularis propria
T_{3a}	Deep invasion of muscularis
T_{3b}	Invasion of perivesical adipose tissue
T_4	Invasion of contiguous organs (e.g., rectum, pelvic sidewall, uterus, or deep prostatic involvement)
N_1	One node positive, <2 cm in diameter
N_2	One node positive, 2–5 cm in diameter, or multiple nodes, all <5 cm in diameter
N_3	Any node(s) >5 cm in diameter
M_1	Distant metastases

18. Which of the above stages correspond to the designation superficial bladder cancer? At initial presentation, what percentage of patients have superficial bladder cancer?

T_{is}, T_a, and T_1 are defined as superficial bladder cancer. Approximately 75–80% of patients present with superficial disease on endoscopic staging and resection.

19. What is the natural history of superficial TCC of the bladder managed by endoscopic resection alone?

Roughly 50–80% of patients with superficial TCC of the bladder suffer a recurrence of tumor within 3 years after initial presentation if not given any adjunctive threapy after endoscopic resection. For grade I tumors, the recurrence rate is 30% at 1 year and 50% at 3 years. For grade III tumors, the recurrence rate is 70% at 1 year and 80% at 3 years.

20. What features of a patient's superficial bladder tumor are predictive of recurrence?

With increasing grade of tumor, the likelihood of tumor recurrence increases. Aneuploidy of the tumor also is suspected to be related to recurrence. Tumors with primarily diploid peaks on the DNA histogram have a low rate of recurrence (roughly 30–40%), whereas tumors with strong aneuploid peaks on the histogram have a 90% rate of recurrence.

Patients with diffuse carcinoma in situ may have a recurrence rate of up to 80%. Patients with a stage T_1 tumor at initial presentation have a 70% incidence of recurrence at 3 years, if they receive no adjuvant therapy after resection. Multiplicity of tumors (>4 tumors at endoscopy) and size of tumor >5 cm also are correlated with a high risk of recurrence.

21. Are there predictors of progression?

Less than 5% of grade I tumors progress to a higher grade, whereas 45% of grade III tumors progress. Multiplicity of tumors is also related to progression. Solitary tumors progress roughly 10% of the time (across all grade categories), whereas approximately 45% of multifocal cases (>3 tumors) progress. Tumors >5 cm progress roughly 35% of the time, whereas tumors <5 cm progress only about 10% of the time. Diffuse carcinoma in situ (CIS) may be related to progression, and aneuploid tumors have been shown to progress up to 60% of the time. T_1 tumors with associated local lymphatic invasion are believed to be at high risk for progression.

Papillary tumors on a narrow stalk appear to progress less frequently, whereas solid tumors on a broad base appear to progress at least 30% of the time. This high rate of progression may be related to the fact that solid tumors are generally of a higher grade.

22. Name four intravesical agents that show activity in the treatment of superficial TCC of the bladder. What key factor is responsible for risk of systemic absorption and subsequent systemic toxicity? Name one unusual toxicity associated with each agent.

In the absence of traumatic catheterization, which allows the direct instillation of the drug into the bloodstream, the molecular weight of the agent is the key factor in absorption through the mucosa and into the bloodstream. Agents with higher molecular weights penetrate the bladder urothelium less readily.

Molecular Weight and Toxicity of Intravesical Agents*

AGENT	MOLECULAR WEIGHT	UNUSUAL TOXICITY
Thiotepa	189 kd	Myelosuppression
Mitomycin C	334 kd	Contact dermatitis
Doxorubicin HCl (Adriamycin)	580 kd	Hypersensitivity reaction
Bacille Calmette-Guérin (BCG)	NA	Disseminated tuberculosis

* Chemical cystitis occurs frequently with all agents.
  kd = kilodaltons; NA = not available.

23. In 1993, what agent has demonstrated the best response rate in the treatment of superficial TCC of the bladder? What results can be expected vis à vis complete eradication of tumor/CIS and prevention of recurrence?

In several carefully conducted, randomized phase III trials, BCG has demonstrated superiority to the majority of the available intravesical chemotherapeutic agents. BCG has been shown to eradicate residual tumor in 60% of cases, to eliminate CIS in 70% of cases, and to prevent recurrence in 80% of appropriately selected cases. At the present time, BCG may be considered the drug of choice for the treatment of superficial bladder cancer with a high likelihood of recurrence or progression.

24. What is the standard induction course for intravesical BCG therapy? How is maintenance therapy administered? Is it effective in prolonging disease-free survival?

The standard induction course for BCG includes 6 weekly instillations, although this recommendation is not founded in scientific fact. BCG causes an ill-defined immune response in the bladder mucosa and lamina propria, which results in tumor cell death. Some patients have a local response (demonstrated usually by irritative urinary symptoms) after 2 or 3 instillations, whereas other patients have no local response even after 6 instillations.

The merits of maintenance therapy are more controversial. One protocol of 3 weekly instillations at 3 months after induction captured an additional 25% of nonresponders into the complete response group at 6-month follow-up. A recently completed trial evaluated the benefits of maintenance therapy at 3 months and 6 months after induction and every 6 months thereafter for a total of 3 years. In this randomized trial, the data suggested that maintenance therapy reduces the rate of tumor recurrence and diminishes the likelihood of cancer progression and death due to bladder cancer.

25. What are the generally accepted absolute contraindications to embarking on an induction course of BCG? Once a patient has begun therapy, what three conditions mandate that BCG must not be instilled on a given day?

BCG is absolutely contraindicated in immunocompromised patients, whether it is due to concomitant systemic chemotherapy, infection with the human immunodeficiency virus (HIV), immunosuppressive doses of steroids, or other immunosuppressed states.

BCG must not be instilled in the face of gross hematuria, traumatic urethral catheterization, or bacterial cystitis. Patients frequently develop irritative urinary symptoms after the second or third instillation of BCG, but culture of the urine is negative. The irritative symptoms are believed to be due to the immune response occurring in the bladder lining.

26. What is the appropriate management of a patient who, in the middle of a 6-week induction course of intravesical BCG, complains of malaise and has a fever of 38.5° C for 2–3 days?

BCG should not be instilled until symptoms abate. The patient should be treated symptomatically with antipyretics, anticholinergics, and antihistamines. Isoniazid (INH), 300 mg daily, should be administered while symptoms persist. INH therapy should be reinstituted 1 day before the next instillation and continued for 3 days after the instillation.

27. What is the recommended treatment of a patient who appears septic from systemic BCG absorption?

Specific therapy includes intravenous prednisolone, isoniazid, and rifampin. Sepsis due to BCG is believed to result partly from a hypersensitivity reaction, and the use of prednisolone is necessary. Supportive therapy of patients in sepsis also is warranted.

28. What is the risk of vascular or lymphatic metastases in superficial papillary TCC and in high-grade CIS?

Roughly 5% of patients with superficial papillary TCC will have metastases, whereas up to 20% with grade III CIS will have metastases.

29. In patients with lymphatic or hematogenous metastases due to bladder cancer, what are the two lymph node chains and the three organs most commonly involved? Give percentages.

Among patients with lymphatic metastases, the obturator node chain is involved roughly 75% of the time and the external iliac lymph node chain about 66% of the time. The most commonly involved organs are the liver (38%), lung (36%), and bone (27%).

30. In 1993, what is the generally accepted first-line therapy for clinically localized, invasive bladder cancer? What is the anticipated 5-year survival of patients treated in this manner (stage T_2 or T_{3a})? What is the 5-year survival of patients treated with second-line therapies?

Radical cystoprostatectomy for men and anterior exenteration for women presently yield the best chance for long-term cancer-free survival. Patients with stage T_2 or T_{3a} TCC of the bladder have a 75% chance for 5-year cancer-free survival.

Definitive external beam radiation therapy (7,000 rads over 7 weeks) results in a 5-year survival rate of about 35% for muscle-invasive disease. In the United Kingdom external beam radiotherapy is used primarily in the management of invasive bladder cancer; patients receive salvage surgery if the cancer recurs after radiation therapy. Unfortunately, only 20% of patients failing radiation are reasonable candidates for salvage cystectomy because of intercurrent illness and metastatic or locally advanced bladder cancer.

Systemic combination chemotherapy with aggressive transurethral resections results in about 50% clinically complete remission. However, roughly one-half of patients with clinically complete remission will have viable cancer when subjected to cystectomy. The appropriate chemotherapy is a combination of methotrexate, vinblastine, Adriamycin, and cisplatin (MVAC).

BIBLIOGRAPHY

1. Atkins MB, Sparano J, Fisher RI, et al: Randomized phase II trial of high-dose IL-2 either alone or in combination with interferon alpha 2B in advanced renal cell carcinoma. J Clin Oncol 11:661–670, 1993.
2. Buzaid AC, Todd MB: Therapeutic options in renal cell carcinoma. Semin Oncol 16(Suppl 6):12–16, 1989.
3. Dayal H, Kinman J: Epidemiology of kidney cancers. Semin Oncol 10:366–371, 1983.
4. Droller MJ (ed): Advanced bladder cancer. Urol Clin North Am 19: 1992.
5. Fradet Y: Biological markers of prognosis in invasive bladder cancer. Semin Oncol 17:533–543, 1990.
6. de Kernion JB, Mukamael E: Selection of initial therapy for renal cell carcinoma. Cancer 60:539–546, 1987.
7. Kiemeney LA, Witjes JA, Heijbroek RP, et al: Predictability of recurrent and progressive disease in individual patients with primary superficial bladder cancer. J Urol 150:60–64, 1993.
8. Lamm DL (ed): Superficial bladder cancer. Urol Clin North Am 19:421–620, 1993.
9. Lum BL, Torti FM: Adjuvant intravesicular pharmacotherapy for superficial bladder cancer. J Natl Cancer Inst 83:682, 1988.
10. Mrstik C, Salamon J, Weber R, et al: Microscopic venous infiltration as predictor of relapse in renal cell carcinoma. J Urol 148:271–274, 1992.
11. Olsson CA, Sawczuk IS (eds): Kidney tumors. Urol Clin North Am 20:193–369, 1993.
12. Rawls WH, Lamm DL, Lowe BA, et al: Fetal sepsis following intravesical BCG administration for bladder cancer. A Southwest Oncology Group Study. J Urol 144:1328, 1990.
13. de la Sanchez MP, Rosell D, Aguera L, et al: Multivariate analysis of progression in superficial bladder cancer. Br J Urol 71:284, 1993.
14. Yagoda A (ed): Chemotherapy of renal cell carcinoma. Semin Urol 7:199–206, 1989.

74. PROSTATE CANCER

Cliff Vestal, M.D., and L. Michael Glode, M.D.

1. What is the incidence of prostate cancer?

The incidence (number of new cases diagnosed) of prostate cancer is 165,000 cases per year. This is now the most common cancer in males besides skin cancers. It ranks second in causes of male cancer deaths.

2. What is the prevalence of prostate cancer?

The prevalence (number of cases existing at any one time) is difficult to obtain. However, in autopsy series, over 30% of men over the age of 50 years had cancer in their prostate. Some studies have shown prostate cancer in greater than 10% of males between the ages of 20 and 40 years in autopsy series.

3. Describe the zones of the prostate.

The fetal prostate consists of the dorsal, ventral, and lateral lobes. In the adult, McNeal's description of the peripheral, anterior, and posterior zones with prostatic periurethral glands is generally accepted.[7] The peripheral zone comprises 65% of total gland size, the central zone 25%, and the transition zone 5–10% of prostatic volume.

4. What are the clinical staging systems for prostate cancer commonly used today?

The two most commonly used systems are the Whitmore system and the TNM system.

Tumor Staging

Whitmore System

A1	One to three foci of well-differentiated tumor or <5% of specimen contains tumor that is well differentiated
A2	Greater than 3 foci of tumor or >5% well-differentiated tumor or any high-grade tumor
B1	Palpable nodule that is 1–1.5 cm in size
B2	Palpable nodule that is >1.5 cm and involving one whole lobe, both lobes, or bilateral nodules
C1	Lateral extension of tumor beyond the prostate gland
C2	Seminal vesicle involvement
C3	Both lateral and seminal vesicle involvement
D1	Local disease rectally, positive pelvic lymph nodes
D2	Nodal disease above the pelvic brim, bone metastases, soft tissue metastases

TNM System

T0a	Focal tumor at prostatectomy
T0b	Diffuse tumor at prostatectomy
T1a	1-cm nodule confined to the prostate
T1b	1-cm nodule confined to one lobe
T1c	Involves both lobes and confined to the prostate
T2	Invades but does not penetrate the capsule
T3	Penetrates capsule with or without seminal vesicle invasion
T4	Fixed to periprostatic side wall or adjacent organs
N1	Single ipsilateral lymph node
N2	Multiple or contralateral lymph nodes involved
N3	Bulky pelvic lymph nodes
N4	Juxtaregional lymph nodes involved
Mx	No metastases found of incomplete assessment
M0	No known metastases
M1	Metastases present

5. Is prostate cancer unifocal or multifocal?

With the addition of whole mount sectioning technique in the microscopic evaluation of the prostate glands, it has been determined that the majority of cancers are multifocal.

6. Define PSA.

PSA stands for prostate-specific antigen. It is a kallikreinlike serine protease and is produced exclusively by the epithelial cells lining the acini and ducts of all types of prostatic tissue. It has recently been demonstrated that some PSA also is produced in the periurethral glands adjacent to the prostate. It is involved in the liquefaction of the seminal coagulum that is formed at the time of ejaculation.

7. What are normal values for PSA?

In 1993, the normal value for all men is <4.0 nanograms per milliliter (ng/ml). Elevations above this level raise the suspicion of malignancy. Mild to moderate elevations may also be due to benign prostatic hyperplasia (BPH).

8. What are the common causes of PSA elevation?
Contrary to popular belief, digital rectal examinations do not raise the PSA. The common causes of PSA elevation include cancer, prostatitis (both chronic and acute), benign prostatic hyperplasia (usually glands that are of significant size), cytoscopy, needle biopsy of the prostate, and transurethral resecton of the prostate (TURP).

9. At what age should screening for prostate cancer be started?
The general recommendation by the American Cancer Society is to screen for prostate cancer after the age of 50 years. In persons with an increased risk (positive family history and black descent), screening should begin at age 40 years. At present, screening includes a digital rectal examination and measurement of PSA level. If either is abnormal, referral to a urologist and subsequent ultrasound and biopsy are usually recommended.

10. Describe the testicular hypothalamic axis in the production of testosterone.

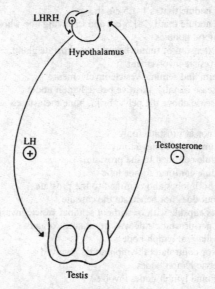

11. Who discovered the relationship between testosterone and prostate cancer?
Huggins and Hodges discovered that hormonal ablation caused regression of metastatic prostate cancer. The Nobel Prize was awarded in 1953 to Huggins for this discovery.

12. Which two methods are most commonly used to decrease testosterone levels produced by the testicles?
Surgical removal of the testicles has been the mainstay of hormonal therapy for metastatic prostate cancer and is a sure way of decreasing 95% of androgens in the male body.

Medical therapy to eliminate testosterone production from the testis involves daily or monthly injections with luteinizing hormone–releasing hormone (LHRH) agonist, which causes a down regulation of luteinizing hormone and therefore decreases the testosterone level to orchiectomy levels. Available formulations include leuprolide (Lupron) and goserelin acetate implant (Zoladex).

13. Name several drugs that inhibit androgenic and/or testicular synthesis of steroids.
Ketoconazole interferes with the P450 cytochrome complex that produces steroid hormones. Side effects include weakness, lethargy, nausea, emesis, and decreased libido. Aminoglutethimide blocks the transformation of cholesterol to pregnenolone by blocking 20-24 desmolase. It requires concomitant administration of corticosteroids to avoid an

addisonian crisis. Spironolactone inhibits 17-α-hydroxylase and 17,20-desmolase, thus decreasing testicular androgen production.

14. What survival benefits does complete androgen ablation afford patients with metastatic cancer of the prostate?
Crawford et al. have shown a survival advantage of >7 months in a randomized clinical trial comparing LHRH alone with LHRH and antiandrogen.[1] Most of the advantage was in low-volume metastatic disease.

15. Name the methods of staging newly diagnosed prostate cancer.
Laboratory staging is essential in evaluating prostate cancer. Studies required include complete blood count (CBC), PSA, serum acid phosphatase, and a complete chemistry profile, including an alkaline phosphatase. The CBC allows evaluation of the hemoglobin and hematocrit. If these values are low, they may suggest bone marrow involvement from prostate cancer. The PSA may have led to the diagnosis of cancer in the first place. Studies have shown that levels of PSA <20 ng/ml in low- to middle-grade tumors rarely show evidence of bony metastasis. An elevated serum acid phosphatase (done by enzymatic method) implies metastatic disease in the majority of patients. In one study of patients with elevated serum acid phosphatase and prostate cancer, 60% of patients had nodal metastasis and 83% developed bony metastases within 2 years. Alkaline phosphatase elevation may also imply bone involvement.

Computed tomography (CT) scanning is quite useful in the staging of tumors thought to be stage D1 with bulky disease. It is quite specific for nodal metastasis. However, CT is a poor test for localized low-stage disease. CT scanning is not able to determine capsular involvement.

Magnetic resonance imaging (MRI) has been used to try and predict capsular involvement of the prostate cancer. Studies have *not* shown increased accuracy of diagnosis with this modality.

Radionuclide bone scanning may detect the areas of metastases to various bony structures. When used with PSA levels, it becomes a highly accurate method of detecting bony lesions. If the PSA level is <20 ng/ml, the chance of a positive bone scan is 0.3%. When the PSA is 15 ng/ml or lower, then a chance of a negative bone scan is virtually 100%. Patients with positive bone scans are considered stage D2.

Pelvic lymph node dissection, either laparoscopic or open, allows one to determine whether there is metastatic disease to the lymph nodes draining the prostate. This procedure should be performed on patients who are candidates for definitive therapy. Elevated levels of PSA or serum acid phosphatase with negative bone and CT scans may lead one to perform a laparoscopic lymphadenectomy in an attempt to avoid a larger operation because of an increased risk of nodal disease. Open lymphadenectomies are performed prior to a radical prostatectomy in patients who are unlikely to have nodal disease.

16. Name the most likely areas of metastasis in prostate cancer.
The most likely areas of metastasis are the lymph nodes draining the prostate. Bone, lung, liver and adrenal glands are less frequently involved.

17. Name the treatment options for stage B1 cancer of the prostate.
Methods of treatment for stage B1 cancer vary. The following modalities are the most commonly used options. Radical prostatectomy is a surgical procedure that removes the prostate gland, the seminal vesicles, and the more distal portion of the ejaculatory ducts. This can be accomplished via a retropubic (abdominal extraperitoneal) or perineal approach. It is often considered the most effective treatment for localized disease. Advances in technique have decreased the rate of incontinence and impotence significantly. The morbidity associated with this procedure includes impotence from 30–50%, depending on

the age of the patient. Incontinence generally ranges from 1–5%. Other complications are those considered inherent in any surgical procedure.

Radiation therapy in the form of external irradiation is currently popular as treatment for prostate cancer. Treatment includes the obturator, hypogastric, and iliac lymph nodes as well as the prostate gland. The incontinence and impotence rates are similar to radical prostatectomy but may take longer to develop. Other complications seen with radiation therapy include radiation cystitis and proctitis.

Brachytherapy, the placement of radioactive substances into the prostate gland, is an option in localized prostate cancer. Techniques include open implantation in combination with a lymph node dissection and ultrasound-guided perineal placement. Substances most often used include iridium-192, gold-198, iodine-125, and palladium-103. Complications are similar to external beam radiotherapy as well as the complications of a pelvic lymph node dissection.

18. What percentage of patients with prostate cancer will have rectal involvement?
Less than 1% of patients will have local extension into the rectum. This is due to Denonvillier fascia, a peritoneal vestige, which lies between the prostate gland and the rectum and usually prevents extension from the gland to the rectum.

19. Administration of estrogens in a man with prostate cancer may cause what significant side effects?
Administration of estrogens to a man increases thromboembolic cardiovascular complications such as stroke and myocardial infarction. It can also cause gynecomastia. The gynecomastia may be prevented by radiotherapy to the breast prior to estrogen therapy.

20. Complete androgen blockage involves removal of all testicular testosterone production and blockade or cessation of adrenal androgen production. Name the drug most commonly associated with complete androgen ablation and its side effects.
Flutamide is the drug most commonly used in the United States to achieve complete androgen blockade. It is given in conjunction with either a surgical or medical orchiectomy. Common side effects of flutamide include diarrhea, nausea, emesis, and occasionally altered liver function tests. When given alone, flutamide may cause gynecomastia.

BIBLIOGRAPHY

1. Crawford ED, et al: A controlled trial of leuprolide with and without flutamide in prostatic carcinoma. N Engl J Med 321:419–424, 1989.
2. Das S, Crawford ED: Cancer of the Prostate. New York, Marcel Dekker, 1993.
3. Garnick MB: Prostate cancer: Screening, diagnosis, and management. Ann Intern Med 118:804–818, 1993.
4. Gillenwater JY, Grayhack JT, Howards SS, Duckett JW (eds): Adult and Pediatric Urology, 2nd ed. St. Louis, Mosby-Year Book, 1991, pp 1277–1394.
5. Huggins C: The effect of castration, of estrogen and of androgen injections on serum phosphatases in metastatic carcinoma of the prostate: Studies on prostate cancer. Cancer Res 1:293–297, 1941.
6. Littrup PJ, Goodman AC, Mettlin CJ: The benefit and cost of prostate cancer early detection. CA 43:134–149, 1993.
7. McNeal JE: Origin and development of carcinoma of the prostate. Cancer 23:24, 1969.
8. Meikle AW, Smith JA: Epidemiology of prostate cancer. Urol Clin North Am 17:709–718, 1990.
9. Pienta KJ, Esper PS: Risk factors for prostate cancer. Ann Intern Med 118:793–803, 1993.
10. Walsh PC, et al (eds): Campbell's Textbook of Urology, 6th ed. Philadelphia, W.B. Saunders, 1992, pp 1159–1221.
11. Whitesel JA, Donohue RE, Mani JH, et al: Acid phosphatase: Its influence on the management of carcinoma of the prostate. J Urol 131:70, 1984.

75. CUTANEOUS MELANOMA

Stephen J. Hoffman, Ph.D., M.D.

1. What is malignant melanoma?
Melanoma is a malignancy of melanocytes and nevus cells. Melanocytes migrate from the neuroectoderm to the skin during the early embryologic period. Melanocytes also migrate to the eye, respiratory tract, and gut. In the skin, they are thought to have the capability of forming nests of cells with a different level of differentiation. These groups of cells are called nevi and appear clinically as moles. Melanoma can arise from a preexisting nevi or spontaneously.

2. Who was Rene Laënnec?
In 1806, the French physician Rene Laënnec first described melanoma as a disease entity. He also was the inventor of the stethoscope, for which he is more well known.

3. Name the warning signs of melanoma.
Typically, melanoma lesions follow the **ABCD**s. They often show **A**symmetry of shape, color or appearance. The **A**ppearance of a new mole in an adult should be evaluated. Their **B**orders are irregular or notched and they occasionally **B**leed. The **C**olor of the mole can be variable with shades of blue, gray, pink, red, or white present in addition to the typical tan or brown color. Any **C**hanging mole should be evaluated. The **D**iameter of most melanomas is >6 mm, but small size should not rule out malignancy.

4. How is melanoma diagnosed?
The diagnosis of melanoma is made histologically. Melanoma is evaluated on the basis of its depth of invasion into the skin and its thickness. **Clark's** level of invasion describes how deep into the skin the tumor has reached. The **Breslow** thickness measures in millimeters the tumor size from the granular layer of the epidermis to the deepest part of the tumor. In general, the deeper and thicker the primary tumor, the more likely it is to have metastasized.

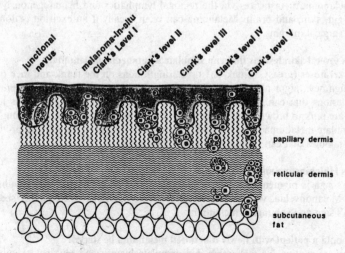

Determination of Clark's levels in primary melanoma.

5. Are there different types of melanoma?
Superficial spreading melanoma is the most common form of tumor, which may arise in preexisting nevi and grow slowly over years. **Nodular melanoma** is the next most common form, and as is implied by the name, is usually a nodule on the skin that is often friable and ulcerated. Nodular melanoma can grow very quickly. **Lentigo maligna melanoma** is similar to the superficial spreading type and generally occurs on the face in elderly patients (this type of melanoma has also been called Hutchinson's melanotic freckle). **Acral lentiginous melanoma** occurs on the palms and soles and sometimes under the nails. This is the more common type of melanoma in nonwhites and generally has a worse prognosis, because the melanoma is not noticed until it becomes fairly thick.

6. How common is melanoma?
According to statistics from the National Cancer Institute, the incidence of melanoma is increasing in the United States at a rate second only to lung cancer in women. The incidence of melanoma in the United States is approximately 14:100,000. The lifetime risk for developing melanoma in the United States is currently ~1:100 for whites. It is too uncommon among those with pigmented skin to estimate risk.

7. Give the most common risk factors for patients developing melanoma.
The incidence of melanoma is approximately equal between men and women. It is generally a disease of young adults (median age ~45 years) and those of northern European ancestry. A personal or family history of melanoma places one in a higher risk group. The most important risk factors, however, are a history of severe sunburning, especially as a child *(use sunscreen!)* and the presence of large numbers of moles, especially atypical ones. If you are reading this book, however, chances are *you* are at risk for melanoma—the incidence of melanoma is statistically correlated with level of education and is increased in people who work primarily indoors but experience short, intense doses of sunlight.

8. What is the natural history of metastatic melanoma?
The most predictable thing about melanoma is its unpredictability. Unlike many malignancies, there is nothing magical about a 5-year disease-free survival. Melanoma can recur for long periods of time after excision of the primary tumor (our clinic recently saw a man with a recurrence of melanoma 37 years after removal of a primary lesion). As a generalization, however, melanoma metastasizes via the regional lymphatics and hematogenously to the liver, lung, gut, skin, and brain. Melanoma can recur locally if an excision is done with insufficient surgical margins.

9. Discuss several skin lesions that can simulate a cutaneous melanoma.
Seborrheic keratoses (greasy, "stuck-on"-appearing lesions on the trunk and face of older adults), benign nevi, pigmented basal cell carcinomas, and solar lentigos ("liver spots") are pigmented lesions that can mimic melanoma. Spitz's nevi, previously known as juvenile melanoma, are pink to brown papules that occur in children, adolescents, and young adults that can simulate melanoma clinically and histologically. Pyogenic granulomas are friable, pink to red nodules that can simulate a nodular melanoma.

10. What is Hutchinson's sign?
Hutchinson's sign is pigmentation of the proximal nail fold associated with a subungual melanoma. Melanonychia, vertical pigmentation of the nail, also is frequently seen with Hutchinson's sign and subungual melanoma.

11. How should a patient with newly diagnosed melanoma be staged?
The hallmark of staging for melanoma is a complete history and physical examination. Because melanoma has propensity to recur on the skin, all cutaneous areas must be fully examined, including the scalp, the palms and soles, and genitals/perineum. Cutaneous

lesions suspicious for second melanomas, atypical nevi, and/or subcutaneous metastases require biopsy. Palpable lymph nodes require histologic sampling by lymph node dissection or fine-needle aspiration. Minimum baseline staging procedures include chest radiographs (with computed tomography [CT], if indicated, to evaluate possible nodules fully) and evaluation of serum liver chemistries. Patients having palpable abdominal masses or complaining of symptoms consistent with visceral metastases may require abdominal/pelvic CT scanning. Patients complaining of central nervous system (CNS) symptoms require brain magnetic resonance imaging (MRI) to rule out intracranial metastases. Based on the depth/thickness of the primary tumor, melanoma is staged by the American Joint Committee on Cancer Staging (AJCCS) criteria.

AJCC Staging Criteria for Cutaneous Melanoma

STAGE	CRITERIA
Ia	Primary melanoma <0.75 mm thick and/or Clark's level II (pT1); no nodal or systemic metastasis (N0, M0)
Ib	Primary melanoma 0.76–1.50 mm thick and/or Clark's level III (pT2); N0, M0
IIa	Primary melanoma 1.51–4.00 mm thick and/or Clark's level IV (pT3); N0, M0
IIb	Primary melanoma >4.00 mm thick and/or Clark's level V (pT4); N0, M0
III	Regional lymph node and/or in-transit metastasis (any pT, N1 or N2, M0)
IV	Systemic metastasis (any pT, any N, M1)

The AJCC Melanoma Committee recommends that tumor thickness takes precedence over Clark's level and should be used for pT (pathologic tumor) staging when differences arise or when Breslow's tumor thickness is unknown or cannot be measured.

12. Describe the treatment for stages I and II melanoma.
The appropriate treatment for stages I and II melanoma is surgical excision of the primary tumor with adequate margins. The current recommendations for surgical margins for excision of primary melanoma are:

Thickness (mm)	Surgical Margins (cm)
In situ	0.5
≤1.0	1.0
≥1.0	2.0

13. What is the role of elective lymph node dissection in melanoma?
This area of melanoma treatment is very controversial. Previously, elective removal of draining regional lymph nodes was performed based on the thought that melanoma metastasized via regional lymphatics and that removal of uninvolved nodes could prevent spread. Melanoma is now known also to metastasize via hematogenous routes. Adequate data now exist from randomized studies to show that elective lymph node dissection has no benefit for patients with primary melanomas of the extremities. For truncal and head/neck melanoma, the case is less clear, although any benefit is marginal and probably limited to patients with primary tumors at high risk to metastasize (e.g., thick or ulcerated tumors).

14. Is there any effective adjuvant therapy for resected melanoma?
Several regimens, including chemotherapy, immunotherapy, radiation therapy, and combinations thereof, have been evaluated with no clear-cut advantage being shown to adjuvant therapy.

15. What is the prognosis for stage I or II melanoma?
In general, the prognosis is inversely proportional to the thickness and depth of the tumor. Total excision of a superficial melanoma, that is, malignant cells limited to the epidermis,

is essentially curative. The 10-year survival rates for Clark's level II melanoma is 96%, level III is 90%, level IV is 67%, and for level V is 26%.[11] Ten-year survival data by stage is 93% for stage I, 68% for stage II, 40% for stage III, and 0% for stage IV disease.

16. Describe how often patients with newly diagnosed melanoma should be evaluated.
We recommend that, at a minimum, patients with melanoma be followed at least every 6 months for the first 2 years after diagnosis. Patients at higher risk for recurrence (e.g., thick primary tumors, primary tumors of the head and neck region, ulcerated primary tumors) should be seen more often, such as every 3–4 months. Complete physical examinations and review of systems should be performed with each evaluation. Follow-up radiologic and laboratory evaluations should be done every 6–12 months or as indicated.

17. What is the treatment for stage III melanoma?
Treatment for stage III disease, that is, in-transit metastases or regional lymph node involvement, is surgical resection of tumor. Patients that advance from stage I/II disease to stage III need to be fully reevaluated to rule out visceral metastases.

18. Discuss the therapeutic options for stage IV melanoma.
Surgery, radiation therapy, chemotherapy, immunotherapy, regional perfusion chemotherapy, and hyperthermia have all been attempted and have some utility in treating the patient with advanced-stage disease.[1] Radiation therapy is generally reserved for palliative treatment of certain tumors, because melanoma is very radioresistant. Surgical excision of isolated visceral tumors is mostly palliative, but in certain cases and in combination with chemotherapy can result in increased disease-free survival. The mainstay of treatment for advanced stage disease is multiagent chemotherapy. Immunotherapy with biologic response modifiers (e.g., interferon alpha, interleukin-2) and/or activated lymphocytes (e.g., lymphokine-activated killer [LAK] cells, tumor-infiltrating lymphocyte [TIL] cells) is under investigation.

19. What is the most effective single chemotherapeutic agent? How is it normally used?
Dacarbazine, or dimethyltriazeno-imidazole carboxamide (DTIC), is the most effective single agent for use in metastatic disease. The most common side effects are gastrointestinal complaints (i.e., nausea, vomiting, and diarrhea) and low-grade fever and chills. DTIC is typically given in combination with cisplatin and tamoxifen. A recent report combining this regimen with interferon alpha and interleukin-2 resulted in a substantially increased response rate for patients with stage IV disease.[10]

BIBLIOGRAPHY

1. Aapro MS: Advances in systemic treatment of malignant melanoma. Eur J Cancer 29A:613–617, 1993.
2. Friedman RJ, Heilman ER, Gottlieb GJ, et al: Malignant melanoma: Clinicopathologic correlations. In Friedman RJ, Rigel DS, Kopf AW, et al (eds): Cancer of the Skin. Philadelphia, W.B. Saunders, 1991, pp 148–176.
3. Friedman RJ, Rigel DS, Silverman MK, et al: Malignant melanoma in the 1990s: The continued importance of early detection and the role of physician examination and self-examination of the skin. CA 41:201–226, 1991.
4. Garbe C, Krasagakis K: Effects of interferons and cytokines on melanoma cells. J Invest Dermatol 100:239S–244S, 1993.
5. Harris MN, Roses DF: Malignant melanoma: Treatment. In Friedman RJ, Rigel DS, Kopf AW, et al: Cancer of the Skin. Philadelphia, W.B. Saunders, 1991, pp 177–197.
6. Ho VC, Sober AJ: Therapy for cutaneous melanoma: An update. J Am Acad Dermatol 22:159–176, 1990.
7. Hoffman SJ, Yohn JJ, Norris DA, et al: Cutaneous malignant melanoma. Curr Prob Dermatol V:1–44, 1993.
8. Koh HK: Cutaneous melanoma (see comments). N Engl J Med 325:171–182, 1991.

9. NIH Consensus conference. Diagnosis and treatment of early melanoma. JAMA 268:1314–1319, 1992.
10. Richards JM, Mehta N, Ramming K, Skosey P: Sequential chemoimmunotherapy in the treatment of metastatic melanoma. J Clin Oncol 10:1338–1343, 1992.
11. Rigel DS, Sober AJ, Friedman RJ: Prognostic factors influencing survival in persons with cutaneous malignant melanoma. In Friedman RJ, Rigel DS, Kopf AW, et al (eds): Cancer of the Skin. Philadelphia, W.B. Saunders, 1991, pp 198–206.
12. Shih IM, Herlyn M: Role of growth factors and their receptors in the development and progression of melanoma. J Invest Dermatol 100:196S–203S, 1993.

76. NONMELANOMA SKIN CANCER

Patrick Walsh, M.D.

1. What is the most common cancer in humans?
Skin cancer. In 1993, it is estim..ted there will be 700,000 cases diagnosed in the United States. It is estimated that 40–50% of people who live to 65 years of age will have at least one skin cancer.

2. What is the second most common cancer in humans?
Skin cancer. Okay, this may be splitting hairs, but it is true. There are several different kinds of skin cancer. Basal cell carcinoma is the most common, accounting for about 75% of skin cancers (this percentage varies with geographic location, being higher in the South and lower in the North). Squamous cell carcinoma is the next most common skin cancer. It is usually more rapidly growing skin cancer and may metastasize.

3. Which type of cancer has the most rapidly increasing incidence rate in the United States?
Skin cancer. Specifically malignant melanoma, which is discussed in the preceding chapter.

4. Define basal cell carcinoma (BCC).
It is a tumor of cells that resemble cells of the basal layer of the epidermis. The epidermis comprises several distinct layers. The basal layer (stratum germinativum) is the bottom layer overlying the dermis and is the only actively dividing layer (regenerative layer) of the epidermis. Above the basal layer is the squamous layer (stratum spinosum), then the granular cell layer (stratum granulosum), and then the cornified, or horny, cell layer (stratum corneum).

5. Describe the appearance of BCC.
There are several different forms and each looks a little different. The most common form is the nodular BCC. This looks like a waxy or translucent bump that often has small dilated blood vessels over the top. As this tumor grows, it often develops raised, rolled borders and a central indentation or ulceration. The pigmented BCC is similar to the nodular BCC but has brown, blue, or black pigment distributed irregularly throughout the lesion. Other more uncommon variants include the superficial BCC, which appears as a well-demarcated red patch, and the morpheaform BCC, which is a poorly demarcated, firm, yellow or waxy plaque.

6. Are there other lesions that look like BCC?
The differential diagnosis includes melanocytic nevus (e.g., an intradermal nevus, especially one that is not making much pigment), fibrous papule or angiofibroma, trichoepithelioma (a benign tumor), and other adnexal tumors.

7. How is BCC treated?

There are several effective treatment modalities. Excision, electrodesiccation and curettage, and cryosurgery are curative in over 90% of cases. Each is destructive to the tumor and its surrounding stroma.

8. What happens if BCC is not treated?

Left untreated, BCCs are usually only locally invasive. As they grow, they can invade and destroy underlying structures (e.g., muscle, nerves, bone). They usually do not travel through blood vessels or lymphatics.

9. Discuss Mohs' surgery and when it is indicated.

Mohs' microscopic surgery is a surgical technique developed by Frederic Mohs. The location and orientation of the tumor are accurately mapped on excision, and the excised tumor is frozen and sectioned in such a way as to allow microscopic analysis of all margins (including the deep margin). Any residual tumor can then be accurately identified and removed. This procedure is curative in >95% of cases. Mohs' surgery is indicated for recurrent skin cancers, skin cancers that occur in certain areas of the body (the so-called embryonic cleavage planes), and for skin cancers that occur in cosmetically sensitive areas. Because only the involved tissue is excised, this is a tissue-sparing technique that is ideal for lesions in cosmetically sensitive areas.

10. Define squamous cell carcinoma (SCC).

It is a tumor composed of cells that resemble (both in terms of appearance and molecularly in terms of keratin expression) cells of the squamous layer of the epidermis. This is the second most common skin cancer.

11. Discuss the appearance of an SCC.

There are several forms with distinctive appearances. Beginning with the earliest, most superficial form, SCC in situ, there are three forms: Bowen's disease, erythroplasia of Queyrat, and bowenoid papulosis. Bowen's disease appears as a red, scaly patch or plaque with sharply defined borders. Erythroplasia of Queyrat is a bright red patch or plaque without scale that occurs on the glans penis. Bowenoid papulosis appears as multiple flat-topped red, brown, or flesh-colored bumps on the external genitalia. The more serious (and potentially metastatic) form of SCC is the invasive form. This form usually appears as an ill-defined, red, scaly bump that may ulcerate or bleed easily with trauma.

12. Are there other lesions that look like SCC?

Actinic keratoses, which are red, scaly patches found on sun-exposed skin, may resemble Bowen's disease but usually have less well-defined borders. Inflammation of the glans penis, which may be caused by a variety of factors and conditions, may resemble erythroplasia of Queyrat. Inflammation can be distinguished by its usually transient character. Condyloma acuminata (venereal warts) may resemble bowenoid papulosis. Indeed, bowenoid papulosis is associated with human papillomavirus (HPV) 16 infection. Keratoacanthomas (KAs), rapidly growing and frequently spontaneously involuting tumors, resemble invasive SCC. Some KAs are impossible to distinguish from well-differentiated SCC.

13. How is SCC treated?

Excision is the treatment of choice with dermatopathologic assessment of margins to ensure completeness of excision. Because of the chance of metastases, the destructive modalities used for BCCs, such as cryotherapy and curettage with electrodesiccation, are usually not used unless a section of surrounding skin/mucosa is obtained after the procedure to allow assessment of completeness of destruction of the tumor. Mohs' surgery is recommended for recurrent SCC in any location and SCCs in cosmetically sensitive areas (because of the tissue-sparing quality of the technique).

14. What factors are associated with metastases of SCC?

Location, etiology, and tumor duration are factors strongly associated with metastases. SCC on the lower lip has an incidence of metastases from 10–20%. SCCs that arise in burn scars, chronic ulcers, and sites exposed to high doses of ionizing radiation are usually less well differentiated and have up to a 20–30% incidence of metastases. Tumors that have been present for long periods of time usually penetrate deeper into the skin, which may mean penetration into lymphatics and superficial vasculature and metastases by these routes.

15. Explain the causes of skin cancer.

There are several risk factors associated with nonmelanoma skin cancer. Ultraviolet radiation is believed to be the most common cause of skin cancer. The source is usually the sun but can also be tanning booths and sun lamps. Nonmelanoma skin cancers usually develop in individuals with fair complexion and blue eyes on chronically sun-exposed surfaces such as the face, ears, neck, and the back of the hands. Exposure to certain chemicals such as coal tars, polycyclic aromatic hydrocarbons, inorganic pentavalent arsenic, tobacco smoke tars, nitrogen mustard, and chromates predispose to the development of nonmelanoma skin cancer. Ionizing radiation also predisposes to skin cancer. Finally, immunosuppression, genetic predisposition, and defective DNA repair mechanisms (as seen in xeroderma pigmentosum) all predispose to the development of skin cancer.

16. Who was Percival Pott?

He was a London physician who accurately identified chemical carcinogenesis as the cause of SCC arising on the scrotum of a chimney sweep in 1775. He realized that the chimney sweep's chronic occupational exposure to chimney soot led to the development of SCC on the scrotum. This analysis of the etiology of SCC of the scrotum is often cited as the beginning of cancer research. It is probably the first accurate identification of a human carcinogen.

BIBLIOGRAPHY

1. Arnold HC, Odom RB, James WD (eds): Andrews' Diseases of the Skin: Clinical Dermatology, 8th ed. Philadelphia, W.B. Saunders, 1990.
2. Fitzpatrick RB, Eisen AZ, Wolff K, et al (eds): Dermatology in General Medicine. New York, McGraw-Hill, 1987.
3. NIH Publication No. 92-1564: What you need to know about skin cancer. Bethesda, MD, US Department of Health and Human Services, 1992.
4. Potter M: Percival Pott's contribution to cancer research. Bethesda, MD, National Cancer Institute, NCI Monograph 10:1–5, 1963.

77. PRIMARY BRAIN TUMORS

Allen L. Cohn, M.D.

1. What are the three most common classes of primary brain tumors?

Most brain tumors can be divided into three classes: gliomas, meningiomas, and neural sheath tumors. Gliomas represent the most frequent type of primary brain tumor and include astrocytomas, ependymomas, oligodendrogliomas, and medulloblastomas. Meningiomas are the next most common class of primary brain tumors. Neural sheath tumors are less common and include schwannomas (neurinomas).

2. Is there any genetic predisposition to brain tumors?
For most patients with brain tumors, there are genetic syndromes predisposing them to these tumors. There are some rare exceptions, including tuberosclerosis, Li-Fraumeni syndrome, Turcot's syndrome, neurofibromatosis (NF-1 and NF-2), and Osler-Weber-Rendu syndrome.

3. Are there any environmental factors that have been associated with brain tumors?
Exposure to vinyl chlorides and the subsequent development of gliomas is the only known association between an environmental factor and brain tumors. This environmental exposure is an etiologic factor in only a very small fraction of patients with primary brain tumors.

4. How are astrocytomas graded histopathologically?
Astrocytomas have been graded by different systems. The most common is the Kernohan and Sayre system. In this system, astrocytomas are graded from I to IV. Grades I and II are considered low-grade astrocytomas and grades III and IV are high grade. Grade III also is referred to as anaplastic astrocytoma. Glioblastoma multiforme is a grade IV astrocytoma in this system.

5. What are the biologic behavior differences between low- and high-grade astrocytomas?
Low-grade astrocytomas typically are slower growing and are more differentiated. The median survival is much longer than with high-grade astrocytomas, which are faster growing and less differentiated. The median survival of patients with high-grade astrocytomas varies from 9 to 14 months.

6. Are any astrocytomas cured?
Although the prognosis for low-grade astrocytomas is much more favorable than for high-grade astrocytomas, very few, if any, are cured. The 10-year survival rates vary between 10% and 20%, depending on which series are reviewed.

7. What role does surgery play in the treatment of astrocytomas?
Surgery is important for two reasons. First, it is oftentimes the means of diagnosis. In the past, this was done with an open craniotomy, but now diagnosis can be achieved with a stereotactic needle biopsy. The other role surgery plays is to debulk as much of the tumor as possible. This allows reduction of the mass effect. Gross total resection is performed if possible.

8. What is the role of radiation therapy in the treatment of astrocytomas?
For low-grade astrocytomas that are incompletely resected, radiation therapy can often prolong survival. There are currently no data to support its use in totally resected low-grade astrocytomas. Many studies have shown an increase in survival for patients with high-grade astrocytomas treated with radiation therapy.

9. Does the addition of chemotherapy to radiation therapy benefit patients with astrocytomas?
There have been studies that show a survival benefit for patients treated with radiation therapy and chemotherapy compared with chemotherapy alone for high-grade astrocytomas. A longer survival benefit was seen for patients with anaplastic astrocytoma than with glioblastoma multiforme. The chemotherapeutic agents varied between studies but included drugs such as BCNU, CCNU, procarbazine, vincristine, and cisplatin.

10. Does chemotherapy help patients with recurrent or progressive astrocytomas?
There are many studies that demonstrate response rates of about 20–30% for various agents such as BCNU, CCNU, cisplatin, and the combination PCV (procarbazine, CCNU, vincristine). The median times to progression vary from 10–30 weeks in these studies.

Patients with anaplastic astrocytomas had higher response rates and longer median time to progression than patients with glioblastoma multiforme.

11. Is the treatment of oligodendrogliomas different from that of astrocytomas?
Overall, the prognosis of oligodendrogliomas is superior to astrocytomas. Surgery is the primary therapy. Radiation is recommended for incompletely resected tumors. The use of radiation remains controversial for individuals with completely resected tumors. The role of chemotherapy is less defined. There have been some responses with various regimens such as PCV.

12. Are meningiomas cured by "complete resections"?
Meningiomas that are totally resected have local relapse rates that vary from 7% at 5 years to 30% at 15 years. Most meningiomas that recur do so locally. It is very unusual for metastatic disease to develop.

13. Is radiation or chemotherapy used in the treatment of meningiomas?
Radiation therapy has no role in completely resected tumors. In patients with incomplete resection, it is controversial whether to use radiation therapy postoperatively or when the patient shows signs of tumor regrowth. There is little evidence to support the use of chemotherapy for meningiomas.

14. What can be done to decrease intracranial swelling caused by brain tumors?
Many studies have shown that the use of glucocorticoids can decrease the swelling induced by intracranial neoplasms. Patients usually experience significant improvement after the administration of these agents.

BIBLIOGRAPHY

1. Bullard DE, Rawlings CE, Phillips B, et al: Oligodendroglioma: An analysis of the value of radiation therapy. Cancer 60:2179, 1987.
2. Cairncross JG, MacDonald DR: Chemotherapy for oligodendroglioma: Progress report. Arch Neurol 48:225, 1991.
3. Cairncross JG, Laperriere NJ: Low grade gliomas: To treat or not to treat? Arch Neurol 46:1238, 1989.
4. Chang CH, Horton J, Schoenfeld D, et al: Comparison of postoperative radiotherapy and combined postoperative radiotherapy and chemotherapy in the multidisciplinary management of malignant gliomas. Cancer 52:997, 1983.
5. DeVita VT, Hellman S, Rosenberg SA: Cancer: Principles and Practice of Oncology, 4th ed. Philadelphia, J.B. Lippincott, 1993.
6. Fazekas JT: Treatment of grade I and II brain astrocytomas: The role of radiotherapy. Int J Radiat Oncol Biol Phys 2:661, 1977.
7. Kernohan JW, Sayre GP: Tumors of the central nervous system. In Atlas of Tumor Pathology. Section 10, Fascicle 35. Washington, DC, Armed Forces Institute of Pathology, 1952.
8. Levin VA, Silver P, Hannigan J, et al: Superiority of postradiotherapy adjuvant chemotherapy with CCNU, procarbazine, and vincristine (PCV) over BCNU for anaplastic gliomas: NCOG 6G61 final report. Int J Radiat Oncol Biol Phys 21:709, 1991.
9. Mirmanoff RO, Dosaretz DE, Linggood RM, et al: Meningioma. Analysis of recurrence and progression following neurosurgical resection. J Neurosurg 62:18, 1985.
10. Moss AR: Occupational exposure and brain tumors. J Toxicol Environ Health 16:703, 1985.
11. Russell DJ, Rubenstein LJ: Pathology of Tumors of the Nervous System, 4th ed. Baltimore, Williams & Wilkins, 1977.
12. Shapiro WR, Green SB, Burger PC, et al: Randomized trial of three chemotherapy regimens and two radiotherapy regimens in post-operative treatment of malignant glioma: Brain tumor cooperative group trial 8001. J Neurosurg 71:1, 1989.
13. Solan MJ, Kramer S: The role of radiation therapy in the management of intracranial meningiomas. Int J Radiat Oncol Biol Phys 11:675, 1985.
14. Wallner KE, Gonzales M, Gheline GE: Treatment of oligodendrogliomas with or without post-operative irradiation. J Neurosurg 68:684, 1988.

78. THYROID AND PARATHYROID CANCER

Daniel H. Bessesen, M.D.

THYROID CANCER

1. How does thyroid cancer present?

Thyroid cancer usually presents as a nodule in the thyroid gland. Thyroid nodules are quite common. The exact prevalence varies depending on the sensitivity of the examination. If normal adults are screened by palpation of the thyroid gland alone, nodules are identified in 3–5%. If on the other hand, the thyroid is examined in 2-mm sections at autopsy, thyroid nodules are found in 50% of all individuals. Thyroid nodules are more common in women, the elderly, and in those who have been exposed to ionizing radiation. Fewer than 5% of clinically apparent thyroid nodules are malignant. Excluding ovarian cancer, thyroid cancer is the most common cause of endocrine cancer (12,100 cases per year) and endocrine cancer death (1,025 cases per year) in the United States. The problem then is to identify which of the many thyroid nodules are likely to be malignant and remove them.

2. Discuss how a solitary thyroid nodule should be evaluated.

In evaluating a thyroid nodule, the goal is to identify nodules with a high likelihood of being malignant. The evaluation of a solitary thyroid nodule has changed in recent years. In the past, after thyroid hormone levels were checked, the next test was usually a radioactive iodine thyroid scan. Although it is true that a "hot" or autonomous nodule is virtually never malignant, "hot" nodules are relatively uncommon, and as a result a thyroid scan usually does not obviate the need for a biopsy of the nodule. Another test that was popular was the thyroid ultrasound. If an ultrasound of the nodule demonstrates a simple, uncomplicated, thin-walled cyst, then the nodule is probably benign. Any other appearance on ultrasound is not reassuring and the next step should be a fine-needle aspiration of the mass. A thyroid scan and ultrasound add substantial cost to the evaluation of a thyroid nodule and rarely are adequate to rule out the possibility of malignancy. Therefore, many endocrinologists now think that the initial steps in the evaluation of a thyroid nodule should be measurement of thyroid-stimulating hormone (TSH) and thyroid hormone level (T4, T3RU) to rule out hyperthyroidism followed by fine-needle aspiration (FNA) biopsy of the nodule.

3. Explain how fine-needle aspiration biopsy is performed and what it shows.

The FNA biopsy is a safe, inexpensive, minimally invasive, simple, outpatient procedure that, when done by an experienced operator, is very accurate in categorizing thyroid nodules as possibly malignant or not. FNA has virtually no complications and is well tolerated by patients. With the patient supine, a 21- to 25-gauge needle attached to a 20-ml syringe is passed multiple times through the nodule applying constant suction. An adequate biopsy contains at least six groups of cells with at least 10 cells in each group. The diagnostic accuracy of the FNA biopsy depends on the skill and experience of the person performing the biopsy and the pathologist interpreting it. The biopsy can be read as either benign (69%), suspicious (10%), malignant (4%), or inadequate/nondiagnostic (17%). An adequate specimen can be obtained about 50% of the time on repeat biopsy when the initial specimen was inadequate. If a "suspicious" result is obtained, most experts would recommend surgical removal of the nodule, as the risk of malignancy is approximately 20%. Autonomous nodules can appear suspicious or malignant on FNA. Therefore, if FNA is used as the initial step in the evaluation of a thyroid nodule, scans must be done on all patients with malignant or suspicious biopsies. This markedly reduces the total number of scans done. If used as the initial test, FNA can reduce the cost of evaluating a thyroid nodule by at least 25% compared with an approach that first utilizes a thyroid scan.

4. Are there different types of thyroid cancer?

The most common types of thyroid cancer arise from thyroid parenchymal cells and are of one of two histologic types: papillary (60–70%) or follicular (15–20%). Some tumors have mixed papillary and follicular histology and behave in a manner that is similar to pure papillary tumors. Medullary carcinoma of the thyroid (MCT) arises from the calcitonin-producing C cells of the thyroid gland. These tumors make up approximately 5% of all thyroid cancers. MCT may occur sporadically, in familial clusters, or as part of the multiple endocrine neoplasia II (MEN IIa and MEN IIb) syndromes. MEN IIa consists of the associated MCT, pheochromocytoma, and less commonly hyperparathyroidism. Individuals with MEN IIb also have mucosal neuromas and a marfanoid habitus. The most malignant and rare of the thyroid cancers are lymphoma of the thyroid (2–5% of all thyroid cancers) and anaplastic thyroid cancer (2–5% of all thyroid cancers). These cancers often present in the elderly as large rock-hard masses in the neck.

5. What factors have prognostic significance in thyroid cancer?

The histologic type of the tumor has prognostic significance. Papillary or mixed tumors have the best prognosis, whereas follicular tumors have a slightly worse prognosis. These types are referred to as "differentiated" thyroid cancers. MCT has a substantially worse prognosis. Anaplastic carcinoma and lymphoma of the thyroid have the worst prognosis, with mean survival of 3–5 months.

The size of the primary tumor also is important. For papillary and follicular cancers, tumors <2.5 cm have the best prognosis. Larger primaries are of more concern. Surprisingly, involvement of regional lymph nodes is not a poor prognostic factor if the histology is papillary. This is not true if the histology is follicular, medullary, anaplastic tumors or lymphoma. Extension of the tumor through the thyroid capsule is a poor prognostic sign, as is a more aggressive histologic grade. The age of the individual at the time of diagnosis also is important. Age <20 years or >60 years confers a worse prognosis. Finally, distant metastases are a poor prognostic sign.

6. Describe the proper initial management of papillary or follicular thyroid cancer.

Surgical resection is the first step in the treatment of thyroid cancer. The surgical resection not only serves to remove all malignant tissue from the neck but sets the stage for future monitoring and treatment. For low-risk cancer (papillary histology, age 20–60, <2-cm primary lesion, no capsular invasion, and absence of nodal or distant metastasis), a simple lobectomy is adequate surgery. For tumors associated with poor prognostic factors, most experts think that ablation of all thyroid tissue in the neck allows for optimal long-term follow-up. If there is no thyroid tissue in the patient, then the detection of a thyroid-specific protein (thyroglobulin) in the serum or radioactive iodine uptake in the body signals recurrent thyroid cancer. If there is still normal thyroid tissue in the patient (as is true when only a lobectomy is done during the initial surgery), then these tests for recurrence are not useful.

Ablation of all normal thyroid tissues begins with a "near-total" thyroidectomy. The goal of a near-total thyroidectomy is to remove, in addition to the primary tumor, almost all normal thyroid tissue in the neck leaving only a small amount of tissue around the parathyroid glands to minimize the risk of iatrogenic hypoparathyrodisim. Following a near-total thyroidectomy, the normal thyroid tissue that has been left behind can be ablated with radioactive iodine.

7. How is the remaining normal thyroid tissue or any metastatic tissue ablated?

Metastatic thyroid cancer and normal thyroid tissue left behind by the surgeon can be ablated with ^{131}I. The standard initial dose of radioactive iodine used to ablate metastatic tumor is 100 to 150 millicuries (mCi). The ^{131}I must be taken up by the tumor to destroy it. A large dose is required for recurrent cancer, because the malignant tissue does not take up iodine as readily as normal thyroid tissue.

The dose necessary to ablate a remnant of normal thyroid tissue left behind after surgery is more controversial. A dose of 100 mCi will work, but it requires that the patient be hospitalized, as the radioactivity excreted in the urine following this high dose exceeds levels that can enter public water treatment facilities. In addition, these high doses expose nonthyroidal tissues in the patient to significant radiation, which may predispose to a second malignancy later in life. A dose of 29.9 mCi has been championed by some, because it is often effective in ablating the normal thyroid tissue left behind following surgery, doesn't require hospitalization (is therefore less expensive), and exposes the patient to less risk of a second malignancy.

8. Discuss the follow-up of the patient with treated thyroid cancer.
Differentiated thyroid cancer is believed to grow in response to the pituitary hormone TSH. For this reason, following adequate initial treatment, all patients with differentiated thyroid cancer should receive lifelong suppression therapy with oral levothyroxine (T4). The dose of levothyroxine should be sufficient to decrease TSH to low or undetectable levels, so as not to stimulate growth of thyroid tissue. Differentiated thyroid cancer is usually very slow growing, and therefore tests for recurrent disease are done every 6 months for 1–2 years and then annually for several years. The two tests that are useful in detecting recurrent thyroid cancer are the serum thyroglobulin level and the total body ^{131}I scan. As mentioned above, these tests are useful only when the patient has had a near-total thyroidectomy followed by radioactive iodine ablation. The sensitivity of these tests is improved if TSH is elevated at the time they are done. To accomplish this, levothyroxine is discontinued and oral T3 therapy is begun (25 μg of liothyronine sodium [Cytomel] two to three times daily) 4 weeks before the studies are performed. The oral T3 is discontinued 7–10 days before the total body scan is done. The sensitivity of the total body scan is a function of the dose of ^{131}I given. A large dose of ^{131}I will reveal more disease than a small dose. Unfortunately, simply visualizing a "spot" of recurrent disease on a total body scan does not mean that enough radioactivity can be delivered to that site to ablate it. For this reason, most endocrinologists use 5–10 mCi as a diagnostic scanning dose. If recurrent disease is identified, 100–150 mCi of ^{131}I is then given to ablate it. Chemotherapy and traditional radiotherapy do not have an important role in the treatment of differentiated thyroid cancer.

9. Are there any risks associated with suppressive therapy with levothyroxine?
It is becoming increasingly clear that suppressive therapy with levothyroxine may cause osteoporosis in some who are predisposed. These include lean, white, postmenopausal women not on estrogen replacement therapy, smokers, and those individuals with a family history of osteoporosis or preexisting osteoporosis.

10. How are medullary carcinoma, anaplastic carcinoma, and lymphoma of the thyroid treated?
The only effective form of therapy for these tumors is complete surgical resection. MCT is usually a more slow-growing tumor than anaplastic cancer or lymphoma of the thyroid, and it can be identified early by screening serum calcitonin levels following calcium or pentagastrin stimulation in predisposed family members. For these reasons, a substantial number of individuals with MCT are cured of their disease. Conversely, anaplastic cancer and lymphoma usually present late and are often not resectable. As a result, the prognosis for these conditions is quite poor.

PARATHYROID CANCER

11. How does parathyroid cancer present?
Parathyroid cancer classically presents with marked hypercalcemia, increased parathyroid hormone (PTH) levels, and a neck mass. Parathyroid cancer probably accounts for <1% of all cases of hyperparathyroidism. Parathyroid cancers are equally distributed between men and women, and are often much larger at presentation than benign parathyroid adenomas. A palpable neck mass is present up to 50% of the time when hyperparathyroidism is caused

by parathyroid cancer. Mean serum calcium levels in those individuals with parathyroid cancer are >14 mg/dl 70% of the time and can be as high as 24 mg/dl. PTH levels are often 5 to 10 times higher than the upper limits of normal in individuals with parathyroid cancer as compared with an elevation of 2 to 3 times normal, which is usually seen in patients with benign adenomas. Virtually all patients with parathyroid cancer are symptomatic at presentation in marked contrast to those with hyperparathyroidism caused by a benign adenoma. Kidneys and bones are most often affected. In one series, 37 of 47 individuals with parathyroid cancer had renal involvement and 34 of 62 had specific radiologic evidence of hyperparathyroid bone disease. In another large series, 84% had renal insufficiency and 91% has some evidence of bone involvement.

12. Discuss the treatment of parathyroid cancer.
Surgical resection is the only effective form of therapy in this condition. En bloc resection of the mass without biopsy is the initial procedure of choice. Intraoperative biopsy of the lesion is often associated with dissemination of malignant cells into the operative field resulting in subsequent local recurrence. The average time between initial surgery and recurrence is 3 years, but intervals as long as 20 years have been reported. When tumor recurs, the most effective form of therapy is repeat surgery. Some patients have had as many as eight operations for recurrent disease. The possibility of surgical cure decreases markedly after the second operation, but subsequent surgery can provide long periods of reduced serum calcium levels and a significant improvement in quality of life. Radiation therapy, combination chemotherapy, calcitonin, mithramycin, and diphosphonates have all been tried in this condition, and none has reliably had any effect on serum calcium or survival. Five-year survival is <50% and 10-year survival is approximately 35%.

BIBLIOGRAPHY

1. Gharib H, Goellner JL: Fine needle aspiration biopsy of the thyroid: An appraisal. Ann Intern Med 118:282–289, 1993.
2. Kaplan MM (ed): Thyroid carcinoma. Endocrinol Metab Clin North Am 19:469–766 , 1990.
3. Mazzaferri EL: Management of a solitary thyroid nodule. N Engl J Med 328:553–559, 1993.
4. Mazzaferri EL: Carcinoma of follicular epithelium. In Braverman LE, Utiger RD (eds): Werner and Ingbar's The Thyroid: A Fundamental and Clinical Text, 6th ed. Philadelphia, J.B. Lippincott, 1991, pp 1138–1165.
5. Obara T, Fujimoto Y: Diagnosis and treatment of patients with parathyroid carcinoma: An update and review. World J Surg 15:738–744, 1991.
6. Robbins J: Thyroid cancer: A lethal endocrine neoplasm. Ann Intern Med 115:133–147, 1991.
7. Shane E, Bilezikian JP: Parathyroid carcinoma: A review of 62 patients. Endocrine Rev 3:218–226, 1982.
8. Wynne AG, Heerden JV, Carney JA, et al: Parathyroid carcinoma: Clinical and pathologic features in 43 patients. Medicine 71:197–205, 1992.

---

79. PITUITARY TUMORS AND ADRENAL CARCINOMA

Michael T. McDermott, M.D.

---

1. What kind of tumors occur in the pituitary gland?
Tumors of the pituitary gland may be nonfunctioning or functioning pituitary adenomas, craniopharyngiomas, carcinomas metastatic to the pituitary, and rarely pituitary carcinomas.

2. Which structures may be damaged by pituitary tumor growth?
Superiorly, pituitary tumors may compress the optic chiasm. Laterally, they can invade the cavernous sinuses and compress cranial nerves III, IV, V, and VI or the internal carotid artery. Inferiorly, they may erode into the sphenoid sinus. These tumors also often compress or destroy the remaining normal pituitary tissue.

3. Discuss the clinical features of nonfunctioning pituitary tumors.
These tumors most often present as space-occupying masses, compressing nearby neurologic and/or vascular structures. Common clinical manifestations include headaches, visual field defects, visual loss, and extraocular nerve palsies. Pituitary compression may further result in adrenal insufficiency, hypothyroidism, hypogonadism, growth failure in children, and diabetes insipidus.

4. What is the treatment for a nonfunctioning pituitary tumor?
The treatment of choice is transsphenoidal surgery, in which access to the pituitary gland is gained through the sphenoid sinus. Because these tumors are usually quite large, surgical resection is often incomplete and postoperative radiation therapy may be advisable.

5. What are the clinical features of functioning pituitary tumors?
Prolactinomas produce galactorrhea and amenorrhea in women and impotence in men. Growth hormone–secreting tumors cause acromegaly in adults and gigantism in children. Corticotropin (ACTH)–secreting tumors produce Cushing's disease. Gonadotropin (LH, FSH)–producing tumors and thyrotropin (TSH)–producing tumors usually cause only mass effects but occasionally result in gonadal dysfunction or hyperthyroidism.

6. How are functioning pituitary tumors treated?
Prolactinomas are treated with bromocriptine or pergolide; surgery is performed if there is an inadequate response. Transsphenoidal surgery is the primary treatment for all other pituitary tumors. Growth hormone–secreting tumors also respond to octreotide, a somatostatin analogue. Radiation therapy may be used for any of these tumors, but its full effects are delayed for years.

7. Which cancers metastasize to the pituitary gland?
Metastatic disease to the pituitary gland occurs in approximately 3–5% of patients with widely disseminated carcinoma. The most commonly reported primary tumors are breast, lung, kidney, prostate, liver, pancreas, nasopharynx, plasmacytoma, sarcoma, and adenocarcinoma of unknown primary site.

8. Discuss the clinical features of pituitary carcinoma.
Pituitary carcinomas, which are extremely rare, expand rapidly and cause mass effects. Some secrete hormones causing endocrine syndromes similar to those seen with adenomas. Metastatic disease to the central nervous system, cervical lymph nodes, liver, and bone are commonly associated. Mean survival is approximately 4 years.

9. What is the treatment for pituitary carcinoma?
Transsphenoidal surgery is the primary therapy followed by postoperative radiation. Prolactin- and growth hormone–secreting carcinomas may partially respond to bromocriptine or pergolide. There has been no significant reported use of chemotherapy for pituitary carcinomas.

10. What types of cancer occur in the adrenal glands?
Adrenal cortical carcinomas
Adrenal medullary carcinomas
Carcinomas metastatic from other sites

11. Discuss the clinical features of nonfunctioning adrenal cortical carcinomas.

Approximately 30–50% of adrenal cortical carcinomas do not produce hormones. They present clinically as abdominal or flank pain or as an incidentally discovered adrenal mass. They are locally invasive and metastasize most commonly to liver and lung. The mean survival is approximately 15 months, and the 5-year survival is about 20%.

12. Discuss the clinical features of functioning adrenal cortical carcinomas.

Adrenal cortical carcinomas may secrete aldosterone, cortisol, and androgens alone or in combination. Aldosterone excess, or Conn's syndrome, causes hypertension and hypokalemia. Cortisol overproduction results in the development of Cushing's syndrome. Androgen excess causes hirsutism and virilization in women and abnormal precocious puberty in children.

13. What is the treatment for an adrenal cortical carcinoma?

The treatment of choice is surgery. Mitotane has produced partial or complete tumor regression, reduced adrenal hormone production and improved survival in nonrandomized noncontrolled trials. Other chemotherapeutic agents and radiation therapy do not appear to be effective.

14. Discuss the clinical features of a malignant pheochromocytoma.

Pheochromocytomas cause hypertension, headaches, sweating, and palpitations. Approximately 10% of pheochromocytomas are malignant. In addition to elevated urinary excretion of vanillylmandelic acid (VMA), metanephrine and catecholamines, malignant tumors often have a disproportionate increase in urinary dopamine and homovanillic acid. These tumors eventually metastasize to the liver, lung, and bone.

15. What is the treatment for a malignant pheochromocytoma?

Surgery is the treatment of choice. Alpha-adrenergic blocking agents such as phenoxybenzamine and prazosin are given preoperatively to control blood pressure and replete intravascular volume. These drugs and alpha-methyl tyrosine, a catecholamine synthesis inhibitor, also are effective long-term therapy for patients with unresectable tumors. Cyclophosphamide, vincristine, dacarbazine, and ^{131}I metaiodobenzylguanidine (MIBG) may cause partial regression of residual tumors.

16. What is the significance of metastases to the adrenal gland from other primary sites?

The vascular adrenal glands are a frequent site of bilateral metastatic spread from other tumors such as lung, breast, melanomas, stomach, pancreas, colon, kidney, and lymphomas. Acute adrenal crisis is rare. However, up to 33% of patients may have subtle adrenal insufficiency and experience improvement in their well-being when given physiologic corticosteroid replacement.

17. How should the incidentally discovered adrenal mass be managed?

Adrenal masses should be evaluated for oversecretion of cortisol, aldosterone, androgens, and catecholamines. Cancer is rare in tumors <6 cm in size. All functioning tumors and nonfunctioning masses ≥ 6 cm should be removed surgically. Some experts recommend a size cutoff of 4.5 cm for surgery. Smaller masses should be reassessed in 3–6 months and then annually. They should be removed if there is growth or if hormone secretion develops.

BIBLIOGRAPHY

1. Branch CL Jr, Laws ER Jr: Metastatic tumors of the sella turcica masquerading as primary pituitary tumors. J Clin Endocrinol Metab 65:469–474, 1990.
2. Brennan MF: Adrenocortical carcinoma. CA 37:348–365, 1987.
3. Copeland PM: The incidentally discovered adrenal mass. Ann Intern Med 98:940–945, 1983.

4. Kaufman B, Arafah B, Selman WR: Advances in neuroradiologic imaging of the pituitary gland: Changing concepts. J Lab Clin Med 109:308–319, 1987.
5. Klibanski A, Zervas NT: Diagnosis and management of hormone-secreting pituitary adenomas. N Engl J Med 324:822–831, 1991.
6. Luton J-P, Cerdas S, Billaud L, et al: Clinical features of adrenocortical carcinoma, prognostic factors, and the effect of mitotane therapy. N Engl J Med 322:1195–1201, 1990.
7. Molitch ME, Russell EJ: The pituitary "incidentaloma." Ann Intern Med 112:925–931, 1990.
8. Mountcastle RB, Roof BS, Mayfield RK, et al: Case report: Pituitary adenocarcinoma in an acromegalic patient: Response to bromocriptine and pituitary testing: A review of the literature on 36 cases of pituitary carcinoma. Am J Med Sci 298(2):109–118, 1989.
9. Schteingart DE: Treating adrenal cancer. Endocrinologist 2:149–157, 1992.

80. CARCINOID SYNDROME AND PANCREATIC ISLET CELL TUMORS

Michael T. McDermott, M.D.

1. What are carcinoid tumors?

Carcinoid tumors are neoplasms that arise from enterochromaffin cells. They are classified as coming from the foregut (bronchus, stomach, duodenum, bile ducts, pancreas), midgut (jejunum, ileum, appendix, ascending colon), or hindgut (transverse colon, descending and sigmoid colon, rectum). They occasionally occur in the gonads, prostate, kidney, breast, thymus, or skin.

2. What is the carcinoid syndrome?

The carcinoid syndrome is a humorally mediated syndrome. It consists of cutaneous flushing (90%), diarrhea (75%), wheezing (20%), endocardial fibrosis (33%), right heart valvular lesions, and occasionally pleural, peritoneal, or retroperitoneal fibrosis. Pellagra may also occur because of diversion of tryptophan from niacin to serotonin synthesis by the tumor.

3. Name the biochemical mediators of the carcinoid syndrome.

Carcinoid tumors produce a variety of humoral mediators, including serotonin, bradykinin, tachykinins, histamine, prostaglandins, neurotensin, and substance P. Diarrhea and fibrous tissue formation are probably caused by serotonin, whereas flushing and wheezing are likely due to kinins, histamine, or prostaglandins.

4. Under what circumstances does a carcinoid tumor cause the carcinoid syndrome?

Carcinoid syndrome results when humoral mediators reach the systemic circulation. Gastrointestinal carcinoids usually do not cause carcinoid syndrome unless there are hepatic metastases that impair metabolism of the mediators or secrete mediators directly into the hepatic vein. Extraintestinal carcinoids may cause carcinoid syndrome in the absence of metastases.

5. How is the diagnosis of carcinoid syndrome made?

The diagnosis depends on the demonstration of increased serum or urinary serotonin, 5-hydroxytryptophan (5-HTP), or 5-hydroxyindoleacetic acid (5-HIAA). Foregut carcinoids frequently make only 5-HTP. Midgut carcinoids often produce serotonin and 5-HIAA. Hindgut carcinoids may not make any of these substances, and their production in extraintestinal carcinoids is variable.

6. Can patients with carcinoid syndrome be cured?
Benign extraintestinal tumors causing carcinoid syndrome may be cured by surgery. Malignant carcinoids with metastases are usually incurable but are slow growing, allowing prolonged survival. Extensive debulking is risky and rarely helpful. Chemotherapy and radiation are relatively ineffective.

7. How can the symptoms of carcinoid syndrome be controlled?
Niacin should be given to prevent pellagra. Flushing may decrease with histamine antagonists, phenoxybenzamine, phenothiazines, or glucocorticoids. Diarrhea may respond to methysergide, cyproheptadine, diphenoxylate, loperamide, or codeine. Octreotide, a somatostatin analogue, often controls both flushing and diarrhea.

8. What are pancreatic islet cell tumors?
These tumors, which arise from the islet cells of the pancreas, cause syndromes as a result of overproduction of hormones such as insulin, gastrin, glucagon, somatostatin, and vasoactive intestinal polypeptide (VIP). Insulinomas are benign in 80–90% of cases, but 40–60% of all other islet cell tumors are malignant.

9. Discuss the clinical manifestations of insulin-producing tumors.
Insulinomas produce excessive insulin causing hypoglycemia, which usually occurs in the fasting state or after exercise. The most common symptoms include confusion, slurred speech, blurred vision, seizures, and coma due to neuroglycopenia or reduced glucose delivery to the brain. Adrenergic symptoms of tremor, sweating, palpitations, headache, and nausea also occur occasionally.

10. How is the diagnosis of insulinoma made?
Hypoglycemia (glucose <55 mg/dl in men, <40 mg/dl in women) with hyperinsulinemia (insulin/glucose ratio >0.33) during a 12- to 72-hour supervised fast is diagnostic. Measurement of C peptide, which is cosecreted with insulin, will help distinguish an insulinoma (high C peptide) from surreptitious insulin administration (low C peptide). The urine should also be screened for sulfonylureas.

11. Describe how to localize an insulinoma.
Imaging procedures such as computed tomographic (CT) scan, ultrasonography, transhepatic portal vein sampling, and splanchnic arteriography may all give the correct location, but some tumors cannot be found prior to surgery. Intraoperative palpation and/or ultrasonography usually provide correct localization in these cases.

12. What is the treatment for an insulinoma?
Solitary benign insulinomas should be removed surgically. Patients with unresectable malignant tumors should be treated with frequent feedings and inhibitors of insulin secretion such as diazoxide, verapamil, propranolol, phenytoin, and octreotide. Chemotherapy with streptozotocin and doxorubicin or 5-fluorouracil increases survival and improves symptoms.

13. Discuss the clinical manifestations of a gastrin-producing tumor.
Gastrinomas secrete excessive gastrin, which stimulates prolific gastric acid secretion. Patients develop severe peptic ulcer disease often associated with secretory diarrhea. Gastrinomas usually arise from the pancreatic islets but also may occur in the duodenum and stomach. This disorder also is known as the Zollinger-Ellison syndrome.

14. Explain how the diagnosis of gastrinoma is made.
The diagnosis is made by demonstrating the presence of gastric acidity (pH <3.0) in association with a fasting serum gastrin level >1000 pg/ml or a moderately elevated value that increases by more than 200 pg/ml within 15 minutes after the intravenous administration of secretin.

15. What is the best way to localize a gastrinoma?
Localization of the tumor may be pursued with a variety of techniques to include CT scan, magnetic resonance imaging (MRI), ultrasonography, endoscopic ultrasonography, transhepatic portal venous sampling, selective arterial secretin infusions, and radioactive octreotide scanning.

16. How is gastrinoma treated?
Most benign and some malignant gastrinomas can be cured by surgery. Otherwise, attention should be directed toward reduction of gastric acid overproduction. High-dose H_2 receptor antagonists, omeprazole, and octreotide effectively decrease acid secretion and symptoms in most patients. Refractory patients may require total gastrectomy for symptom relief.

17. Discuss the characteristics of glucagon-secreting tumors.
Glucagonomas cause diabetes mellitus, weight loss, anemia, and a skin rash known as necrolytic migratory erythema. The diagnosis depends on an elevated serum glucagon level (>500 pg/ml). Treatment options include surgery for localized disease, octreotide to reduce glucagon secretion, and chemotherapy with streptozotocin, 5-fluorouracil, and dacarbazine.

18. Discuss the characteristics of somatostatin-secreting tumors.
Somatostatinomas cause diabetes mellitus, weight loss, steatorrhea, and cholelithiasis. The diagnosis is made by finding an elevated serum somatostatin level. Surgery is the treatment of choice. When surgery is not possible, streptozotocin may reduce somatostatin secretion and tumor size.

19. What are the characteristics of vasoactive intestinal polypeptide–secreting tumors (VIPomas)?
VIPomas cause watery diarrhea, hypokalemia, and achlorhydria (WDHA syndrome or pancreatic cholera). The diagnosis is made by finding an elevated serum VIP level. Surgery is the treatment of choice. Octreotide effectively reduces diarrhea in most patients. Radiation therapy, streptozotocin, and interferon alpha also may reduce diarrhea and tumor size.

BIBLIOGRAPHY

1. Feldman JM: The carcinoid syndrome. Endocrinologist 3:129–135, 1993.
2. Friesen SR: Tumors of the endocrine pancreas. N Engl J Med 306:580–590, 1982.
3. Godwin JD II: Carcinoid tumors: An analysis of 2837 cases. Cancer 36:560–569, 1975.
4. Krejs GJ, Orci L, Conlon M, et al: Somatostatinoma syndrome: Biochemical, morphologic and clinical features. N Engl J Med 301:285–292, 1979.
5. Kvols LK, Moertel CG, O'Connell MJ, et al: Treatment of the malignant carcinoid syndrome: Evaluation of a long-acting somatostatin analogue. N Engl J Med 315:663–666, 1986.
6. Leichter SB: Clinical and metabolic aspects of glucagonoma. Medicine 59:100–113, 1980.
7. Moertel CG, Lefkopoulo M, Lipsitz S, et al: Streptozocin-doxorubicin, streptozocin-fluorouracil, or chlorozotocin in the treatment of advanced islet-cell carcinoma. N Engl J Med 326:519–523, 1992.
8. Scully RE, Galdabini JJ, McNeely BU: Case records of the Massachusetts General Hospital: Case 22-1981. N Engl J Med 304:1350–1356, 1981.
9. Service FJ, McMahon MM, O'Brien PC, Ballard DJ: Functioning insulinomas—Incidence, recurrence, and long-term survival of patients: A 60-year study. Mayo Clin Proc 66:711–719, 1991.
10. Wolfe MM, Jensen RT: Zollinger-Ellison syndrome: Current concepts in diagnosis and management. N Engl J Med 317:1200–1209, 1987.

81. OSTEOGENIC SARCOMA

Kyle M. Fink, M.D., Louis Bair, D.O., and Ross Wilkins, M.D., M.S.

1. Who does osteosarcoma affect?
Osteosarcoma is the most common malignant primary bone tumor in childhood and adolescents and of all age groups with the exception of myeloma. Its highest prevalence is in males ages 10 to 22 years.

2. How common are malignant tumors of bone?
Only about 4,000 new cases are seen every year in the United States. This represents only about 0.2% of primary cancers.

3. In what bone(s) is osteosarcoma most commonly found?
In children and adolescents, osteosarcoma is usually found in the distal femur and proximal tibia. Those diagnosed in the elderly population are associated with Paget's disease and are found in the humerus, pelvis, and proximal femur.

4. How do patients with osteosarcoma present?
The typical symptoms are pain, tenderness, and enlargement of a localized area. There is usually a decreased range of motion of an adjacent joint and many patients have pain, particulary at night.

5. Do osteosarcomas frequently metastasize?
Yes. Over 80% of patients have micrometastatic disease secondary to hematogenous spread at diagnosis. The first recognizable site of metastases is the lungs. Regional lymph node spread is rare, although bone metastases can occur.

6. What are osteosarcomas composed of histologically?
They arise from primitive mesenchymal cells—usually malignant osteoblasts and spindle cells that produce immature fragments of trabecular bone often erratically located in the bone.

7. What imaging studies of osteosarcoma are important?
The diagnosis of osteosarcoma is usually confirmed on plain roentgenographs. CT and MRI help in defining the osseous and soft tissue extent of the tumor and its involvement with adjacent joints and neurovascular structures. These images are particularly important in comparison before and after chemotherapy. Imaging is vital in determining local recurrence and metastatic disease. Radionuclide bone scanning is helpful in locating bone metastases.

8. How are osteosarcomas staged?
Staging is based on grade, compartmentalization of the tumor, and metastases.

Surgical Staging of Bone Sarcomas

STAGE	GRADE	SITE
IA	Low	Intracompartmental
IB	Low	Extracompartmental
IIA	High	Intracompartmental
IIB	High	Extracompartmental
III	Low or High	Regional or distant metastasis

From Enneking WF, Spanier SS, Goodman MA: A system for the surgical staging of musculoskeletal sarcoma. Clin Orthop 153:106–120, 1980, with permission.

9. How are suspected osteosarcomas biopsied?
Open biopsy is preferred to sample these heterogenous tumors adequately. The biopsy should be done by the surgeon, who makes the ultimate decision regarding future operative procedures.

10. Is there a standard regimen for successful treatment of osteosarcomas?
Currently, patients undergo preoperative chemotherapy and in many protocols incorporate intra-arterial or intravenous chemotherapy using cisplatinum. After maximum response, the patient then undergoes limb-sparing surgery, if possible. Ninety percent of patients now retain their limb when the tumor involves the extremity, with only 10% having to undergo amputation. Based on the tumor kill at the time of resection, the patient then receives further postoperative adjuvant chemotherapy. If the tumor kill is >90%, the same chemotherapy is used postoperatively, usually for three to four cycles. If there is <90% tumor kill, different chemotherapeutic agents are used postoperatively versus those preoperatively. Radiation therapy is generally only used for unresectable tumors.

11. What chemotherapeutic agents are commonly used?
The most effective agents are Adriamycin, cisplatin, and high-dose methotrexate with leucovorin rescue. Recently, ifosfamide has also been shown to be a highly effective drug for osteosarcoma.

12. What is the overall survival for osteosarcomas?
With the advent of multidrug chemotherapy (used both pre- and postoperatively) in combination with surgical resection, the 5-year survival has risen from approximately 20% to over 80%. Unfortunately, if patients with osteosarcoma already have metastatic disease, particulary in the lung, long-term survival is usually nil. However, late pulmonary metastasis can be wedge resected for curative intent in about 20–25% of patients, which is the same as in soft tissue sarcomas.

BIBLIOGRAPHY

1. DeVita VT Jr, et al (eds): Cancer: Principles and Practice of Oncology. Philadelphia, J.B. Lippincott, 1989.
2. Fink K, Wilkins R: Intra-arterial chemotherapy and limb preservation in osteosarcoma in children (abstract). American Society of Clinical Oncology, 1991, p 1126.
3. Fletcher BD: Response of osteosarcoma and ewing sarcoma to chemotherapy: Imaging evaluation. Am J Roentgenol 157:825–833, 1991.
4. Holleb AI, et al (eds): Clinical Oncology. Atlanta, American Cancer Society, 1991.
5. Jaffe N: Chemotherapy for malignant bone tumors. Orthop Clin North Am 30:487–499, 1989.
6. Klein MR, Kenan S, Lewis MM: Osteosarcoma: Clinical and pathological considerations. Orthop Clin North Am 20:327–345, 1989.
7. Meyer WH, Malawer MM: Osteosarcoma: Clinical features and evolving surgical and chemotherapeutic strategies. Pediatr Clin North Am 38:317–348, 1991.
8. Seeger LL, Gold RH, Chandnani VP: Diagnostic imaging of osteosarcoma. Clin Orthop Rel Res 270:254–263, 1991.
9. Sim FH, Bowman WE, Wilkins RM, Choa EYS: Limb salvage in primary malignant bone tumors. Orthopedics 8:574–581, 1985.
10. Wilkins RM, Sim FH: Evaluation of bone and soft tissue tumors. In D'Ambrosia (ed): Musculoskeletal Disorders: Regional Examination and Differential Diagnosis, 2nd ed. Philadelphia, J.B. Lippincott, 1986.

82. SOFT TISSUE SARCOMAS

Kyle M. Fink, M.D., Louis Bair, D.O. and Ross Wilkins, M.D., M.S.

1. What is a soft tissue sarcoma?

This refers to a large group of malignant tumors arising embryonically from the primitive mesoderm. The primitive mesenchyme within the mesoderm differentiates into the various connective tissues of the body, that is, tendon, ligament, muscle, and bone. Tumors of these tissues are referred to as soft tissue sarcomas. Because of imprecise differentiation, some sarcomas have ectodermal and epithelial origins.

2. How common are soft tissue sarcomas?

They account for an estimated 5,700 cases a year, with an incidence similar to testicular cancer and slightly less frequent than Hodgkin's disease. Approximately 3,100 people die of the disease annually.

3. Where do soft tissue sarcomas arise?

The most common site is the lower extremities but they also are found in various other body sites.

Anatomic Sites of Soft Tissue Sarcomas

SITE	INCIDENCE (%)
Lower extremity	38.9
Retroperitoneal/intra-abdominal	15.2
Trunk	12.9
Upper extremity	10.9
Genitourinary	7.2
Visceral	5.4
Head and neck	4.8
Other	4.6

From Posnar MC, Brennan MF: Soft tissue sarcomas. In Holleb AI, et al (eds): Clinical Oncology. Atlanta, American Cancer Society, 1991, with permission.

4. What is the clinical presentation of sarcoma?

Sarcomas in the extremities are usually painless, slow-growing masses. Retroperitoneal sarcomas are typically asymptomatic until late in their course when patients generally complain of an abdominal mass with associated abdominal fullness, vague abdominal pain, or early satiety. They may also have initial symptoms of diffuse retroperitoneumlike low back pain. This is a constant boring pain even at rest, particularly at night, which is relieved by sitting up or even motion. Occasionally, pain is associated with signs of peripheral or nerve root compression.

5. What predilections do soft tissue sarcomas have?

Soft tissue sarcomas show no predilection for any group or sex. A database study done by Memorial Sloan-Kettering Cancer Center from July 1982 to December 1987 of 1,091 patients with soft tissue carcinomas showed a median age of 50 years, 54% to 46% male to female ratio; 90% of patients were Caucasian.

6. Are there risk factors for soft tissue sarcomas?

No clear etiologic factor has been defined. Patients with neurofibromatosis (von Recklinghausen's disease) have a 10–15% risk of developing neurofibrosarcomas. Chronic lymphedema, particularly in the arms after radical mastectomy and radiotherapy (Steward-Treves syndrome), has resulted in cases of lymphangiosarcomas. Radiation injury and chemical carcinogen exposure also appear to be responsible for a small number of sarcomas. The *majority* of soft tissue sarcomas arise spontaneously.

7. Where do sarcomas metastasize?
The lung is the most frequent site of metastatic involvement. A few histopathologic types have regional lymph node involvement.

8. Which imaging studies are useful in the diagnosis and work-up of a patient with a soft tissue sarcoma?
Recently, when compared with computed tomography (CT) and angiography, magnetic resonance imaging (MRI) has proved to be superior in assessing soft tissue tumors because of better resolution and enhanced distinction between normal and abnormal tissue.

9. Describe how soft tissue sarcomas are staged.
Staging is based on histologic grade, tumor size, regional lymph node involvement, and presence of metastases. However, tumor *grade* is the best prognostic indicator. Grading criteria to type a sarcoma high-grade or low-grade are listed below.

Guidelines to Histologic Grading of Sarcomas

LOW GRADE	HIGH GRADE
Good differentiation	Poor differentiation
Hypocellular	Hypercellular
Much stroma	Minimal stroma
Hypovascular	Hypervascular
Minimal necrosis	Much necrosis
<5 mitosis/10 hpf	>5 mitosis/10 hpf

hpf = high-power field.

10. How are soft tissue sarcomas biopsied for diagnosis?
The procedure of choice is an open biopsy for extremity lesions. The biopsy must be done with an awareness of the subsequent treatment plan if the tissue is malignant. Incisional biopsy should be oriented longitudinally in the extremity for a possible subsequent limb preservation surgical procedure.

11. What is the definitive treatment of soft tissue sarcomas?
Surgery is the primary treatment of all soft tissue sarcomas. In extremity lesions, the goal is limb-sparing surgery if the tumor can be removed and a functional extremity remains. If the surgeon cannot remove the entire tumor, the tumor, in general, cannot be cured with irradiation or chemotherapy alone. If there is already metastatic disease present, particularly in the lungs at the time of presentation of a primary soft tissue sarcoma, cure is almost always impossible.

12. Explain the roles that chemotherapy and radiation play in the treatment of soft tissue sarcoma.
Irradiation may allow less aggressive surgery in selected cases when used as a local adjuvant. The role of systemic chemotherapy for soft tissue sarcomas has not been well defined, particularly in the adjuvant setting. Chemotherapy is currently reserved for palliation of metastatic disease. Generally, if the surgeon does not adequately resect the disease in soft tissue sarcomas, the disease then recurs and treatment becomes palliative with chemotherapy and radiation therapy.

13. Which chemotherapeutic agents are used in the treatment of soft tissue sarcomas?
The most common agent used is doxorubicin (Adriamycin). Other agents used are cyclophosphamide, DTIC, and most recently, ifosfamide.

14. Are patients with pulmonary metastases potentially curable?
If the primary site has been deemed disease free, up to 20–25% of patients with resected pulmonary metastases have been alive and disease free at 5 years in numerous trials. The major factors for their prognosis include tumor doubling time >20 days, disease-free interval >12 months, and the presence of less than four nodules. The two surgical procedures being used are lateral thoracotomy and, more recently, median sternotomy.

15. What is the risk of local recurrence following treatment of soft tissue sarcomas?
Local recurrence remains a problem, with rates as high as 40–50% for head, neck, and truncal sarcomas and 75% for retroperitoneal sarcomas. Extremity sarcomas, however, have shown more favorable results of 25% or less owing to multimodality therapy.

16. List the factors predictive of the likelihood of a local recurrence.

Age >50 years	Certain specific histopathologies
Presentation with recurrent disease	Inadequate margins in resection
High-grade tumor	Size (particularly ≥10 cm)

17. What factors are predictive of likelihood to metastasize?
Size of the tumor appears to be a major predictor, with the greater the size the more likely to metastasize. Other predictors include high-grade tumors and proximal site on an extremity.

18. List the factors predictive of decreased survival.

Age >50 years	Size ≥10 cm
High tumor grade	Regional lymph node involvement
Painful mass at presentation	Inadequate margins
Proximal site	Amputation

BIBLIOGRAPHY

1. DeVita VT Jr, et al (eds): Cancer: Principles and Practice of Oncology. Philadelphia, J.B. Lippincott, 1989.
2. Eilber FR, et al (eds): The Soft Tissue Sarcomas. Orlando, FL, Grune & Stratton, 1987.
3. Geer RJ, Woodruff J, Casper ES, et al: Management of small soft-tissue sarcoma of the extremity in adults. Arch Surg 127:1285–1289, 1992.
4. Hoekstra HJ, Schraffordt KH, Molenaar WM, et al: A combination of intraarterial chemotherapy, preoperative and postoperative radiotherapy, and surgery as limb-saving treatment of primarily unresectable high-grade soft tissue sarcomas of the extremities. Cancer 63:59–62, 1989.
5. Holleb AI, et al (eds): Clinical Oncology. Atlanta, American Cancer Society, 1991.
6. Jaffe KA, Morris SG: Resection and reconstruction for soft-tissue sarcomas of the extremity. Orthop Clin North Am 22:151–176, 1991.
7. Sondak VK, Economou JS, Eilber FR: Soft tissue sarcomas of the extremity and retroperitoneum: Advance in management. Adv Surg 24:333–359, 1991.
8. Springfield DS: Introduction to limb-salvage surgery for sarcomas. Orthop Clin North Am 22:1–5, 1991.
9. Wilkins RM, Sim FH: Evaluation of bone and soft tissue tumors. In D'Ambrosia R (ed): Musculoskeletal Disorders: Regional Examination and Differential Diagnosis, 2nd ed. Philadelphia, J.B. Lippincott, 1986, pp 189–217.

83. CANCER OF UNKNOWN PRIMARY SITE

Kerry Scott Fisher, M.D.

1. How do you know the primary site is unknown?
When a histologically confirmed cancer is identified in a site not consistent with a primary tumor in that organ and no primary site is apparent after a reasonable search, this is considered carcinoma of unknown primary site.

2. Is cancer of unknown primary site a common problem?
Yes. It accounts for 4–15% of histologies in all cancer patients with solid tumors and is the eighth most common form of cancer. It is a disease that usually affects older individuals, with an average age at diagnosis of 60 years.

3. How does the biology of cancer of unknown primary site differ from cancer where the primary site is known?
When the primary site is established during the patient's life or at autopsy in patients with unknown primary site, the tumor is often found in an organ not expected from the common patterns of spread in known primary tumors. If the primary site is identified, the pattern of metastasis is often unexpected for that cancer. Aside from lung cancer, cancers that occur commonly in the general population make up only a small percentage of unknown primary tumors.

4. What is the most common histology and the usual sites of presentation of cancer of unknown primary site?
Adenocarcinoma and undifferentiated carcinoma account for >75% of these cases. Most will present below the diaphragm.

5. When a primary site is eventually found, which sites are most common?
A primary tumor in the pancreas will account for about 25% of cases and lung cancer will be diagnosed in 20%. Stomach, colorectal, and kidney primary tumors will account for a smaller but significant percentage.

6. Which diagnostic studies are most helpful in cancer of unknown primary site?
The "shotgun" approach is out! Extensive, expensive, and uncomfortable evaluations are diagnostic of the primary site in only 5–30% of patients. Even if the primary site is suspected, the antemortem diagnosis will be found at autopsy to be wrong in 25% of cases. Most diagnoses are made on follow-up when specific symptoms direct diagnostic evaluations. The goal in evaluating these patients is to identify those patients with treatable tumors, anticipate complications, and avoid low-yield, invasive, or costly procedures. The most productive evaluation will consist of a thorough history and physical examination, routine laboratory evaluation, and a chest radiograph.

7. How can the pathologist help in the diagnosis of a cancer of unknown primary site?
The importance of direct communication with the pathologist cannot be overemphasized. Precise histologic diagnosis is essential in evaluating these patients. Morphologic clues may suggest certain anatomic sites. The distinction between adenocarcinoma, squamous carcinoma, and undifferentiated carcinoma also narrows the diagnostic possibilities. Providing the pathologist with clinical clues can result in the optimal use of special stains, histochemistry, flow cytometry, and electron microscopy.

8. Is electron microscopy useful in finding a cancer of unknown primary site?

A small percentage of patients with poorly differentiated carcinoma and an unknown primary site will be found with electron microscopy to have neuroendocrine features. The pathognomonic finding is the "dense-core granule." This subset of patients is especially important to recognize, as they tend to respond well to cisplatin-based chemotherapy regimens and a small number (10–20%) are actually cured!

9. Are any clues from the history and physical examination helpful in finding the primary site of a tumor?

Findings from a detailed history and physical examination can direct subsequent diagnostic and staging evaluation. The review of systems may identify sites that deserve further diagnostic evaluation. Careful examination of the thyroid, breasts, prostate, testis, and skin may yield a primary diagnosis. Rectal and pelvic examinations are often wrongly overlooked.

10. If the tumor presents in the cervical nodes, what should you do?

Suspicious nodes should never be biopsied until a complete diagnostic examination is performed. A careful endoscopic examination of the upper respiratory tract and computed tomographic (CT) scans of the neck are required. Of patients with squamous carcinoma in cervical nodes, 30–40% will have potentially curable cancers.

11. Which laboratory studies are indicated in diagnosing a primary tumor?

Routine laboratory tests can help in diagnosing a primary tumor (e.g., red cells in the urine suggest renal cell carcinoma) and in determining the extent of metastatic spread.

12. Are tumor markers helpful in cancer of unknown primary site?

Although assays for a number of tumor-associated markers are available, lack of specificity limits their usefulness. A few specific markers do exist, however. Prostate-specific antigen can suggest prostate cancer in a man with carcinoma of unknown primary site. Young men with unknown primary sites, especially those with mediastinal masses, should be screened for germ cell tumors with beta human chorionic gonadotropin and alpha-fetoprotein. Women with adenocarcinomas should have material submitted for hormone receptor analysis, which may correctly identify breast cancer. These studies may have diagnostic and therapeutic implications.

13. What is the prognosis of a patient with a tumor of unknown primary site?

The prognosis of these patients is not affected by correctly identifying the primary tumor. Patients who present with upper cervical nodes have a 5-year survival of 30–50%. Metastasis at any other site is associated with a median survival of 3–5 months and 5-year survival of <5%.

14. What is the best treatment for such patients with a tumor of unknown primary site?

Most patients who present with cancer of unknown primary site will have tumors that are not curable with chemotherapy. Your evaluation should be directed at diagnosing treatable malignancies such as breast, germ cell, or prostate cancer. Performance status is the most important predictor of response to treatment. About 20% of patients with adenocarcinoma of unknown primary site will respond to fluorouracil, but survival is not affected. Patients should be chosen who will benefit from the palliative effects of this treatment. The most important exceptions are suspected germ cell tumors and tumors with neuroendocrine features; these patients are generally treated with cisplatin-containing regimens, and 20% of such patients may be cured.

BIBLIOGRAPHY

1. Gaber AO, Rice P, Eaton C, et al: Metastatic malignant disease of unknown origin. Am J Surg 145:493–497, 1983.

2. Greco FA, Vaugn WK, Hainsworth JD: Advanced poorly differentiated carcinoma of unknown primary site: Recognition of a treatable syndrome. Ann Intern Med 104:547–553, 1986.
3. Grosbach AB: Carcinoma of unknown primary site: A clinical enigma. Arch Intern Med 142:357–359, 1982.
4. Hainsworth JD, Greco FA: Managing carcinomas of unknown primary site. Oncology 2:43–52, 1988.
5. Hainsworth JD, Johnson DH, Greco FA: Poorly differentiated neuroendocrine carcinoma of unknown primary site. Ann Intern Med 109:364–371, 1988.
6. Nystrom JS, Weiner JM, Wolf RM, et al: Identifying the primary site in metastatic cancer of unknown origin: Inadequacy of roentgenographic procedures. JAMA 241:381–383, 1979.
7. Osteen RT, Kopf G, Wilson RF: In pursuit of the unknown primary. Am J Surg 135:494–498, 1978.
8. Pasterz R, Savaaj N, Burgess M: Prognostic factors in metastatic carcinoma of unknown primary. J Clin Oncol 4:1562–1565, 1986.
9. Robert NJ, Garnick MB, Frei E: Cancers of unknown origin: Current approaches and future perspectives. Semin Oncol 9:526–530, 1982.
10. Schildt RR, Kennedy PS, Chen TT et al: Management of patients with metastatic adenocarcinoma of unknown origin: A Southwest Oncology Group Study. Cancer Treat Rep 67:77–79, 1983.

84. WILMS' TUMOR

Edythe A. Albano, M.D.

1. Estimate the frequency of occurrence of Wilms' tumor in the United States.

Wilms' tumor occurs at a rate of 7.5 cases per million white children and 7.8 cases per million black children each year (<15 years of age). This represents approximately 460 new cases annually in the United States. Wilms' tumor accounts for 5–6% of cancers diagnosed in children <15 years of age.

2. Which chromosome abnormality has been linked to Wilms' tumor?

Although most patients with Wilms' tumor are karyotypically normal, those with congenital aniridia frequently have a constitutional deletion at the 11p13 locus. This deletion has also been found in Wilms' tumor cells of patients without aniridia and who have a normal constitutional (or germline) karyotype.

Kaneko Y, Eques MC, Rowley JD: Interstitial deletion of short arm of chromosome 11 limited to Wilms' tumor cells in a patient without aniridia. Cancer Res 41:4577–4578, 1981.

3. What congenital anomalies are associated with Wilms' tumor?

Congenital Anomalies Associated with Wilms' Tumor

CONGENITAL ANOMALY	PREVALENCE IN GENERAL POPULATION (per 1000)	PREVALENCE IN PATIENTS WITH WILMS' TUMOR (per 1000)
Aniridia	0.02	7.6
Hemihypertrophy	0.03	32.6
Genitourinary malformations*	10	62.5

* For example, cryptorchidism, hypospadias, gonadal dysgenesis, pseudohermaphroditism, and horseshoe kidney.

Other congenital syndromes have an increased association with the development of Wilms' tumor and include Beckwith-Wiedemann syndrome (visceromegaly, macroglossia, omphalocele, hemihypertrophy, mental retardation), Drash's syndrome (glomerulopathy and genital abnormalities), WAGR sydrome (Wilms', Aniridia, ambiguous Genitalia, mental Retardation; deletion 11p13).

4. How does a patient with Wilms' tumor usually present?

An asymptomatic abdominal mass or abdominal swelling noted by the child's parent brings most children to medical attention (83%). Other presenting complaints include fever (23%) and hematuria (21%). Approximately 25% of children with Wilms' tumor will be hypertensive at presentation.

5. At what age is a child typically diagnosed with Wilms' tumor?

The median age at diagnosis is related to gender and laterality of kidney involvement. Wilms' tumor is uncommon over 6 years of age.

	Unilateral tumor (months)	Bilateral tumor (months)
Female	43	30
Male	36	23

6. What is the differential diagnosis of congestive heart failure in a patient undergoing evaluation for Wilms' tumor?

Severe hypertension secondary to hyperreninemia

Tumor thrombi in the pulmonary arteries or extension of tumor into the right atrium causing tamponade

7. To which sites does Wilms' tumor metastasize?

Lung, liver, and regional nodes. Eighty percent of patients with stage IV tumors will have lung metastases and 15% will have liver metastases.

8. How can a Wilms' tumor be distinguished from an abdominal neuroblastoma?

Neuroblastoma, which arises from the adrenal gland or parasympathetic ganglia, displaces the kidney, whereas Wilms' tumor, being intrarenal, distorts the kidney. On imaging, calcifications are frequently seen with neuroblastoma ($\geq$50%) but are uncommon in Wilms' tumor (10–15%).

Neuroblastoma is the most common retroperitoneal malignancy in childhood and is the most common misdiagnosis in the preoperative assessment. In a recent study, neuroblastoma was the incorrect preoperative diagnosis one-third of the time.

9. Which diagnostic imaging studies are essential for evaluating the child suspected of having a Wilms' tumor?

Ultrasonography or computed tomography (CT). The radiographic examination should establish the presence of an intrarenal mass. It is essential also to evaluate the contralateral kidney for presence and function, as well as synchronous Wilms' tumor. The inferior vena cava (IVC) needs to be evaluated for presence and extent of tumor propagation. The liver should also be imaged and the presence or absence of metastatic disease ascertained. A plain radiograph of the chest (four view) should be obtained to determine if pulmonary metastases are present or absent.

10. What are the histologic features of a classic Wilms' tumor?

A Wilms' tumor, also called nephroblastoma, is composed of three elements: blastema, epithelium, and stroma. The ratio of these components varies among tumors. This is the classic triphasic Wilms' tumor.

Multiple tissues of neonatal types, including skeletal muscle, squamous epithelium, cartilage, and neuroglia, may also be seen in Wilms' tumors.

11. To what does unfavorable histology refer?

It refers to anaplasia, clear cell sarcoma of the kidney (CCSK), and rhabdoid tumor of the kidney (RTK). Although CCSK and RTK are no longer thought to be Wilms' tumor variants, these three unique histologies were identified in early Wilms' tumor studies as being associated with a markedly worse outcome when compared with favorable-histology Wilms' tumor. Anaplasia is defined by extreme nuclear atypia. Only one or a few small foci of anaplasia in a Wilms' tumor is sufficient to impart a markedly worse prognosis in patients with stages II, III, and IV tumors.

12. How is Wilms' tumor staged?
The clinical stage is decided on by the surgeon in the operating room and confirmed by the pathologist.

Stage I:	Tumor limited to the kidney and complete excised.
Stage II:	Tumor extends beyond the kidney but is completely excised. There is no residual tumor beyond the margins of excision.
Stage III:	Residual nonhematogenous tumor confined to the abdomen.
IIIa:	Lymph nodes are found to be involved.
IIIb:	Diffuse peritoneal contamination by tumor.
IIIc:	Peritoneal implants are found.
IIId:	Tumor beyond surgical margins (microscopic or gross).
IIIe:	Unresectable tumor infiltrating into vital structures.
Stage IV:	Hematogenous metastases (e.g., lung, liver).
Stage V:	Bilateral renal involvement at diagnosis.

13. Name four factors that independently predict the likelihood of relapse-free survival in Wilms' tumor.
1. Favorable histology
2. Lymph nodes negative for tumor
3. Age <24 months at diagnosis
4. Tumor weight <250 gm

Breslow R, Sharples K, Beckwith JB, et al: Prognostic factors in nonmetastatic, favorable histology Wilms' tumor. Cancer 68:2345–2353, 1991.

14. What is the National Wilms' Tumor Study (NWTS)?
It is a cooperative clinical trial carried out in the United States, Canada, and several overseas countries. Clinical trials began in 1969 with NWTS 1. Much of the progress in the treatment of Wilms' tumor has resulted from these large multinational randomized studies that could not have been realized in a single or a small group of institutions.

15. How is Wilms' tumor treated in the United States?
The treatment begins with surgical exploration of the abdomen. A transabdominal approach allows for:
1. Inspection and palpation of the contralateral kidney for tumor involvement (one-third of patients with bilateral disease have no evidence of this on preoperative imaging studies)
2. Inspection and biopsy of suspicious liver and periaortic nodes
3. En bloc resection of tumor and involved kidney

This cannot all be accomplished from a flank incision. Following surgical excision and pathologic examination, the patient is assigned a stage that defines further therapy.

16. What is the role of radiotherapy in the treatment of Wilms' tumor?
NWTS 3 was designed to determine what dose of radiotherapy as well as which stage of Wilms' tumor would benefit from radiotherapy. Results of this study show that nonirradiated patients with stage II/FH (favorable-histology) tumors fared no worse than their irradiated counterparts. The outcome results for children with stage III tumors were similar whether they received 1000 or 2000 cGy.

Thomas PRM, Tefft M, Compaan PJ, et al: Results of two radiation therapy randomizations in the Third National Wilms' Tumor Study. Cancer 68:1703–1707, 1991.

17. When should radiotherapy begin?
Within 10 days of nephrectomy.

18. Which chemotherapeutic agents are used in the treatment of Wilms' tumor?
Vincristine and actinomycin D are used in the treatment of patients with Wilms' tumor; doxorubicin (Adriamycin) is administered to patients with stages III and IV tumors. In NWTS 3, cyclophosphamide as a fourth agent was not shown to offer a survival advantage to patients with stage IV tumors over the standard three-drug regimen.

19. Typically, when is chemotherapy begun after nephrectomy?
It is started on postoperative day 5, with the day of surgery being day 0.

20. What is the survival of patients with Wilms' tumor 4 years from diagnosis by stage and histology?

Four-Year Survival of Patients with Wilms' Tumor

STAGE/HISTOLOGY	EVENT-FREE SURVIVAL (%)	SURVIVAL (%)
I/FH	90.4	96.5
II/FH	88	92.2
III/FH	79	86.9
IV/FH	74	82.5
I–III/UH	64.7	68
IV/UH	55.6	55.7
Overall	**83.3**	**89.1**

FH, favorable histology; UH, unfavorable histology.

21. What long-term complications of Wilms' tumor therapy do survivors face?
Musculoskeletal abnormalities (e.g., scoliosis atrophy) in patients treated with radiation, cardiovascular abnormalities in patients who received Adriamycin, and second malignant neoplasms (5 of 623 patients) were reported as the more common late effects of treatment by the National Wilms' Tumor Study Group.

Evans AE, Norkool P, Evans I, et al: Late effects of treatment for Wilms' tumor. Cancer 67:331–336, 1991.

BIBLIOGRAPHY

1. Breslow R, et al: Prognostic factors in nonmetastatic, favorable histology Wilms' tumor. Cancer 68:2345–2353, 1991.
2. D'Angio GJ, Breslow N, Beckwith JB, et al: Treatment of Wilms' tumor: Results of the Third National Wilms' Tumor Study. Cancer 64:349–360, 1989.
3. Evans AE, et al: Late effects of treatment for Wilms' tumor. Cancer 67:331–336, 1991.
4. Ganick DJ: Wilms' tumor: Cancer in children. Hematol Oncol Clin North Am 1:695–719, 1987.
5. Green DM, D'Angio GJ, Beckwith JB, et al: Wilms' tumor (nephroblastoma, renal embryoma). In Pizzo PA, Poplack DG (eds): Principles and Practice of Pediatric Oncology. Philadelphia, J.B. Lippincott, 1993.
6. Kaneko Y, et al: Interstitial deletion of short arm of chromosome 11 limited to Wilms' tumor cells in a patient without aniridia. Cancer Res 41:4577–4578, 1981.
7. National Wilms' Tumor Study Committee: Wilms' tumor: Status report, 1990. J Clin Oncol 9:877–887, 1991.
8. Thomas PRM, Tefft M, Compaan PJ, et al: Results of two radiation therapy randomizations in the Third National Wilms' Tumor Study. Cancer 68:1703–1707, 1991.

85. CHILDHOOD ACUTE LYMPHOBLASTIC LEUKEMIA

Linda Stork, M.D.

1. What is acute leukemia?

Acute leukemia is defined as the presence of 30% or more hematopoietic blasts in a bone marrow smear. It is an uncontrolled proliferation of white blood cells at an early stage òf maturation.

2. Name the types of acute leukemia that occur in childhood.

Acute lymphoblastic leukemia (ALL) is the most common acute childhood leukemia, representing about 80% of cases. Acute nonlymphocytic (ANLL), or acute myelogenous leukemia (AML), accounts for the remaining 20%. ALL is treated very differently from ANLL (AML), and thus the distinction between the two is very important.

3. Give the incidence of acute leukemia in childhood.

Acute leukemia is the most common malignancy of childhood. New cases are diagnosed in about 2,500 children each year in the United States, with an incidence of about 1 in 25,000 children per year (<15 years of age).

4. How is ALL distinguished from ANLL (AML)?

The clinical presentations of ALL and ANLL (AML) are generally similar. The morphology of blasts on a bone marrow aspirate stained with Wright/Giemsa distinguishes the majority of cases of ALL from ANLL (AML). Lymphoblasts are typically small, with cell diameters equal to that of approximately two red blood cell (RBC) diameters. They have a scant amount of cytoplasm, usually without granules. The nucleus usually contains none or one small indistinct nucleolus. Blasts of the myeloid leukemias are usually much larger than two RBC diameters and have more cytoplasm surrounding the nucleus than do lymphoblasts. Granules are often present in the cytoplasm of an ANLL blast, and the nucleus usually contains one or more distinct nucleoli. Cytochemical stains also distinguish ALL from ANLL blasts. The latter cells stain with myeloperoxidase and/or nonspecific esterase, whereas the former cells do not.

5. What cell type is the blast of ALL?

Immunophenotyping of ALL blasts, using monoclonal antibodies and flow cytometry, has helped us understand the heterogeneity of ALL. About 80% of cases are of B-cell lineage and 20% T-cell lineage. Lymphoblasts of B-cell lineage are found at various stages of B-cell development, but the majority are at an early stage of B-cell maturation before the synthesis of immunoglobulins. However, some B-lineage lymphoblasts have immunoglobulin chains within their cytoplasm and, very rarely, immunoglobulins on their surface. In general, the lymphoblasts of T-cell lineage are found at a stage before helper or suppressor T-cell functions are expressed.

6. Discuss the usual presenting clinical findings in ALL.

Signs and symptoms of patients presenting with ALL include those related to decreased bone marrow production of RBCs, white blood cells (WBCs), and platelets. Pallor and easy bruisability with purpura or petechiae are seen in over 50% of cases. Intermittent fevers are common owing to the leukemia itself or to infections secondary to a decreased number of functioning WBCs. About 25% of patients experience bone pain, especially of the pelvis, vertebral bodies, and legs. Signs and symptoms may also be related to leukemic infiltration of extramedullary (outside the bone marrow) sites. Generalized lymphadenopathy, hepato-megaly, and splenomegaly occur in over 50% of cases. Some patients, particularly those with T-cell leukemia, present with a mediastinal mass that may cause respiratory distress, orthopnea, and airway compromise.

The differential diagnosis of ALL initially includes juvenile rheumatoid arthritis, infectious mononucleosis, idiopathic thrombocytopenic purpura (ITP), and aplastic anemia.

7. What are the laboratory abnormalities found at diagnosis in ALL?

The complete blood cell count (CBC) with differential is the most useful initial laboratory test for determining if a patient has ALL. Ninety-nine percent of patients have decreased numbers of at least one cell type (leukopenia, neutropenia, thrombocytopenia, or anemia), and the majority of patients have decreased numbers of two blood cell types. The WBCs are low or normal (WBCs $<10,000/\mu l$) in about 50% of patients, but a differential often shows neutropenia (absolute neutrophil count $<1000/\mu l$) along with a small percentage of blasts amid normal lymphocytes. In 30% of patients, the WBC is $>10,000/\mu l$ and in 20% of cases it is $>50,000/\mu l$, occasionally $>300,000/\mu l$. Blasts are usually readily identifiable on peripheral smears of patients with elevated WBCs. Blasts on peripheral blood smears may not look identical to those in bone marrow aspirates, but the lymphoid versus myeloid nature of these blasts usually can be recognized.

The majority of patients with ALL have decreased platelet counts ($<150,000/\mu l$) and decreased hemoglobin ($<11g\%$) at diagnosis, although cases with normal platelet counts and hemoglobin do occur.

Several serum chemistries, particularly uric acid and lactate dehydrogenase (LDH), are often elevated at diagnosis in patients with ALL. Uric acid and LDH are intracellular products released after cell breakdown. Liver function tests may be mildly abnormal as well because of leukemic infiltration.

8. Define the tumor lysis syndrome (TLS). How is it managed?

TLS results from rapid cell breakdown once chemotherapy has been initiated for ALL or T-cell and B-cell lymphomas. Chemotherapy causes lymphoblasts to release cellular contents into the bloodstream. Uric acid, a purine metabolite, can precipitate in the kidneys as chemotherapy is initiated and cause acute renal failure.

Patients are always treated with oral allopurinol prior to and during initial chemotherapy. Allopurinol inhibits the synthesis of uric acid from xanthine and hypoxanthine and helps prevent uric acid nephropathy. Patients are always treated with hydration to maintain high urine output (approximately 1.5 × the hourly maintenance rate) along with sodium bicarbonate alkalinization, since uric acid is more soluble in alkaline than acidic urine. Intracellular phosphates also are released following initiation of chemotherapy, potentially resulting in phosphate deposition in kidneys. Hyperphosphatemia may be accompanied by hypocalcemia and tetany. To prevent hyperphosphatemia, oral phosphate binders like Amphojel (aluminum hydroxide) may be helpful. Once hyperphosphatemia is present, urine should no longer be alkalinized, because phosphates are poorly soluble in alkaline urine. Intracellular potassium also is released from the blasts and hyperkalemia can result, requiring dialysis to prevent a fatal arrhythmia. Intravenous fluids during initial chemotherapy should not contain K+ unless the serum level is less than normal. Dialysis may also be required for hyperphosphatemia with tetany or fluid overload. TLS usually is at its worst 3 days into chemotherapy and diminishes thereafter.

9. What is the current treatment for ALL?

A number of chemotherapeutic agents in combination are used to treat ALL. Treatment is generally divided into three phases. The first month of therapy consists of induction, at the end of which over 95% of patients exhibit remission bone marrows. Consolidation is the second phase of treatment, during which intrathecal chemotherapy and sometimes cranial irradiation is given to treat lymphoblasts that may be present in the meninges of the central nervous system (CNS). Maintenance therapy is the third phase of treatment and usually has fewer acute side effects than the other two phases. Short courses of intensive chemotherapy may be interspersed among the maintenance chemotherapy treatment.

Chemotherapeutic agents most commonly used in induction include oral prednisone, intravenous vincristine, intramuscular L-asparaginase, intrathecal methotrexate, and intravenous daunorubicin. For T-cell ALL, intravenous cyclophosphamide is given in induction as well. Maintenance treatment of ALL generally includes oral daily 6-mercaptopurine (6MP), weekly oral or intramuscular methotrexate, and monthly pulses of intravenous vincristine and oral prednisone. Intrathecal chemotherapy, either with methotrexate alone or combined with cytarabine and hydrocortisone, is usually administered every 2–3 months. In the Children's Cancer Group protocols, girls are currently treated for about 2 years and boys for about 3 years, because previous statistical analyses found that boys required longer treatment than girls for an equivalent cure rate.

10. Can ALL be cured?

The chance of cure depends to some degree on specific prognostic features that are present at diagnosis of ALL. The two most important prognostic features include WBC count and age. In the 1970s, it became clear that children with WBCs $<50,000/\mu l$ had a much better chance of cure than did children with WBCs $>50,000/\mu l$ receiving the same chemotherapy. Children from ages 2 to 9 years have a better chance of cure than do younger or older patients. Certain chromosome abnormalities present in the leukemic blasts at diagnosis also have prognostic significance. Patients with a translocation between chromosomes 9 and 22:t(9;22) have a very poor chance of cure even with intensive therapy. Patients with a translocation between chromosomes 4 and 11:t(4;11) generally have a poorer chance of cure than do other patients with ALL. On the other hand, patients whose blasts are hyperdiploid (contain >50 chromosomes instead of the normal 46) have a better chance of cure than do patients without hyperdiploidy.

Treatment for ALL currently is tailored to prognostic groups. A child between the ages of 2 and 9 years with WBCs at diagnosis of $<10,000/\mu l$ and without t(9;22) or t(4;11) would be treated with less intensive therapy than a patient with WBCs $>50,000/\mu l$ or a patient >10 years. This treatment approach has significantly increased the cure rate among patients with the less favorable prognostic features while minimizing treatment-related toxicities in those with favorable prognostic features. The overall chance of cure for ALL is now at least 70%.

11. What is meant by "extramedullary relapse"?

The CNS and the testes are considered sanctuary sites of extramedullary leukemia. Systemic chemotherapy does not penetrate these tissues as well as it penetrates most organs. "Prophylactic" intrathecal chemotherapy is a critical part of all ALL treatment protocols to prevent leukemic relapse in the CNS. Before the institution of such therapy in the 1970s, the CNS was a major site of initial leukemic relapse. Lymphoblasts are presumed to be present in the CNS at diagnosis in all patients with ALL even if not detected in spinal fluid samples. Lymphoblasts probably reach the CNS via hematogenous spread by migrating out of blood vessels into meninges or by direct extension from cranial bone marrow into the arachnoid. Now about 10% of patients with ALL have leukemic relapse in the CNS. Symptoms suggestive of CNS disease include headache, nausea and vomiting, irritability, nuchal rigidity, and cranial nerve palsies.

Up to 15% of boys experience leukemic relapse in their testes after completion of standard chemotherapy, usually presenting with unilateral painless testicular enlargement. The incidence of testicular relapse has decreased significantly as treatment for ALL has intensified, suggesting that more chemotherapy may be penetrating the "blood-testes" barrier. Routine follow-up of boys on treatment and off treatment includes examination of the testes.

12. Is there a role for bone marrow transplant in ALL?
Bone marrow transplant is rarely used as initial treatment following induction of remission for ALL, because the majority of patients are cured without it. However, patients with certain chromosome abnormalities in their leukemic blasts, like t(9;22), appear to have a much better cure rate with early bone marrow transplantation from an HLA-DR-matched sibling donor than with intensive chemotherapy. Bone marrow transplant does play a role for patients who have relapsed with ALL, particularly if the relapse is during the course of treatment or within several months of completion. For these patients, virtually the only chance of cure is with a bone marrow transplant once a second remission has been achieved with chemotherapy.

13. What medical problems may develop in long-term survivors of ALL?
The majority of patients treated for ALL will have normal gonadal function and fertility. Boys who received testicular radiation for testicular relapse will be infertile and some may need testosterone replacement. Patients, especially those <10 years old, who received cranial irradiation as "prophylaxis" or treatment of CNS leukemia will probably develop some learning disabilities as a result. Patients who received spinal radiation for CNS leukemia may lose several centimeters of expected height. CNS radiation may also cause endocrinopathies, including hypothyroidism and growth hormone deficiencies, both of which can be corrected with hormone replacement. Cardiac failure has been reported in patients who received high cumulative doses of anthracyclines (daunorubicin, doxorubicin) as treatment for ALL. Aside from brain tumors after cranial irradiation, second malignancies have been reported infrequently in long-term survivors of ALL. As these children are followed into their fourth and fifth decades, more medical problems secondary to the treatment of ALL may surface.

BIBLIOGRAPHY

1. Bennett JM, Catorsky D, Daniel MT, et al: Proposal for the classification of acute leukemia. Br J Haematol 33:451, 1976.
2. Beyer WA, Poplack DG: Prophylaxis and treatment of leukemia in central nervous system and other sanctuaries. Semin Oncol 12:121, 1985.
3. Borowitz MJ: Immunologic markers in childhood acute lymphoblastic leukemia. Hematol Oncol Clin North Am, 1990.
4. Cohen LF, Balow JE, Magrath IT: Acute tumor lysis syndrome: A review of 37 patients with Burkitt's lymphoma. Am J Med 68:486, 1980.
5. Meadows AT, Silber J: Delayed consequences of therapy for childhood cancer. Cancer 35:271, 1985.
6. Poplack DG: Acute lymphoblastic leukemia. In Pizzo PA, Poplack DG (eds): Principles and Practice of Pediatric Oncology. Philadelphia, J.B. Lippincott, 1993.
7. Ribeiro RC, Abromowitch M, Raimondi SC, et al: Clinical and biologic hallmarks of the Philadelphia chromosome in childhood acute lymphoblastic leukemia. Blood 70:948, 1987.
8. Sanders JE, Thomas ED, Buckner D, et al: Marrow transplantation for children with acute lymphoblastic leukemia in second remission. Blood 70:324, 1987.

86. OSTEOGENIC SARCOMA AND EWING'S SARCOMA IN CHILDREN

Brian S. Greffe, M.D.

1. When does the peak incidence of osteogenic sarcoma and Ewing's sarcoma occur in childhood?

The second decade of life is usually the peak incidence for osteogenic sarcoma (OS). This is the time of the adolescent growth spurt. Interestingly, there may be a relationship between this period of growth and the development of OS. The disease occurs at an earlier age in girls than in boys, corresponding to their more advanced skeletal age and earlier adolescent growth spurt. OS also has a predilection for the metaphyseal portions of the most rapidly growing bones in adolescents.

Ewing's sarcoma (ES) is seen most commonly in the early to midportion of the second decade of life and rarely occurs in children less than 5 years old or in adults older than 30 years. It is extremely uncommon in blacks and Chinese.

2. What are the most common sites of presentation for OS and ES?

OS usually involves the long bones. These tumors can be found most commonly in the distal femur and proximal tibia. The proximal humerus and mid and proximal femur also are frequently involved. Involvement of the axial skeleton (such as the pelvis) accounts for only 10% of cases in the pediatric age group.

ES, on the other hand, is seen most commonly in the pelvis and frequently involves the axial skeleton. It also commonly occurs in the humerus and femur.

3. What are the clinical manifestations of OS and ES?

The most common symptoms for both tumors at the time of presentation include pain and swelling of the involved bone and surrounding tissue. In newly diagnosed cases of OS, 10–20% of patients will have gross metastatic disease at the time of presentation. Up to 30% of patients with ES will have macrometastatic disease at diagnosis. The most common sites of metastatic disease include lung (OS, ES) and bone marrow (ES). Multifocal disease is present in 1–3% of patients with OS at presentation. Patients with metastatic disease may present with fever, respiratory distress, and, in the case of bone marrow involvement, pancytopenia.

4. What radiographic studies are important in the diagnosis of ES and OS?

Plain films of the involved area are usually the first radiographic studies obtained. In ES, the area of the tumor usually shows a moth-eaten pattern of bony destruction. An onion-skin appearance secondary to elevation of the periosteum may also be present. In OS, the bony destruction seen on radiography is usually accompanied by periosteal new bone formation and lifting of the cortex with formation of Codman's triangle.

A radionuclide bone scan is helpful in defining the extent of the primary tumor and, in the case of OS, can also be useful in identifying "skip lesions" that are seen infrequently in these patients. Computed tomography (CT) scanning can be helpful in defining the extent of the primary tumor in the medullary cavity and soft tissues. Magnetic resonance imaging (MRI) may be more sensitive in this regard and in some centers is replacing CT. CT scan of the chest and chest radiography are necessary in order to identify pulmonary lesions.

5. Which laboratory tests should be considered in patients with newly diagnosed bone malignancies?

There are no specific tumor markers identified as yet for OS and ES. Serum levels of lactate dehydrogenase (LDH) and alkaline phosphatase, however, may be of prognostic value in patients with OS. Those patients with either of these markers elevated at the time of diagnosis appear to have a worse outcome. Erythrocyte sedimentation rate (ESR) can be elevated at the time of diagnosis in patients with ES and may be of value in following response to therapy and monitoring for recurrence in these patients. Bone marrow examination (bilateral aspirates and biopsies) is essential in patients with ES prior to the initiation of therapy.

6. What are the histologic considerations in evaluation of a biopsy specimen in these patients?
The presence of osteoid formation on biopsy combined with a connective tissue stroma containing large, atypical, spindle-shaped cells that are highly malignant with irregular nuclei and abnormal mitotic figures usually confirms the diagnosis of OS.

In ES, electron microscopy is essential in confirming the diagnosis, as this tumor must be differentiated from other tumors comprising small blue cells, including lymphoma, neuroblastoma, rhabdomyosarcoma, and peripheral neuroepithelioma.

7. What are the tumor cytogenetic abnormalities seen in OS and ES?
In the majority of patients with ES, a translocation of chromosomes 11 and 22 is seen in the tumor cells. This translocation also is seen in peripheral neuroepithelioma, another small blue cell tumor. This chromosomal abnormality is characterized by the translocation of the c-*sis*-oncogene from chromosome 22 to chromosome 11. C-*sis* appears not to be expressed; however, the oncogene c-*ets,* located near the breakpoint on chromosome 11, is variably expressed.

In OS, analysis of the DNA content of the tumor cells has shown that patients whose tumors contain a low percentage of diploid cells and an aneuploid peak are more likely to develop metastatic disease.

8. What are the prognostic factors that are important in patients with bone malignancies?
The site of primary disease without metastases is an important prognostic variable in patients presenting with ES. Pelvic and sacral sites appear to have the least favorable outcome.

In both OS and ES, the presence of metastatic disease at the time of diagnosis portends a poor outcome. In OS, patients who present with pulmonary metastatic disease can expect to have a disease-free survival of only 11–40% at 5 years. Ten to twenty percent of patients with metastatic ES will be cured of their disease. OS presenting with multifocal bony metastases is uniformly fatal.

In patients with OS, the level of LDH and alkaline phosphatase at the time of diagnosis appear to have prognostic implications. Individuals presenting with high LDH or alkaline phosphate levels have a worse outcome. Patients with primaries of the axial skeleton and poor tumor kill (<90%) with preoperative chemotherapy also have a poor prognosis.

9. What role does surgery play in the treatment of OS and ES?
Surgery plays a very important role in both of these bone malignancies. In order to prevent local recurrence, it is essential to remove all gross and microscopic tumor. Surgery is usually performed after several courses of preoperative chemotherapy have been given. The chemotherapeutic agents are useful in making the primary tumor more amenable to resection, as well as controlling micrometastatic disease. Micrometastatic disease, principally in the lung, is usually present at the time of diagnosis.

Surgery for primary bone tumors can be accomplished either with an amputation or a limb-salvage procedure. Amputation provides removal of all gross and microscopic tumor with clean margins and good local control. Limb-salvage procedures are reserved for those tumors that can be removed en bloc with a margin of normal tissue and do not have a large extramedullary component. Once the tumor has been removed, restoration of the structural integrity of the involved extremity is obtained using biologic materials such as cadaveric allografts or autologous grafts and metallic endoprosthetic devices. Patients who have not yet achieved their full growth potential may not be ideal candidates for a limb-salvage procedure, as they may develop a leg length discrepancy later on in life.

10. What chemotherapeutic agents are useful in patients with OS or ES?
Chemotherapy plays a role in both the preoperative and postoperative phases of therapy in these patients. Response to preoperative chemotherapy (as measured by the percentage of tumor kill in the resected specimen) is in fact an important prognostic factor particularly in OS. Patients whose tumors demonstrate greater than 90% tumor kill with preoperative therapy are more likely to survive disease free.

Chemotherapeutic agents effective in OS include cisplatin, doxorubicin (Adriamycin), methotrexate, vincristine, and ifosfamide. Selected pediatric oncology centers are currently using intra-arterial cisplatin in preoperative patients in order to deliver intense chemotherapy directly into the tumor, potentially maximizing tumor kill.

ES responds to a variety of agents such as cyclophosphamide, Adriamycin, vincristine, etoposide, and ifosfamide, which are all given by the standard intravenous route.

11. What is the indication for radiation therapy in the treatment of these bone malignancies?
Radiation therapy plays an important role in the local control phase of treatment in patients with ES. Although the tumor is sensitive to radiation, high doses (>5000 cGy) are usually needed to achieve adequate control. It is important to realize that radiation therapy can interfere with growth potential in young children, and surgery in fact may be the local control measure of choice in these patients. Individuals with ES metastatic to the lungs may achieve limited benefit from radiation therapy. The maximum amount of total radiation to the lungs, however, cannot exceed 2000 cGy, which is below the amount of radiation needed to achieve adequate control (usually between 4000 and 5000 cGy).

Radiation therapy plays a small role in the treatment of OS, as this tumor is not particularly radiosensitive.

12. Does bone marrow transplant play a role in the treatment of bone malignancies?
Patients with poor prognosis ES at the time of diagnosis (pelvic primaries, metastatic disease) have been treated with intensive chemotherapy, total body irradiation, and autologous bone marrow transplant. This approach to therapy is currently limited to certain pediatric oncology centers. The majority of institutions use a multimodality approach (chemotherapy, surgery, radiation therapy) for treatment of these patients.

13. What is the therapy for patients who develop pulmonary metastases after treatment for OS?
Patients who develop pulmonary nodules greater than 1 year following initial surgery for OS still have a chance for cure when compared with those individuals who develop pulmonary nodules within 6 months of the surgery. Once metastatic disease is diagnosed, a thorough search for other metastatic sites should be undertaken using CT scan and radionuclide bone scan. The primary tumor site should also be evaluated radiologically for evidence of local recurrence if a limb-salvage procedure has been performed. In patients with resectable disease, a surgical procedure such as a thoracotomy or median sternotomy should be performed in order to remove all evidence of disease. Patients with three nodules or less may have long-term survival with surgery alone. Adjuvant chemotherapy should be considered for patients with more than three nodules, incompletely resected metastatic disease, or evidence of disruption of the pleura by tumor.

BIBLIOGRAPHY

1. Gehan EA, Nesbit ME, Burget EO, et al: Prognostic factors in children with Ewing's sarcoma. Natl Cancer Inst Monogr 56:273–278, 1981.
2. Glass AG, Fraumeni JF: Epidemiology of bone cancer in children. J Natl Cancer Inst 44:187, 199, 1970.

3. Huvos A: Bone Tumors: Diagnosis, Treatment and Prognosis. Philadelphia, W.B. Saunders, 1979.
4. Knudson AG: Hereditary cancer, oncogenes, and antioncogenes. Cancer Res 45:1437–1443, 1985.
5. Mankin H, Conner J, Schiller A, et al: Grading of bone tumors by analysis of nuclear DNA content using flow cytometry. J Bone Joint Surg 67:404–413, 1985.
6. Meyers PA: Malignant bone tumors in children: Osteosarcoma. Hematol Oncol Clin North Am 4:655–665, 1987.
7. Meyers PA: Malignant bone tumors in children: Ewing's sarcoma. Hematol Oncol Clin North Am 4:667–673, 1987.
8. Meyers PA, Heller G, Healey J, et al: Chemotherapy for nonmetastatic osteosarcoma: The Memorial Sloan-Kettering experience. J Clin Oncol 10:5–15, 1992.
9. Miser JS, Steis R, Longo DL, et al: Treatment of newly diagnosed high risk sarcomas and primitive neuroectodermal tumors (PNET) in children and young adults. Proc ASCO 4:C-935, 1985.
10. Pizzo PA, Poplack DG: Principles and Practice of Pediatric Oncology. Philadelphia, J.B. Lippincott, 1993.
11. Price C: Primary bone-forming tumours and their relationship to skeletal growth. J Bone Joint Surg 40:574–593, 1958.
12. Young JL, Miller RW: Incidence of malignant tumors in U.S. children. J Pediatr 86:245–258, 1975.

87. CHILDHOOD BRAIN TUMORS

Lorrie F. Odom, M.D.

1. How common are brain tumors in children?

Brain tumors are next in frequency only to acute leukemias in children, thus being the second most common type of childhood cancer and the most common solid tumor of childhood. Brain tumors account for about 20% of all pediatric malignancies. In the United States, brain tumors are the third leading cause of death in children under 16 years of age. There are about 1500 new malignant central nervous system tumors in children under 15 years of age each year, or an incidence of 2 to 3 per 100,000 children at risk per year.

2. Where is the most common location for childhood brain tumors to arise and what symptoms are usually present at diagnosis?

Over 75% of brain tumors in children arise in the posterior fossa and include medulloblastomas, cerebellar astrocytomas, brain stem gliomas, and fourth ventricle ependymomas. The most common symptoms at diagnosis are usually related to increased intracranial pressure and include headaches, morning vomiting, and lethargy. These symptoms may also be associated with unsteadiness of gait and diplopia.

3. What are the most common types of childhood brain tumors?

Almost 70% of childhood central nervous system (CNS) tumors are of astrocytic origin, with 80–90% of these being low-grade astrocytomas (LGA). Thus, LGA represent overall the largest group of CNS tumors. They are a heterogeneous group of tumors varying in incidence, biologic behavior, and microscopic features. The group includes juvenile pilocytic, fibrillary and protoplasmic astrocytomas, oligodendrogliomas, gangliogliomas, and low-grade mixed gliomas. In the currently favored classification system, there are two other subgroups of childhood astrocytoma—anaplastic astrocytoma and glioblastoma multiforme.

4. In what locations do *axial* LGA commonly occur?

These tumors commonly occur in optic pathways, the suprasellar region, and brain stem. Degeneration into a malignant neoplasm may occur in approximately 5–6% of the patients.

5. How common is neuraxis dissemination at the time of diagnosis of malignant brain tumors in children?

Reports of neuraxis dissemination at diagnosis vary from 10% to 46% of children with primary CNS tumors. Such spread is most common in children with medulloblastoma, other malignant embryonal tumors (cerebral primitive neuroectodermal tumor [PNET] and pineoblastoma), and malignant gliomas (such as anaplastic astrocytoma or glioblastoma multiforme), as well as in children under 5 years of age at diagnosis. Leptomeningeal involvement may be determined by obtaining cerebrospinal fluid (CSF) cytology (cytocentrifuge examination of spinal fluid). Neuraxis "drop metastases" may be diagnosed by gadolinium-enhanced magnetic resonance imaging (MRI) of the neuraxis to include sagittal and axial views and/or myelography.

6. What is the most common malignant brain tumor in children and at what age does it usually occur?

Medulloblastoma (considered to be synonymous with PNET) is the most common malignant tumor of the brain in children. Medulloblastoma (MB) or PNET usually occurs within the first decade of life, with a peak incidence between 5 and 10 years of age and a 2.1 to 1.3 female to male ratio. These tumors commonly arise in the posterior fossa in the midline cerebellar vermis with variable extension into the fourth ventricle. MB or PNET, therefore, usually causes brain stem or cerebellar dysfunction and is often associated with blockage of the fourth ventricle and hydrocephalus. Affected children typically present with symptoms of increased intracranial pressure, including vomiting, lethargy, and morning headaches. They may also have unsteadiness of gait and diplopia. If the tumor occurs under the age of 1 year, the clinical presentation may be different and consist of increasing lethargy and head size.

7. What outcome of treatment for children with MB or PNET can currently be expected?

"Favorable" MB or PNET is considered grossly resected tumor without neuraxis dissemination. Standard radiation therapy (5400 cGy to the posterior fossa tumor bed and 3600 cGy to the remaining neuraxis) yields about a 70% 5-year disease-free survival (DFS).

"Unfavorable" tumors are those with neuraxis dissemination at the time of diagnosis. Other adverse factors, although probably less important, are size of primary tumor >3 cm, usually resulting in subtotal resection, age under 4 years, or histologic presence (within the tumor) of foci of glial, ependymal, and/or neuronal cell differentiation.

Prognostic Factors in Children with MB or PNET

	FAVORABLE	UNFAVORABLE
Extent of disease	Nondisseminated	Disseminated
Size of primary tumor	≤3 cm (completely resected)	>3 cm
Histology	Undifferentiated	Foci of glial, ependymal or neuronal differentiation
Age	≥4 years	<4 years

It is unclear whether the effect of large tumor size at diagnosis can be negated by the extent of resection. It is clear that patients with locally extensive disease or metastatic disease at diagnosis have improved outcome with the addition of chemotherapy. Treatment that incorporates radiotherapy, especially to a young child, often results in significant neurologic, endocrinologic, and intellectual sequelae.

8. What other posterior fossa/brain stem tumors occur in childhood?

Brain stem gliomas represent the third most common posterior fossa tumor of childhood and occur most frequently between 5 and 10 years of age. Although more aggressive approaches to treatment are being investigated, mean survival remains <1 year, with <25% 3-year survival.

Ependymomas are the least common posterior fossa neoplasm and represent 8–10% of CNS tumors of childhood. Over half of these tumors occur in children <3 years of age. About 70% of these tumors arise from ependyma of the fourth ventricle and grow to fill that ventricle. Using microsurgical techniques, gross total resection can be accomplished in 30–40% of children. Good prognostic factors correlating with 80% to 85% 5-year relapse-free survival are gross total resection, no evidence of leptomeningeal dissemination, and age >2–3 years. Less favorable prognostic factors, associated with <40% relapse-free survival at 5 years, are subtotal surgical resection, leptomeningeal dissemination, and young age.

9. Are there differences in the clinical presentation of the various childhood posterior fossa/brain stem tumors?
Children with MB or PNET usually have symptoms of relatively short duration, with the majority of patients being symptomatic for less than 4 months prior to diagnosis. Ependymomas of the posterior fossa are most likely to mimic MB or PNET in their clinical presentation. However, symptoms caused by ependymomas tend to be present for a longer period of time (6–12 months), and cranial nerve palsies tend to be more frequent with ependymomas. Cerebellar astrocytomas tend to present with limb ataxia and nonspecific unsteadiness. Symptoms may be present for up to 2 years before diagnosis, although they are more commonly present 6–12 months.

10. What imaging studies are useful in diagnosis of brain tumors in children?
In infants whose fontanel has not closed, head sonography through the fontanel is a good screening study. Supratentorial tumors are usually well visualized by CT scan of the head with and without contrast, whereas posterior fossa tumors are better imaged by a gadolinium-enhanced MRI scan. Diagnosis of neuraxis "drop metastases" can be accomplished by conventional myelography or more recently and less invasively by gadolinium-enhanced MRI scan. Less widely available imaging techniques that are likely to become more accessible in the future are positron emission tomography (PET) and single positron emission computed tomography (SPECT) scanning. PET scanning, using 18F-fluorodeoxyglucose, localizes areas of altered metabolism. It can help distinguish necrosis due to radiation or chemotherapy (hypometabolic) from recurrent tumor (hypermetabolic). Thalium SPECT scanning has been helpful in the evaluation of recurrent neoplasm in adults. Although early pediatric experience has been less promising, MR spectroscopy shows potential and is currently undergoing clinical trials.

11. What new approaches are available for the management of low-grade astrocytomas of childhood?
In the past, low-grade astrocytomas of childhood were treated with excision of as much tumor as possible and irradiation of visible residual tumor. More recently, it became apparent that children with cerebellar astrocytomas may do very well even with incomplete excision of their tumors and no irradiation. The growth of certain infiltrative LGA may arrest, in some cases spontaneously and in others after subtotal excision. Management of axial LGA presents a particular challenge, and for many decades, extreme conservatism dominated the neurosurgical attitude toward these tumors. In recent years, many technologic advances have greatly increased the safety of an open surgical approach to these midline tumors. Resection of LGA in the brain stem was pioneered by neurosurgeon Fred Epstein, MD. Additionally, clinical studies have shown the efficacy of chemotherapy such as vincristine, etoposide, and carboplatinum in these LGA. The use of these agents may prove to be of particular value in the treatment of young children, in whom it is advisable to delay irradiation to the brain as long as possible or omit it altogether.

12. When should radiotherapy be used to treat residual LGA in children?
Radiotherapy should be restricted to patients with LGA who are older than 5 years, can be treated only by biopsy, have tumors that show evidence of progressive growth despite

resection, or have tumors that are significantly interfering with either visual or neurologic function. As evidence of the efficacy of certain chemotherapeutic agents for these tumors mounts, it may become advisable to offer an initial trial of chemotherapy in an effort to further delay or omit radiotherapy.

13. What is the current approach to the management of high-grade gliomas in children?
If a child is suspected of having a high-grade glioma, initiating supportive treatment with high-dose decadron, prophylactic antiseizure medication, and an H_2 blocker is indicated. Treatment with steroids for 3–4 days prior to surgery usually results in better tolerance of the procedure by the patient. Impact of the extent of surgical resection has been debated, but on balance, studies in adults indicate that length of survival directly correlates with extent of resection and inversely with amount of residual tumor seen on postoperative scan.

There appears to be benefit from postsurgery adjuvant radiotherapy (RT) as established in two large, multiinstitutional randomized trials in adults. The use of 6000 cGy extended median survival over 5000 cGy.

The role of chemotherapy in the treatment of high-grade gliomas in children is evolving. The Childrens Cancer Group (CCG) demonstrated prolongation of median survival with the administration of postoperative lomustine (CCNU), vincristine, and prednisone in addition to radiotherapy. Currently, the use of much more intensive adjuvant chemotherapy is under investigation.

14. Does the dose of dexamethasone (Decadron) make a difference in the symptomatic management of patients with brain tumors?
Clinical experience with dexamethasone indicates there is a dose dependency in patients with brain tumors. Occasionally, patients deteriorate neurologically or functionally while the steroid dose is being tapered. A temporary boost in dosage followed by a slower taper usually reverses this pattern. Some patients may have a particular threshold below which clinical deterioration becomes a repetitive problem.

15. What specific neurosurgical technologic advances have taken place in recent years?
Advances include the magnification and illumination of the operating microscope, the gentleness of the ultrasonic tissue aspirator and CO_2 laser, and the accuracy of computerized stereotactic resection. The Viewing Wand (ISG Technologies, Toronto), a jointed robotic position-sensing arm, is now undergoing clinical testing. Using this technique, prior to surgery the patient undergoes a CT and/or MRI scan from which a three-dimensional (3-D) color image of the brain, skull, and scalp is reconstructed, clearly differentiating tumor from healthy tissue. Precise measurements of distance, angles, volumes, and densities are taken, and the image is rotated to explore different approaches preoperatively. The data are transferred to the Viewing Wand in the operating room. This device functions as an imaging computer with a mechanical position-sensing arm attached to the side of the operating table integrating the information of the patient's position with that from the previously obtained 3-D image, providing the surgeon with a 3-D picture of the tumor and surrounding brain. This technique makes possible eliminating unnecessary damage to the brain by avoiding manipulation of healthy tissue, particularly the motor cortex or other eloquent areas.

16. What new techniques are available for more precise delivery of local treatment to children with brain tumors?
With advances in computer technology and treatment planning, it is now possible to treat the tumor and surrounding brain while sparing distant brain from unnecessary radiotherapy (RT). A new method for delivering RT precisely to gliomas and other tumors, 3-D conformal RT, is currently undergoing trials. The technique involves shaping the isodose surface of an RT plane to conform to the tumor's 3-D anatomic boundaries. Its advantages include the following:

1. Minimizing RT exposure of surrounding healthy tissue (e.g., 30% to 50% reduction in amount of surrounding brain tissue irradiated)
2. Safely delivering higher-dose RT to the tumor than was previously possible
3. Ability to reirradiate a tumor at recurrence

Following standard RT, stereotactic radiosurgery (SRS) or brachytherapy (BT) may be used to boost the total tumor dose resulting in improved local control and survival. With SRS, multiple arcs in 3-D are used to focus single-fraction high-dose RT delivery within a precisely localized target volume.

BIBLIOGRAPHY

1. Albright AL: Pediatric brain tumors. CA Cancer J Clin 43:272–288, 1993.
2. Ammirati M, Vick N, Liao I, et al: Effect of the extent of surgical resection on survival and quality of life in patients with supratentorial glioblastomas and anaplastic astrocytomas. Neurosurgery 21:201, 1987.
3. Austin EJ, Alvord EC Jr: Recurrences of cerebellar astrocytoma: A violation of Collin's law. J Neurosurg 68:41–47, 1988.
4. Coleman RE, Hoffman JM, Hanson MW, et al: Clinical application of PET for the evaluation of brain tumors. J Nucl Med 32:616, 1991.
5. Duffner PK, Horowitz ME, Krisher JP, et al: Postoperative chemotherapy and delayed radiation in children less than three years of age with malignant brain tumors. N Engl J Med 328:1725–1731, 1993.
6. Epstein F, McLeary EL: Intrinsic brainstem tumors of childhood: Surgical indications. J Neurosurg 64:11–15, 1986.
7. Kovnar EH, Kellie SJ, Horowitz ME, et al: Preirradiation cisplatin and etoposide in the treatment of high-risk medulloblastoma and other malignant embryonal tumors of the central nervous system. J Clin Oncol 8:330–336, 1990.
8. Laurent JP, Chang CM, Cohen ME: A classification system for primitive neuroectodermal tumors (medulloblastoma) of the posterior fossa. Cancer 56:1807–1809, 1985.
9. Loeffler JS, Alexander E III, Wen PY, et al: Results of stereotactic brachytherapy used in the initial management of patients with glioblastoma. J Natl Cancer Inst 82:1918, 1990.
10. McIntosh S, Chen M, Sartain PA, et al: Adjuvant chemotherapy for medulloblastoma. Cancer 56:1316–1319, 1985.
11. Pons M, Finlay J, Walker R, et al: Chemotherapy with vincristine (VCR) and etoposide (VP-16) in children with low-grade astrocytoma. J Neuro-Oncol 14:151–158, 1992.
12. Raimondi AJ, Tomita T: The advantage of total resection of medulloblastoma and disadvantages of whole brain postoperative radiation therapy. Child's Brain 5:585–590, 1979.
13. Renaudin J, Fewer D, Wilson CB, et al: Dose dependency of Decadron in patients with partially excised brain tumors. J Neurosurg 50:361, 1979.
14. Schneider JH Jr, Raffel D, McComb JG: Benign cerebellar astrocytomas of childhood. Neurosurgery 30:58–63, 1992.
15. Silverberg E, Lubera JA: Cancer statistics 1988. CA 38:5–22, 1988.
16. Suc E, Kalifa C, Brauner R, et al: Brain tumors under the age of three: The price of survival. Acta Neurochir 106:93–98, 1990.
17. Walker MD, Alexander E Jr, Hunt WE, et al: Evaluation of BCNU and/or radiotherapy in the treatment of anaplastic gliomas. J Neurosurg 49:333, 1978.
18. Walker MD, Green SB, Byar DP, et al: Randomized comparisons of radiotherapy and nitrosoureas for the treatment of malignant glioma after surgery. N Engl J Med 303:1323, 1980.

88. AIDS-ASSOCIATED NON-HODGKIN'S LYMPHOMAS

Jill Lacy, M.D.

1. What is the incidence of non-Hodgkin's lymphoma (NHL) in patients with acquired immunodeficiency syndrome (AIDS)?

The exact incidence of NHL in human immunodeficiency virus (HIV)–infected patients is uncertain. Among a cohort of 55 patients followed at the National Cancer Institute since 1985, 14.5% have developed lymphoma. Other studies place the incidence at 2% to 5%. The incidence of NHL in HIV-infected patients is apparently increasing in part because of longer survival made possible by antiretroviral agents and improved treatment and prophylaxis of infections.

2. Which patients with HIV infection are at risk for developing NHL?

Virtually any patient with HIV infection is at risk for the development of NHL, including asymptomatic patients as well as those with overt AIDS. In contrast to Kaposi's sarcoma, which is seen almost exclusively in homosexual males, AIDS-associated NHL is encountered in all HIV risk groups.

3. Describe the clinical features of AIDS-associated NHL.

It is a biologically aggressive tumor, and patients typically present with advanced-stage disease. Involvement of extranodal sites is common, occurring in the majority of patients (>75%). Although the most frequent extranodal sites of involvement are bone marrow, liver, brain, leptomeninges, and gastrointestinal (GI) tract, virtually any site can be involved (e.g., myocardium, urethra, common bile duct). "B" symptoms (fevers, night sweats, weight loss) occur in about 50% of patients.

4. Are AIDS-associated lymphomas usually T- or B-cell lymphomas?

Virtually all are B-cell tumors.

5. Describe the pathologic subtypes of NHL associated with AIDS.

AIDS-associated NHLs are one of three pathologic subtypes:
1. Burkitt-like small noncleaved cell (high grade)
2. Immunoblastic sarcoma (high grade)
3. Diffuse large cell (intermediate grade)

Interestingly, the latter two subtypes occur more frequently in the later stages of HIV infection (median CD4 counts <100), whereas Burkitt's lymphoma occurs more frequently in earlier stages of the disease (median CD4 count >200). Low-grade lymphomas do not occur with increased frequency in patients with AIDS.

6. Which human herpesvirus is implicated in the etiology of AIDS-associated NHL?

Epstein-Barr virus (EBV). EBV is present in about half of the AIDS-associated NHLs; tumor cells carry EBV DNA and express viral proteins. Interestingly, all of the primary central nervous system (CNS) lymphomas encountered in patients with AIDS are EBV positive.

7. What is the characteristic cytogenetic abnormality that occurs in about half of the AIDS-associated NHLs?

The t(8;14) chromosomal translocation that juxtaposes the heavy chain immunoglobulin locus with the c-*myc* oncogene.

8. What is the overall prognosis of patients with AIDS-associated NHL?

The majority of patients with AIDS-associated NHL have a poor prognosis, with an overall median survival in the range of 4–7 months. The two major causes of death are opportunistic infection (50% to 70%) and progressive lymphoma (30% to 50%).

9. What is the single most important prognostic factor for survival in AIDS-associated NHL?

The CD4 count. Patients with CD4 counts >100 have a median survival of 24 months versus 1 to 2 months for CD4 counts <100. Importantly, about half of the patients with AIDS-associated NHL have a CD4 count >100 at presentation. Additional prognostic factors for survival include no prior AIDS-defining illness, no prior opportunistic infections, and a good performance status.

10. Describe the appropriate staging evaluation in patients diagnosed with AIDS-associated NHL.

The staging evaluation in patients with AIDS-associated NHL is similar to the evaluation performed in immunocompetent patients with lymphoma and includes the following: careful history and physical examination with special attention to GI and CNS signs and symptoms; chest radiograph or chest computed tomographic (CT) scan; abdominal and pelvic CT scan; and bilateral bone marrow biopsies. In addition, because of the high incidence of leptomeningeal disease, a lumbar puncture should be performed routinely. The presence of GI symptoms or heme-positive stools may indicate lymphomatous involvement of the GI tract, necessitating an upper GI series or endoscopy. A brain CT scan or MRI should be performed in any patient with cognitive changes or focal neurologic signs. In addition to the staging evaluation, patients with fever should be thoroughly evaluated for concurrent opportunistic infections. If identified, such infections should be treated prior to treatment with chemotherapy.

11. Describe the clinical features of primary CNS lymphoma in patients with AIDS.

They present with lymphomatous involvement of the brain with or without leptomeningeal involvement. These patients are usually profoundly immunocompromised with low CD4 counts and have an extremely poor prognosis with an exceedingly short survival (median <2 months). The most common presenting symptom is cognitive changes that can be readily confused with AIDS-related dementia. Other presenting signs and symptoms include focal neurologic signs, seizures, and cranial nerve palsies.

12. What difficulties are encountered in the diagnosis of AIDS-associated primary CNS lymphoma?

The diagnosis of AIDS-associated NHL is often problematic because radiographic evaluation (brain CT scan or MRI) cannot reliably distinguish the mass lesion(s) of lymphoma from toxoplasmosis or, on occasion, progressive multifocal leukoencephalopathy. Thus, a reasonable approach to the patient with a mass lesion and HIV infection is to check toxoplasmosis titers. If the titers are positive, the patient is given therapy for toxoplasmosis; if there is no improvement clinically and radiographically after 1 week of therapy, a brain biopsy is performed. If toxoplasmosis titers are negative, a stereotactic brain biopsy should be performed immediately.

13. How is AIDS-associated primary CNS lymphoma treated?

Whole brain radiation therapy with dexamethasone (Decadron). The majority of patients will experience improvement in symptoms with radiation therapy, and about half will achieve a radiographic complete remission. Nonetheless, survival remains poor, with opportunistic infections a major cause of death in these profoundly immunocompromised patients. Systemic chemotherapy is not routinely recommended, because it is unlikely to affect overall survival in the setting of severe immunodeficiency.

14. Multidrug chemotherapy is highly effective treatment for intermediate- and high-grade NHLs in immunocompetent patients. What is the role of chemotherapy in AIDS-associated NHL?

If untreated, the AIDS-associated NHLs are rapidly fatal. Thus, the majority of patients should be treated with cytotoxic drugs. The standard multidrug chemotherapy regimens that are effective in the treatment of intermediate- and high-grade NHL in immunocompetent patients (e.g., cyclophosphamide, hydroxydaunomycin, Oncovin [vincristine], prednisone [CHOP], M-BACOD [methotrexate, bleomycin, doxorubicin, cyclophosphamide, vincristine, and dexamethasone]) are also highly effective in the treatment of AIDS-associated NHL. Response rates are about 50–70%, with 30–50% of patients achieving a complete remission. Most patients derive significant palliation from the administration of multidrug chemotherapy. Although about 15% of patients will have a durable remission (>2 years), relapses are frequent and occur early (25–50% of complete responders relapse within 6 months of completing therapy) and overall median survival is short (4–7 months).

15. What are some of the reasons for the poor outcome of chemotherapy in the treatment of AIDS-associated NHL compared with NHL in immunocompetent patients?

Several factors contribute to the poor outcome of AIDS-associated NHL, including:

1. Death due to non–lymphoma-related complications of AIDS (e.g., opportunistic infections, wasting syndrome)

2. Failure to administer full doses of chemotherapy drugs on schedule owing to impaired hematologic reserve and intercurrent opportunistic infections

3. Advanced stage of disease at presentation

16. Explain the role of colony-stimulating factors in the management of AIDS-associated NHLs.

Severe and prolonged neutropenia is a frequent complication of chemotherapy in patients with AIDS. The use of colony-stimulating factors (granulocyte CSF or granulocyte-macrophage CSF) reduces both the severity and duration of neutropenia and its associated infectious sequelae in these patients. In addition, the administration of full doses of chemotherapy is often possible when the CSFs are used.

17. Should patients with AIDS-associated NHL receive the standard doses of cytoxic drugs used in the treatment of NHL in immunocompetent patients or should they receive reduced doses of drugs?

Definitive recommendations with respect to the optimal dose of chemotherapy in patients with AIDS await the outcome of ongoing clinical trials. Early experience in the treatment of AIDS-associated NHL with standard doses of chemotherapy (without the use of CSFs) was associated with severe neutropenia and opportunistic infections. Indeed, a retrospective analysis suggested that the use of higher doses of chemotherapy was actually associated with a poorer overall survival. Thus, investigators explored the use of low-dose chemotherapy (modified M-BACOD with CNS prophylaxis) without CSFs and observed a complete response rate of about 50%. It is not known whether the use of standard-dose chemotherapy with CSFs will, in fact, improve on the results obtained with low-dose chemotherapy. An ongoing cooperative group study comparing standard-dose M-BACOD (with GM-CSF) and low-dose M-BACOD may resolve the issue of optimal doses of cytotoxic drugs in the treatment of AIDS-associated NHL.

18. Should patients continue on antiretroviral therapy while receiving chemotherapy?

The most widely used antiretroviral agent azidothymidine (AZT) is marrow suppressive and markedly enhances the marrow toxicity of cytotoxic drugs. Thus, AZT should not be administered routinely to patients who are receiving chemotherapy. The non-marrow-suppressive antiretrovirals (e.g., dideoxyinosine [ddI]) can be administered with chemotherapy, although careful attention to additive toxicities (e.g., peripheral neuropathy from ddI and vincristine) is important.

19. Should patients routinely receive *Pneumocystis carinii* prophylaxis while on systemic chemotherapy?

Yes. These patients should receive *P. carinii* prophylaxis regardless of CD4 counts, because standard cytotoxic agents and prednisone are likely to cause further immunosuppression.

20. What is the role of intrathecal chemotherapy in the management of AIDS-associated NHL?

Given the propensity for AIDS-associated NHL to involve the leptomeninges, it is common practice to administer prophylactic intrathecal chemotherapy with either cytosine arabinoside (ara-C) or methotrexate weekly or biweekly for 4–6 doses. Patients who have overt involvement of the leptomeninges at presentation (i.e., positive CSF cytology) should receive a more prolonged course of intrathecal chemotherapy, as well as whole brain irradiation.

BIBLIOGRAPHY

1. Ambinger RF: AIDS lymphomas. In Niederhuber JE (ed): Current Therapy in Oncology. 1993, pp 611–616.
2. Baumgartner JE, Rachlin JR, Beckstead JH, et al: Primary central nervous system lymphomas: Natural history and response to radiation therapy in 55 patients with acquired immunodeficiency syndrome. J Neurosurg 73:206, 1990.
3. Gill PS, Levine AM, Krailo M, et al: AIDS-related malignant lymphoma: Results of prospective treatment trials. J Clin Oncol 5:1322, 1987.
4. Gill PS, Levine AM, Meyer PR, et al: Primary central nervous system lymphoma in homosexual men: Clinical, immunologic, and pathologic features. Am J Med 78:742, 1985.
5. Hamilton-Dutoit SJ, Palleson G, Franzman MB, et al: AIDS-associated non-Hodgkin's lymphoma: Histopathology, immunophenotype, and association with Epstein-Barr virus as demonstrated by in situ nucleic acid hybridization. Am J Pathol 138:149, 1991.
6. Kaplan LD, Abrams DI, Feigal E, et al: AIDS-associated non-Hodgkin's lymphoma in San Francisco. JAMA 261:719, 1989.
7. Kaplan LD, Kahn JO, Crowe S, et al: Clinical and virologic effects of recombinant human granulocyte-macrophage colony stimulating factor in patients receiving chemotherapy for human immunodeficiency virus-associated non-Hodgkin's lymphoma: Results of a randomized trial. J Clin Oncol 9:929, 1991.
8. Levine AM: Lymphoma in AIDS. Semin Oncol 17:104, 1990.
9. Levine AM, Wernz JC, Kaplan L, et al: Low-dose chemotherapy with central nervous system prophylaxis and ziduvudine maintenance in AIDS-related lymphoma. JAMA 266:84, 1991.
10. MacMahon EME, Glass JD, Hayward SD, et al: Epstein-Barr virus in AIDS-related primary central nervous system lymphoma. Lancet 338:969, 1991.
11. Meeker TC, Shiramizu B, Kaplan L, et al: Evidence for molecular subtypes of HIV-associated lymphoma: Division into peripheral monoclonal, polyclonal, and central nervous system lymphoma. AIDS 5:669, 1991.
12. Moore RD, Kessler H, Richman DD, et al: Non-Hodgkin's lymphomas in patients with advanced HIV infection treated with zidovudine. JAMA 265:2208, 1991.

89. KAPOSI'S SARCOMA

Adam M. Myers, M.D.

1. What is Kaposi's sarcoma (KS)?

It is a dermal malignancy that is multifocal in origin. Lesions may be flat or raised and are typically of purplish color. Histopathologically, lesions comprise spindle cells and vascular structures with lymphocytic, macrophage, and plasma cell infiltration. Fibrosis is variably present.

2. How is KS diagnosed?

Traditionally, cancer lesions should be confirmed by biopsy. However, biopsy of lesions for KS is not uniformly necessary, although it is sometimes done to confirm the clinical impression. Kaposi's lesions, when characteristic and multiple, are hard to confuse with another process. For example, an experienced bronchoscopist who visualizes typical KS lesions in the endobronchial tree can note these without biopsy. The vascular nature of the lesion can result in significant hemorrhage if biopsied. There have been occasional reports of *single* lesions being misidentified. In one case, for instance, *Pneumocystis carinii* involvement of the skin was mistaken for KS.

3. Who gets KS?

KS has been seen in three populations at risk:

1. Elderly men of eastern European or Mediterranean descent ("classic")
2. Equatorial Africa ("endemic")
3. Organ transplant recipients, where the increased risk of KS has been reportedly 400–500-fold.

These forms of KS are usually indolent in their course. Since the AIDS epidemic, however, a new variety of KS with significantly more aggressive biologic activity has been encountered. This form of KS is considered "epidemic." It remains the most common malignancy associated with human immunodeficiency virus (HIV) infection, occurring in approximately 10–15% of gay or bisexual men with AIDS.

4. How does KS behave? Does it truly metastasize?

KS is thought to be a multicentric disease. Metastases in the true sense of the word do not occur. KS in the epidemic variety has been described to involve at one time or another most organ sites. The central nervous system, however, is generally spared, with just a few cases being reported in which KS has involved that site.

5. What are the complications of KS?

KS is commonly asymptomatic. However, cutaneous lesions might be associated with mild to moderately severe edema, especially if those lesions are confluent and periorbital in location or are on the lower extremities. Patients with marked edema often are found to have lymph node involvement by KS. Lesions that are protuberant or ulcerative in the mouth or gingiva can severely compromise deglutition and worsen the patient's nutritional status. The worst stage of KS is when visceral sites are involved. It is then that the morbidity of KS, such as seen with diffuse involvement of the gastrointestinal (GI) tract or pleuropulmonary areas, might be the cause of or significantly contribute to the death of the patient. This stage of the disease necessitates the use of combination chemotherapy. Otherwise, although a morbid complication of AIDS, KS is not commonly the primary cause of death.

6. Is KS encountered in all individuals with AIDS?

KS is rarely seen in individuals who contract AIDS as a result of the transfusion of blood products (i.e., hemophiliacs). It also is significantly less common in women who have AIDS as a result of heterosexual contact or intravenous drug use (IVDU). Ninety-five percent of cases of KS occur in homosexual or bisexual men.

7. Why is KS primarily seen in gay men?

Chronic immune system activation probably plays a role in the pathogenesis of KS. The lifestyle of homosexual men exposes them to multiple infections that results in chronic antigen stimulation. An exact reason for this association is yet unexplained. Lifestyle changes as a result of health education and/or fear of contracting AIDS might explain in part the drop in reported cases of AIDS with KS from 30–40% at the beginning of the epidemic to 10–15% more recently.

8. How is KS documented?
It is important to describe the presence of KS carefully prior to therapy. Standard body diagrams can be used to record lesions when they are diffuse. Polaroid photographs also can be taken to document the appearance of lesions prior to therapy. Lesions should be described as to their color, whether or not they are raised or ulcerated, if there is associated edema, and if the lesions are associated with "halos." A yellow halo around a lesion represents heme products leaking from lesions and may indicate active growth. Usually three to five lesions are chosen to monitor as "target" lesions.

9. How do you determine the extent of KS involvement?
It is important to document the extent of KS so that treatment outcomes can be assessed and clinical comparisons drawn. It is reasonable to estimate the numbers of KS lesions present as to none, 1 to 10, >10 but <50, or >50 lesions rather than attempt an exact count that would be hard to duplicate on subsequent visits. A thorough physical examination is essential, including examination of the gingiva and mouth. The presence of gingival and palatal lesions is associated with a greater risk for mucosal lesions to be present at sites such as the GI tract and the respiratory tree. Aside from a chest radiograph and routine laboratory tests, including the determination of the CD4 cell count, more extensive and invasive studies are not routinely justified. The identification of the patient's immune status as measured by CD4 cell count at time of diagnosis of KS has significant implications as to therapeutic options.

10. Is there any specific significance to the medical history in regard to therapy?
Yes! Patients who have had AIDS-related opportunistic infections (OIs) or who have KS-related "B" symptoms are generally not candidates for therapy with interferon alpha (INFα).

11. How do I organize this information to make it more meaningful?
How about considering the time-honored staging approach? (I know, questions shouldn't be answered with questions!) The following will help you to categorize a patient's disease and develop guidance for decisions about therapy. Tumor extent and location, immune status, and the presence or absence of symptoms all have therapeutic implications.

Suggested Staging Classification

Tumor (T)	1. Good risk—minimal cutaneous*
	2. Intermediate risk—diffuse cutaneous or nodal involvement
	3. Poor risk—visceral sites (i.e., GI tract or lung)
	Also, any tumor associated edema, halos around lesions, or extensive oral KS[†]
Immune (I)	1. Good risk—CD4 cells ≥200 cells/μl
	2. Intermediate risk—CD4 cells ≥100 <200 cells/μl
	3. Poor risk—CD4 cells <100 cells/μl
Symptoms(S)	1. Good risk—absence of symptoms
	2. Intermediate risk—h/o OIs
	3. Poor risk—tumor related symptoms[‡]

* Lesions confined to one or two geographic sites, with <25 lesions total.
[†] Nodular KS or KS not confined to the hard palate.
[‡] Unexplained fevers, night sweats, >10% unexplained weight loss.

12. How is KS treated?
It is best to consider treatment as being either *local* or *systemic* (see question 14). Let's discuss local therapies first. These include radiation therapy, cryotherapy (with liquid nitrogen), the injection of lesions with a dilute solution of an antineoplastic agent (i.e.,

vinblastine), or painting with dinitrochlorobenzene (DNCB) in sensitized patients. Less-studied therapies include topical retinoids and intralesional (INFα) injections. Except for radiotherapy, these treatments should not be used on facial lesions or lesions on the soles of the feet. With topical therapies, lesions are treated weekly until an appropriate inflammatory reaction develops and then the patient is observed to assess the status of the lesions when the inflammation resolves. This approach should be used for light-skinned people only. Intralesional injections are done every 2 weeks for up to three injections total. Patients with painful gingival lesions can have those lesions injected with a 3% sodium tetradecyl sulfate solution. Probably the most effective local therapy remains radiation therapy. Again, the intention for radiotherapy is to treat confluent areas of disease or painful single geographic sites or to facilitate effective cosmetic control. This usually results in reduction of pain or swelling and will often lead to the flattening and fading of lesions. Lesions rarely completely disappear. Radiation therapy to diffuse areas in the lower extremities might be complicated during the latter course of disease should KS recur in the radiated site. Tense edema with poor tissue quality as a result of radiation damage might lead to ulceration with development of secondary infection. This is an extremely morbid complication of KS. Of course minimal and asymptomatic disease might be observed, if there are no investigative protocols, and not treated.

13. Wait a minute! No therapy for a known cancer? That sounds like oncologic heresy!
Remember, we are treating for palliation. It is difficult to palliate an asymptomatic patient, especially when theapies have potentially significant side effects.

14. What about systemic therapy for KS?
Good-risk patients, i.e., CD4 cells ≥200 cells/μl and asymptomatic, are good candidates for INFα, usually in conjunction with an antiretroviral agent (which is started when the CD4 count is <500 cells/μl). Otherwise, poor-risk patients can be considered for systemic therapy with antineoplastic agents. Antineoplastic chemotherapy using single agents such as vinblastine, vincristine, bleomycin, or doxorubicin or combinations of these are used. Oral VP-16 also is effective and has the advantage of oral administration. Combination therapy, however, is usually necessary. Intermediate-risk patients also are usually treated with systemic antineoplastic agents. Less aggressive therapy with single agents, such as bleomycin with or without vincristine, might afford reasonable palliation. The most difficult decision is whether or not to treat. Patients may have asymptomatic KS lesions and yet have other clinical conditions associated with AIDS that are causing significant morbidity. In this situation, antineoplastic chemotherapy might actually increase the risk for opportunistic infections to develop or worsen these coexistent conditions by further depressing immunity. Antineoplastic chemotherapy is generally marrow suppressive. This toxicity might complicate the use of necessary treatments with agents that are also marrow toxic, i.e., azidothymidine (AZT), ganciclovir. Therefore, close observation without therapy may be appropriate with therapy initiated if symptoms develop related to KS and/or a more aggressive tumor biology ensues, i.e., there are rapidly increasing numbers of lesions.

15. Is it true that KS sometimes spontaneously regresses?
KS can wax and wane in its appearance, particularly in patients whose immune status, when KS develops, is relatively preserved, i.e., CD4 cell count >400 cells/μl. This clearly supports the contention that KS behaves like an opportunistic malignancy in immune compromised patients. Perhaps the most dramatic example of KS regression has been seen in KS developing in individuals who are given immunosuppressive therapy to enable them to engraft a renal transplant. In this situation, if organ engraftment fails and immunosuppressive therapy is discontinued, KS has been seen to spontaneously resolve.

16. Are there any new thoughts about the pathogenesis of KS?
Some think that KS, at least in its early stages, might not be a true malignancy. KS has a

low mitotic activity histologically, a low S-phase fraction with flow cytometry, and when studied KS has always been found to be diploid. The tumor's growth often is seen microscopically to push through involved tissue and not truly to "invade." These are features more characteristic of benign growth.

17. Does this suggest that alternative therapies for KS should be evaluated?
The growth of KS in patients with AIDS involves a complex interaction between many cytokines. Because of this, there may be a role in the therapy of KS for antiangiogenic agents or growth factor inhibitors. Combining a retinoid, such as 13-cis-retinoic acid or all-transretinoic acid, with INFα and an antiretroviral agent theoretically might be effective therapy.

BIBLIOGRAPHY

1. Biggar RJ: Cancer in acquired immunodeficiency syndrome: An epidemiological assessment. Semin Oncol 17(3):251–260, 1990.
2. Fukanaga M, Silverberg S: Kaposi's sarcoma in patients with acquired immune deficiency syndrome. A flow cytometric DNA analysis of 26 lesions in 21 patients. Cancer 66:758–764, 1990.
3. Gill PS, Rarick M, McCutchan JA, et al: Systemic treatment of AIDS-related Kaposi's sarcoma: Results of a randomized trial. Am J Med 90:427–433, 1991.
4. Krown SE: Interferon and other biologic agents for the treatment of Kaposi's sarcoma. Hematol Oncol Clin North Am 5(2):311–322, 1991.
5. Krown SE, Metroka C, Weinz JC: Kaposi's sarcoma in the acquired immune deficiency syndrome: A proposal for uniform evaluation response and staging criteria. J Clin Oncol 7(9):1201–1207, 1989.
6. Muzyka BC, Glick M: Sclerotherapy for the treatment of nodular intraoral Kaposi's sarcoma in patients with AIDS. N Engl J Med 328:210–211, 1989.
7. Schwartz JJ, Muskowski PL: New treatments for Kaposi's sarcoma. The AIDS Reader July/August:129–134, 1992.
8. Stribling J, Weitzner S, Smith GV: Kaposi's sarcoma in renal allograft recipients. Cancer 42:442–446, 1978.

INDEX

Page numbers in **boldface** type indicate complete chapters.